D1605443

ENVIRONMENTAL
PATHOLOGY

ENVIRONMENTAL PATHOLOGY

Edited by

N. KARLE MOTTET, M.D.
Professor of Pathology and Environmental Health
University of Washington School of Medicine

New York   Oxford
OXFORD UNIVERSITY PRESS
1985

Oxford University Press

Oxford   London   New York   Toronto
Delhi   Bombay   Calcutta   Madras   Karachi
Kuala Lumpur   Singapore   Hong Kong   Tokyo
Nairobi   Dar es Salaam   Cape Town
Melbourne   Auckland

and associated companies in
Beirut   Berlin   Ibadan   Mexico City   Nicosia

Copyright © 1985 Oxford University Press, Inc.

Published by Oxford University Press, Inc.
200 Madison Avenue
New York, New York 10016

All rights reserved. No part of this publication may be reproduced,
stored in a retrieval system, or transmitted, in any form or by any
means, electronic, mechanical, photocopying, recording, or otherwise, without the prior permission of Oxford University Press.

Library of Congress Cataloging in Publication Data
Main entry under title:
Environmental pathology.
Bibliography: p.
Includes index.
1. Environmentally induced diseases.   2. Pathology.
I. Mottet, N. Karle, 1924–
RB152.E578   1984   616.9′8   83-23831
ISBN 0-19-503427-9

Printing (last digit):   9 8 7 6 5 4 3 2 1

Printed in the United States of America

*To the students of Pathology, Toxicology,
Environmental Health and Occupational Medicine*

Preface

It has long been recognized that the occurrence of most diseases results from the interaction of an exogenous etiologic agent with a susceptible individual. Perhaps it was the recognition of this fact that led Rudolf Virchow (1821–1902), the scientist who first related clinical disease to cellular pathology, to devote so much of his time to the development of public health laws in Germany. It was his view that "the ultimate task of medicine is the constitution of society on a physiological basis." Even at the time of Virchow's death, seven of the ten leading causes of death in the United States of America were infectious (biotic) agents (bacterial, viral, parasitic, or fungal). After the battle against infectious diseases was won by public health measures, improved nutrition and living standards, and antibiotics in medicine, the leading causes of fatal diseases in industrial countries changed dramatically. Chronic diseases came to the fore, especially cancer and cardiovascular disease, and questions were raised about environmental and occupational exposures to chemical and physical agents. Population growth and the development of industrial structures sufficient to support the population increased exposures to unusual concentrations and new forms of chemicals as well as radiation.

The goal of this book is to bring together for the first time a comprehensive synthesis of information about the increasingly important non-biotic etiologic agents of human disease. The book is intended to serve as a text and reference for pathologists, toxicologists, veterinarians, occupational physicians, and environmental health scientists seeking further understanding of the role of environmental chemical and physical agents in the pathogenesis of human disease. Much of the relevant information has developed within these sciences.

Because of the diverse origins of the book's subject matter, the contributing authors include toxicologists, pathologists, veterinarians, clinical physicians, and environmental health scientists. All have emphasized human disease and have sought to make their disciplines understandable to others in related fields. The authors' occupations include industrial, governmental, research, and administrative positions, which attests to the breadth of this new field.

Although this is a "pathology" text, it deals as much with subcellular and molecular effects of chemical and radiation exposures as with the more conventional histopathology. Etiology and pathogenesis are the focus rather than differential diagnosis. The book is divided into two parts: (1) four chapters that present pathologic processes affecting the body as a whole and (2) ten chapters based on organ systems. It is hoped that this organization will enable the reader to quickly find sought-after information.

Even on brief perusal of the book, it will be apparent that the state of knowledge about environmental pathology varies considerably from one organ system to another. The disease processes caused by environmental chemicals in the respiratory, urinary, and nervous systems have been much more extensively studied than those of the immune and gastrointestinal systems. I was unable to justify chapters on the endocrine and musculoskeletal systems and pancreas because of similar limitations.

Almost a decade ago I organized and began teaching a course in environmental pathology at the University of Washington. It was taken by medical, dental, and public health students, as well as graduate and postgraduate students in the environmental sciences. Several of the authors have partici-

pated in the course. The approach the book takes is, in part, an outgrowth of our experience teaching the course. I am most grateful for the many useful suggestions made by the students. Their positive response to the course served as a stimulus to develop the book.

Finally, I wish to thank all of those who contributed to this book as chapter authors and in other ways. My wife, Nancy, assisted greatly in the preparation of the prospectus and draft outlines of the overall plan, format, and index. Mr. Ralph L. Body spent much of his spare time doing library searches to confirm references and develop background information. Mrs. Maureen K. Levell worked on the organization, manuscript development, and galley and page proofs. Many others contributed in different ways. To all who helped I express thanks.

London, England   N.K.M.
January, 1985

Contents

Contributors

Ellsworth C. Alvord, M.D.
Professor of Pathology
Department of Pathology
University of Washington
Seattle, Washington 98195

Robert Burrell, Ph.D.
Professor of Microbiology
Department of Microbiology
The Medical Center
West Virginia University
Morgantown, West Virginia 26506

Robert L. Dixon, Ph.D.
Director, Office of Health Research
U.S. Environmental Protection Agency
Washington, D.C. 20460

Robert A. Ettlin, M.D.
F. Hoffmann-La Roche & Co. Ltd.
Biological Pharmaceutical Research
Department
Basel, Switzerland

Robert A. Goyer, M.D.
Deputy Director
National Institute of Environmental Health
Sciences
Research Triangle Park, North Carolina 27709

Thomas W. Huang, M.D.
Associate Professor of Pathology
Department of Pathology
University of Washington
% Veterans Administration Hospital
Seattle, Washington 98118

Atiya B. Khan, M.D.
Department of Pediatric Oncology
The Johns Hopkins Oncology Center
Baltimore, Maryland 21205

Brigid G. Leventhal, M.D.
Department of Pediatric Oncology
The Johns Hopkins Oncology Center
Baltimore, Maryland 21205

Lawrence A. Loeb, M.D., Ph.D.
Professor of Pathology
Department of Pathology
University of Washington
Seattle, Washington 98195

Howard I. Maibach, M.D.
Professor
Department of Dermatology
University of California Hospital
University of California at San Francisco
San Francisco, California 94143

Mary Treinen Moslen, M.D.
Department of Pathology
University of Texas Medical Center
Galveston, Texas 77550

N. Karle Mottet, M.D.
Professor of Pathology and Environmental
Health
Department of Pathology
University of Washington
Seattle, Washington 98195

Carl J. Pfeiffer, Ph.D.
Professor
Division of Veterinary Biology
Virginia-Maryland Research College of
Veterinary Medicine
Virginia Tech
Blacksburg, Virginia 24601

Dennis D. Reichenbach, M.D.
Professor of Pathology
Department of Pathology
University of Washington
Seattle, Washington 98195

(Late) Edward S. Reynolds, M.D.
Professor and Chairman
Department of Pathology
University of Texas Medical Center
Galveston, Texas 77550

(Late) John D. Scribner, Ph.D.
Program Head for Carcinogenesis
Pacific Northwest Research Foundation
Seattle, Washington 98104

Cheng-Mei Shaw, M.D.
Professor of Pathology (Neuropathology)
Department of Pathology
University of Washington
Seattle, Washington 98195

John R. Silber, Ph.D.
University of California, San Francisco
Veterans Administration Hospital
4150 Clement Street
San Francisco, California 94121

Arthur C. Upton, M.D.
Professor and Chairman
Institute of Environmental Medicine
New York University Medical Center
New York, New York 10016

Ronald C. Wester, Ph.D.
Department of Dermatology
University of California
School of Medicine
San Francisco, California 94143

I

General Reactions to Injury by Environmental Agents

1

The Molecular Basis of Environmental Mutagenesis

John R. Silber and Lawrence A. Loeb

Concern has been mounting during the last decade about the possible deleterious effects of the introduction of an increasing number of exobiotic substances into the environment. It has been estimated that approximately 50,000 chemical compounds are presently used for industrial and domestic purposes, and that this number is increasing by 1000 new compounds yearly (Ames, 1979). The growing ubiquity of these compounds can be appreciated when it is realized that the introduction of many of them into the environment, either as manufactured goods or polluting waste products, is measured in the millions of pounds.

The toxicologic properties of most of these compounds as well as many natural substances are only now beginning to be evaluated. It has been found that many of these compounds as well as ionizing and ultraviolet radiation from man-made and natural sources can chemically alter DNA. The alterations produced, called DNA damage, can lead to two deleterious consequences. First, the damage can grossly interfere with the essential functioning of DNA to such an extent as to cause cell death. Second, in some instances the damage is an intermediate in the production of mutations. This is an immediate concern, because mutations have been implicated in the pathogenesis of many inherited and somatic human disease states.

The danger to human health from mutagenic environmental agents is best perceived in their possible etiologic role in the causation of cancer. It is currently argued that the majority of human cancers are due to environmental factors. The finding that many mutagens are also carcinogens has increased the trepidation about the increasing presence of toxicologic agents in the environment. More importantly, mutations in germ cells cause deformations at birth and increase the incidence of inherited disease. These consequences of mutagenesis are more costly to society than diseases such as cancer that primarily afflict older individuals.

This chapter will introduce mechanisms by which environmental agents can produce mutations. Special emphasis will be placed on the repair of DNA damage, because much mutagenesis by exogenous agents in experimental systems has been found to be the result of deficient or faulty DNA repair. Possible mechanisms of mutagenesis due to alterations in the fidelity of DNA replication by exogenous agents also will be detailed.

The Primacy of DNA

In order to define clearly what a mutation is, it is first necessary to elucidate briefly some of the structural and functional properties of DNA molecules.

DNA is an informational molecule. It contains all of the instructions necessary to define the total behavioral repertoire of a cell. Considering its important role, DNA is a surprisingly simple molecule composed of two strands wound about each other forming a double helix. Each strand of the helix is made up of only four deoxyribonucleotides covalently bound together by phosphodiester linkages. The nucleotides differ by containing either a purine base, adenine or guanine, or a pyrimidine base, thymine or cytosine. The two strands are held together by weak hydrogen bonding between complementary base pairs. As shown in Figure 1-1, the complementarity of the bases is highly specific, with adenine hydrogen bonding with thymine, and guanine bonding with cytosine. Complementarity enables a DNA molecule to act as a template to direct its faithful replication by DNA polymerases and the synthesis of RNA transcripts by RNA polymerases.

The information in a DNA molecule is contained in the linear sequence of its nucleotides on each strand. For this information to be biologically expressed, the sequence of nucleotides of a gene must be converted into the sequence of amino acids of a protein. The translation of the one sequence into the other requires a complementary RNA transcript of the gene to direct the protein-synthesizing machinery of the cell and a genetic code that allows only four different nucleotides to specify for the 20 amino acids from which proteins are constructed. The genetic code is composed of sets of three nucleotides, call triplet codons, each of which corresponds to an amino acid. Of the 64 possible codons, 61 specify an amino acid, which necessitates some amino acids being represented by more than one codon. The three remaining codons code for no amino acids and act as stop signals to denote the termination of an amino acid chain.

The primacy of DNA in the scheme of life should be apparent from this short discussion. In its nucleotide sequences resides the information to build the characteristic amino acid chains of the proteins whose enzymatic and structural properties determine all cellular behavior. The template properties afforded to DNA by base pair complementarity allow this information to be accurately expressed as well as duplicated for future generations. The dominant role that DNA plays in the expression and perpetuation of life, however, designates it as the critical target for the action of mutagenic environmental agents.

Mutations

A mutation is a change in the nucleotide sequence of a gene. The change can come about by one of two processes, which are outlined in Table 1-1.

Line A of Table 1-1 lists the nucleotide sequence of a hypothetical gene coding for a protein composed of six amino acids. The sequence has been grouped as triplet codons with the abbreviations for the corresponding amino acids listed beneath them. A simple way to create a mutation in this sequence is to substitute guanine for cytosine in the third triplet; the codon for the amino acid leucine has been converted into that for phenylalanine. The simple act of replacing one nucleotide in the sequence with another has resulted in an alteration of the amino acid sequence of the protein. Another consequence of a single nucleotide substitution is shown in line C. When the adenine at the second position of the third codon is replaced with thymine, a premature stop signal is introduced into the gene,

Table 1–1. Possible Modes of Nucleotide Sequence Mutation

(A)	TAC	AGA	AAC	TGT	GTG	TGT	ATC
	MET	SER	LEU	THR	HIS	THR	STOP
(B)	TAC	AGA	AAG	TGT	GTG	TGT	ATC
	MET	SER	PHE	THR	HIS	THR	STOP
(C)	TAC	AGA	ATC	TGT	GTG	TGT	ATC
	MET	SER	STOP	THR	HIS	THR	STOP
(D)	TAC	AGA	AAC	GTG	TGT	GTA	TC
	MET	SER	LEU	HIS	THR	HIS	—

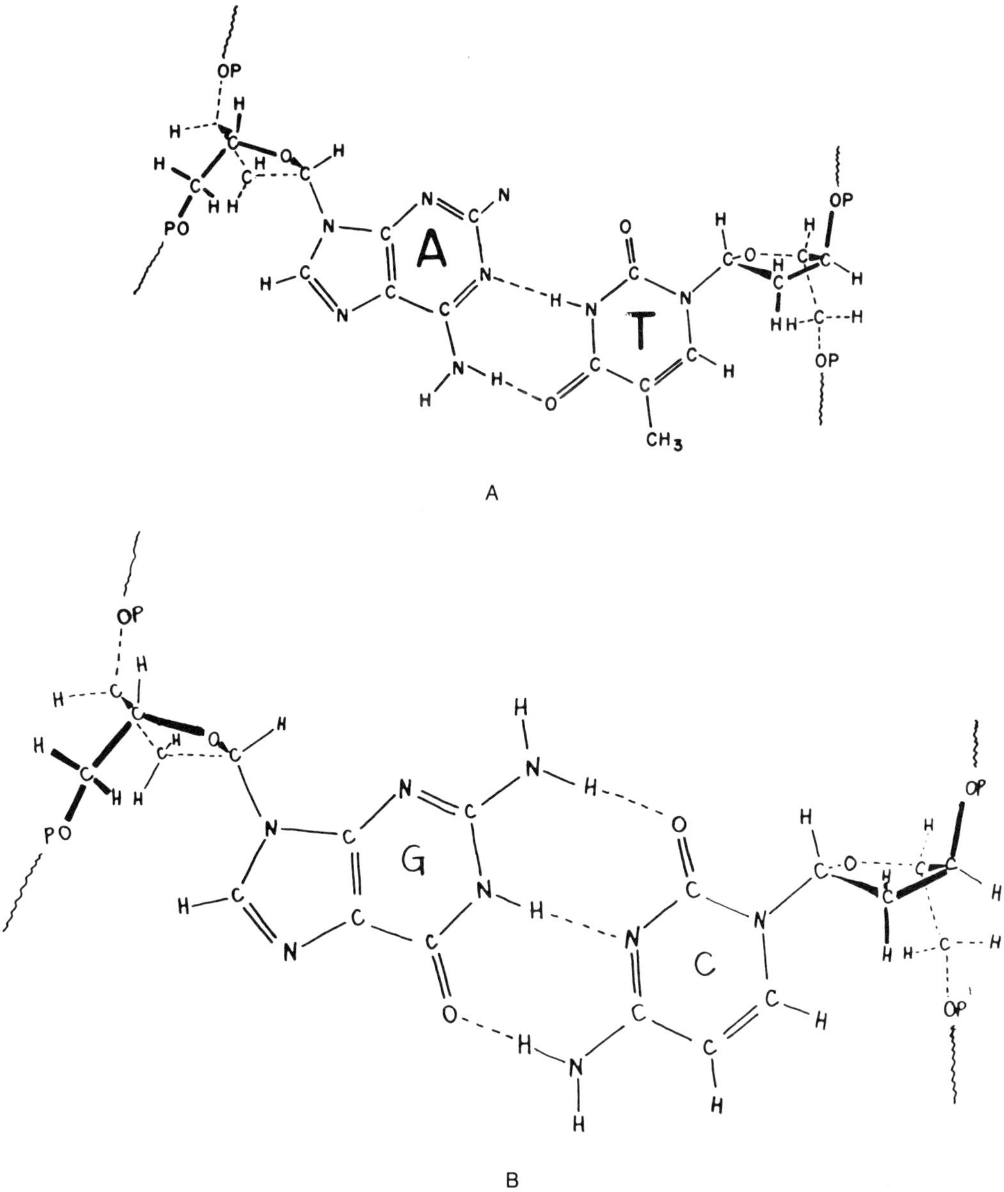

Figure 1–1. Complementary base-pairing (A) between adenine and thymine, and (B) between guanine and cytosine.

which now codes for a trucated protein of only two amino acids.

The other way to produce a mutation is to alter the frame in which the nucleotides of a gene are read as triplet codons. Frameshift mutations are created by adding or deleting one or more nucleotides in the sequence of the gene. The result of deleting the thymine in the first position of the fourth codon from the nucleotide sequence coding for the hypothetical protein of Table 1-1 is shown in line D. With one less nucleotide, the reading frame of the gene after the third codon will be shifted to the right to re-establish a sequence of codons. The result of this is to change the sequence of the final three amino acids of the protein, and to destroy the termination codon.

Although a mutation is always produced when the nucleotide sequence of a gene is changed, all changes are not biologically expressed. Mutations may be silent. This is most easily understood for single-base substitutions. The substitution of one amino acid for another may have no effect on a protein if the change has no effect on its functional properties. The same may be true for substitutions that produce premature termination signals if the abbreviated amino acid chain can still form a biologically active protein. It is also possible that a base substitution will convert one triplet into another that codes for the same amino acid. Frameshift mutations can be unexpressed if the addition or deletion of a limited number of nucleotides at one position can be compensated by a similar event elsewhere in the nucleotide sequence, which will re-establish an amino acid sequence that is still biologically active.

There are no absolute rules that limit the changes that can occur to a sequence of nucleotides. A purine nucleotide may be substituted for another purine, or may be substituted for by a pyrimidine nucleotide. Frameshift mutations may be the result of the addition or deletion of a single nucleotide or many. In some instances, a significant fraction of a chromosome may be relocated from one position to another. The addition to or the loss from the genome of an entire chromosome is also possible. Regardless of how a change is effected, it is conserved and is normally propagated from one generation to the next.

Considering the permanency of mutations, it is of interest to know how frequently they occur. During normal DNA replication, spontaneous single-nucleotide changes are estimated to occur at a frequency of less than one for every 10^9 nucleotides replicated (Loeb et al., 1979). Alteration of the nucleotide sequence of DNA, therefore, is an exceedingly rare event, and under normal circumstances, the sequence is highly conserved. However, there are environmental agents that interact with DNA and increase the frequency of mutagenesis by orders of magnitude. These agents are mutagens and are the topic of the next section.

Mutagens and DNA Damage

The number of mutagenic agents from both natural and man-made sources in the environment is enormous. Table 1-2 lists a variety of mutagens that might be encountered in everyday life. From this list, it is apparent that even seemingly innocuous endeavors can bring one in contact with a great diversity of mutagenic substances.

Mutagens vary greatly in their form and mutagenic potential. They are classified somewhat arbitrarily as either physical or chemical in nature. Examples of physical mutagens include heat, ultraviolet light, and ionizing radiation such as X rays and γ rays. Chemical mutagens include substances as simple as inorganic salts of metals to complex polycylic aromatic compounds. Regardless of their heterogeneity, most mutagens (but not all) share a common property of being able to interact chemically with DNA. The production of new chemical structures in a DNA molecule, DNA dam-

Table 1–2. Common Environmental Mutagens

Mutagen	Source
Ultraviolet light	Sunlight
Ionizing radiation	Cosmic rays, medical X rays
Aflatoxin B$_1$	Fungi-contaminated peanuts and grains
Flavonoids (quercetin kaempferol)	Fruits and vegetables
Chloroform	Chlorinated water
Nitrosamines	Beer and whiskey
Pyrolysis products of tryptophan	Broiled meat
Nickel	Metal alloys, mines
Saccharin	Sweeteners
Hydrazine	Cigarettes and wood smoke
Benz[a]pyrene	Cigarettes and wood smoke
Vinyl chloride	Plastics
Benzidine	Textile dyes; manufacture of leather and paper
2-Naphthylamine	Textile dyes; manufacture of leather and paper
Imuran	Anticancer drugs
Nitrogen mustards	Anticancer drugs
Cyclophosphamide	Anticancer drugs

age, can have profound effects on its biologic functions.

The variety of DNA damage produced by
mutagenic compounds is extremely large.
This reflects the large number of mutagens
that react with DNA and the diversity of
products that result from these reactions.
Experimental evidence suggests, however,
that alterations of the purine and pyrimidine bases of DNA are responsible for most
of the biologic consequences of DNA damage. Five classes of altered base damage,
along with mutagens that produce them, are
discussed below (Setlow and Setlow, 1972;
Cerruti, 1975; Miller, 1978; Lindahl, 1979;
W. Harm, 1980).

1. *Small adducts.* Some chemical mutagens such as methylmethane sulfonate, dimethylnitrosamine, and ethylnitrosourea can
transfer a short aliphatic chain to a base.
Figure 1-2A shows two possible adducts that
are formed when dimethylnitrosamine reacts
with guanine. A single methyl group from
the mutagen is covalently bound to either
the N-7 or 0-6 position of guanine. The addition of a small group to a base may cause
it to be unable to hydrogen-bond properly
with its complementary base. Usually,
however, a small adduct will create only a
minor distortion in the double-helical
structure of DNA (Cerruti, 1975). Physical
mutagens are also capable of producing
small adducts in bases. One example is
shown in Figure 1-2B, in which the double
bond of thymine has been saturated by
water. This type of damage can be induced
by ultraviolet light and γ rays.

2. *Large adducts.* Other chemical mutagens including benz[a]pyrene, aflatoxin B₁,
and 3-methylcholantherene can add large
chemical structures to bases. This is shown
in Figure 1-3A and B, in which aflatoxin B₁
and benz[a]pyrene have formed adducts at
two different positions on guanine. The addition of such a large chemical moiety cannot be accomodated by the DNA helix. Such
lesions destroy the base-pairing specificity
of the altered base and disrupt hydrogen
bonding of adjacent base-paired nucleotides (Cerruti, 1975).

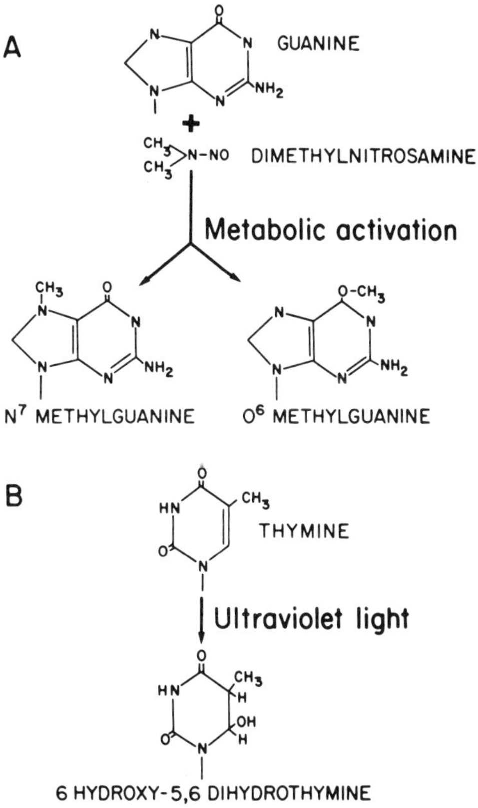

Figure 1–2. Small adducts produced by chemical and physical mutagens. (A) Methyl group
adducts at the N-7 or O-6 positions of guanine
caused by reaction with metabolically activated
dimethylnitrosamine. (B) Saturation of the double bond of thymine with water, induced by ultraviolet light.

Notice in Figure 1-3 that the original
chemical structure of benz[a]pyrene has been
modified prior to its binding to guanine.
Many chemical mutagens will not react with
the DNA unless they are first metabolically
activated into a more electrophilic or elec-
tron-seeking compound (Miller, 1978). The
activated compound will readily react with
the many electron-rich nucleophilic sites on
a DNA molecule. Metabolic activation is
performed by cellular enzymes, which normally detoxify the cell of endogenous and
exogenous substances. There are a variety
of activating enzymes generically referred to
as mixed-function oxidases, which are found
in a great many cell types. The activation of
chemical mutagens is a consequence of these

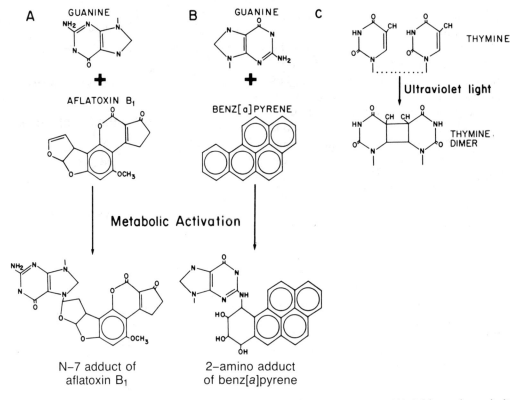

Figure 1–3. Large adducts produced by chemical and physical mutagens. (A) Adduct of metabolically activated aflatoxin B₁ at N-7 position of guanine. (B) Adduct of metabolically activated
benz[a]pyrene at the 2-amino position of guanine. (C) Ultraviolet light–induced thymine–thymine
dimer.

enzymes performing the normal detoxification of the cell.

Physical mutagens also are capable of
producing large adducts. The classic example in this case shown in Figure 1-3C is the
ultraviolet light–induced pyrimidine dimer
(Setlow and Setlow, 1972). In this example,
adjacent pyrimidine bases on the same strand
of DNA undergo a reaction that covalently
binds each to the other. The pyrimidine dimer is a model example of a large adduct
and is the most studied lesion of this class
of damage.

3. *Cross-links.* Certain chemical mutagens, such as mitomycin C, nitrogen mustard, and light-activated psoralins can link
one chemical moiety to two bases on opposing strands of a DNA molecule. Cross-
links covalently bind the two strands together and create large distortions in the
structure of the double helix, although the

exact structure of the strand-to-strand DNA
cross-links is not known (W. Harm, 1980).

4. *Nucleotide analogs.* These lesions are
produced when base analogs such as 5-
bromouracil and 2-aminopurine are incorporated in the place of thymine and adenine, respectively, during DNA replication.
Such analogs may also arise via the deami-
nation by heat or chemical treatment of cytosine or adenine to produce nucleotides
containing uracil or hypoxanthine (Lindahl, 1979). Many analogs produce noncomplementary base-paired nucleotides in
DNA that result in only minor distortions
of the double helix.

5. *Missing bases.* Depurination, the loss
of the purine bases adenine and guanine from
a DNA strand, probably is the most frequently occurring type of DNA base damage. It is the result of the breaking of the
glycosylic linkage between the purine base

and the deoxyribose moiety of the nucleotide. This damage is very stable, having a half-life of 200 hours. Heat is a causative agent of depurination. It is estimated that at physiologic temperatures, as many as 10,000 purines may be lost from the genome of a mammalian cell in one generation (Lindahl, 1979). Furthermore, the addition of alkyl and large chemical groups can increase the rate of depurination 1000 to 10,000 times. It is possible that depurination is the common fate of many diverse types of adducted bases. Depyrimidization also occurs but at a rate 100- to 1000-fold less than that of depurination.

From the standpoint of biologic effect, it is useful to reclassify DNA base damage as consisting of either blocking or nonblocking lesions (Cerruti, 1975). Blocking lesions cause large distortions in the DNA molecule, such as those produced by the benz[a]pyrene adduct of guanine or by ultraviolet light–induced dimers. These lesions interfere with the template function of DNA by blocking the progress of DNA polymerases during replication and RNA polymerases during transcription (Moore et al., 1981). It has been proposed that DNA polymerases are blocked by this type of lesion as a result of the damaged base not being able to properly base-pair with any other nucleotide (Radman, 1974, 1975; Radman et al., 1978). During synthesis, the DNA polymerase randomly incorporates a nucleotide opposite the noncoding damaged nucleotide in the template strand. Before the polymerase continues its synthesis, a proofreading function excises the newly incorporated nucleotide (Burtlag and Kornberg, 1972). The role of the proofreading function is to guarantee that during DNA synthesis each newly incorporated nucleotide is properly hydrogen-bonded with its template complement before replication can continue. Because any nucleotide incorporated opposite the noncoding damaged base will not be correctly base-paired, the proofreading function removes it. The polymerase then incorporates another nucleotide at the same site, only to have it also excised by

proofreading. Evidence for such a mechanism has come from studies with bacteria.

Whereas the blockage of RNA polymerase at the damaged site in the gene may be absolute, the DNA polymerase will only hesitate temporarily at the site of the blocking lesion before skipping over it to reinitiate synthesis farther along on a template strand (Hanawalt et al., 1979). This produces a single-strand gap as large as several thousand nucleotides in the newly synthesized DNA molecule. The gap represents lost genetic information. The DNA strand opposite the gap is also susceptible to being broken and degraded by nucleases. This will cause the loss of the genetic information in this DNA strand, disrupt the physical continuity of the DNA molecule, and possibly inhibit the coordinate expression of genes on the two separated pieces of DNA. The fragmentation of the DNA molecule is assured if the gapped strand is used as a template for subsequent DNA replication. The presence of a single-strand gap, therefore, can be of very grave consequence to a cell.

Nonblocking lesions do not prohibit synthesis by DNA and RNA polymerases (Saffhill, 1974). These lesions are usually the result of the incorporation or formation of base analogs in a DNA molecule or are the result of the addition of small groups to a base. Some small adducts are innocuous and produce no biologic consequences. Other adducts as well as nucleotide analogs change the base-pairing specificity of the damaged base. This can have two consequences. The first is unfaithful gene expression during transcription. The presence of a miscoding lesion in the DNA sequence of a gene will change the sequence of its messenger RNA transcript (Singer and Kröger, 1979). The transcript will direct the synthesis of an altered protein that could have deleterious effects on normal cellular behavior. The second consequence comes into being when the DNA strand containing the miscoding lesion is replicated. The newly synthesized DNA strand will contain a nucleotide that is complementary to the miscoding lesion rather than to the original, undamaged base. Thus, an altered nucleotide sequence is created. This is the first example by which mutagen-induced DNA damage can cause a mutation.

The severe consequences that can result when environmental agents interact with DNA make the survival of any cell very unlikely if it cannot mitigate the effects of DNA damage. Enzymatic repair systems exist that allow the cell to overcome the challenge of mutagen-induced damage in its DNA. (For reviews see Grossman et al., 1975; Witkin, 1976; Hanawalt et al., 1979; Lindahl, 1979; and Schendal, 1981.)

The function of DNA repair is to restore the physical integrity of damaged DNA molecules so that they can serve as templates for DNA replication and RNA transcription. Because the consequences of DNA damage caused by mutagens do not occur until either ongoing RNA or DNA synthesis encounters the lesion, a competition between repair and replication exists. There are mechanisms of DNA repair that specifically act at lesions only before or after replication has had to deal with the damage.

Of the prereplicative repair systms, photoactivation, diagrammed in Figure 1-4, is the simplest (Rupert, 1975; H. Harm, 1976). This process is catalyzed by a single enzyme that recognizes and binds only to ultraviolet light–induced pyrimidine dimers. In the presence of visible light, the enzyme splits the covalent bonds, linking the two adjacent pyrimidines, and the DNA helix regains its original, undamaged conformation.

Figure 1–4. Schematic representation of the photoreactivation of an ultraviolet light–induced pyrimidine dimer in DNA.

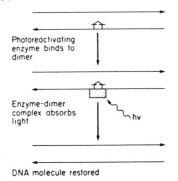

Photoreactivation has been detected in a wide variety of prokaryotic and eukaryotic cells. It is interesting to note that photoreactivation has been observed experimentally to occur in the cells of tissues and organs that are never exposed to ultraviolet light.

The adaptive response is another prereplicative repair system that, like photoreactivation, does not involve the disruption of the physical structure of the DNA molecule (Schendal, 1981). This type of repair has been extensively studied in bacteria, and there is circumstantial evidence to suggest its existence in eukaryotic cells. This repair system is not constitutively expressed in the cell. It is expressed only after cellular DNA is damaged by alkylating agents such as N-methyl-N-nitrosourea that produce small miscoding adducts. Experimental evidence suggests that a protein is synthesized that binds to the alkyl group adducted to the base in the DNA molecule. The bond between the adduct and the base is then broken, restoring the base to its original undamaged configuration while the adduct remains bound to the protein. The identity and nature of the protein involved in the adaptive response is unknown, but it is known that expression of this repair system makes the cell transiently more resistant to the killing and mutagenic effect of subsequent exposures to alkylating agents.

Another prereplicative repair mechanism is excision repair (Grossman et al., 1975; Lindahl, 1979). The first step of this process, shown in Figure 1-5A, is the recognition of the lesion, probably by an endonuclease, which makes an incision in the DNA strand immediately adjacent to the damaged nucleotide. The incision is recognized by an exonuclease, which excises the damaged nucleotide by degrading a portion of the DNA strand containing it. A double-stranded DNA molecule with a single-strand gap of varying size is created. The gap is filled by a DNA polymerase, which uses the intact complementary strand opposite the gap as a template for resynthesizing the DNA. The final step is the enzymatic ligation of the newly synthesized DNA to the preexisting strand. Excision repair restores

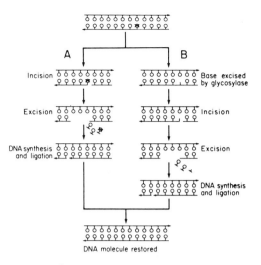

Figure 1–5. Schematic representation of excision repair. (A) Nucleotide excision repair. (B) Base excision repair.

the original structural and functional integrity of a damaged DNA molecule by physically removing the damaged nucleotide.

Excision repair of damaged nucleotides has been studied in many organisms. A wide variety of excision repair pathways exist that differ primarily in the type of DNA damage they recognize. The specificity of excision repair pathways is a function of the first incision step. Some excision repair endonucleases will incise only at lesions, such as large chemical adducts or pyrimidine dimers, that create major helix distortions, whereas others cleave only nucleotides containing small adducts. Endonucleases have been discovered that will act only at depurinated sites. For the most part, however, the degree of DNA helix deformation, rather than the chemical nature of the damage, determines which excision repair endonuclease will cleave at the damaged nucleotide.

A variation of nucleotide excision repair, shown in Figure 1-5B, is base excision repair. Specific base analogs or bases containing small alkyl groups are recognized by glycosylases, which cleave the covalent bond between the base and deoxyribose, creating a depurinated nucleotide (Lindahl, 1979). The depurinated site can then be repaired by a nucleotide excision repair pathway specific for such lesions. Recent evidence

suggests that an enzyme exists that can replace the missing base of the apurinic nucleotide (Deutsch and Linn, 1979). This mechanism would eliminate the need for excision repair of the depurinated nucleotide. Reconsider the consequences of a DNA polymerase encountering a damaged base. If the damage causes only minor distortions in the steric configuration of the template strand, DNA synthesis can proceed. If the damage is a large, blocking lesion, the DNA polymerase temporarily hesitates at the lesion before skipping past it to reinitiate synthesis farther along on the template strand. The result is a single-strand gap opposite an intact DNA strand containing a damaged base. This damage cannot be removed by excision repair mechanisms, because they will break the intact strand, thereby fragmenting the DNA molecule. However, two postreplication mechanisms exist that fill the single-strand gap.

The first of these is recombinational postreplicational repair. Figure 1-6 shows that the replication of a DNA molecule containing a blocking lesion in one strand produces a daughter molecule with a single-strand gap and another intact daughter

Figure 1–6. Schematic representation of a probable pathway of postreplicational recombinational repair. Heavy lines represent original template DNA strands. Lighter lines represent newly synthesized DNA.

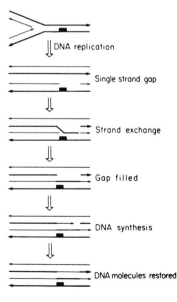

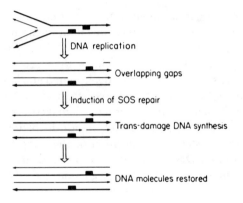

Figure 1-7. Schematic representation of SOS repair.

molecule. The original template strand of the intact daughter molecule contains a segment of DNA that is complementary to the DNA opposite the gap. Recombinational repair—by an as yet undefined process—transfers the homologous piece of DNA into the gap and ligates it to the preexisting strand of DNA (Hanawalt et al., 1979). This leaves the other DNA molecule with a single-strand gap that can be closed by a DNA polymerase using the opposite strand as a template. The original damage is now contained in a double-stranded DNA molecule and can be removed by excision repair. The mechanism of recombinational repair does not remove lesions from DNA as it mediates the closure of single-strand gaps. The closing of the gaps, however, is a preliminary step in establishing a DNA structure conducive to the removal of damage by excision repair.

Now consider the consequence of both strands of a DNA molecule containing a blocking lesion in close proximity to one another as shown in Figure 1-7. Replication of this molecule results in each daughter molecule containing a single-strand gap. There is no complete complementary segment of DNA on either of these molecules to fill the gap on the other. Subsequent replication of these molecules will result in fragmentation of half of the daughter DNA molecules with attendant dire consequences for the cell. Damage of this sort leads to a conditional, replicative repair response that is usually referred to as SOS repair (Witkin, 1976; Radman et al., 1978).

SOS repair is unusual in several respects. Like the adaptive response previously discussed, it is not constitutively present in the cell. It is believed that several of the proteins that participate in this repair mechanism are synthesized only after DNA has been damaged. These proteins also have a transient existence in the cell. Evidence also has been presented that—like recombinational repair—SOS repair promotes the tolerance of DNA damage rather than its removal. SOS repair apparently utilizes a DNA-synthesizing activity that can successfully incorporate nucleotides opposite noncoding DNA damage. The ability to perform trans-damage synthesis enables SOS repair to fill single-strand gaps opposite blocking lesions. Once this is done, it is possible for excision repair to remove the damage and restore the physical and functional integrity of the DNA molecules.

Evidence is accumulating that SOS repair may involve other mechanisms of dealing with DNA damage in addition to trans-damage synthesis (Clark and Volkert, 1978). Genetic analysis of the bacterium *Escherichia coli* indicates that the SOS repair response may be mediated in part by novel mechanisms involving proteins normally involved in excision and recombinational repair. This contention has been supported by the recent finding that damaging conditions, which induce SOS repair, also cause the enhanced expression of proteins involved in constitutive excision repair.

Fidelity of DNA Repair

From the previous section, it is apparent that repair mechanisms can effectively restore the structural integrity of damaged DNA molecules. The restoration of physical integrity alone, however, does not completely determine the efficacy of a DNA repair mechanism in dealing with mutagen-induced damage. The fidelity of DNA repair—how faithfully the original nucleotide sequence is conserved during repair—must also be examined.

The concept of fidelity is extremely important in biology, because it is a measure of how accurately biologic information is expressed and perpetuated. This importance is exemplified by the great lengths taken during DNA replication to ensure a level of faithful synthesis estimated to be less than one incorrect nucleotide for every 10^9 incorporated (Loeb et al., 1979). Base pair complementarity, which defines the template properties of DNA, is insufficient to account for the observed fidelity of DNA replication, because it could provide an accuracy of one incorrect nucleotide for only every 100 incorporated. Active selection by the DNA polymerase of the proper nucleotide to be inserted into the growing DNA chain, and the proofreading of each newly added nucleotide to check for correct base-pairing, enhances the fidelity of DNA synthesis by orders of magnitude (Brutlag and Kornberg, 1972). The fidelity of DNA polymerases is enhanced further by the attachment of DNA-binding proteins to the DNA template (Kunkel, Meyer, and Loeb, 1979). A final editing system may exist that can remove incorrect nucleotides that have escaped detection by proofreading functions and have become stably incorporated into the growing DNA strand (Radman et al., 1978). There is evidence from prokaryotic and eukaryotic cells that a repair system recognizes the small distortions produced in a DNA molecule by two opposing noncomplementary nucleotides. This repair system apparently is capable of delineating the original template strand of a DNA molecule from the newly synthesized daughter strand. After identifying the mismatched nucleotides, the incorrect nucleotide is excised from the newly synthesized strand, and the resulting gap is filled by a DNA polymerase, using the correct original strand as a template. The removal of mismatched nucleotides is analogous to excision repair, with the exception that the object of repair is an incorrect nucleotide sequence rather than DNA damage.

It is not clear to what extent these fidelity-enhancing mechanisms or others participate in assuring the faithfulness of DNA repair. Photoreactivation and the adaptive response are in principle incapable of causing changes in nucleotide sequences, and experimentation with bacteria has confirmed this expectation. Additional information derived from bacterial mutants defective in the different repair mechanisms has shown excision repair and recombinational repair both to be very faithful processes (Witkin, 1976). The same processes that ensure the high fidelity of DNA replication probably are active during excision repair, because DNA synthesis plays a major role in its course. Unknown mechanisms must operate during recombinational repair to guarantee a high degree of complementarity between nucleotide sequence opposite a single-strand gap and the piece of DNA that fills it.

The hypothetical mechanism of SOS repair involving the random insertion of nucleotides opposite noncoding base damage suggests that it would result in changes in the nucleotide sequence of the repaired strand of DNA. Studies with bacteria and eukaryotic cells have shown SOS repair to be an error-prone process relative to other repair mechanisms (Witkin, 1976; Radman et al., 1978). Further experimentation has demonstrated that the expression of SOS repair in a cell can lower the fidelity of DNA synthesis on undamaged DNA. This finding favors the hypothesis that SOS repair is made possible in part by the relaxation of mechanisms such as proofreading, which guarantee fidelity during normal DNA synthesis. The nonspecific mutagenic effect on DNA synthesis by the expression of SOS repair may explain why it is an inducible rather than constitutive part of the DNA repair machinery. SOS repair has a limited lifetime after its induction, approximately 1 hour in bacteria. This is probably a safety mechanism to ensure that mutagenesis due to this repair mechanism altering the fidelity of DNA synthesis does not become overwhelming.

Because DNA damage can induce error-prone DNA repair mechanisms, a competition between faithful and unfaithful repair processes can be envisioned. Photoreactivation, excision repair, recombinational repair, and the adaptive response are antimutagenic. They either remove miscoding lesions from the DNA template or prevent the formation of overlapping strand gaps that lead to the induction of mutagenic SOS repair. When damage is present that cannot be repaired by faithful mechanisms, error-prone SOS repair gains the upper hand in the competition. Because these lesions represent such a dire threat to the continued proper functioning of the DNA molecule, an accommodation between survival and mutagenesis must be made.

Mutagens and DNA Replication

The two mechanisms of mutagenesis previously considered require the interaction of DNA damage with DNA replication, which either produces a mutation directly or induces the synthesis of an error-prone DNA repair system. Environmental agents might also exert mutagenic effects by altering DNA polymerases, either transiently or permanently, in such a way as to lower their intrinsic level of fidelity of DNA replication. So far, there has been only limited evidence for covalent binding of chemical mutagens to DNA polymerases or other replicating proteins. However, transient interactions may be the basis for mutagenesis by many common metals.

Metals have been shown to be mutagenic in both prokaryotic and eukaryotic organisms. These include salts of arsenic, chromium, copper, iron, and manganese (Zakour et al., 1979). The mechanism by which metals cause mutations is not known; however, their effects on fidelity suggest that metal mutagenesis may involve increased misincorporations during DNA replication (Sirover and Loeb, 1976). So far, about 40 metal compounds have been added to in vitro assays that measure the fidelity of DNA synthesis. In Figure 1-8, the results of assays using polynucleotide templates are shown. Most known metal mutagens and/or carcinogens have been shown to increase the frequency of misincorporation by DNA polymerases when added to assays in the form of soluble divalent ions. In contrast, nonmutagenic metals have little effect on fidelity. The interactions of the metal ions with either the DNA template or the DNA polymerase could provide a mechanism for increased misincorporation.

FIDELITY ASSAY
SCREEN FOR MUTAGENS AND/OR CARCINOGENS

In Vitro Assay

Template poly $\left[d(A-T)\right]$
Correct Substrates: dATP + $\left[\alpha-^{32}P\right]$ dTTP

Incorrect Substrate: $\left[^3H\right]$ dGTP
DNA Polymerase
Mg^{2+}

+ Exogenous Agents
(Metal Cations)

Known Carcinogens and/or Mutagens	Increased Misincorporation	No Change in Fidelity
Ag	Ag	Al
Be	Be	Ba
Cd	Cd	Ca
Co	Co	Fe
Cr	Cr	K
Cu	Cu	Rb
Mn	Mn	Mg
Ni	Ni	Na
Pb	Pb	Sr
		Zn

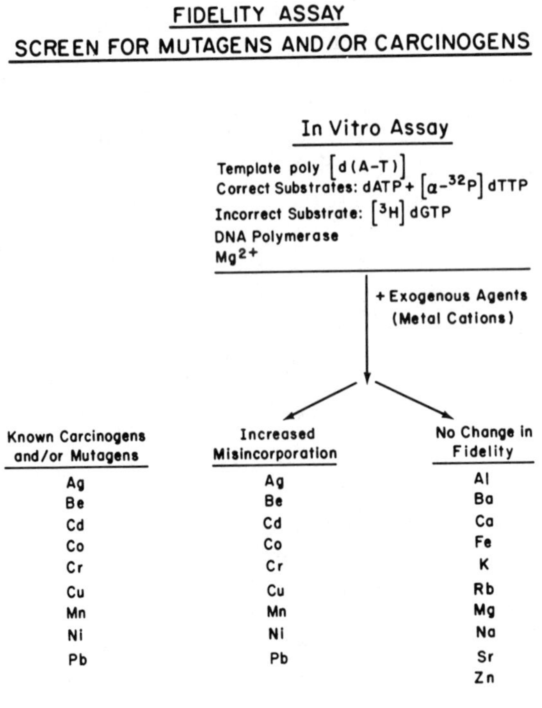

Figure 1-8. Scheme for determining the effect of metals on the fidelity of synthesis by DNA polymerases and classification of metals tested.

Mutagens and Altered Nucleotide Pools

The accuracy of copying DNA using purified DNA polymerases (Battula and Loeb, 1974) and crude extracts from animal cells has been shown to be a function of the relative concentration of the different deoxynucleoside triphosphate substrates. Increasing the concentration of the incorrect nucleotide results in an increased frequency of misincorporation; conversely, increasing the concentration of the correct nucleotide reduces the frequency of misincorporation. This dependency provides a new mechanism for mutagenesis. Agents that alter nucleotide pools may increase the frequency of single-base substitutions during DNA replication and repair. It is surprising that eukaryotic cells do not have overwhelming mechanisms to militate against fluctuations in nucleotide concentrations. In fact, the addition of nucleosides to cells in tissue culture results in increased cellular concentrations of the corresponding deoxynucleoside triphosphate. Infidelity at the level of DNA polymerization could be central to toxicity and mutagenicity by a variety of agents that affect the metabolism of nucleotides. This concept could underlie toxic effects of thymidine on cells in tissue culture, mutagenesis by bromodeoxyuridine (a thymidine analog) (Davidson and Kaufman, 1978), enhancement of mutagenesis by alkylation agents (Peterson et al., 1978), as well as manifestations of diseases with inherited dysfunctions in nucleotide metabolism.

Summary

There are a great number of environmental agents that produce mutations. Many of these compounds, after proper metabolic activation, react with the bases of DNA to form covalently bound adducts. Small adducts change the base-pairing specificity of the damaged base that can lead directly to a mutation on replication. Large adducts destroy the base-pairing specificity of the damaged base altogether. This type of damage will block DNA replication, which in turn induces the expression of a mutagenic DNA repair system. Some environmental agents may exert a mutagenic effect by lowering the ability of DNA polymerases to perform accurate DNA synthesis. This may be done either by physically altering the DNA polymerase itself or by disturbing the relative intracellular concentrations of the nucleotide precursors of DNA replication. In all instances, however, mutagenesis is dependent on DNA replication. Mutagenesis cannot occur by the mechanisms described in this chapter in nondividing cells that are not actively replicating their DNA.

DNA damage does not inevitably lead to mutagenesis in dividing cells. Most DNA repair systems are antimutagenic in that they remove DNA damage before it interacts with replication or eliminate the mutagenic consequences of it after replication has encountered it. Only in instances when DNA damage cannot be repaired by antimutagenic repair systems is error-prone repair expressed as a last resort to ensure cell survival.

Acknowledgments

Support for the preparation of this report was provided by grants from the National Institutes of Health (CA-24845, CA-24498, and AG-0751) and the National Science Foundation. J.R.S is a postdoctoral fellow of the National Institutes of Health (CA-06395).

REFERENCES

Ames, B. 1979. Identifying environmental chemicals causing mutations and cancer. *Science* 204:387–393.

Battula, N., and Loeb, L. A. 1974. The infidelity of avian myeloblastosis virus deoxyribonucleic acid polymerase in polynucleotide replication. *J. Biol. Chem.* 249:4086–4093.

Brutlag, D., and Kornberg, A. 1972. Enzymatic synthesis of deoxyribonucleic acid. XXXVI. A proofreading function for the 3'-5' exonuclease activity in deoxyribonucleic acid polymerases. *J. Biol. Chem.* 247:241–248.

Cerutti, P. A. 1975. Repairable damage in DNA: overview. In *Molecular mechanisms for repair of DNA*, part A, eds. P. C. Hanawalt and R. B. Setlow, pp. 3–11. New York: Pleunum Press.

Clark, A. J., and Volkert, M. R. 1978. A new classification of pathways repairing pyrimidine dimer in DNA. In *DNA repair mech-*

anisms, eds. P. C. Hanawalt, E. C. Fried-berg, and C. F. Fox, pp. 57–72. New York: Academic Press.

Davidson, R. L., and Kaufman, E. R. 1978. Bromodeoxyuridine mutagenesis in mammalian cells is stimulated by thymidine and suppressed by deoxycytidine. *Nature* 276:722–724.

Deutsch, W. A., and Linn, S. 1979. Further characterization of a depurinated DNA purine base insertion activity from cultured human fibroblasts. *J. Biol. Chem.* 254:12099–12103.

Grossman, L., Braun, R., Feldberg, R. and Mahler, I. 1975. Enzymatic repair of DNA. *Ann. Rev. Biochem.* 44:19–43.

Hanawalt, P. C., Cooper, P. K., Ganesan, A. K., and Smith, C. A. 1979. DNA repair in bacteria and mammalian cells. *Ann. Rev. Biochem.* 48:783–836.

Harm, H. 1976. Repair of UV-irradiated biological systems: Photoreactivation. In *Photochemistry and photobiology of nucleic acids*, Vol. 2, ed. S. Y. Wang, New York: Academic Press.

Harm, W. 1980. *Biological effects of ultraviolet radiation.* Cambridge: Cambridge University Press.

Kunkel, T. A., Meyer, R., and Loeb, L. A. 1979. Single-strand binding protein enhances the fidelity of DNA synthesis *in vitro. Proc. Natl. Acad. Sci. U.S.A.* 76:6331–6335.

Lindahl, T. 1979. DNA glycosylases endonucleases for apurinic-apyrimidinic sites and base excision repair. *Prog. Nucleic Acid Res. Mol. Biol.* 22:135–192.

Loeb, L. A., Weymouth, L. A., Kunkel, T. A., Gopinathan, K. P., Beckman, R. A., and Dube, D. K. 1979. On the fidelity of DNA replication. *Cold Spring Harbor Symp. Quant. Biol.* 43:921–929.

Miller, E. C. 1978. Some current perspectives on chemical carcinogenesis in humans and experimental animals. Presidential address. *Cancer Res.* 38:1479–1496.

Moore, P. D., Bose, K. K., Radkin, S. D., and Strauss, B. S. 1981. Sites of termination of *in vitro* DNA synthesis on ultraviolet and N-acetylaminofluorine treated ΦX174 templates by prokaryotic and eukaryotic polymerases. *Proc. Natl. Acad. Sci. U.S.A.* 78:110–114.

Peterson, A. R., Landolph, J. R., Peterson, H., and Heidelberger, C. 1978. Mutagenesis in Chinese hamster cells is facilitated by thy-midine and deoxycytidine. *Nature* 276:508–510.

Radman, M. 1974. Phenomenology of an inducible mutagenic DNA repair pathway in *Escherichia coli:* SOS repair hypothesis. In *Molecular and environmental aspects of mutagenesis*, eds. L. Prakash, F. Sherman, M. W. Miller, C. M. Lawrence, and H. W. Taber, pp. 128–142. Springfield, Ill: Charles C Thomas.

Radman, M. 1975. SOS repair hypothesis: Phenomenology of an inducible DNA repair which is accompanied by mutagenesis. In *Molecular mechanisms for repair of DNA*, part A, eds. P. C. Hanawalt, and R. B. Setlow pp. 355–367. New York: Plenum Press.

Radman, M., Villani, G., Boiteux, S., Kinsella, A. R., Glickman, B. W., and Spadari, S. 1978. Replicational fidelity: Mechanisms of mutation avoidance and mutation fixation. *Cold Spring Harbor Sump. Quant. Biol.* 43:937–946.

Rupert, C. S. 1975. Enzymatic photoreactivation: Overview. In *Molecular mechanisms for repair of DNA*, part A, eds. P. C. Hanawalt and R. B. Setlow, pp. 73–88. New York: Plenum Press.

Saffhill, R. 1974. The effect of ionizing radiation and chemical methylation upon the activity and accuracy of *E. coli* polymerase I. *Biochem. Biophys. Res. Commun.* 61:752–758.

Schendal, P. F. 1981. Inducible repair systems and their implications for toxicology. *CRC Crit. Rev. Toxicol.* 7:311–362.

Setlow, R. B., and Setlow, J. K. 1972. Effects of radiation on polynucleotides. *Ann. Rev. Biophys. Bioengineering* 1:293–346.

Singer, B., and Kröger, M. 1979. Participation of modified nucleosides in translation and transcription. *Prog. Nucleic Acid. Res. Mol. Biol.* 23:151–194.

Sirover, M. A., and Loeb, L. A. 1976. Infidelity of DNA synthesis *in vitro:* Screening for potential metal mutagens or carcinogens. *Science* 194:1434–1436.

Witkin, E. 1976. Ultraviolet mutagenesis and inducible DNA repair in *Escherichia coli. Bacteriol. Rev.* 40:869–907.

Zakour, R. A., Loeb, L. A., Kunkel, T. A., and Koplitz, R. M. 1979. Metals, DNA polymerization and genetic miscoding. In *Trace metals in health and disease*, ed. N. Kharasch, pp. 135–153. New York: Raven Press.

2

Chemical Carcinogenesis

John D. Scribner

OBSERVATIONS IN HUMANS

Occupational Hazards
(Kipling, 1976)

It has been known for more than 200 years that some occupations represent risk factors for some forms of cancer. At the risk of repeating unnecessarily a fact that has been cited to the state of boredom, I note that an English physician, Percival Pott, first reported the occurrence of an occupational cancer in 1776. He cited the frequent occurrence of cancer of the scrotum among chimney sweeps, a disease common enough to have been given a street name ("soot wart"), and suggested that it was directly due to infiltration of soot into the rugae of the scrotum. Well before experimental work was begun on chemical carcinogenesis, the Danish parliament required chimney sweeps to bathe daily, and thus directly reduced the incidence of scrotal cancer. Other occupational exposures to tars and oils have included fishing and working in textile factories. Fishermen, of course, have tarred their nets far back into history, whereas the risk associated with textile factories is due to a specific occupation, tending the mule spinners, the machines used to spin cotton. The spindles of the mule spinners were lubricated with shale oil, which sprayed onto the groin area of the workman as he leaned over the machine, leading in this occupation also to scrotal cancer. Metal-working operations involving extensive use of lubricants have also led to high incidences of skin cancer. The active agents in such tar- and soot-induced cancers appear to be various polycyclic aromatic hydrocarbons, in that carcinogens of this type were first isolated from coal tar, but other components of the mixture may be important factors in determining the rate of tumor development (see sections on tumor promotion and cocarcinogenesis).

The next important occupational hazard to be recognized was the high risk of bladder cancer associated with working in the dye industry (Parkes, 1976). This was first associated with aniline, an aromatic amine common to dye factories, but aniline was later found not to be a risk factor, although it is toxic. In a classic epidemiologic study, Case et al. (1954) investigated numerous cases of bladder cancer in England and Wales, and showed not only that aniline was not a risk factor, but that benzidine, 1-naphthylamine, and 2-naphthylamine were important bladder carcinogens in humans. Simply working in the dye industry increased the risk of developing bladder cancer 30-fold, while working with 2-naphthylamine increased the risk by 87 times. In later studies in this country, 4-aminobiphenyl has been found to be possibly the most potent industrial bladder carcinogen. While production of these compounds has been severely curtailed or forbidden in England, benzidine is still made in large quantities in the United States, and until very recently with no protective measures for the workers. A remarkable situation has now arisen in which another industrial intermediate has been found experimentally to be at least as potent a bladder carcinogen as benzidine, but is being processed in numerous small factories throughout the United States without significant protection of either the workers or the surrounding communities. Methylene-bis(2-chloroaniline) (MOCA) is used as a curing agent in polyurethane manufacture, and in some factories inspection has revealed that MOCA dust visibly settled on many of the work surfaces. This compound has been found to be a potent carcinogen in rats and mice, and has produced a 100% incidence of bladder cancer in dogs in a test carried out in the DuPont toxicology laboratory (Stula et al., 1977). Because its use has been begun relatively recently, we have not yet seen a new epidemic of industrial bladder cancer. Because of lack of regulation (a proposed standard was invalidated by the courts for technical reasons), its use continues with little control. Thus, MOCA may represent a significant test of our ability to predict an occupational hazard from experimental data.

Vinyl chloride is a human carcinogen (IARC, 1974, 1979). By the summer of 1974, 13 cases of angiosarcoma of the liver had been discovered in a population of 20,000 vinyl chloride workers (i.e., the total of all workers to date), but only about twice that many cases were expected among the entire population of the United States for the same period. Thus, these figures alone suggested an increased risk of 400-fold. However, the risk factor in one plant was about 1 in 20,000. For vinyl chloride, as for the aromatic amines, the average latent period for tumor induction in the factory workers was about 20 years.

The industrial production of synthetic resins has resulted in an excess risk of lung cancer (Nelson, 1976). This was associated with the use of bis(chloromethyl) ether (BCME) as a cross-linking agent. In one group of 18 testing laboratory workers exposed to BCME, 6 developed lung cancer, while in the same factory 2 more cases were found among 50 production workers. Of these 8 cases, 5 were oat cell carcinoma. Among chloromethyl methylether (CMME) workers, who are also exposed to BCME as an impurity in the CMME, 14 cases of lung cancer were found in an exposed group of 111, including 12 cases of oat cell carcinoma. Since the latter represents only a third of all cases of lung cancer, it was clear that a specific hazard was associated with these workplaces, a conclusion that also followed from the overall lung tumor incidence in these studies of 12%.

Cole and Goldman (1975) have summarized a number of other occupational cancers, some of which have been linked with reasonable certainty to specific agents, but including others which are, at best, associated only with the occupation. Mesothelioma may be unique in its association with asbestos. Miners, textile workers, insulation workers, and shipyard workers have all developed this disease, which is rare in the general population. Lung cancer, however, develops excessively only in asbestos workers who also smoke. This is probably the clearest example in humans of a cocarcinogenic effect (Selikoff and Hammond, 1975).

Another possible cocarcinogenic effect may be the interaction of sulfur dioxide with arsenic in and around smelters. It is clear now that arsenic is a hazard, responsible for lung cancer, but there is still no experimental system that reproduces this phenomenon in animals. Recently, however, sulfur dioxide has been shown to be a comutagen in short-term assays. This may indicate that both arsenic and sulfur dioxide must be present to produce lung cancer; in industry, arsenic is usually accompanied by sulfur dioxide.

In the past, cancer epidemiology has dealt primarily with the occurrence of the disease, and then with the search for its cause. Recently, however, we have seen the beginnings of an effort to investigate occupations associated with compounds found to be potential hazards by various screening procedures. This can be represented by a search for excess cancer risk among beauticians, based on the finding that 85% of the hair dyes available to the general public are mutagenic to *Salmonella typhimurium*. In two separate studies, a sixfold and a twofold excess risk of lung cancer were found among female beauticians (Garfinkel et al., 1977; Menck et al., 1977). In one of these, a twofold increase in risk for thyroid cancer was also found, but the number of cases was too small for the result to be statistically significant. It is hoped that there will be more epidemiologic efforts along these lines.

Cultural Associations

One such effort (actually several efforts) has been concerned with determining the hazard to the general public from use of artificial sweetners. Both saccharin and sodium cyclamate had been in wide use for a number of years until testing of a standard commercial mixture by implantation of a pellet into the lumen of the rat bladder yielded a significant incidence of bladder tumors. Saccharin was generally considered to be safe, with the result that cyclamate was removed from the market. There was little public objection because saccharin remained available, until this too was found to produce a low incidence of bladder tumors in a two-generation high-dose feeding test. Public pressure demanded legislative obstruction of regulation that would have removed saccharin from the market as well. As a result, several epidemiologic studies were undertaken in an attempt to determine whether a carcinogenic effect of artificial sweetners could be detected in humans. All were retrospective, at various levels of sensitivity. Smaller studies, involving 300–500 bladder cancer patients, were unable to detect any effect. However, in an effort that involved about 3000 cancer patients and about 6000 controls, excess risk of bladder

cancer was detected in otherwise low-risk subjects who reported use of both diet drinks and tabletop artificial sweetners *and* used one of these heavily (Hoover and Strasser, 1980). There was also a suggestion of increase in risk in smokers who also used artificial sweetners.

Smokers, of course, are already at excess risk of cancer at various sites, including the bladder. Eight different thorough prospective studies have established that there is a dose-related risk of lung cancer due to cigarette smoking, with the highest risk in these studies found to be 32 times greater than that for people who had never smoked (Levin et al., 1974). Other sites of direct exposure are also at risk—the lip, the oral cavity, and the esophagus.

A high risk of oral cancer has also been found in those who combine heavy smoking with heavy drinking (Rothman, 1975). The combination of two packs of cigarettes per day with more than 1.5 ounces of alcohol results in a risk of oral cancer 6 times higher than for either by itself, and 15 times higher than for those who neither smoke nor drink.

Various drugs are associated with human cancer or neoplasia. Phenacetin has been widely used as an analgesic, and is associated with both bladder and kidney tumors in humans (Carro-Ciampi, 1978). Remarkably enough, acetaminophen (a major metabolite of phenacetin) has not shown any tumorigenic or mutagenic potential in experimental animals, nor has a putative activated metabolite, N-hydroxyacetaminophen. Thus, while an overdose of acetaminophen may be lethal, it appears that this compound is not likely to exert any long-term genotoxicity.

Compounds with hormonal activity have been associated with human cancer. The most clear-cut case is the transplacental induction of vaginal adenocarcinoma or cervical clear cell adenocarcinoma in women (Herbst, et al., 1977). In the daughters of women given diethylstilbestrol (DES) during pregnancy, there is about 0.1% absolute risk of developing one of these forms of cancer. These diseases, like angiosarcoma of the liver in vinyl chloride workers, demonstrate the ease of recognizing a hazard if it induces a rare disease. Such vaginal tumors were virtually unknown in young women before 1965; thus the diagnosis of only eight cases within 4 years was enough to raise a warning flag. In the age-specific incidence rates that have since been established, there is a sharp peak at age 19, with almost all of the distribution falling between the ages of 13 and 24. Estrogenic hormones have been associated with tumors of the liver and of the uterine endometrium. The first gross association between uterine cancer and estrogens came from the observation that this type of cancer was increasing dramatically in the early 1970s (Weiss, 1977). A 62% increase was seen in San Francisco in 4 years, while the rate doubled in New Mexico in just 3 years, with the greatest change generally being seen in the 45–64 age group. This effect is not correlated with an increased use of estrogens in the early 1950s, but with an increase in the sale of noncontraceptive estrogens in the 1960s (fourfold increase between 1963 and 1973). Instead of the 20-year latent period seen for DES carcinogenesis, many forms of industrial carcinogenesis, and tobacco-induced lung cancer, this early response to estrogen use (5- 10-year latent period) suggests that a different mechanism of tumor induction is being manifested.

The association between the use of oral contraceptives and the development of liver adenomas is stronger than the association developed for endometrial cancer and noncontraceptive estrogens (Pike et al., 1977). Since the mid-1960s there has been a sharp increase in the number of these liver tumors, which was found to be related to the dose of contraceptive. Women who used contraceptives for more than 9 years had a risk of tumor development 20-fold greater than those who had used these drugs for a year or less. Here too, a relatively short latent period for tumor induction was observed; in most cases, the women with tumors were still using the contraceptives at time of diagnosis.

The examples cited above, and those mentioned by Cole and Goldman (1975) represent substances for which there is already epidemiologic evidence of a carcinogenic effect. It might as well be noted here that the success of screening procedures designed to protect human beings from carcinogens can only be established if the screens fail or if the will of the public fails, in responding to positive indications from screening tests. That is, epidemiology can only tell us about the consequences of those substances that are allowed into the environment. Consequently, if a perfect screening system is established, and we act according to its information, we will never be able to show that it was effective. Thus our end point must be experimental animals, and must be accepted to be experimental animals. With this in mind, let us review the carcinogenesis studies carried out in lower mammals.

OBSERVATIONS IN EXPERIMENTAL SYSTEMS

From Crude Mixtures to Pure Compounds
(Clayson, 1962)

Not only were tars and soot the first recognized human carcinogens, but coal tar was also used in the first experimental induction of cancer. Yamagiwa and Ichikawa, in 1918, reported the formation of benign tumors, followed by cancer, following repeated application of coal tar to the ears of rabbits. This regimen was followed by the demonstration that similar painting of the backs of mice also produced benign and malignant tumors, an advance that allowed improvement in statistical evaluation (because larger numbers of animals could be entered into experiments) and reduction in latent period. This development of an appropriate animal model was accompanied by the isolation of pure compounds from coal tar with carcinogenic activity, and the synthesis of carcinogenic compounds based on similarity of properties with known carcinogens. The first, and historically most important, carcinogen isolated from coal tar was benzo[a]pyrene. This compound was isolated specifically because it had a fluorescence spectrum that could be followed through the lengthy isolation procedure. It was pure good fortune, of course, that the fluorescent compound also had carcinogenic activity. Tars and soots contain numerous other polycyclic aromatic hydrocarbons, some more potent carcinogens than benzo[a]pyrene and many less so. Thus, the experimental importance of benzo[a]pyrene rests on two factors: history and the fact that it is the smallest (and therefore most easily synthesized) unsubstituted polycyclic aromatic hydrocarbon that will produce tumors easily in experimental animals.

With only chemists and pathologists to investigate chemical carcinogenesis, in that molecular biology did not exist, the avenues open for investigating the mechanism(s) of carcinogenesis were limited. The chemists chose their area of expertise and began making compounds.

Structure–Activity Studies

In an English school and at Harvard, numerous polycyclic aromatic hydrocarbons were synthesized and tested for their ability to induce skin cancer in mice. Although the efforts at Harvard have long since ceased, the work at the Chester Beatty Research Institute in London has continued uninterrupted to the present. The early skin tumor induction experiments reported by the British group are a model of detailed reporting of such experiments, but the unifying thread sought from these studies has yet to be found. Chemical and theoretical studies on the polycyclic aromatic hydrocarbons led to what might be cited as a classic example of misdirection in scientific research, the pursuit of the notorious "K region." It is remarkable that the British group was never as persuaded of the usefulness of this concept as were some others, and finally showed that it very likely is irrelevant to explanation of hydrocarbon carcinogenicity.

A second important area of structure–activity studies was begun as a result of the finding in Japan that a common food coloring ("butter-yellow"—N,N-dimethyl-4-aminoazobenzene, or DAB) is a fairly potent hepatocarcinogen in rats. The Millers and their associates at the University of Wisconsin, as well as other various groups, synthesized numerous analogous azo dyes and tested them for carcinogenic activity. In addition, they also synthesized and tested many other aromatic amines and amides, based on the known human carcinogenicity of such compounds, and on the finding that the potential insecticide 2-acetamidofluorene was found to be a mutipotent carcinogen in rats.

Nitrosamines have been studied exhaustively in Germany and the United States. It is only in this class that relatively clear structure–activity relationships have been elucidated, presumably because of the relative simplicity of the activating metabolism required. In recent years, ostensibly highly sophisticated computer-based correlation schemes have been applied to the study of structure and activity for chemical carcinogens, but it seems safe to say that, except for some of the work on nitrosamines, these schemes have not added to our knowledge of carcinogenic mechanisms.

Metabolic Studies

Early views of carcinogenesis imagined that the unmodified compound itself interacted with biologic organization in some fashion such as to alter growth control. However, the studies with aromatic amines, which showed that tumors usually arose distant from the point of first exposure, suggested to the Millers and others that metabolic activation of the nonreactive precarcinogen was essential for carcinogenic activity. Long and patient study by the Millers established the concepts of "proximate" and "ultimate" carcinogens, substances resulting from metabolism that are closer to (in metabolic sequence) or are the species that can react nonenzymatically with a crucial target in the cell. Such studies have become such a predominant part of carcinogenesis research that a tendency has arisen to consider metabolic studies as investigations into the mechanism of carcinogenesis. A moment's reflection will reveal, of course, that such studies *may* show why certain tissues or organisms resist carcinogenesis, but they do not tell us how an ultimate carcinogen attacks its target, they do not identify which target is more critical than others, and they do not relate the event of attack to the process of transformation from a normal cell to tumor cell. While indispensable in developing a rational basis for risk assessment, metabolic studies are not studies on the mechanism of carcinogenesis.

Carcinogen Chemistry

Elucidation of the chemical events that occur when an activation-requiring carcinogen attacks cellular targets is a relatively recent entry into the study of carcinogenesis mechanisms. The first adduct between a carcinogen other than a simple alkylating agent and a cellular macromolecule was identified in 1965, an adduct of N-methyl-4-aminoazobenzene with methionine in protein. The first adduct with DNA was reported in 1967, a product from 2-acetamidofluorene and guanine. A product from a polycyclic aromatic hydrocarbon requiring metabolic activation was finally identified in 1975, with the report of an adduct between benzo[a]pyrene and guanine. Since these studies, the chemistry of polycyclic hydrocarbon adducts has proved to be remarkably consistent from compound to compound, while the chemistry of aromatic amine adducts has been heavily dependent on the position of substitution of the nitrogen atom and on the aromatic system. Compounds in other classes of carcinogens are usually found to be activated to alkylating agents. This includes particularly the nitrosamines and aflatoxin. The chemistry of the aromatic amine and polycyclic hydrocarbon ultimate carcinogens is such that one could say that *all* of the principal classes of carcinogens are converted to what could formally be called alkylating agents.

Biochemistry and Molecular Biology

Knowing the nature of chemical attack of carcinogens on cellular macromolecules is

also not equivalent to knowing the mechanism(s) of carcinogenesis. This requires knowing the consequences of such attack, or at least establishing a complete logical chain of events between such attack and the formation of a transformed cell. Historically, before carcinogen chemistry was understood, numerous studies on tumor enzymology had been undertaken. Out of these arose the preliminary ideas of, first, anaerobic glycolysis, and later, the common enzyme complement as characteristic of tumors. Both seemed useful generalizations at the times of their formations, but it has since been found that neither is required for malignancy. In recent years, various enzymes, either in their induction or deletion, have been proposed as markers for tumors, but the mechanistic significance of these enzymes is not obvious.

Molecular biology has been approached gingerly from the other aspect of carcinogenesis, the characterization of early events in the carcinogenic process. A strong qualitative correlation has been established between mutagenicity and carcinogenicity, and under certain carefully defined conditions, strong quantitative correlations have been shown. Proof that carcinogenicity depends on mutagenicity is lacking, however. Some powerful promoters of mouse skin tumorigenesis and transformation in vitro are known to alter differentiation in numerous model systems, and to induce the synthesis of various enzymes associated with DNA synthesis. What relationship these effects have on tumor promotion, and what the chemical mechanisms of their induction are remain unknown.

Multistep Models of Carcinogenesis

Tumor promotion itself is a process widely misunderstood phenomenologically. Early studies, which have been repeated many times, showed that the process of tumor induction in mouse skin by repeated application of carcinogen could be replaced by a procedure in which a single dose of carcinogen was followed by repeated doses of a noncarcinogenic promoter. After many years of being widely ignored as a useful model for carcinogenesis, this regimen and its implications for human cancer have been taken to heart, the result being a new dogma that all carcinogenesis proceeds by a combination of "initiation" and "promotion." In fact, proof for such a position is lacking, and mechanistic characterizations of the two steps remain murky, at best. Extension of the two-step regimen to other tissues has been successful, but there is no evidence that the initiation steps, or promotion steps, in the various systems consist of the same molecular events. With all these caveats in mind, let us move on to more detail.

Experimental Induction of Neoplasia

THE NCI BIOASSAY
(Saffiotti and Page, 1977)

Feeding of suspect compounds at high doses for a lifetime to rats and mice has become for many the minimum acceptable test for carcinogenic activity. The model regimen for such studies is the bioassay schedule established by the Carcinogenesis Testing Program of the United States National Cancer Institute (NCI). For a single compound, such a test requires, on the average, about 40 months. Three months are required just for planning the resources, obtaining the animals, and obtaining the compound for test. Included in this time is analysis (and possibly purification) of the test substance. If the substance is a commercial product that results from a specific production scheme, the crude material may be tested. Otherwise, an attempt is normally made to test the purest material possible.

This introductory period is then followed by prechronic toxicity testing, to determine the doses to be used in the actual long-term testing. Acute toxicity is first determined, followed by feeding for several weeks at high doses. It is at this point in the program that a maximum tolerated dose (MTD) is determined. The MTD is the maximum dose that permits survival and normal growth for at least 90% of the animals over a feeding period of 3 months. The normal growth criterion is worth emphasizing, as this assures that the animals used in the long-term test-

ing will not be suffering from overt toxicity, contrary to what is often suggested in the popular and uninformed scientific press.

The full carcinogenesis assay itself normally involves 50 animals of each sex, of each species, at each of two doses, the MTD and MTD/2. Feeding is carried out for 24 to 30 months, unless a high tumor incidence is discovered earlier. Control groups, of course, are maintained for the full period. Occasionally, the MTD found in the subchronic testing proves too high for feeding longer than 3 months, as detected by weight loss or other signs of toxicity. The dose is then reduced by about 10% to 20%, to permit the test to continue for the full planned period.

It must be emphasized that there are several pitfalls to this approach. The first is that it is of objective value only for the exhaustive evaluation of the carcinogenicity of inadequately tested compounds that are intended to be used routinely by humans. The cost of such an assay alone, estimated to be hundreds of thousands of dollars, is sufficient to restrict its use for such compounds. However, the fact that a compound has not been subjected to such a test is a poor criterion for acceptibility in any studies intended to determine the value of other, quicker assay methods in risk assessment.

A second problem is that the animals used must be carefully chosen. A potent human carcinogen, 4-aminobiphenyl, was found to be inactive in rats in the NCI bioassay. Aminobiphenyl has indeed been found to be carcinogenic in the outbred Sprague-Dawley rat, with its primary target being the mammary gland of the female. The rat used in the NCI bioassay, however, is the F344 inbred rat, which is particularly resistant to mammary carcinogenesis by aromatic amines. It appears that there is no particular virtue to the F344 rat other than its being inbred, so that one must wonder how many other compounds found negative, and tested only in the NCI bioassay, are in fact noncarcinogenic. From both the analytic and public health points of view, then, the NCI bioassay is not a guarantor of noncarcinogenicity. This also follows from another consideration—some compounds may be carcinogenic on local application but noncarinogenic on feeding.

LOCAL APPLICATION

Application of compounds to the skin of rabbits and mice is the oldest method of carcinogenicity testing. As noted earlier, coal tar was shown to be carcinogenic on local application to the ears of rabbits, and all of the extensive studies on polycyclic aromatic hydrocarbons carried out in the 1920s and 1930s were performed by painting on the backs of mice. This procedure may appear to be more time-consuming than feeding, but when the time involved in mixing diets and filling diet cups is reckoned, together with the better control of dose and reduced hazard involved in skin painting, it is clear that the latter is actually a relatively undemanding application procedure. In the past, skin "painting" was actually that, the application of a solution of compound to the skin with an artist's brush. The literature contains numerous references to specific-sized camel's hair brushes. Now, however, use is made of any of the numerous commercially available thumb-operated micropipettes with disposable tips, which offer much more reproducible doses than brushes. In studies on the mouse (and any other species for which the experimenter wishes to apply compound to a normally furry area of the body), judgments must be made regarding whether to shave the animal at the beginning of the experiment, and whether to shave repeatedly during the experiment. In the induction of squamous cell tumors (papillomas and carcinomas) on mouse skin, failure to shave the animal repeatedly would seem to reduce the effective dose, since much of the compound applied may be absorbed by hair. However, any wounding produced by repeated shaving, particularly of animals already bearing tumors, may alter the kinetics of tumor induction in unknown fashion. Our practice has been to shave once before any application of compound, without any further shaving. Detention of the induction of melanomas in hamster skin, however, absolutely requires repeated shaving, just to see the affected area and observe the tumors.

Local application, of course, is not restricted to skin painting. It also includes subcutaneous or intramuscular injection into the leg or other local tissue (such as under mammary glands in female rats). Such application is usually used for mechanistic studies or to conserve small amounts of difficultly prepared compound. In certain instances it has been used as an alternative to feeding for compounds that produce high systemic toxicity. For a few compounds, it has proved to be the only method of detecting carcinogenicity. Various metallic compounds make up the bulk of this latter class. Compounds have also been administered by gavage, with their effects appearing in the tissues of the digestive tract, representing here too a form of local application.

INITIATION AND PROMOTION
(Scribner and Süss, 1978)

The use of skin painting as the routine assay for carcinogenic activity was probably an important factor in Berenblum's decision to determine whether irritation per se is a carcinogenic influence (Berenblum, 1929a, 1929b, 1930, 1931) Inflammation and hyperplasia induced by a number of agents could be observed directly in the skin, and comparisons made with the carcinogenic activity or lack of it for each compound. It was soon clear that irritating agents were not necessarily carcinogenic agents. Berenblum then tested whether they might be cocarcinogenic agents by alternating application of benzo[a]pyrene and the test agent. Again, he established that irritating ability was not intrinsically associated with cocarcinogenic ability. However, among the agents tested was croton oil, which had a powerful cocarcinogenic effect. Berenblum was able to show that through the combination of benzpyrene and croton oil tumors could be made to appear even though the total dose of benzpyrene used was itself noncarcinogenic. Some further development finally led to the regimen (Mottram, 1944) in which the carcinogen is administered only once, followed by repeated treatment with croton oil. This represents the ideal initiation–promotion regimen.

For many years, the initiation–promotion regimen was considered a rather special case of tumor induction, applicable only to mouse skin carcinogenesis. However, since 1970 a variety of systemic initiation–promotion systems has developed. Most resembling the mouse skin system in the clarity of results in the induction of bladder carcinoma in rats. In this system, as in mouse skin, a subthreshold dose of carcinogen (in this case, methylnitrosourea) could be established, which did not lead to tumors without promotion, but which resulted in 50% to 60% carcinoma induction following promotion (with either saccharin or cyclamate). In the rat liver, initiation could be accomplished by feeding 2-acetamidofluorene (AAF) to weanling rats for 3 weeks, followed by promotion with either phenobarbital or DDT. This system has been expanded tremendously in recent years, with variations in both the initiator (diethylnitrosamine, 3′-methyl-N,N-dimethyl-4-aminoazobenzene) and the promoter (polychlorinated biphenyls, 2,3,7,8-tetrachlorodibenzo-p-dioxin), as well as numerous modifications in the administration regimens (see below). While other two-stage systems have been developed (colon, lung, tissue culture), the predominant ones for mechanistic studies remain mouse skin, rat bladder and rat liver.

Cocarcinogenesis
(Van Duuren and Goldschmidt, 1975)

Following the development of the initiation–promotion system, a systematic investigation of the phenomenon of cocarcinogenesis fell by the wayside. Cocarcinogenesis in this respect refers to repeated administration of both carcinogen and cocarcinogen. However, Van Duuren revived study of this phenomenon with experiments that showed that there are several compounds (notably including some components of cigarette smoke) that are cocarcinogenic with benzpyrene, but that do not have promoting ability. That is, when administered repeatedly after a single dose of benzpyrene, these compounds did not induce tumors; if given in alternation with extremely small doses of benzpyrene, however, these substances led to tumors with the otherwise noncarcinogenic total dose of benzpyrene. These experiments thus showed that promotion and cocarcinogenesis are distinct phenomena, as further demonstrated by the observation that some weak promoters, such as phenol, lacked cocarcinogenic activity. Thus, it is now clear that in some pollutant mixtures to which humans are exposed, there are substances that are carcinogenic in animals, substances with promoting activity, and substances with cocarcinogenic activity. This combination can lead to a risk of tumor development far greater than would be anticipated simply from the content of carcinogen alone.

Biologic Studies on Initiation and Promotion

Reversibility and Irreversibility

Following the early studies of Berenblum and Mottram that led to the initiation–promotion model, an important next step was to investigate the properties of these two stages in more detail. It was soon established that initiation is an irreversible, permanent event. Promotion could be delayed as long as a year without markedly reducing the eventual tumor yield (Scribner and Süss, 1978, Scribner, 1969). This observation has been repeated in several laboratories since then, most recently in the author's group. Using the SENCAR strain (selected for sensitivity to initiation and promotion), we found that delaying promotion by 12-O-tetradecanoylphorbol-13-acetate (TPA, the most potent component of croton oil) for 40 weeks had absolutely no effect on the average number of tumors per mouse induced by initiation with 7,12-dimethylbenz[a]anthracene (DMBA, the most potent polycyclic hydrocarbon skin carcinogen) (Figure 2-1). The effects of two other initiators (di-

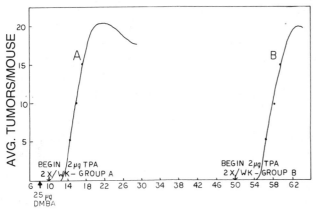

Figure 2–1. Effect of delaying tumor promotion by TPA after initiation by DMBA in SENCAR strain mice. All mice received DMBA on week 5. Group A began receiving TPA (2 μg twice a week) on week 10, group B on week 50.

benz[a,c]anthracene and 7-bromomethylbenz[a]anthracene) were also found to be permanent in the same experiment. This permanence suggests additivity, and such additivity has been demonstrated by Boutwell (1964), using DMBA, and in our work, using dibenz[ac]anthracene (Scribner and Scribner, 1980). Such permanence and additivity imply a remarkable stability in the stem cell lineage of mouse skin, because the epidermis turns over many times during such experiments.

In contrast, Boutwell has shown that a given total dose of croton oil must be appropriately distributed over time in order to achieve promotion (Boutwell, 1964). A high dose given infrequently or a very low dose given several times a week fails to promote. We have observed a similar phenomenon with 7-bromomethylbenz[a]anthracene (7-Br-Me-BA) used as a promoter (Figure 2-2). The demonstration of reversibility of promotion is only possible if promotion with a high dose of promoter can be achieved early in the lifetime of the animal. Thus, with TPA, a 50% response to optimum level of promoter can be obtained within 6 to 8 weeks. Effective promotion of liver tumors or bladder tumors in rats, however, requires 6–12 months. Therefore, one cannot reduce the dose of promoter (e.g., phenobarbital or saccharin) greatly and expect to observe a significant tumor incidence within the life-

time of the animal, even if the promoting effect were additive.

It is obvious, then, that it is impossible in principle to determine whether the effects of weak promoters are additive or not. If one is fortunate, the dose–response curve may drop so sharply that simply halving the dose would result in a loss of promoting activity. Experiments published to date, however, have not indicated this occurs. The eventual conclusion, as unsatisfactory as it may be, is that we cannot determine experimentally whether there is a threshold of promoting acitvity for weak promoters. If we are so fortunate as to determine the acute processes induced by these promoters that are responsible for promotion, a demonstration that there is a threshold dose for these processes would imply a threshold for promoting activity itself. This fact alone justifies research on the mechanism of promotion.

SEQUENCING THE CARCINOGENIC PROCESS

If tumors can be induced in mouse skin and other tissues through a two-step regimen combining initiation by a carcinogen with promotion by a noncarcinogen, it follows that the carcinogenic process induced by a single compound might consist of the steps induced separately by initiators and promoters. This eminently logical and reason-

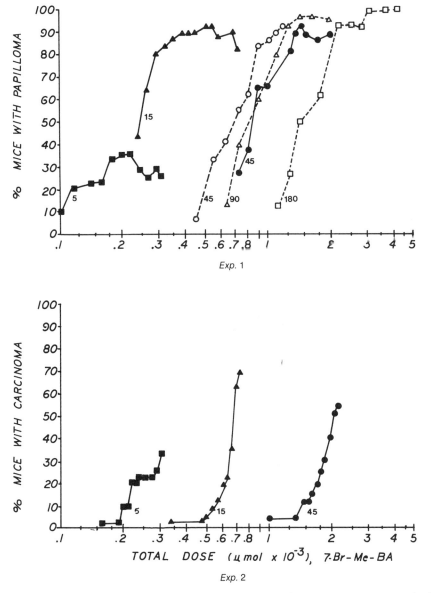

Figure 2–2. Reversibility of promotion shown by decreasing dose. Exp. 1: ○ 45 nmol/wk, △ 90 nmol/wk, □ ⊕⊖⊡ nmol/wk. Exp. 2: ■ 5 nmol/wk, ▲ 15 nmol/wk, ● 45 nmol/wk.

able conclusion has already been largely supplanted by the illogical conclusion that complete carcinogenesis *must* consist of initiation plus promotion. In any case, it is reasonable to address this issue experimentally: what are the events that occur during complete carcinogenesis? Identifying such events, even without identifying their causes, has proved to be a monumental task. Most

information of value has come from studies on rat liver and mouse skin, despite the fact that these tissues have little relevance to the human cancer problem (hepatomas being rare in humans and skin cancer being readily treatable).

In the mouse skin system, initiation has generally been considered to be a very rapid, single event, having all of the properties of a mutation. Yet, in a repeated experiment, Boutwell (1964) has shown that there is a threshold total dose for initiation. These two statements are not necessarily in conflict, but Boutwell's experimental design belies the idea of a single event being the substance of initiation. He found that four 0.25-µg doses of DMBA, separated by 2-week intervals, yielded the same number of tumors as one 1-µg dose (30 papillomas in 20 mice). This result, of course, demonstrates only additivity of initiating doses. However, a single 0.25-µg dose of DMBA did not yield proportionately fewer tumors; rather, it gave no tumors at all. Because four such doses had the same effect as a single dose of 1 µg, it is clear that the single lower dose is not a "no-effect" dose. Because no tumors appeared, however, it is also clear that more than one event had to take place to initiate papillomas.

Because of the characteristics of the mouse skin system, the word "initiation" is not being used rather indiscriminately to describe carcinogenic processes generally. However, it is now clear that there are significant differences between initiation in mouse skin and what is operationally initiation in other tissues. The dose of methylnitrosourea used to initiate rat bladder tumors, while inadequate to produce cancer by itself, still is sufficient to produce significant local toxicity and subsequent regenerative hyperplasia (Hicks and Chowaniec, 1978). In contrast, skin papillomas can be initiated by doses of DMBA that produce no detectable change in the tissue, either histologic or biochemical. Initiation of liver tumors similarly seems to require administration of necrogenic doses of carcinogen, or partial hepatectomy (Columbano et al., 1981; Ying et al., 1981). Such differences in the level of insult required for initiation in different tissues suggest that the promoters act in the respective tissues may also have different levels, that is, that different promoters differ not only in degree of induction of various processes, but also in the kinds of processes they influence.

One example may be instructive. It has been found that an essential enzyme in po-

lyamine synthesis, ornithine decarboxylase, is induced several hundredfold in mouse skin by doses of TPA that are optimum for tumor promotion (O'Brien, 1976). In contrast, the normal dose of phenobarbital used for promoting rat liver tumors is without detectable effect on this enzyme. Even high doses given by injection produced only a small increase. Saccharin, a promoter of rat bladder tumors at extremely high doses (5% of diet), was inactive in several investigations of its ability to produce alterations in the bladder. A hyperplastic influence was finally detected through the use of the labeling index (Fukushima and Cohen, 1980). Further critical research remains to be done to determine whether there are indeed qualitative differences among various promoters. The results summarized above suggest that this may be the case.

For many years it has been believed that there are compounds that might be considered pure initiators, and others that are pure promoters. By this is meant that pure initiators, regardless of total dose, would not induce tumors by themselves. The same applies to pure promoters. It now seems unlikely that either exists operationally, and likely that strong promoters must be capable of inducing tumors theoretically, as well as operationally. Urethane has been considered to be a pure initiator in mouse skin, because no single dose of urethane has ever been found to lead to skin tumors without promotion. A second example is perhaps more rigorous. The hydrocarbon dibenz[a,c]anthracene is a tumor initiator in mouse skin that has been tested directly for promoting activity, and found inactive (N. K. Scribner and J. D. Scribner, 1980). Yet, repeated administration of dibenz[a,c]anthracene for a long enough period resulted in a high incidence of skin cancer (Lijinsky et al., 1970).

This example, plus others, make it questionable to assert that all carcinogenesis consists of a combination of initiating and promoting processes. An indirect suggestion of the adequacy of repeated initiation alone as a carcinogenic process was found in comparing the susceptibility of initiation and complete carcinogenesis by 3-methyl-cholanthrene to inhibition by dexamethasone (Slaga and Scribner, 1973). The latter compound can completely suppress promotion by TPA and has a modest inhibitory effect on methylcholanthrene initiation. Its effect on complete carcinogenesis by methylcholanthrene could be completely accounted for by addition of individually inhibited initiating events. Thus, both direct and indirect evidence support the idea that complete carcinogenesis by some compounds can take place without promotion.

Such a statement implies that promotion really is different from initiation. While this may be true in the ideal mouse skin situation, it may not be so in other experimental systems. To judge whether the two processes are different, one must be able to determine other events induced by various initiators and promoters, and establish whether the essential events really differ in character for the two processes. In other words, one must determine the mechanisms of initiation and promotion.

MUTAGENESIS AND HYPERPLASIA

It has become fashionable to synthesize a mechanism of carcinogenesis through fusion of the two oldest durable theories of carcinogenesis—Virchow's irritation hypothesis and Bauer's mutation hypothesis. Because initiation (at least in mouse skin) has the properties of a mutation, and because croton oil is irritating, initiation has been considered to be equivalent to mutagenesis, while promotion has been thought to consist of selection of initiated cells through hyperplastic stress. Probably the most that can be said about these two positions is that they represent part of the truth. It has been easy to show that many carcinogens are mutagenic, both in bacteria and in mammalian cells. There is a high quantitative correlation between mutagenicity of polycyclic aromatic hydrocarbons in V79 cells in culture and initiating potency in mouse skin. The correlation between initiating potency and mutagenic activity in bacteria (*Salmonella* tester strains) is not

good at all, but is improved markedly (to the level of the mammalian cell correlations) by introduction of the octanol–water partition coefficients for the hydrocarbons into the regression analysis. This suggests that the lack of correlation is due to factors unrelated to the basic mechanistic question. (One might note here that many structure–activity correlations in the literature depend on factors probably unrelated to the actual mechanism of action of the drug or toxin series under investigation.)

The idea that initiation equals mutagenesis is countered by tissue culture studies that find in many instances that the frequency of a specific detectable mutation is far lower than the transformation frequency in the same cell line. For those who believe that transformation is due to mutagenesis, the traditional defense has been that the target for transformation in such cell lines is much larger than the target for an arbitrarily chosen mutation. It has also been found that two of the cell lines best suited for detecting transforming ability of carcinogens are tumorigenic in whole animals simply on being inoculated together with plastic films, although they are not tumorigenic without the films (Boone and Jacobs, 1976). This suggests that the transformation seen in such cultured cells on treatment with carcinogen is simply due to the last of a series of steps necessary for the process, and that transformation in culture is not a good model for initiation in vivo. To be sure, initiation and promotion have also been carried out in culture, but there is no evidence that the two steps coincide with the steps observed in mouse skin.

Two separate studies, using X radiation and methylcholanthrene as transforming agents, have shown that transformation is a random event that occurs rarely in a population of cells that are ostensibly identical (Mondal and Heidelberger, 1970; Kennedy and Little, 1980). Effectively, what was observed in both studies was that when single cells were selected from carcinogen-treated colonies, then grown up into complete colonies, only one or a few transformed colonies were observed in each dish. Subsequent cloning of normal cells from these dishes gave rise to the same transformation frequencies in subsequent colonies. These data were used as evidence for the proposition that transformation is not a mutagenic process. They can equally well be considered evidence for the opposite viewpoint, that a mutagen is necessary for both the permanent ability to be transformed at a constant, albeit low rate, and the random appearance of transformation. An epigenetic alteration could be responsible for either of these properties, but it seems unlikely that it could result in both.

Pathologists have sometimes treated promotion as simply hyperplasia, and it is true that most promoters, possibly all, do stimulate growth of their target tissues. TPA, as the most potent of these agents, produces a severalfold increase in the number of cell layers in mouse epidermis, whereas, as mentioned above, the effect of saccharin in rat bladder is detectable only by determination of the labeling index. The fact that many agents that produce hyperplasia in mouse skin lack promoting activity has been used as the primary argument for the proposition that promotion consists of more events. This argument may have two fallacies. The first is that hyperplasia is normally measured as a response to a single application of irritant. If the tissue adapts to repeated applications, then there will not be a sustained hyperplasia. Such adaptation has been reported for hamster skin and TPA. Thus, the hyperplasia determined in a short-term experiment may not represent the effect over a longer period.

The second possible fallacy is that the events essential to promotion may vary with the initiating agent used and the tissue response during the initiation process. That is, it may prove that only hyperplasia is required as a promoting stimulus if numerous other events have already taken place during the treatment with initiator. Even in mouse skin, regenerative hyperplasia produced by repeated abrasion has had a modest promoting effect (Argyris, 1980). This was obtained, however, by complete removal of the interfollicular epidermis, re-

quiring complete replacement of the epidermis by outgrowth from the hair follicles. It is not clear what relationship there may be between such a process and the hyperplasia produced by TPA or by nonpromoting agents, such as ethylphenylpropiolate. Earlier work showed a correlation between hyperplasiogenic potency and promoting ability for several agents, but the dose of initiator was high enough that one could imagine it to be very close to the threshold of complete carcinogenic activity. Recent work with TPA analogs has identified compounds with inflammatory potency that produce extensive hyperplasia, as well as other biochemical changes also produced by TPA, which lack promoting activity. A single dose of TPA before chronic treatment with either of these agents (mezerein, 12-O-retinoylphorbol-13-acetate), however, did result in high yields of papillomas, suggesting both that there is more than one event in promotion and that hyperplasia is an important part of the process (Slaga et al., 1980; Berry et al., 1981).

THE VARIETY OF INITIATION–PROMOTION SYSTEMS
(Scribner and Süss, 1978)

As mentioned above, the initiation–promotion model has been extended to a number of systems. Initiators in mouse skin have included numerous polycyclic aromatic hydrocarbons, alkylating agents, urethane, and N-arylhydroxylamines, covering a 100,000-fold range in potency. In addition, it has been shown that feeding 2-acetamidofluorene, which is inactive on local application, results in initiation of skin tumors in mice. Not so remarkable, but with some experimental advantages, is the finding that a single oral dose of DMBA can also initiate skin tumors. Transplacental initiation has been demonstrated, with numerous tissues other than skin being additional targets. The most effective promoters in skin are TPA and analogs of comparable molecular weight with the same location of substitution of fatty acid side chains. Closely following in potency is the aromatic alkylating agent 7-bromomethylbenz[a]anthracene (N. K. Scribner and J. D. Scribner, 1980). Because of the carcinogenic properties of many alkylating agents, they have not been tested directly for promoting ability. However, it seems likely that β-propiolactone and a few other alkylating agents also possess promoting activity. This judgment is based on comparison of the initiating potencies and complete carcinogenic potencies of such agents. It is suggested that initiation may be a poor index of complete carcinogenic activity, because the potency as a complete carcinogen would presumably be markedly enhanced by significant intrinsic promoting ability.

Other promoters in mouse skin are significantly weaker than those already mentioned. The most active of the others are certain high-molecular-weight phenols, notably anthralin and 2-hydroxybenzpyrene. Phenol itself and some of its ring-substituted derivatives are weak promoters, much less active than anthralin.

The rat bladder is being investigated increasingly as a target for initiation and promotion. Either the original system of a single local application of methylnitrosourea or restricted feeding of the nitrofuran derivative FANFT has allowed the ideal system in which no tumors are obtained without promotion. Most effort is currently being given to the study of the nitrofuran derivatives, with tryptophan and saccharin being used as promoters. Detailed scanning electron-microscopic studies have been carried out on the progression of preneoplastic changes in the bladders of rats fed FANFT, in an attempt to discern what changes, if any, are part of the initiation process.

Several laboratories in the United States, Canada, and Japan are feverishly developing new methods for sequencing hepatocarcinogenesis. Following Peraino's (1973) original demonstration of initiation by feeding 2-acetamidofluorene to weanling male rats, and promotion by feeding phenobarbital, efforts have been made not only to test other compounds in this basic regimen, but also to alter the regimen and the end point themselves. Because early foci of enzymatic alteration and later hyperplastic

nodules can be observed before hepatocellular carcinoma actually appears, efforts have been made to determine the significance of the temporal relationship among these different levels of toxicity. Because the enzyme alterations (induction of γ-glutamyltranspeptidase, deficiency in adenosine triphosphatase, deficiency in glucose 6-phosphatase) are almost uniformly observed in hyperplastic nodules and carcinomas, foci of cells that are distinguished only by these alterations have been taken to be indicative of early preneoplastic changes. Although these enzyme changes are usually coincident with each other, about 10% of the time they are not. While counting significant numbers of one type of focus would seem to be a reliable indicator of an event that induces all three, therefore, any single focus would have only a 90% chance of being representative. The number of hyperplastic nodules that appears later is lower than the number of early foci by orders of magnitude, with the number of carcinomas further reduced. This has been considered evidence that early transformation of certain cells does not result in the final tumor cell that needs only to reproduce, but rather requires further rare events in this and successively altered populations to produce cancer. The nature of these events is not known, and as yet has not even been concretely imagined. Whether they are to be assigned to the initiation process or to promotion is unknown, and it is not even clear that such an assignment would be useful. Because some investigators have observed early stages of malignancy in hyperplastic nodules, it may be reasonable to believe that the latter are direct precursors of cancer. In contrast, recent evidence obtained in mouse skin with DMBA as initiator and bromomethylbenzanthracene as promoter suggests that papillomas and carcinomas in mouse skin arise from different cell populations.

Other initiation–promotion systems have offered little insight into mechanistic aspects of carcinogenesis, but they have pointed out the possibilities of a variety of environmental hazards, as well as the possibilities for dietary prevention of promotion. The mammary gland of the rat has been found to be susceptible to tumor initiation by DMBA and promotion by phorbol (the parent alcohol of the croton oil esters). Tumors initiated in mouse liver by dimethyl-nitrosamine have also been promoted by phorbol. The liver of the rainbow trout is sensitive to tumor initiation by aflatoxin and promotion by methyl sterculate, a fatty acid ester found in cottonseed oil. Bile acids have been shown to enhance the tumor yield in the rat colon following a single intrarectal dose of N-methyl-N'-nitro-N-nitrosoguanidine. This effect was significant only for benign tumors (polypoid adenomas), with no increase in the number of carcinomas over the level found in control animals. This result resembles that obtained with bromomethylbenzanthracene as promoter in mouse skin, in that cancer risk in both instances was unrelated to benign tumor incidence.

The nature of the tumors obtained in the various initiation–promotion systems represents a final question mark on the issue of whether this model is the same in the different systems. In the DMBA–TPA system on mouse skin, cancer appears well after the maximum number of papillomas has been reached, whereas in the rat bladder system, for example, mostly malignant tumors are found, with the same pattern of progression as that found without promoter. The fact that only benign colon tumors appear in response to bile acids (although the authors did report signs of malignancy in a few of the adenomas) may be an artifact of the time of sacrifice, but otherwise suggests that the promotion observed in this case has little to do with risk of cancer. Similar questions may be directed to the promotion observed in the mouse lung using butylated hydroxytoluene or saccharin as promoter. The tumors observed (initiated with urethane) are all benign, and no attempt has been made to determine whether these regimens lead to cancer with any higher frequency than that obtained without promotion.

COMMITMENT AT INITIATION AND PROTECTIVE PROMOTION

Farber (1980) suggested that benign tumors (at least in the liver) may be a protection mechanism, in that such lesions are relatively resistant to the acute toxicity of carcinogens, and may regress in the absence of toxic stress. The experiments with DMBA as initiator and bromomethylbenzanthracene as promoter suggest the further possibility that mouse skin papillomas evoked by promotion of DMBA-initiated skin with TPA or bromomethylbenzanthracene represent a protective pathway induced by the promoter acting on cells in the earliest stages of initiation. By this shunt into a new pattern of genetic expression, the promoter may protect these cells from changes that would produce malignancy. Because some cells treated with initiator may have been altered beyond these early stages, they are no longer subject to a protective shunt, and may respond differently to the same promoter, leading directly to cancer, or first to papillomas that are microscopically different from the majority of papillomas. The evidence is strongest for the idea that cancer and papillomas arise from different populations, but all of these ideas are testable. We may find in the future that the strongest promoters produce effects that are generally irrelevant, while weak promoters lose their activity at levels of environmental exposure.

RELEVANCE TO COMPLETE CARCINOGENESIS

Thus, we are brought back to an essential question: is the two-stage system relevant to complete carcinogenesis (determined experimentally) or to environmental carcinogenesis? We have shown that at least one carcinogen possesses promoting activity, but that there are others that do not. If, as Boutwell has shown, initiating activity is irreversible and cannot be titrated out, if complete carcinogenic activity can be achieved through addition of initiating events, and if promoting activity can be titrated out, then the essential activity of environmental agents may lie exclusively in their initiating activity. It should be recalled that all known human carcinogens have been identified because of massive exposure of some part of the population to these carcinogens. Thus, although promoting effects may have played a significant role in these cases, they may well be inconsequential in accidental, trace exposure.

In contrast, experimental studies carried out with high doses of carcinogen may give tumor induction kinetics governed predominantly by promoting effects, so that both mechanistic inferences regarding early stages of carcinogenesis and environmental relevance are questionable on the basis of such studies. The Druckrey principle suggests, in contrast, that environmental relevance at least is not affected by the use of high doses. Druckrey has shown for a variety of carcinogens and carcinogen types that reduction of the unit dose in a complete carcinogenesis experiment usually does not cause a proportionate increase in the latent period for tumor induction (Druckrey, 1967). Rather, lower unit doses behave as if they are more effective. Such studies have been carried out over only a 30-fold range of unit doses, however, and a greater range may be necessary to titrate out promoting effects. Obviously this issue is still largely in the dark.

The matter of environmental promoters as a real risk is similarly a matter of conjecture. As was pointed out earlier, it appears impossible to establish directly whether weak promoters have reversible effects or no effect at low doses. If this is the case, then environmental promotion may be a nonissue. It remains to be shown that this is so, and considerable research effort needs to be directed along these lines.

Structure–Activity Studies

Hydrocarbon Carcinogenesis and the K Region Theory
(Dipple, 1976)

As a result of the extensive work and tumor induction experiments carried out in En-

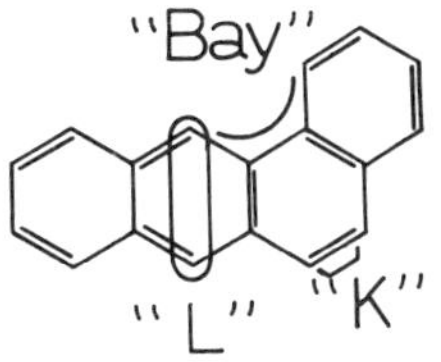

Figure 2–3. K, L, and bay regions in benz[a]anthracene.

gland before World War II, it was possible to ask whether there were any structural features of the many tested polycyclic hydrocarbons that governed carcinogenic activity. Possibly the earliest suggestion of a common feature was Schmidt's identification of the so-called K region as a carcinogenic feature. This K region is represented by the 9,10-double bond in phenanthrene (Figure 2-3). In 1954, Badger reported that there are remarkable differences among polycyclic hydrocarbons in their susceptibility to osmium tetroxide addition at the K region, and that benzpyrene was relatively highly reactive. Using elementary molecular orbital theory, it was possible to calculate the relative susceptibilities of many alternant hydrocarbons with fairly high accuracy. It soon became evident that K region reactivity alone was not well correlated with carcinogenic activity. The Pullmans then suggested that the reactivity at this position was better characterized by a combination of addition and substitution parameters, and that susceptibility to reaction at the "L region" (the 9,10 atoms of anthracene, calculated similarly) was a detoxication process that should be included (Pullman and Pullman, 1955). Because activity would presumably depend on the balance of reaction rates at these two sites, the activation energy for K region attack would have to be sufficiently low for reaction to take place sufficiently often to lead to tumors, whereas activation at the L region would have to be sufficiently difficult to prevent detoxication. Working from this logic, the Pullmans chose values for these two activation energies that permitted the best fit between observed and predicted carcinogenic activities. This done, there re-

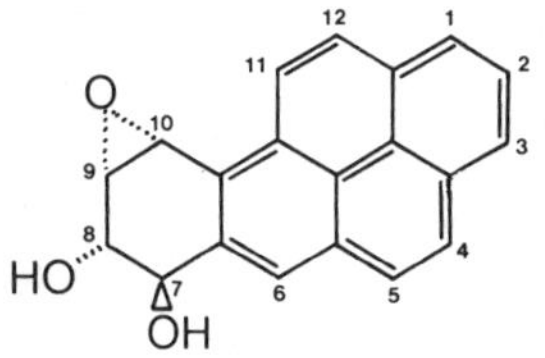

Figure 2–4. Structure of benz[*a*]pyrene-7, 8-dihydrodiol-9, 10-epoxide.

mained 11 exceptions out of a group of 37 compounds. Further work showed that if the K and L regions are of importance, calculation of the activation energies for simple substitution reactions at these positions could produce an equally good correlation, suggesting that there was no need to invoke addition reactions. Various other approaches over the years have involved correlations with ionization potentials and electron affinities of the hydrocarbons, as well as similarly related parameters, but none of these has proved useful. Once a reaction with DNA was identified, however, new correlations based on known chemistry could be attempted. As discussed below, the major metabolite of benzpyrene leading to attack on DNA is one in which the 7,8-double bond is oxidized and hydrated, and the 9,10-double bond is oxidized to an epoxide (Figure 2-4). Calculations could then be made regarding the rates of each of these steps, as well as the rate of ring opening of the epoxide. A new jargon was created as well, in which the necessary metabolism was believed to take place on a benzo-ring adjacent to the "bay region" (Figure 2-3), the concavity in a hydrocarbon opposite a K region. Further, the final epoxide must be adjacent to the bay region. Substitution in the K region directly adjacent to the initial oxidation site appears to depress activity, while substitution *in* the bay region (but not at the site of the final epoxide) enhances activity. Correlations for the unsubstituted hydrocarbons have been highly successful, even quantitatively, using either Hückel molecular orbital theory (the simplest form) or extended Hückel theory (Smith et al., 1978). A slight improvement of the initial correlation was obtained by correcting for

the degree of charge delocalization in the cation formed by opening of the diol epoxide.

At the moment, it seems that there are no major advances to be made in theoretical structure–activity correlations for the polycyclic aromatic hydrocarbons. There remain numerous problems in determining the roles of the known adducts in mutagenesis by the various hydrocarbons, to say nothing of understanding their role in tumor initiation and carcinogenesis.

AZO DYES AND OTHER AROMATIC AMINES
(Clayson and Garner, 1976)

Although aromatic amines were the first chemical class associated with human cancer, experimental induction of cancer with aromatic amines began about 10 years after the beginning of the studies on polycyclic hydrocarbons. Three compounds gave rise to three lines of investigation that did not really merge until about 30 years later. In 1936, a Japanese worker showed that *N,N*-dimethyl-4-aminoazobenzene (DAB) induces liver tumors in male rats. In 1938, an American group found that 2-naphthylamine induced bladder cancer in dogs, and in 1941 a group at the U.S. Department of Agriculture published the finding that 2-acetamidofluorene is a mutipotent carcinogen in rats. Subsequently, many structure–activity studies were published on substituted DAB derivatives. These culminated, for all practical purposes, in a summary paper in 1957 in which it was proposed that an unsubstituted 2-position was necessary for activity (Miller et al., 1957). Fifteen years later, in unpublished work, it was found that application of computer-based pattern recognition methods to an expanded list of DAB derivatives led to exactly the same conclusion. In the interim, of course, studies on metabolic activation and the identification of chemically reactive and mutagenic metabolites had come to fruition, and it was clear that there was no obvious relationship between the unsubstituted 2-position and the mechanism of activation. In the original paper by Hansch and Fujita (1964) regarding the use of the octanol–water partition coefficient as a predictor of biologic activity, a good correlation was obtained between partition coefficient and carcinogenicity for DAB and its "prime" ring-substituted derivatives. As yet, however, no structure–activity relationships have been established with mechanistic significance.

The demonstration that 2-naphthylamine could induce tumors experimentally led primarily to extensive metabolic studies on a few aromatic amines. There does not seem to have been any attempt to follow the classical pattern of preparing numerous substituted derivatives and determining their biologic activities. This may be because the first target animal was the dog, which requires vastly greater resources than rats or mice for tumor induction experiments. Instead, comparative studies were undertaken on a few unsubstituted aromatic amines in several species of animals, in an attempt to associate metabolic patterns with susceptibility to carcinogenesis. From this approach arose the concept of a substituted para (to the amino group) position being necessary for carcinogenesis. As with the azo dyes, the eventual elucidation of the mechanism of metabolic activation produced no obvious significance to the earlier structure–activity conclusions, so that there is still no obvious predictor of carcinogenic activity for aromatic amines. For any of these compounds, as well as those to be discussed below, it seems safe to say that highly polar substituents tend to detoxify them. Thus, sulfonates and carboxylic acids, and possibly even phenols, are noncarcinogenic aromatic amines (e.g., methyl orange).

Structure-activity studies and metabolic studies were also carried out based on 2-acetamidofluorene. Here, as with the azo dyes, numerous substituted derivatives were prepared, as well as compounds with altered ring structures and the insertion of heteroatoms. A major distinguishing feature of many of these compounds is that they were prepared and administered to animals as acetamides. This thus altered the kinetics of tumorigenesis and in some cases the

targets of the carcinogen. In the end, however, the increased stability of the amides and the high selectivity and reactivity of 2-acetamidofluorene metabolites led to the first identification of an in vivo adduct between carcinogen and cellular macromolecule. Ten years lapesed between the first identification of an aromatic amine adduct and the first identification of a polycyclic hydrocarbon adduct.

One of the characteristics of aromatic amine carcinogenesis that fragmented the field for so long was the variety of targets. While the target of polycyclic hydrocarbon carcinogenesis seems to depend only on the method of application, major differences have been observed among the aromatic amines. DAB derivatives, for example, appear to act only on the liver of the male rat when administered in the diet. 2-Naphthylamine, which induces bladder tumors in humans and dogs, appears to be inactive in the rat (but may be weakly active toward the bladder). 2-Acetamidofluorene attacks the liver, ear duct gland, kidney, bladder, intestine, salivary glands, thyroid, and breast. 2-Acetamidophenanthrene is carcinogenic toward the ear duct gland, the breast, and the intestine, and causes leukemia but does not induce liver tumors. The variety of targets of aromatic amines, and the observation that amides in some instances are more effective than the amines, and in other areas are not, indicates that a satisfactory explanation of the many carcinogenic effects of aromatic amines may require a long struggle yet. The polycyclic hydrocarbons, in contrast, appear to act locally (and have been studied primarily in the skin) or to induce mammary tumors when injected into female rats at sensitive points in their maturation.

NITROSAMINE CARCINOGENICITY AND LIPOPHILICITY
(Magee, et al., 1976)

The nitrosamines, as a rule, are much simpler compounds than the aromatic amines or polycyclic hydrocarbons. Metabolism of dimethylnitrosamine has only four atoms to work with; this fact alone suggests that structure–activity studies with the nitrosamines ought to be simpler than with the aromatic carcinogens. The ease of synthesis of nitrosamines has also contributed to the synthesis and testing of numerous compounds in this class. In their review, Magee et al. (1976) summarize the biologic data for 130 different N-NO compounds or compounds that yield N-NO compounds by hydrolysis. There are two basic subdivisions of this class: the dialkylnitrosamines, which require metabolism to become chemically active, and the acylalkylnitrosamines, which react spontaneously in aqueous medium. As will be obvious from reviewing the metabolism of the dialkylnitrosamines, there must be at least one primary or secondary carbon attached to the amino group, to be oxidized or eliminated. Beyond the requirement for an oxidizable carbon, the potency of the nitrosamine is related both to partition coefficient, as evaluated in a Hansch analysis, and to susceptibility to oxidation. Neighboring groups or large groups at more remote carbon atoms may interfere with oxidation, which also reduces potency. The ultimate reactive species is formally a carbocation, which is more susceptible to detoxication by the solvent (water) the more stable it is. Such stability is usually associated with increasing substitution on the reacting carbon. A cation relatively resistant to solvolysis will also tend to react more at positions of DNA that are now believed to play little part in mutagenesis or carcinogenesis. Thus, we can see that there is an optimum partition coefficient for a nitrosamine, that increasing size of functional groups inhibits metabolic activation to an ultimate carcinogen, and that there is an optimum degree of substitution of the ultimate carcinogen. Conceivably these three factors can be treated together in a quantitative fashion. So far, however, only the partition coefficient has been dealt with in a logical, directed fashion. Other factors have only been extensively dealt with in the context of pattern recognition techniques, which have not treated them using the rationale suggested here. One study, however, has addressed the problem of calculating the susceptibility to oxidation of the α carbon, but based only on electronic factors.

Nitrosamines also have a variety of targets, with a different spectrum of activity from either the hydrocarbons or aromatic amines. The liver is a major target, but other frequent targets include the kidney, the nasal cavities, the respiratory tract, and the esophagus. Pancreatic tumors can be induced with a few nitrosamines, and these seem to represent the only good animal model for such tumors. Several nitrosamides are powerful nervous system carcinogens, without producing any tumors in the liver. The class as a whole offers a choice of numerous experimental models, many of which can be produced largely exclusively of other tumors in a given experiment by a judicious choice of compound and regimen.

Metabolism of Carcinogens

ACTIVATION OF AROMATIC AMINES

Metabolic studies were undertaken on azo dyes, 2-acetamidofluorene (Figure 2-5), and 2-naphthylamine almost from the moment their carcinogenic activities were demonstrated. One working hypothesis that was the driving force for much of the early azo dye work was the "split-product" hypothesis, the idea that metabolic reduction of the azo group would produce smaller aromatic amine derivatives, including phenylenediamines, which would be the active compounds. Numerous products of this type were isolated, including free amines, hydroxylated amines, amides, and hydroxylated amines. All were synthesized, if they were not already known compounds commercially available, and all were tested for carcinogenic activity. Several basic observations concerning the mode of metabolism arose from these early studies, however. Other than the reduction process, which was unique to the azo compounds and other N-oxidized compounds, metabolism of these compounds consisted of oxidation, acylation, and conjugation. These principles hold for all of the carcinogens studied since then.

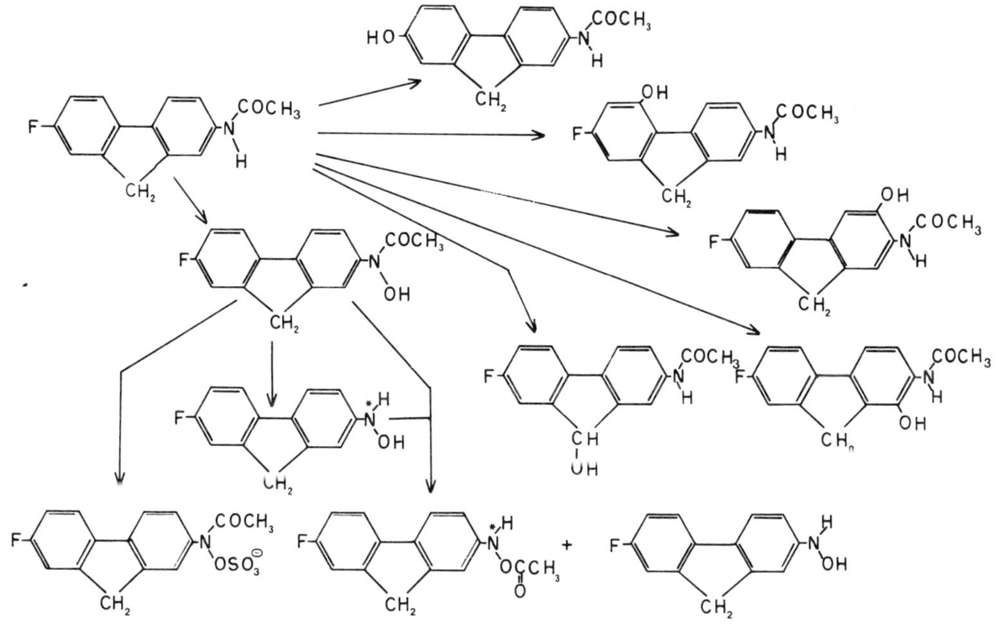

Figure 2–5. Metabolites of 7-fluoro-2-acetamidofluorene (AAF).

Aromatic or aliphatic carbon atoms may be oxidized, to form phenols or alcohols. Primary or secondary amines may be acetylated. This particular process does not take place in the dog, and polymorphism for rate of acetylation has been noted in rabbits and humans. For those compounds depending on free amino groups for carcinogenic activity, this particular process may be of considerable importance in determining individual susceptibility. Conjugation consists of further derivatizing either amino or hydroxy groups to increase greatly the water solubility of the compounds. The usual conjugates of these groups observed in urinary or biliary metabolites are sulfate esters of phenols, or glucuronic acid glycosides of phenols or amines. Also observed in early studies were mercapturic acids, polar compounds in which a thiol-containing amino acid (cysteine or the peptide glutathione) was attached directly to an aromatic ring adjacent to a hydroxy group.

Similar metabolites were observed in the studies on 2-naphthylamine. From these studies, including comparative studies on species of differing susceptibilities to naphthylamine carcinogenesis, the ortho-hydroxylation hypothesis was developed. This hypothesis proposed that metabolic activation consisted of oxidation of the carbon adjacent to the amino group, and that this was general for aromatic amines. Related to this was the requirement for a substituted para-position, because, if this position were available, oxidation would take place there preferentially, and detoxify the compound. This hypothesis was tested through the use of a test in which pellets of compound in cholesterol were implanted directly into the lumen of the rat bladder. Under these conditions, 1-hydroxy-2-naphthylamine was indeed more carcinogenic than 2-naphthylamine. Other ortho-hydroxyamines were not active in this test, however, and even 1-hydroxy-2-naphthylamine was inactive when administered by mouth. Thus, while this hypothesis may have accounted for a few facts, it clearly was not general.

Work with 2-acetamidofluorene led slowly to what is now felt to be a generally valid hypothesis for activation of aromatic amines (Miller and Miller, 1976). As with the azo dyes and 2-naphthylamine, numerous phenols were isolated. All were synthesized and tested, and all were noncarcinogenic. In 1960, however, a new metabolite was reported, N-hydroxy-2-acetamidofluorene under several conditions of test. In the years since then, N-hydroxyderivatives of many representative amines and amides have been synthesized and found to be metabolites, and all have been found to be more carcinogenic than their parent compounds. In a few cases, N-hydroxy derivatives of inactive compounds have also been found to be carcinogenic.

It was known, however, that azo dyes and 2-acetamidofluorene chemically attacked protein and nucleic acid, and it was felt that this chemical attack was related to their carcinogenic activity. None of the metabolites so far isolated were chemically reactive at neutrality, although the hydroxylamines are susceptible to oxidation in air to azoxy compounds. Thus, the search was not felt to be concluded. A "proximate" carcinogen had been identified, but not an "ultimate" carcinogen. With the discovery and identification of a 1:1 azo dye–amino acid adduct (3-methylmercapto-N-methyl-4-aminoazobenzene) from rat liver, a product was in hand that could serve as a reference for any proposed ultimate carcinogen. This came soon after, with the discovery that, first, N-benzoyloxy-N-methyl-4-aminoazobenzene, then N-acetoxy-2-acetamidofluorene could react with methionine or methionine-containing protein to give similar compounds. Because N-hydroxy-2-acetamidofluorene was chemically unreactive, it was clear that the esterified compounds were the reactive species, and were not simply generating N-hydroxy compounds in situ. N-Acetoxy-2-acetamidofluorene has since become a popular model compound for studies on the reactions between carcinogens and nucleic acid. The actual ultimate carcinogen in vivo was imagined to be the sulfate ester, rather than the acetate ester, and several correlation studies confirmed this supposition, for the liver of the male rat.

It has since become clear that this metabolite does not explain the carcinogenicity of 2-acetamidofluorene for other tissues, or the carcinogenicity of other aromatic amines. The necessary sulfotransferase was found to be absent in target tissues such as the mammary gland or the ear duct gland, and the nucleic acid adducts found (as well as the largest proportion of 2-acetamidofluorene adducts in rat liver DNA) lacked the acetyl group. A new soluble enzyme was discovered, which is present in many more tissues, that catalyzes transfer of an acetyl group from a molecule of N-hydroxy-2-acetamidofluorene to the oxygen of a molecule of N-hydroxy-2 aminofluorene. The consequent N-acetoxy-2-aminofluorene is a highly unstable species (in water) that reacts with DNA to give the known major adducts obtained after feeding 2-acetamidofluorene to rats. Although further adduct studies are required to establish the generality of this hypothesis, it seems likely that the necessary metabolic studies on aromatic amines are at an end. What governs the relative potencies and targets of these compounds is still not known.

ACTIVATION OF POLYCYCLIC AROMATIC HYDROCARBONS
(Clayson, 1962c)

The history of polycyclic hydrocarbon metabolic studies is one of having almost the right answer for about 25 years. It was established early, as for the aromatic amines, that the aromatic ring can be oxidized. In addition to phenols, however, the aromatic hydrocarbons also yielded dihydromonoalcohols, dihydrodiols, and quinones. The latter represent further oxidation of the phenols. Mercapturic acids have also been found as metabolites of hydrocarbons. Also, as found with the aromatic amines, none of the phenols was carcinogenic. Among the methylated hydrocarbons, oxidation was often found to take place at the methyl group. In these instances, the resulting hydroxymethyl derivatives have initiating or carcinogenic activity about like that of the parent compound. However, the clear increase in activity that one would expect for a proximate carcinogen (as found for N-hy-droxyamines and N-hydroxyamides) was never noted. Usually direct comparison would show that the hydroxymethyl compound was somewhat less active than the parent.

One outgrowth of Clyason's work was the notion that a metabolic Intermediate in the activation of the hydrocarbons would be an epoxide. This could explain the formation of the dihydrodiols (by hydration) and the mercapturic acids, as well as the observation that hydrocarbons are bound chemically to proteins in mouse skin (and to DNA, as shown after Boyland's suggestion). Even by 1962, however, Boyland's proposal was still being treated as "one further speculation." Several K region epoxides were synthesized, however, and tested for carcinogenic activity. It was in this period that a little knowledge became a dangerous thing. The K region epoxides were found to be inactive as initiators in mouse skin (Dipple, 1976). In tissue culture systems, however, they were powerful transforming agents, much more powerful than the parent compounds (Dipple, 1976). In addition, careful in vitro metabolic studies permitted the isolation of some K region expoxides, because these compounds are not highly reactive at neutrality (Dipple, 1976). Thus, it was clear that such metabolites could be produced in the animal, they could transform fibroblasts in culture to neoplastic cells, but they were not carcinogenic in whole animals. The inconsistency of these findings led to some "crank-turning" while people waited for inspiration. The inspiration came from two studies carried out in England and the United States. The chemistry of DNA adducts in mouse skin and mouse cells in culture was compared for three closely related compounds: 7-methylbenzanthracene, 7-methylbenz-thracene-5-6-oxide (the K region epoxide), and 7-bromomethylbenzanthracene. The latter compound was imagined to be a model for ester-mediated reactions of 7-hydroxymethylbenzanthracene. To simplify the story slightly, each of these three compounds gave different adducts with DNA (Baird et al.,

1973). Thus, it was demonstrated that neither K region oxidation nor methyl group oxidation was responsible for the adducts formed from 7-methylbenzanthracene. In the other study, different known metabolites from benzpyrene were incubated with hamster liver microsomes and DNA, and the amount of hydrocarbon attached to the DNA was measured (Borgen et al., 1973). In this study, most of the metabolites did not bind at all, but the 7,8-dihydrodiol was bound to a much greater extent than benzpyrene itself (Figure 2-6).

The final experiment was carried out in London in the group descended directly from Kennaway's (1925) original group (Sims et al., 1974). An epoxide was prepared from metabolically obtained benzpyrene-7,8-diol, the 7,8-diol-9,10-epoxide. When this was mixed with DNA, the products obtained were the same as those that were formed in mouse skin on application of benzpyrene. Thus, Boyland's proposal of the intermediacy of an epoxide proved correct, although not in quite the manner that he had imagined. In fact, the 7,8-diol is formed by hydration of an initial epoxide, and control of the necessary enzyme (epoxide hydratase) can control the carcinogenicity of unmetabolized hydrocarbon. Remarkably, the epoxide diol is a poor substrate for epoxide hydratase, so that any influence that increases the activity of the enzyme can only increase the concentration of epoxide diol, and presumably increase carcinogenic susceptibility.

The epoxide diol usually (depending on the hydrocarbon) fulfills the requirements of an ultimate carcinogen. It is highly reactive, highly active in tissue culture transformation and mutagenesis assays, and more carcinogenic in whole animals than are the parent compounds. The latter criterion is the one most dependent on the compound. The benzpyrene epoxide diol is clearly less active than benzpyrene (although the 7,8-diol is more active), but benzanthracene-1,2-oxide-3,4-diol is about 25 times more active than benzanthracene. As with the aromatic amines, it appears that the necessary metabolic studies are near the end, but that

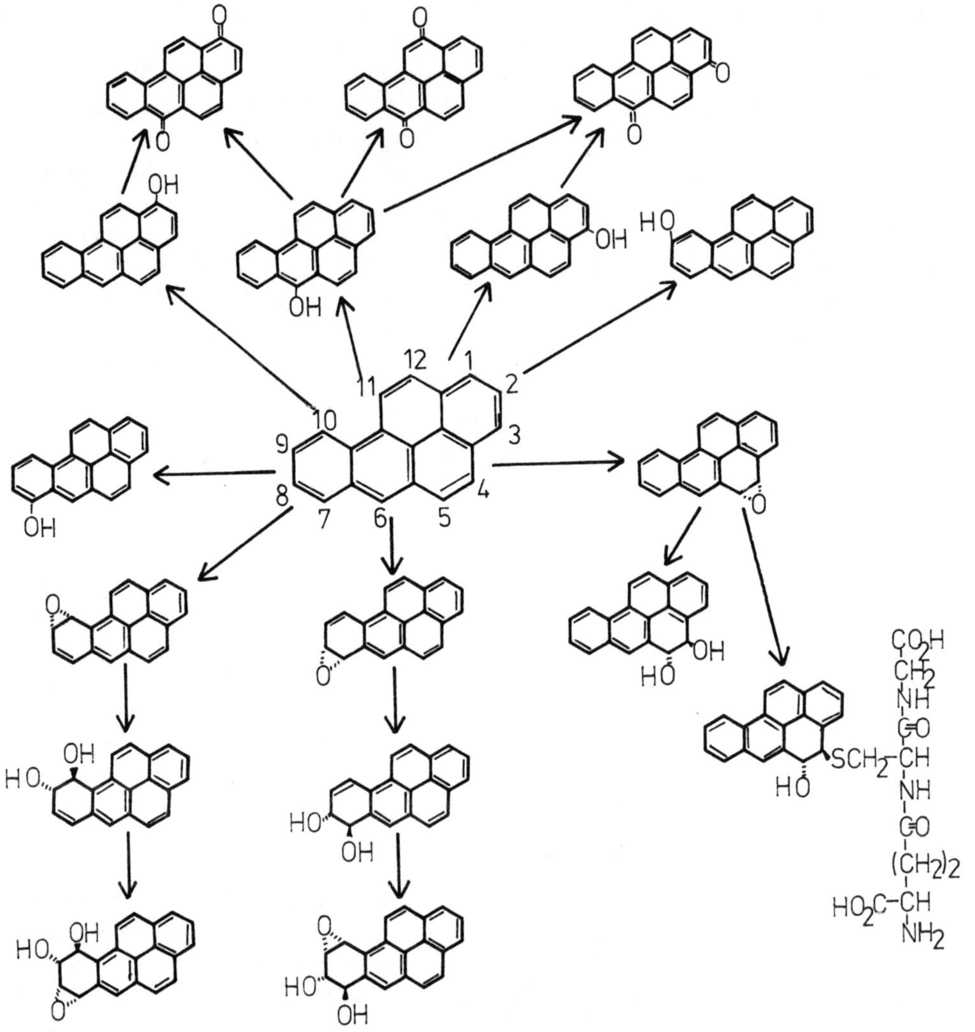

Figure 2–6. Metabolic activation of benz[*a*]pyrene.

the factors that govern carcinogenic activity remain unknown.

One might ask why all of the known metabolites were not tested in animals, as was done for the aromatic amines. It seems that the answer is simply one of feasibility. Synthetic methods were far simpler for the aromatic amine derivatives and for the hydrocarbon phenols. If the diols had been tested, success in identifying the proximate and ultimate metabolites might have come years sooner. Thus, in some cases persistence and technical expertise may sur-

mount obstacles with which imagination cannot deal because of lack of a sufficient data base.

ACTIVATION OF NITROSAMINES
(Magee et al., 1976)

Metabolic studies on nitrosamines have not had the difficulties and romance that are part of the history of aromatic amine and polycyclic hydrocarbon carcinogenesis research. This is so simply because of the simplicity of the molecules and the recency of

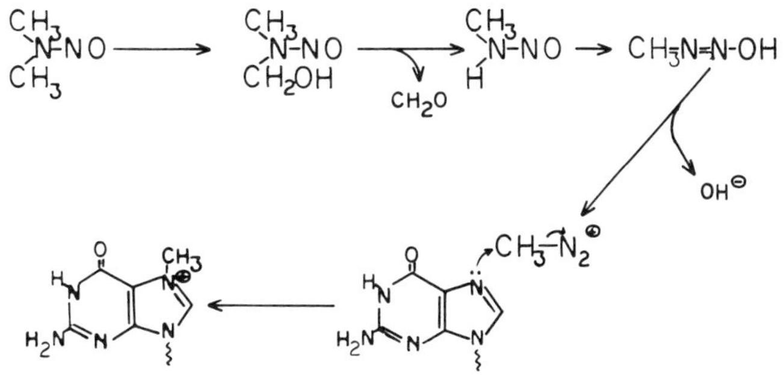

Figure 2–7. Metabolic activation of nitrosamines.

recognition of their hazard. One of the most respected laboratory manuals for organic chemistry, published in a corrected third edition in 1956, describes preparations of dimethyl-and diethylnitrosamine in 40-g quantities using open distillation. Even by 1962, Clayson devoted only a page to nitrosamines in his book, *Chemical carcinogenesis* (pp. 279–280). Thus, by the time serious investigations had begun in nitrosamine metabolism, most of the principles had been established. By 1968, it had already been shown not only that dialkylnitrosamines alkylated DNA, but also that the methyl group from dimethylnitrosamine is transferred to (say) the 7-position of guanine intact. Conversion of a large proportion of administered dimethylnitrosamine to CO_2 had been demonstrated, and one required only a mechanism that could produce both oxidation of methyl groups and release of intact methyl group. The generally accepted mechanism consists of oxidation of one of the methyl groups to a hydroxymethyl group, which can depart nonenzymatically as formaldehyde and be further oxidized. The remaining methyldiazohydroxide can then decompose to water and methyldiazonium ion, the latter reacting either with water, to form methanol (and formaldehyde and CO_2), or with high-molecular-weight nucleophiles, such as nucleic acids and proteins, to give methylated products (Figure 2-7). As with the more complex carcinogens, it is not obvious what factors lead to tumors induced by these compounds. The metabolic and chemical studies have shown how damage to the genetic material may be produced by these compounds. It is clear, however, that such

knowledge is most inadequate for determining whether such damage is necessary to the carcinogenic process, and it is inadequate for determining how general toxicity is induced, and whether the latter is involved in carcinogenesis.

THE MIXED-FUNCTION OXIDASES
(Nebert and Jensen, 1979)

Consistent with the observation that a limited number of processes is involved in carcinogen metabolism is the observation that a limited number of enzymes is involved. Unfortunately, the oxidizing enzymes are in an insoluble lipoprotein matrix, the endoplasmic reticulum, so that purification and mechanistic studies have been severely handicapped. These oxidases, which appear capable of modifying a wide variety of xenobiotics, as well as some endogenous species, are characterized primarily by their possession of a ferro-home type of active site, usually referred to as cytochrome *P*-450. Recent work has identified at least 12 different cytochromes *P*-450, and much work has shown that there are different substrate specificities and inducibilities among these species. Cytochrome *P*-450–mediated monoxygenases have been shown to catalyze oxidation of aliphatic carbon, aromatic carbon, alkyl-substituted nitrogen, aromatic nitrogen, and sulfur, and thereby also to catalyze N-, O-, and S-dealkylation. Different positions on the same substrate can be attacked by different species of *P*-450, as shown by enzyme induction experiments. Enzymes induced by 3-methylcholanthrene in rat liver oxidize the 2-position of biphenyl, the C-6 of estrone, the 2-position of bromobenzene, and the 7,8,9,10-positions of benzpyrene. Induction by phenobarbital leads to preferential oxidation of the 4-position of biphenyl, the C-16 of estrone, the 4-position of bromobenzene, and the K region of benzpyrene. Because of these varying patterns of induction, administration of agents that selectively induce one pathway or another is often used in mechanistic studies of carcinogen metabolism, and may be a feasible strategy for dietary prevention of carcinogenesis.

The mechanism of oxidation appears to involve binding of the substrate to oxidized cytochrome (Fe^{3+}), followed by reduction of the cytochrome, binding of molecular oxygen to the complex, protonation to form a peroxide species, then release of water and the oxidized substrate. In the case of aromatic carbon, an epoxide appears to be the preferred first product, if allowed by the structure of the immediate environment. This is true for oxidation of the aromatic rings in aromatic amines as well. Depending on the relative stabilities of the successive intermediates, this epoxide may rearrange directly to a phenol or be hydrated to a dihydrodiol. Glutathione S-epoxide transferase may catalyze formation of a mercapturic acid from glutathione and the epoxide. Enzymatic reduction would lead to dihydromonoalcohols. In the case of rearrangement, it has been noted that a large fraction of the protons originally present on the eventual phenolic carbons are retained on the adjacent carbon after rearrangement. This is the phenomenon referred to as the NIH shift, and it can be considered direct evidence for epoxidation preliminary to the formation of isolated phenols.

Carcinogen Chemistry

REACTIONS OF AROMATIC AMINES WITH NUCLEIC ACIDS AND PROTEINS
(Miller and Miller, 1969; Kreik and Westra, 1979)
(Figure 2-8)

In 1947, it was reported that livers from rats fed N,N-dimethyl-4-aminoazobenzene turned pink in trichloracetic acid. This might not have been too remarkable, but the protein obtained by alcohol precipitation of liver homogenate, followed by hot alcohol extraction, still gave pink solutions when dissolved in formic acid. Remarkably, the tumors obtained by feeding the dye did not have dye bound to the protein. Thus, it was found that carcinogenic azo dye attacks chemically protein in its target tissue, by some mechanism not involving loss of the azo group. Some 15 years later, using radioactive azo dye, another group demonstrated the binding of dimethylaminoazobenzene to nucleic acid as well. When N-benzoyloxy-N-methyl-4-aminoazobenzene, and later N-hydroxy-N-methyl-4-aminoazobenzene sulfate had been synthesized, it became possible to investigate these reactions in depth. As mentioned above, an adduct of N-methyl-4-aminoazobenzene with methionine had already been identified directly from rat liver, and a similar adduct from 2-acetamidofluorene was identified later. The nature of the adducts and the necessity for the ester groups for the reactions suggested that electron-deficient nitrogen represented the essential starting point for imagining a mechanism. This was confirmed by the observation that the product of reaction between guanosine and N-acetoxy-2-acetamidofluorene is 8-(N-2-fluoroenylacetamido)guanosine, a product that is also obtained from RNA of rats fed or injected with 2-acetamidofluorene. The unstable intermediate from reaction of N-acetoxy-2-acetamidofluorene can then be considered the N-2-fluorenyl-N-acetylnitrenium ion, a delocalized positive ion, resulting from loss of acetate ion. A second adduct found only in DNA, in vivo or in vitro, results from attack of the 2-NH_2 group of guanine on the 3-position of the nitrenium ion. This adduct appears to lie in the narrow groove of DNA without causing significant distortion (however, see comments regarding benzpyrene effects on DNA conformation). The major adduct with DNA on administration of 2-acetamidofluorene to rats is the 8-(N-2-fluorenylamino)guanine adduct. The deacetylated compound appears to accumulate in rat liver during

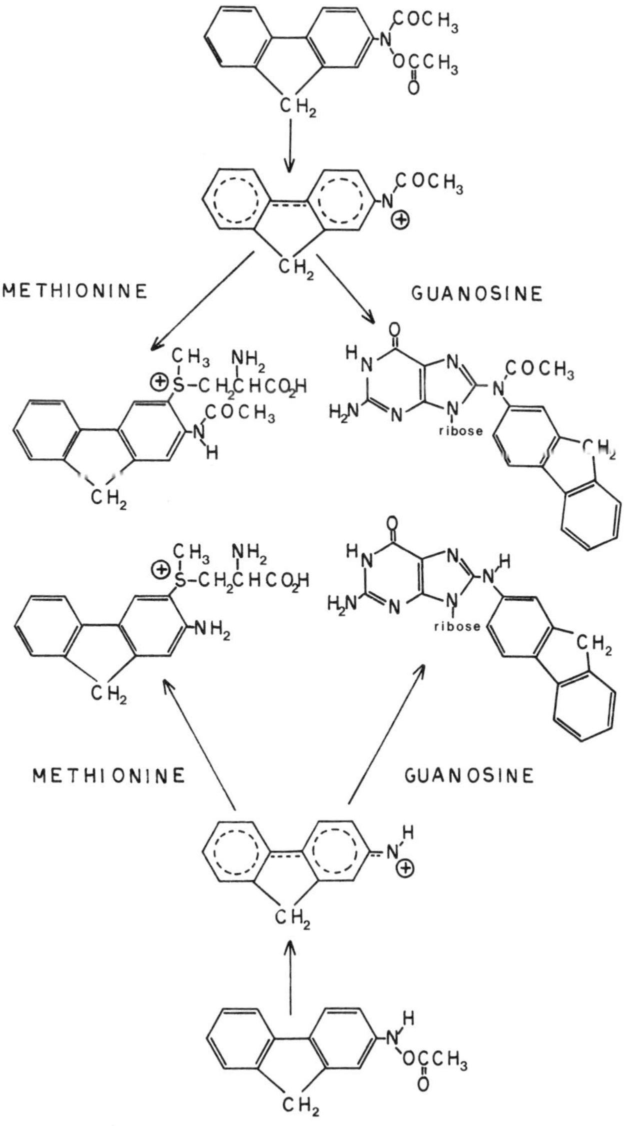

Figure 2–8. Reactions of aromatic amines with nucleic acids.

prolonged feeding of 2-acetamidofluorene, whereas the corresponding acetylated adduct is lost, with a half-life of about 7 days. In fact, prolonged feeding of 2-acetamidofluorene rapidly destroys the capacity of the rat liver to produce acetylated adduct, but has no effect on the level of nonacetylated adducts in male rats (Scribner et al., 1982). Extensive enzymatic and physical studies on acetamidofluorene-modified DNA show that the guanine-C-8 acetylated adduct causes strand separation and probably an inversion such that the fluorene ring is inside the helix and the gua-

nine ring outside (Grunberger and Weinstein, 1979).

Comparable reactions have been studied with N-acetoxy derivatives of 2-acetamidophenanthrene and 4-acetamidostilbene. The phenanthrene derivative reacts with guanosine as does N-acetoxy-2-acetamidofluorene, but reacts equally well with adenodule, at the 6-amino group, and the same product distribution is found in the in vitro reaction between DNA and N-acetoxy-2-acetamidophenanthrene. Other products were also found, but have not yet been identified. In vivo, no acetylated adducts with

DNA or RNA were found (after injecting 2-acetamidophenanthrene) (Scribner and Koponen, 1979). Thus, it appears likely that all of the adducts found were mediated by the acetyltransferase reaction. As yet, however, no structures have been identified, so that this supposition remains to be confirmed.

Studies with N-acetoxy-4-acetamidostilbene gave an entirely different picture. No adducts involving the nitrogen atom were found, and guanosine, adenosine, and cytidine were attacked equally well (Scribner et al., 1979). The products eventually identified resulted from alkylation of the bases (N-1, O^6 of guanosine; N-1, N^6 of adenosine; N^3 of cytidine) by the β-carbon (postulated first intermediate) of the ethylene bridge in the stilbene moiety. Theoretical calculations (see below) indicated that this was consistent with the picture of a delocalized nitrenium ion developed from the 2-acetamidofluorene studies. In vivo studies gave results slightly more illuminating than those obtained with 2-acetamidophenanthrene. A small fraction of the adducts isolated were identical to the known compounds; however, most of the in vivo adducts remain unknown, and are probably deacetylated adducts (Gaugler et al.,

1979). These and the aminophenanthrene adducts are now under investigation.

Adducts of 1- and 2-naphthylamine with DNA in vivo and in vitro have also been investigated (Kadlubar et al., 1978, 1980; Figure 2–9). The primary adduct of 1-naphthylamine in vivo or 1-naphthylhydroxylamine in vitro (pH 4) is the O^6-(N-1-naphthylamino)guanine adduct, while the primary 2-naphthylamine adduct is the 8-(N-2-naphthylamino)guanine compound. Note that in both cases, it is the nitrogen atom from aromatic amine that is attached to the base. It is also worth noting here that, although 1-naphthylamine is apparently noncarcinogenic, its N-hydroxy derivative is more potent than N-hydroxy-2-naphthylamine. Again, as shown below, the products isolated from these compounds are consistent with the hypothesis of a delocalized nitrenium ion.

Adducts with peptides and proteins have been relegated to the back burner in the conviction that studies on nucleic acid reactions will lead more directly to an understanding of carcinogenesis. Since the first structure identification of 2-methylmercapto-N-methyl-4-aminoazobenzene, further studies have identified the complete methionine adduct, oxidation

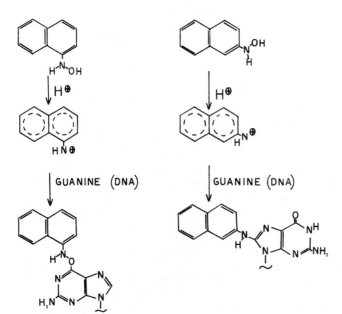

Figure 2–9. Reactions of naphthylamines with DNA guanine.

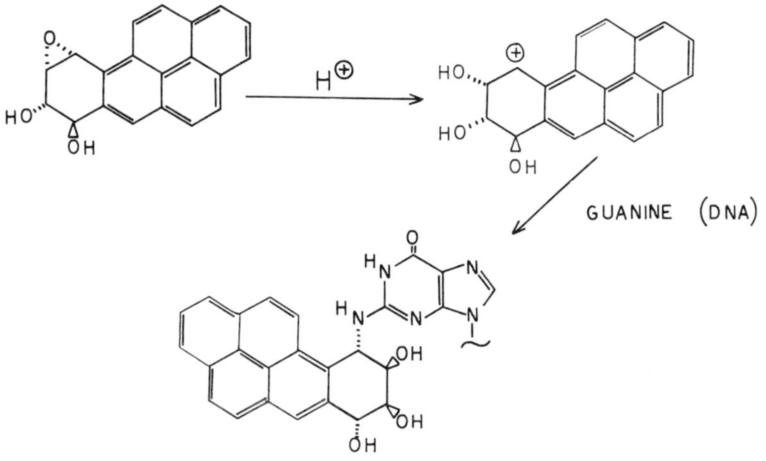

Figure 2–10. Reaction of benz[a]pyrene diol epoxide with DNA guanine.

products thereof (sulfone, sulfoxide), and tyrosine adducts. Studies of glutathione adducts with azo dyes have recently been published, but no further chemical knowledge has been gained. Perhaps as new knowledge regarding the control of gene expression is gained, there will be justification and impetus to return to the study of reactions of aromatic amines with proteins.

REACTIONS OF BENZPYRENE
(Phillips and Sims, 1979)

It is not widely appreciated that the same workers first reported both the binding of azo dyes to liver protein (Miller and Miller, 1947) and the binding of a polycyclic hydrocarbon to mouse skin protein (Miller, 1951). Subsequent studies by others established a high correlation between carcinogenic potency of a series of hydrocarbons in mouse skin and their level of binding to a basic mouse skin protein (Abell and Heidelberger, 1962). A similar correlation had been established earlier for azo dyes in rat liver. Later work showed a quantitative correlation between initiating activity and binding of the hydrocarbons to mouse skin DNA (Scribner and Süss, 1978). With the observation that the epoxide diol of benzpyrene was the ultimate carcinogen responsible for the detectable adducts of benzpyrene with DNA, synthetic methods

for this epoxide diol and those of other hydrocarbons were developed, allowing preparative scale reactions and kinetics studies for these ultimate carcinogens. The major nucleic acid reaction found in vivo and in vitro is attack of the 10-position by the 2-amino group of guanine (Figure 2–10). Comparable reactions are found for the 6-amino group of adenine and the 4-amino group of cytosine, but the levels are much lower. Consideration of a space-filling model of DNA shows that the reaction with guanine may take place without much distortion of the DNA double helix, but that a significant amount of unwinding is required for reactions at the large-groove amino groups.

Physicochemical and enzymatic studies on benzpyrene-modified DNA have led to conflicting views of the actual nature of the alterations in conformation induced by the hydrocarbon (Grunberger and Weinstein, 1979). Some evidence has been considered to support intercalation of the hydrocarbon, while other findings suggest that the hydrocarbon does indeed lie in the narrow groove, without any major effect on conformation. The most recent work, with relatively short, rigid DNA strands, suggests that indeed intercalation is involved, producing a kink or bend in the DNA (Hogan et al., 1981).

The only other hydrocarbon epoxides investigated chemically to any extent are benzanthracene epoxide diols, and the K region epoxide of DMBA. These also react predominantly at the 2-amino group of guanine. However, minor reactions of the DMBA–5,6-oxide with OH groups of the ribose in RNA, and with C-8 of guanine have also been detected.

ALKYLATION
(Singer, 1975; Lawley, 1976)

Direct alkylating agents or metabolically activated nitrosamines may attack any of the oxygen or nitrogen atoms in nucleic acids. The first known alkylation products were the result of attack on N-7 of guanine and N-3 of adenine. It is now clear that, while these positions are major targets, there is little evidence to suggest that they are critical for either mutagenesis or carcinogenesis. In contrast, alkylation at O^6 of guanine seems well correlated with both mutagenic and carcinogenic potency. It is important to realize that the apparent importance of O^6-alkylation may be purely historical. This reaction was the first attack at oxygen to be recognized, and is usually the major reaction at oxygen on the bases. However, attack at O^2 of cytosine and thymine, and at O^4 of thymine has been shown, and the relative effectiveness of these different modifications for introducing mutations has not been established, particularly when the size of the alkyl group is altered. In fact, there is a great deal of mechanistic work to be done in this respect, because the precise mutagenic effects, if any, of most alterations of DNA by carcinogens are not known.

The most important reaction quantitatively for several alkylating agents (e.g., ethylnitrosourea) is alkylating of phosphate in DNA, leading to phosphotriesters. Because such lesions are stable in DNA (although not in RNA) and are not involved in base-pairing, little attention has been given to them. Neutralization of the charge locally, as well as unknown steric effects, could significantly alter the interaction of the DNA with other chromatin components, however. Such effects have not been examined, but could markedly affect gene expression.

THEORETICAL ASPECTS OF CARCINOGEN CHEMISTRY
(Scribner, 1979)

Despite the early correlation studies on the polycyclic aromatic hydrocarbons, theoretical studies of actual known reactions of carcinogens did not begin in earnest until 1970, with the publication of Hückel molecular orbital calculations for the decomposition of N-acetoxy-N-arylacetamides (Scribner et al., 1970). In this work it was shown that the relative rates of reaction of these compounds could be determined, but that these rates were not correlated either with carcinogenicity or with the yield of adduct from guanosine or methionine. Similarly, the most reactive sites on the nitrenium ions could be identified, but how these were related to adduct yields could not be determined, nor did they enable any predictions of targets. Further experimental work with adduct formation added to the information necessary to provide an adequate theoretical picture. Application of polyelectronic perturbation theory later enabled correct identification of the major adduct with guanosine for six aromatic amines and the benzylic compound 7-bromomethylbenzanthracene (Scribner and Fisk, 1978). This work was still at the simplest level of molecular orbital theory, and was inadequate for extension to the study of alkylating agents, to the minor adducts, and to determination of selectivity (solvent competition). Increased support for such studies has recently enabled work at advanced levels of molecular orbital theory, permitting studies on reaction pathways (which will give more reliable results than perturbation theory) and on solvation energy (the major feature that distinguishes carcinogen–nucleoside reactions from those usually studied by theoretical chemists). It is likely that valuable new insights in these areas will be available by the time this book is published.

Theoretical studies of hydrocarbon chemistry are among the oldest in molecular orbital theory, but the most neglected in carcinogen chemistry. Because of the simple structure of the polycyclic aromatic hydrocarbons, simple molecular orbital theory, even on a pnecil-and-paper basis, could produce large amounts of information regarding relative reaction rates and sites of attack. Such approaches have been applied to the diol epoxides, but only at correlation level. The work of most interest in this area was the use of perturbation theory to predict the relative rates of rearrangement (to phenols) and hydration (to diols) of a series of epoxides, and to predict the predominant phenol after rearrangement (Fu et al., 1978). No work has yet appeared, other than the perturbation study on 2-bromomethylbenzanthracene, which deals with the targets of hydrocarbon attack on nucleic acids, or with the degree of solvent competition for the ultimate carcinogen. A few papers have reported calculations on minimum energy conformations of benzpyrene epoxide diol, but these have produced no insight into the reactivity of this type of compound.

At the moment, one of the most exciting areas is the calculation of transition states for a series of alkyldiazonium ions. It is already known experimentally that the ratio of alkylation products obtained from ethylnitrosourea differs markedly from that obtained from methylnitrosourea (Singer, 1975). Yet the traditional "Swain-Scott constants" represent only a correlation device, the explanatory power of which breaks down in dealing with adduct ratios obtained in the reactions of DNA with different alkylating agents. Recent calculations have shown, however, that the transition states for reaction of ethyldiazonium ion with various nucleophiles vary significantly (the nucleophile–ethyl bond is much longer) from those for the same reactions of methyldiazonium ion (G. P. Ford and J. D. Scribner, 1983). The results obtained so far appear sufficient to explain the major shift toward oxygen alkylation found with ethylating agents.

Recent experimental findings with di-*n*-propylnitrosamine (in rat liver) and *n*-propylnitrosourea (with guanosine in vitro) hold promise of establishing a critical experimental model for determining the reliability of any predictive level of molecular orbital calculations. In either system, it is found that the major or sole adduct at N-7 of guanine is *n*-propylguanine, but that the only detectable adduct at O-^{6} of guanine is isopropylguanine (J.D. Scribner and G. P. Ford, 1982). It thus seems clear that one cannot refer to such alkylation reactions as being simply unimolecular or bimolecular, but must develop a deeper understanding of the transition states in order to explain adequately the chemistry of alkylation of DNA.

Mechanistic Studies

MUTAGENESIS

In 1926 it was proposed that cancer is a consequence of a mutation(s) in a somatic cell(s). Proof of this hypothesis has been extraordinarily hard to obtain, and it may still be argued that a change in the genetic code is not the critical event in chemical carcinogenesis. Most evidence to date has been correlative. Two approaches of this sort stand out, either for sheer volume of publication or degree of correlation. Tester strains of *S. typhimurium* have been developed that are sensitive to base substitutions, frameshifts, or deletions (Ames et al., 1975). Sensitivity has been increased in these bacteria by deletion of their repair capacities and the introduction of a mutation which resulted in loss of part of the bacterial membrane. The latter change increases permeability of the bacteria to many more xenobiotics, particularly larger molecules such as polycyclic aromatic hydrocarbons. As usually presented in the literature, two of the tester strains (TA 1535 and TA 1538) are said to be sensitive to base pair substitution and frameshifts, respectively, while two other strains (TA 100 and TA 98), which are TA 1556 and TA 1538 containing a plasmid pKM 101, are said to have increased sensitivity to the same types of mutations. In fact, there is no evidence supporting the latter assertion. There are indeed many compounds that produce much higher mutation rates in TA 100 than they do in TA 1535, but relatively few that produce significantly higher mutation rates in TA 98 than in TA 1538. Based on the evidence regarding the ability of pKM 101 to increase rec A–lex A repair in host bacteria, it seems that the high sensitivity of TA 100 to certain compounds is due to error-prone repair resulting from interruption of DNA synthesis. This interpretation is supported by evidence from several laboratories, while the proposal of greater sensitivity toward base pair substitution is specifically contradicted by a study on a series of alkylating agents that produced the same mutation frequencies in TA 1535 and TA 100 (Bartsch et al., 1980).

The correlation between mutagenicity in the *Salmonella* assay (the "Ames test") and carcinogenic activity is questionable. Original reports claimed qualitative correlations as high as 90%. However, many of the negative controls were structurally different from most of the carcinogens. More recent work using blind samples and structurally related positive and negative samples has given correlations of nearer 50%. Ames has taken the position that this reflects the inadequacy of the whole-animal tests used to determine carcinogenicity. This viewpoint is representative of an attitude (expressed by Ames) that anything that produces a response in the mutagenesis assay is a hazard, not only as a mutagen but also as a carcinogen, despite the artificial sensitivity of the tester strains.

In contrast with the questionable correlations obtained in large studies based on a variety of whole-animal systems, quantitative correlation for a series of tumor initiators, corrected for partition coefficient, is quite good (Scribner et al., 1980). This might suggest that an essential event in initiation is indeed mutagenesis. However, this first correlation must be tested with a wider variety of compounds, and still remains at best a correlation. It is confirmed by mutagenesis studies in a permanent line of Chinese hamster fibroblasts, the so-called V79 line. In this work, a high quantitative correlation between mutagenicity and tumor-initiating activity has been obtained for an extensive list of compounds, without the need for correction by added physical properties (Scribner et al., 1980).

From such correlations, one can conceptually leap to the ultimate proof that carcinogenesis is a consequence of mutagenesis, by isolating a gene product resulting from a mutation (or showing that a specific gene product is lost) and showing that addition (or subtraction) of this gene product leads to a transformed cell. Such a proof has not been achieved, but with modern genetic technology it now appears realizable, if the correct gene product were to be identified. What has been achieved is transformation of nontransformed fibroblast cell lines by transfection with DNA from cells transformed with chemical carcinogen (Shih et al., 1979). While this is evidence that the information needed for transformation is encoded in the DNA, it is not proof that this information consists of an altered base sequence. It is now known that cytosine in DNA can be methylated in situ, and that this methylation also proceeds in a template-dependent fashion (Ehrlich and Wang, 1981). Furthermore, it has been shown that treatment of cells with alkylating agent results in altered methylation of the daughter strands at the time of DNA synthesis (Boehm and Drahovsky, 1981). Because such methylation may control genetic expression, it is clear that this is another possible mode of encoding information in DNA, without altering the base-pairing rule (i.e., both C and 5-methyl-C code for G on DNA synthesis.) Such enzymatic methylation of DNA and its alteration thus represent a mode of introducing a permanent, heritable change in DNA without changing the code itself. In recent work, Yuspa and Morgan (1981) have found that initiation of mouse skin with DMBA gives rise to cells that can be detected by their resistance to terminal differentiation induced by high Ca^{2+} concentration in culture. This result thus suggests a consequence of the chemical events of initiation, but does not identify these events.

EFFECTS OF PROMOTERS

What promoters do depends on which promoter one is looking at. The most thorough investigations have been undertaken with the croton oil promoter (one of many) 12-O-tetradecanoylphorbol-13-acetate (TPA). In 1972 it was reported that TPA produces a marked selective induction of high-molecular-weight proteins in mouse skin (Scribner and Boutwell, 1972). This induction was found to be correlated with promoting ability of a series of phorbol esters, but not with the inflammatory potency of the same compounds. Other laboratories have made similar observations since then. Ornithine decarboxylase (ODC) and S-adenosylmethionine (SAM) decarboxylase are two enzymes involved in polyamine synthesis and are believed to be involved intimately in DNA synthesis. Levels of these enzymes are also elevated in a number of tumors, so it seems reasonable to ask whether they are affected by TPA. It was found that the maximum tolerated dose of TPA caused about a sevenfold induction in SAM decarboxylase, and a 400-fold induction in ODC (O'Brien, 1976). This high induced level of ODC dropped rapidly, while the increased level of SAM decarboxylase returned to control level much more slowly. Agents which produce hyperplasia in mouse skin but fail to promote were found to induce SAM decarboxylase in correlation with their hyperplasiogenic activity, but to induce ODC only to the same level as SAM decarboxylase, and with comparable kinetics. It seemed that a marker for promoting ability had been identified. However, another natural product, mezerein, as well as a synthetic TPA analog, retinoylphorbol acetate, both induced high levels of ODC, but lack promoting ability. Also, as mentioned above, the liver promoter phenobarbital does not induce ODC at the normal promoting dose. Thus, some compounds are known that induce ODC but do not promote, while there are others that promote but do not induce ODC. An attractive solution would be to propose that promotion involves a series of steps, of which ODC induction is early, but not the first, and that some initiation (e.g., in rat liver with 2-acetamidofluorene) carries the tissue through the ODC stage. This proposal has not been directly tested in the liver case yet, but has been tested in mouse skin. A single dose of TPA is sufficient to carry out the effects of which TPA, but not mezerein or retinoylphorbol acetate, is capable. Successive treatment with either of the latter agents results in promotion at levels approaching that obtained from continuous treatment with TPA.

Numerous examples of alteration in differentiation produced by TPA are now in the literature (Diamond et al., 1978). It seems pointless to review the individual examples, but it is important to note that differentiation can be inhibited or accelerated by TPA, depending on the cell type and the culture conditions. There is evidence, of course, that differentiation in mouse skin is also altered by TPA, in that primitive embryonic cells have been found to increase greatly in number on TPA application. The effect of mezerein is somewhat less in this regard, although the difference between TPA and mezerein is not as great as has been claimed.

Two other effects of promoters in culture are worth mention. TPA and other phorbol-related promoters (and also mezerein) induce production of the protease plasminogen activator in cells in culture (Wigler and Weinstein, 1976). This observation, combined with the observation that protease inhibitors can inhibit tumor promotion in mouse skin, may be considered evidence that induction of proteases is an important event in promotion. Very little further evidence is available to support this viewpoint, nor has a model for the role of proteases been proposed that would suggest other experiments. Another effect of promoters worthy of note is inhibition of metabolic cooperation (Trosko et al., 1982). Metabolic cooperation consists of the passing of a metabolite produced in one cell to other cells in the same milieu, apparently by direct transfer through cell–cell junction. The effect can be demonstrated by the failure to recover thioguanine-resistant mutants from a culture of thioguanine-sensitive cells in the presence of thioguanine, and can be counteracted by addition of TPA to the medium. A wide variety of promoters has produced this effect, at doses well correlated with their effective doses in vivo, including phenobarbital and saccharin. Because mezerein produces this effect at the same dose as TPA, it appears that if this phenomenon is part of the promotion process, it is a later event in the progression, a possibly necessary process to isolate transformed cells from the growth- and architecture-controlling influences of the neighboring normal cells.

It thus becomes possible to imagine a series of events induced by promoters, each of which occurs each time promoter is applied, but which is effective only when some cell population has appeared that can take advantage of that particular alteration. Mutagenesis may be the only event peculiar to initiation, while all other events described here, as well as other unmentioned or unknown, may be caused either by initiators or promoters. Specific interference with certain genes may occur, or (more likely) wide-scale pleiotropic effects may cause massive changes in genetic expression, small segments of which may, by accident or because of a mutation, fail to revert to their normal state. A specific case of such an event remains to be demonstrated.

Conclusions

The Electrophilic Hypothesis

In recent years, a so-called electrophilic hypothesis of carcinogenesis has arisen, based on the numerous studies that lead to the conclusion that metabolic activation of carcinogens leads to ultimate forms that may formally be considered alkylating agents (i.e., electrophiles). Such a conclusion seems valid and is better buttressed than virtually any other explanation regarding any aspect of chemical carcinogenesis. In the end, however, it is a hypothesis regarding the nature of the chemical species that acts in the cell to produce cancer. In this respect, it does rule out the effects of nonelectrophilic metabolites of carcinogens, a corollary that has not been subject to rigorous test. It also leaves completely open the nature of the consequences of electrophilic attack by carcinogen on the cell. It is assumed that the principal consequence is mutagenesis, but the specific immediate consequence of any

lesion other than a few resulting from simple alkylation is unknown. Most of the consequences intermediate between mutagenesis and gross tumor are unknown. Toxicity produced by electrophilic attack on targets other than DNA has not been investigated systematically at all. Rather, there are merely occasional demonstrations that toxic effects occur catastrophically when the protective mechanism (e.g., glutathione level) of a tissue is overcome. It is clear, then, that most of carcinogenesis remains unknown territory. If toxicity and subsequent regenerative hyperplasia are promoting effects, how do they differ from normal high rates of cell growth, as seems to be the case? Numerous further questions might be posed by the reader.

Does Multistep Mean Initiation–Promotion?

Studies on the human condition show that for many tumors, risk of cancer is highly age dependent, in some cases a function of the sixth power of age. Mathematical models that have been developed to account for this have depended on a multistage model for carcinogenesis, which has its most obvious experimental support in the initiation–promotion model. We have shown, however, that the property of being able to promote DMBA-initiated tumors in mouse skin is not necessary for a compound to be able to induce cancer in mouse skin. Because most of the properties associated with promoters appear to have a threshold, and to occur to the same extent in all identical exposed cells, it seems likely that promotion as understood experimentally may be inconsequential among members of the human population who "live a clean life." Detailed epidemiologic studies on phenobarbital and saccharin, the two most widespread of the known experimental promoters, have failed to show any increased cancer risk associated with the use of these compounds, with the possible exception of bladder cancer risk among the very heaviest users of saccharin. Even the latter possibility is at a relatively low confidence level. There have been suggestions that high-fat diets have a promoting effect on colon and breast cancer, but there is a lack of agreement on this. Based on the Druckrey experiments and the data showing that pure initiators can be carcinogenic in mouse skin, it seems that human cancer (with the exception of that induced by tobacco smoke and industrial exposure) may well be due to constant exposure to initiating processes. If we assume that initiation in its simplest form consists of mutagenesis, repeated mutations in highly active tissue (e.g., colon, breast) can easily be imagined to be sufficient to lead to tumors.

THE RARITY OF TUMORS

After all, even in the person who develops cancer, this is a rare event. Although it need occur only once to be fatal, once in the lifetime of a human being is a most infrequent event. For polycyclic hydrocarbons, it has been calculated that only one tumor develops in a population of mice for every 5 billion hits on DNA, and this is under conditions in which carcinogen is being deliberately applied to the animal. It is not difficult to imagine that comparable exposure can accumulate in individuals exposed only to unavoidable insults. The final question may well be, why does only one individual in four develop cancer? People are tougher than they think.

Acknowledgment

The author's work described herein, and the preparation of this chapter, were supported by the National Cancer Institute, National Institutes of Health, United States Public Health Service.

REFERENCES

Abell, C. W., and Heidelberger, C. 1962. Interaction of carcinogenic hydrocarbons with tissues. VIII. Binding of tritium-labeled hydrocarbons to the soluble proteins of mouse skin. *Cancer Res.* 22:931–946.

Ames, B. N., McCann, J., and Yamasaki, E. 1975. Methods for detecting carcinogens and mutagens with the salmonella/mammalian-microsome mutagenicity test. *Mutat. Res.* 31:347–364.

Argyris, T. S. 1980. Tumor promotion by abrasion induced epidermal hyperplasia in the skin of mice. *J. Invest. Dermatol.* 75:360–362.

Badger, G. M. 1954. Chemical constitution and carcinogenic activity. *Advances Cancer Res.* 2:73–127.

Baird, W. M., Dipple, A., Grover, P. L., Sims, P., and Brookes, P. 1973. Studies on the formation of hydrocarbon-deoxyribonucleoside products by the binding of derivatives of 7-methylbenz[a]anthracene to DNA in aqueous solution and in mouse embryo cells in culture. *Cancer Res.* 33:2386–2392.

Bartsch, H., Malaveille, C., Camus, A.-M., Martel-Planche, G., Brun, G., Hautefeuille, A., Sabadie, N., Barbin, A., Kuroki, T., Drevon, C., Piccoli, C., and Montesano, R. 1980. Validation and comparative studies on 180 chemicals with *S. typhimurium* strains and V79 Chinese hamster cells in the presence of various metabolizing systems. *Mutat. Res.* 76:1–50.

Berenblum, I. 1929a. The modifying influence of dichloroethyl sulphide on the induction of tumors in mice by tar. *J. Path. Bacteriol.* 32:425–434.

Berenblum, I. 1929b. Tumor formation following freezing with carbon dioxide. *Brit. J. Exp. Pathol.* 10:179–184.

Berenblum, I. 1931. The anticarcinogenic action of dichlorodiethyl sulphide. *J. Pathol. Bacteriol.* 34:731–746.

Berenblum, I. 1930. Further investigations on the induction of tumors with carbon dioxide snow. *Br. J. Exp. Pathol.* 11:208–211.

Berry, D. L., Fürstenberger, G., Sorg, B., and Marks, F. 1981. 12-O-Retinoylphorbol-13-acetate: A new, synthetic, non-promoting phorbol diester with biological properties similar to 12-O-tetradecanoylphorbol-13-acetate. *Proc. Amer. Assoc. Cancer Res.* 22:127.

Boehm, T. L. J., and Drahovsky, D. 1981. Hypomethylation of DNA in Raji cells after treatment with N-methyl-N-nitrosourea. *Carcinogenesis* 2:39–42.

Boone, C. W., and Jacobs, J. B. 1976. Sarcomas routinely produced from putatively nontumorigenic BALB/3T3 and C3H/10T½ cells by subcutaneous inoculation attached to plastic platelets. *J. Supramol. Struct.* 5:131–137.

Borgen, A., Darvey, H., Castagnoli, N., Crocker,

T. T., Rasmussen, R. E., and Wang, I. Y. 1973. Metabolic conversion of benzo-[*a*]pyrene by Syrian hamster liver microsomes and binding of metabolites to deoxyribonucleic acid. *J. Med. Chem.* 16:502–506.

Boutwell, R. K. 1964. Some biological aspects of skin carcinogenesis. *Prog. Exp. Tumor Res.* 4:207–250.

Carro-Ciampi, G. 1978. Phenacetin abuse: A review. *Toxicology* 10:311–339.

Case, R. A. M., Hosker, M. E., McDonald, D. B., and Pearson, J. T. 1954. Tumors of the urinary bladder in workmen engaged in the manufacture and use of dyestuff ingredients in the British chemical industry. *Br. J. Ind. Med.* 11:213–216.

Clayson, D. B. 1962. *Chemical carcinogenesis.* London: Churchill.

Clayson, D. B., and Garner, C. 1976. Carcinogenic aromatic amines and related compounds. In *Chemical carcinogens*, ed. C. E. Searle, pp. 366–461. Washington, D.C.: American Chemical Society.

Cole, P., and Goldman, M. B. 1975. Occupation. In *Persons at high risk of cancer*, ed. J. F. Fraumeni, Jr. pp. 167–184. New York: Academic Press.

Columbano, A., Rajalakshmi, S., and Sarma, D. S. R. 1981. Requirement of cell proliferation for the initiation of liver carcinogenesis as assayed by three different procedures. *Cancer Res.* 41:2079–2083.

Diamond, L., O'Brien, T. G., and Rovera, G. 1978. Tumor promoters: Effects on proliferation and differentiation of cells in culture. *Life Sci.* 23:1979–1988.

Dipple, A. 1976. Polynuclear aromatic carcinogens. In *Chemical carcinogens*, ed. C. E. Searle, pp. 245–314. Washington, D.C.: American Chemical Society.

Druckrey, H. 1967. Quantitative aspects in chemical carcinogenesis. In *Potential carcinogenic hazards from Drugs*, ed. R. Truhaut, pp. 60–78. Berlin: Springer.

Ehrlich, M., and Wang, R. Y. H 1981. 5-Methylcytosine in eukaryotic DNA. *Science* 212:1350–1357.

Farber, E. 1980. The sequential analysis of liver cancer induction. *Biochem. Biophys. Acta* 605:149–166.

Ford, G. P., and Scribner, J. D. 1983. A theoretical study of gas-phase methylation and ethylation by diazonium ions and rationalization of some aspects of DNA reactivity. *J. Am. Chem. Soc.* 105:349–354.

Fu, P. P., Harvey, R. G., and Beland, F. A. 1978. Molecular orbital theoretical prediction of the isomeric products formed from reactions of arene oxides and related metabolites of polycyclic aromatic hydrocarbons. *Tetrahedron* 34:857–866.

Fukushima, S., and Cohen, S. M. 1980. Saccharin-induced hyperplasia of the rat urinary bladder. *Cancer Res.* 40:734–736.

Garfinkel, J., Selvin, S., and Brown, S. M. 1977. Possible increased risk of lung cancer among beauticians. *J. Natl. Cancer Inst.* 58:141–143.

Gaugler, B. J. M., Neumann, H. -G., Scribner, N. K., and Scribner, J. D. 1979. Identification of some products from the reaction of *trans*-4-aminostilbene metabolites and nucleic acids in vivo. *Chem. Biol. Interact.* 27:335–352.

Grunberger, D., and Weinstein, I. B. 1979. Conformational changes in nucleic acids modified by chemical carcinogens. In *Chemical carcinogens and DNA*, vol. 2, ed. P. L. Grover, pp. 59–93. Boca Raton, Fla.: CRC Press.

Hanseh, C., and Fujita, T. 1964. A method for the correlation of biochemical activity and chemical structure. *J. Am. Chem. Soc.* 64:1616–1626.

Herbst, A. L., Scully, R. E., Robboy, S. J., Welch, W. R., and Cole, P. 1977. Abnormal development of the human genital tract following prenatal exposure to diethylstilbestrol. In *Origins of human cancer*, eds. H. H. Hiatt, J. D. Watson, and J. A. Winsten, pp. 399–412. Cold Spring Harbor, N.Y.: Cold Spring Harbor Laboratory.

Hicks, R. M., and Chowaniec, J. 1978. Experimental induction, histology, and ultrastructure of hyperplasia and neoplasia of the urinary bladder epithelium. *Int. Rev. Exp. Pathol.* 18:199–280.

Hogan, M. E., Dattagupta, N. and Whitlock, J.P. 1981. Carcinogen-induced alteration of DNA structure. *J. Biol. Chem.* 256:4504–4513.

Hoover, R. N., and Strasser, P. H. 1980. Artificial sweeteners and human bladder cancer. *Lancet*, 837–840.

International Agency for Research on Cancer. 1974. *IARC monographs on the evaluation of carcinogeneic risk of chemicals to man*, vol. 7. Lyons, France: IARC, pp. 291–318.

Kadlubar, F. F., Miller, J. A., and Miller, E. C. 1978. Guanyl O^6-arylamination and O^6-arylation of DNA by the carcinogen

N-hydroxy-1-naphthylamine. *Cancer Res.* 38:3628–3638.

Kadlubar, F. F., Unruh, L. E., Beland, F. A., Straub, K. M., and Evans, F. E. 1980. In vitro reaction of the carcinogen N-hydroxy-2-naphthylamine with DNA at the C-8 and N^2 atoms of guanine and at the N^6 atom of adenine. *Carcinogenesis* 1:139–150.

Kennaway, E. L. 1925. Experiments on cancer producing substances. *Br. Med. J.* ii, 1–4.

Kennedy, A. R., and Little, J. B. 1980. Investigation of the mechanism for enhancement of radiation transformation *in vitro* by 12-O-tetradecanoylphorbol-13-acetate. *Carcinogenesis* 1:1039–1047.

Kipling, M. D. 1976. Soots, tars and oils as causes of occupational cancer. In *Chemical carcinogens*, ed. C. E. Searle, pp. 315–323. Washington, D.C.: American Chemical Society.

Kriek, E., and Westra, J. G. 1979. Metabolic activation of aromatic amines and amides and interactions with nucleic acids. In *Chemical carcinogens and DNA*, vol. 2, ed. P. L. Grover, pp. 1–28. Boca Raton, Fla.: CRC Press.

Lawley, P. D. 1976. Carcinogenesis by alkylating agents. In *Chemical carcinogens*, ed. C. E. Searle, pp. 83–244. Washington, D.C.: American Chemical Society.

Levin, D. L., Devesa, S. S., Godwin, J. D., and Silverman, D. T. 1974. *Cancer rates and risks*, Washington, D.C.: U.S. Government Printing Office.

Lijinsky, W., Garcia, H., and Saffiotti, U. 1970. Structure–activity relationships among some polynuclear hydrocarbons and their hydrogenated derivatives. *J. Natl. Cancer Inst.* 44:641–649.

Magee, P. N., Montesano, R., and Preussmann, R. 1976. N-Nitroso compounds and related carcinogens. In *Chemical carcinogens*, ed. C. E. Searle, pp. 491–625. Washington, D.C.: American Chemical Society.

Menck, H. R., Pike, M.C., Henderson, B. E., and Jing, J. S. 1977. Lung cancer risk among beauticians and other female workers. *J. Natl. Cancer Inst.* 59:1423–1425.

Miller, E. C. 1951. Studies on the formation of protein-bound derivatives of 3,4-benzpyrene in the epidermal fraction of mouse skin. *Cancer Res.* 11:100–108.

Miller, E. C., and Miller, J. A. 1947. The presence and significance of bound aminoazo dyes in the livers of rats fed *p*-dimethylaminoazobenzene. *Cancer Res.* 7:468–480.

Miller, E. C., and Miller, J. A. 1969. Studies on the mechanism of activation of aromatic amine and amide carcinogens to ultimate carcinogenic electrophilic reactants. *Ann. N.Y. Acad. Sci.* 163:731–750.

Miller, E. C., and Miller, J. A. 1976. The metabolism of chemical carcinogens to reactive electrophiles and their possible mechanisms of action in carcinogenesis. In *Chemical carcinogens*, ed. C. E. Searle, pp. 737–762. Washington, D.C.: American Chemical Society.

Miller, J. A., Miller, E. C., and Finger, G. C. 1957. Further studies on the carcinogenicity of dyes related to 4-dimethylaminoazobenzene. The requirement for an unsubstituted 2-position. *Cancer Res.* 17:387–398.

Mondal, S., and Heidelberger, C. 1970. In vitro malignant transformation by methylcholanthrene of the progeny of single cells derived from C3H mouse prostate. *Proc. Natl. Acad. Sci. U.S.A.* 65:219–225.

Mottram, J. C. 1944. Developing factor in experimental blastogenesis. *J. Pathol. Bacteriol.* 56:181–187.

Nerbert, D. W., and Jensen, N. M. 1979. The *Ah* locus: genetic regulation of the metabolism of carcinogens, drugs, and other environmental chemicals by cytochrome P-450–mediated monooxygenases. *CRC Crit. Rev. Biochem.* 6:401–437.

Nelson, N. 1976. The chloro ethers: Occupational carcinogens. A summary of laboratory and epidemiology studies. *Ann. N.Y. Acad. Sci.* 271:81–90.

O'Brien, T. G. 1976. The induction of ornithine decarboxylase as an early, possibly obligatory, event in mouse skin carcinogenesis. *Cancer Res.* 36:2644–2653.

Parkes, H. G. 1976. The epidemiology of the aromatic amine cancers. In *Chemical carcinogens*, ed. C. E. Searle, pp. 462–480. Washington, D.C.: American Chemical Society.

Peraino, C., Fry, R. J. M., Staffeldt, E., and Kisieliski, W. E. 1973. Effects of varying exposure to phenobarbitol on its enhancement of 2-acetylaminofluorene-induced hepatic tumorigenesis. *Cancer Res.* 33:2701–2705.

Phillips, D. H., and Sims, P. 1979. Polycyclic aromatic hydrocarbon metabolites: Their reactions with nucleic acids. In *Chemical carcinogens and DNA*, vol. 2, ed. P. L. Grover, pp. 29–57. Boca Raton, Fla.: CRC Press.

Pike, M. C., Edmondson, H. A., Benton, B., and

Henderson, B. E. 1977. Liver adenomas and oral contraceptives. In *Origins of human cancer,* eds. H. H. Hiatt, J. D. Watson, and J. A. Winsten, pp. 423–428. Cold Spring Harbor, N.Y.: Cold Spring Harbor Laboratory.

Pullman, A., and Pullman, B. 1955. Electronic structure and carcinogenic activity of aromatic molecules. *Adv. Cancer Res.* 3:117–169.

Rothman, K. J. 1975. Alcohol. In *Persons at high risk of cancer,* ed. J. F. Fraumeni, Jr. pp. 139–150. New York: Academic Press.

Saffiotti, U., and Page, N. P. 1977. Releasing carcinogenesis test results: Timing and extent of reporting. *Med. Pediatr. Oncol.* 3:159–168.

Scribner, J. D. 1969. Formation of a sigma complex as a hypothetical rate-determining step in the carcinogenic action of unsubstituted polycyclic aromatic hydrocarbons. *Cancer Res.* 29:2120–2126.

Scribner, J. D. 1979. Molecular orbital theory in carcinogenesis research. In *Aspects of cancer research 1971–1978,* ed. J. C. Bailar III, pp. 341–345. Washington, D. C.: National Cancer Institute.

Scribner, J. D., and Boutwell, R. K. 1972. Inflammation and tumor promotion: Selective protein induction in mouse skin by tumor promoters. *Eur. J. Cancer* 8:617–621.

Scribner, J. D., and Fisk, S. R. 1978. Reproduction of major reactions of aromatic carcinogens with guanosine, using HMO-based polyelectronic perturbation theory, *Tetrahedron Lett.* 4759–4762.

Scribner, J. D., and Koponen, G. 1979. Binding of the carcinogen 2-acetamidophenanthrene to rat liver nucleic acids: lack of correlation with carcinogenic activity, and failure of the hydroxamic acid ester model for in vivo activation. *Chem. Biol. Interact.* 28:201–209.

Scribner, J. D., Miller, J. A., and Miller, E. C. 1970. Nucleophilic substitution on carcinogenic N-acetoxy-N-arylacetamides. *Cancer Res.* 30:1570–1579.

Scribner, J. D., and Scribner, N. K. 1982. Is the initiation–promotion regimen in mouse skin relevant to complete carcinogenesis? In *Cocarcinogenesis and biological effects of tumor promoters,* eds. E. Hecker, N. Fusenig, and W. Kunz, pp. 13–18. New York: Raven Press.

Scribner, N. K., and Scribner, J. D. 1980. Separation of initiating and promoting effects of the skin carcinogen 7-bromomethylbenz[a]anthracene. *Carcinogenesis* 1:97–100.

Scribner, J. D., and Ford, G. P. 1982. n-Propyldiazonium ion alkylates O^6 of guanine with rearrangement but alkylates N-7 without rearrangement. *Cancer Lett.* 16:51–56.

Scribner, J. D., Scribner, N. K., and Koponen, G. 1982. Metabolism and nucleic acid binding of 7-fluoro-2-acetamidofluorene in rats: oxidative defluorination and apparent dissociation of 8-(N-arylamide) guanine adducts on DNA from hepatocarcinogenesis. *Chem. Biol. Interact.* 40:27–43.

Scribner, J. D., and Süss, R. 1978. Tumor initiation and promotion. *Int. Rev. Exp. Pathol.* 18:137–198.

Scribner, N. K., and Scribner, J. D. 1980. Separation of initiating and promoting effects of the skin carcinogen 7-bromomethylbenz[a]anthracene. *Carcinogenesis* 1:97–100.

Scribner, N. K., Scribner, J. D., Smith, D. L., Schram, K. H., and McCloskey, J. A. 1979. Reactions of the carcinogen N-acetoxy-4-acetamidostilbene with nucleosides. *Chem. Biol. Interact.* 26:27–46.

Scribner, N. K., Woodworth, B., Ford, G. P., and Scribner, J. D. 1980. The influence of molecular size and partition coefficients on the predictability of tumor initiation in mouse skin from mutagenicity in *Salmonella typhimurium. Carcinogenesis* 1:715–719.

Selikoff, I. J., and Hammond, E. C. 1975. Multiple risk factors in environmental cancer. In *Persons at high risk of cancer,* ed. J. F. Fraumeni, Jr., pp. 467–483. New York: Academic Press.

Shih, C., Shilo, B.-Z., Goldfarb, M P., Dannenberg, A., and Weinberg, R. A. 1979. Passage of phenotypes of chemically transformed cells via transfection of DNA and chromatin. *Proc. Natl. Acad. Sci. U.S.A.* 76:5714–5718.

Sims, P., Grover, P. L., Swaisland, A., Pal, K., and Hewer, A. 1974. Metabolic activation of benzo[a]pyrene proceeds by a diol-epoxide. *Nature* 252:326–328.

Singer, B. 1975. The chemical effects of nucleic acid alkylation and their relation to mutagenesis and carcinogenesis. *Prog. Nucleic Acid Res.* 15:219–284; 330–332.

Slaga, T. J., Fischer, S. M., Nelson, K., and Gleason, G. L. 1980. Studies on the mechanism of skin tumor promotion: Evidence for several stages in promotion. *Proc. Natl. Acad. Sci. U.S.A.* 77:3659–3663.

Slaga, T. J., and Scribner, J. D. 1973. Inhibition of tumor initiation and promotion by anti-inflammatory agents. *J. Natl. Cancer Inst.* 51:1723–1725.

Smith, I. A., Berger, G. D., Seybold, P. G., and Servé, M. P. 1978. Relationships between carcinogenicity and theoretical reactivity indices in polycyclic aromatic hydrocarbons. *Cancer Res.* 38:2968–2977.

Stula, E. F., Barnes, J. R., Sherman, H., Reinhardt, C. F., and Zapp, J. A. 1977. Urinary bladder tumors in dogs from 4,4'-methylene-bis (2-chloroaniline) (MOCA). *J. Environ. Pathol. Toxicol.* 1:31–50.

Trosko, J. E., Yotti, L. P., Warren, S., and Chang, C. C. 1982. Inhibition of cell–cell communication by tumor promoters. In *Cocarcinogenesis and biological effects of tumor promoters*, eds. E. Hecker, N. Fusenig, and W. Kunz. New York: Raven Press 7:565–585.

Van Duuren, B. L, and Goldschmidt, B. M. 1975. Cocarcinogenic and tumor-promoting agents in tobacco carcinogenesis. *J. Natl. Cancer Inst.* 56:1237–1242.

Vogel, A. I. 1956. *A textbook of practical organic chemistry.* Longmans, Green & Co. p. 426.

Weiss, N. S. 1977. Exogenous estrogens and the incidence of neoplasm in tissues of müllerian origin. In *Origins of human cancer*, eds. H. H. Hiatt, J. D. Watson, and W. A. Winsten, pp. 413–422. Cold Spring Harbor, N.Y.: Cold Spring Harbor Laboratory.

Wigler, M., and Weinstein, I. B. 1976. Tumor promoter induces plasminogen activator. *Nature* 259:232–233.

Yamagiwa, K., and Ichikawa, K. 1918. Experimental study of the pathogenesis of carcinoma. *J. Cancer Res.* 3:1–29.

Ying, T. S., Sarma, D. S. R., and Farber, E. 1981. Role of acute hepatic necrosis in the induction of early steps in liver carcinogenesis by diethylnitrosamine. *Cancer Res.* 31:2096–2102.

Yuspa, S. H., and Morgan, D. L. 1981. Mouse skin cells resistant to terminal differentiation associated with initiation of carcinogenesis. *Nature* 293:72–74.

3

Injury by Ionizing Radiations

Arthur C. Upton

Within months after Roentgen's discovery of the X ray, in 1895, injurious effects of this newly found form of energy were reported. Among the first to encounter such effects was the pioneer Pierre Curie, who intentionally exposed the skin of his own arm to observe its reaction (Glasser, 1933). So rapidly and enthusiastically was experimentation with radiation undertaken that scores of investigators injured themselves before the hazards were adequately recognized (Brown, 1936).

In the intervening years, study of radiation injury has received continuing impetus from the expanding use of radioisotopes and radiologic techniques in science, medicine, industry, nuclear energy, and defense. Apprehension about the long-term effects of growing levels of radiation in the environment has led to the formation of national and international committees to provide ongoing assessment of the risks to the general population (UN, 1977; NAS, 1980).

In view of the vast amount of effort devoted to the study of radiation injury during the past century, it may be concluded that the effects of radiation are better understood than those of any other physical or chemical agent. To this extent, it is useful to review our experience with radiation in addressing health problems associated with other environmental agents.

Nature, Types, and Measurement of Ionizing Radiation

Ionizing radiations are customarily subdivided into two broad types: electromagnetic and particulate. The former include those radiations of the electromagnetic spectrum that are characterized by relatively short wavelength and high frequency (Figure 3-1). The particulate radiations consist of electrons, protons, neutrons, α particles, and other subatomic particles of varying mass and charge.

Levels of radiation exposure and dosage are measured in various units (ICRU, 1980). The oldest unit is the *roentgen* (R), which denotes a quantity of ionization induced by radiation in a standard volume of air. It is, therefore, a unit of exposure rather than of absorbed dose. The units for expressing absorbed dose are the *rad* (1 rad = 100 ergs/tissue) and the *gray* (1 Gy = 1 joule/kg tissue = 100 rad). Because, in general, the dose imparted to tissue by exposure to 1 roentgen approximates 1 rad, the two units have sometimes been considered to be roughly equivalent.

One rad of particulate radiations generally produces greater injury than 1 rad of X rays. Hence, additional units, the rem and the sievert (Sv), have been introduced into radiologic protection to enable doses of dif-

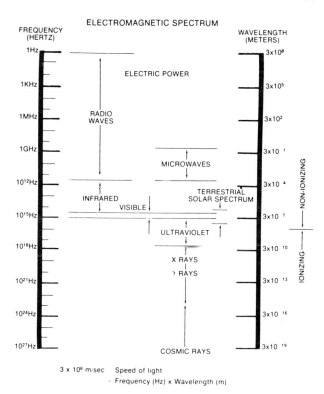

Figure 3–1. Radiations of the electromagnetic spectrum. (From U.S., Dept. of HEW, 1977, p. 135.)

ferent radiations to be normalized. One *rem*, defined loosely, is that dose of any radiation that produces a biologic effect equivalent to 1 rad of X rays or γ rays. One *sievert* is that amount of any radiation that produces a biologic effect equivalent to 1 gray of X rays or γ rays (1 Sv = 100 rem). Because the rem and the sievert are frequently inconveniently large units for radiologic protection purposes, the millirem (1 mrem = 1/1000 rem) is also used. The unit used for expressing the collective dose to a population is the *person-rem*, which is the product of the number of people exposed times the average dose per person (e.g., 1 rem to each of 1000 people = 1000 person-rem).

The units that are used for measuring the amount of radioactivity contained in given sample of matter are the curie (Ci) and the becquerel (Bq); 1 *Ci* is that quantity of a radioactive nuclide in which there are 3.7 × 10^{10} atomic disintegrations per second, and 1 *Bq* is that quantity of a radioactive nuclide in which there is one atomic disintegration per second (1 Bq = 2.7 × 10^{-11}

Ci). Because radionuclides decay exponentially with time, each element at its own rate, the time required for a given quantity of a radionuclide to lose one-half of its radioactivity is called its *physical half-life.*

Elimination of a radionuclide from tissue, through excretion or biologic transfer, may approximate an exponential process, so that such loss of the nuclide can be expressed in terms of the *biologic half-life* of the element.

The dose of radiation delivered by an internally deposited radionuclide will depend on the quantity of radioactivity remaining in situ. The rate at which this decreases determines the *effective half-life* of the nuclide, which varies as the resultant of the physical half-life and the biologic half-life (Figure 3-2).

Sources and Levels of Radiation in the Environment

The major sources of radiation to which the human population is exposed are man-made as well as natural (Table 3-1).

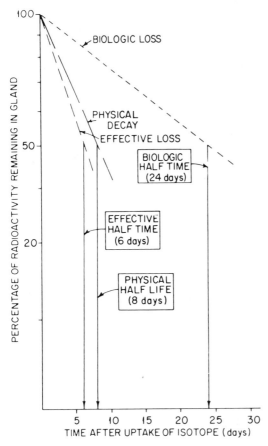

Figure 3–2. Rate of loss of radioactive iodine-131 after maximal uptake in the human thyroid gland. The rate of biologic loss is plotted as exponential, although it is actually somewhat more rapid initially than at later times after uptake. (From Andrews, 1957.)

Table 3–1. Estimates of Annual Whole-Body Radiation Doses to the U.S. Population

Source of radiation	Average dose rates (mrem/year)
Natural	
Environmental	
Cosmic radiation	28 (28–130)[a]
Terrestrial radiation	26 (30–115)[b]
Internal radioactive isotopes	26
Subtotal	80
Man-made	
Environmental	
Technological enhancements	4
Global fallout	4
Nuclear power	0.2
Medical	
Diagnostic procedures	78
Radiopharmaceuticals	14
Occupational	1
Miscellaneous	5
Subtotal	106.2
Total	186.2

[a] Values in parentheses indicate range over which average levels for different states vary with elevation.

[b] Range of variation (shown in parentheses) attributable largely to geographic differences in the content of potassium-40, radium, thorium, and uranium in the earth's crust.

Sources: From U.S., Dept. of HEW (1979); NAS (1980); Langham (1967).

Natural background radiation comes from three main sources: (1) cosmic rays, (2) thorium, radium, and other radionuclides in the earth's crust, and (3) potassium-40, carbon-14, and other naturally occurring radioactive elements in the body (Table 3-1). Collectively, the average dose received from these sources by a person living at sea level is about 80 mrem per year. It will be noted, however, that doses at least twice as large are received by populations living at higher elevations, where cosmic rays are more intense, and in areas where there is an increased content of radioactive material in the soil and subterranean rock.

In addition to natural background radia-

tion, man-made sources are estimated to contribute an average of 106 mrem per year to the dose received by each member of the population (Table 3-1). The largest of the man-made contributions comes from medical diagnostic procedures. Lesser contributions come from "technologically enhanced" sources—such as the use of phosphate fertilizers and building materials containing trace amounts of radioactivity—global fallout from atmospheric testing of atomic weapons, nuclear power, high-altitude jet flight, occupational exposure, and consumer products (color TV sets, smoke detectors, luminescent clock and instrument dials, etc.).

In comparison with the average annual dose to the general population from cosmic radiation, which approximates 28 mrem, the average dose to the thorax of an individual from a standard X-ray examination of the chest is of the order of 10 mrem. Other diagnostic procedures may entail substantially larger doses; for example, the average dose to the bone marrow of an individual from a barium enema examination of the colon is of the order of 500 to 800 mrem.

Interaction of Radiation with Tissue

When radiation penetrates matter, it loses its energy through a series of interactions with atoms in its path. These interactions, which involve the removal of electrons from atoms and collisions between impinging particles and atomic nuclei, result in the formation of ions and reactive radicals. These, in turn, cause damage to molecules in their vicinity by breaking chemical bonds and other chemical alterations.

In general, the density of ionization events along the path of an impinging radiation— or its rate of linear energy transfer (LET)— increases with increasing mass and charge of the radiation, and with decreasing energy of the radiation. X Rays, for example, tend to deposit relatively little energy along their paths and to penetrate deeply; α particles, in contrast, are densely ionizing and penetrate relatively poorly. Because the biologic effects of radiation result from chemical changes that are caused by ionization of atoms and molecules, traversal of a cell by a high-LET radiation, such as an α particle, involves a higher probability of damage than traversal by a low-LET radiation, such as an X ray.

Types of Radiation Injury

Ionizing radiation can cause a wide variety of effects. Any living organism can be killed by radiation if exposed to a large enough dose, but the effects in a given organism depend on the conditions of exposure.

Heritable effects on germ cells are expressed in the descendants of exposed individuals. In contrast, *somatic* effects are expressed in the exposed individuals themselves. Among somatic effects, some may appear soon after irradiation—such as mitotic inhibition—whereas others may not become manifest until after decades (e.g., radiation-induced cancer).

The various types of injury include *stochastic* effects, which vary in frequency, but not severity, with dose, and *nonstochastic* effects, which vary in both frequency and severity with dose. Included among the former are mutagenic, carcinogenic, and teratogenic effects. These are thought to be inducible by subtle injury to only one or few cells of the body, damaged singly. Hence, no threshold for these effects is presumed to exist.

Nonstochastic effects, in contrast, are attributed to gross tissue damage, involving injury of many cells. For such effects, therefore, a practical threshold is assumed to exist.

Effects of Radiation on the Cell

Ionizing radiation can cause many types of cellular injury, including mitotic inhibition, chromosome aberrations, mutation, interphase death, reproductive death, endomitosis, neoplastic transformation, apoptosis, and various other degenerative changes associated with necrobiosis (Rubin and Casarett, 1968; Cole et al., 1980; and Kerr and Searle, 1980). Although there is still uncertainty about the identity of the macromolecular targets involved in each of the various forms of radiation injury, it is generally accepted that damage to DNA plays a critical role in most of the effects in question (Cole et al., 1980).

The *changes in DNA* ascribed to radiation include base alteration, base destruction, sugar–phosphate bond cleavage, chain breakage (single-strand, double-strand), cross-linking of strands (intrastrand, interstrand), DNA–protein cross-links, and degradation (Cerutti, 1974). While complex damage is likely to occur when a high-LET particle traverses a DNA molecule, simpler lesions, such as single-strand breakage or base damage, are more likely to occur on traversal by a low-LET radiation (Figure 3-3).

Because of repair processes, the cell may be able to survive a relatively large number of lesions in DNA; for example, the mean lethal dose of X rays for dividing cells causes

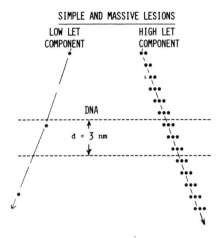

SIMPLE AND MASSIVE LESIONS

Figure 3–3. Representative distributions of energy events for traversals of a DNA molecule by particles with low and high LET. A 0.5-nm hydration sheath, which contributes active radicals, is added to the 2-nm DNA diameter to form a 3-nm diameter sensitive cylinder. The asterisks symbolize average energy exchanges of about 60 eV, each of which is capable of inducing simple lesions such as a backbone scission or sugar or base damage. (From Cole et al., 1980.)

hundreds of single-strand breaks and dozens of double-strand breaks in the DNA of each cell (Cole et al., 1980; Elkind, 1980). What ultimately determines whether there is permanent damage to DNA is the product of a sequence of reactions, the outcome of which may depend as much on the effectiveness of repair of lesions as on the nature of the primary lesions themselves. Studies with α-particle beams imply that the most sensitive sites of DNA damage, insofar as lethality and division delay are concerned, are localized in the periphery of the nucleus, closely beneath the nuclear membrane (Cole et al., 1980).

Mitotic inhibition was one of the first biologic effects of radiation to be investigated. It varies in magnitude and duration with the dose and conditions of exposure, as well as with the type and condition of exposed cells. Typically, the mitotic rate falls promptly after irradiation, remains depressed for a dose-dependent interval, and then returns to normal following a transitory period of overshooting (Figure 3-4). The effect cannot be elicited by irradiation of the

cytoplasm alone but requires exposure of the cell nucleus (Cole et al., 1980).

Chromosome damage is frequently evident in dividing cells at the time of mitotic recovery. The changes may include clumping of chromosomes, chromosome bridges, tripolar mitoses, and other abnormalities. The breakage of chromosomes by radiation and the repair of such breaks have been studied extensively. When two or more breaks are produced close together in space and time, the broken ends from one breakpoint may be joined incorrectly with those from another, giving rise to translocations, inversions, rings, dicentrics, deletions, and other types of chromosome rearrangements (Gaulden, 1973).

The yield of such "two-event" aberrations increases as a linear function of the dose and is virtually independent of the dose rate with high-LET irradiation. With low-LET irradiation, however, it increases less steeply, as a linear quadratic function of the dose. At low doses and low dose rates, the linear dose term predominates, whereas at high doses and high dose rates, the quadratic term predominates (Figures 3-5 and 3-6). From these dose–effect relationships, it is inferred that a two-event chromosome aberration has a small probability of being produced by low-LET irradiation unless two or more radiation tracks traverse a given region of the cell nucleus closely enough together in space and time that the separate DNA lesions caused by each track can interact with one another. Conversely, with each traversal of a high-LET radiation track, lesions are caused that tend to interact with one another independently of those caused by other traversals.

The majority of chromosome aberrations are "unstable," in that they cause death of the affected cell. Hence, their frequency decreases with time after irradiation in cells having a high rate of turnover, In tissues having a low rate of cell turnover, such as the liver, the aberrations may continue to be observed at high frequency long after irradiation if cells are recruited into division by appropriate stimulation (e.g., partial hepatectomy). Such aberrations may also be

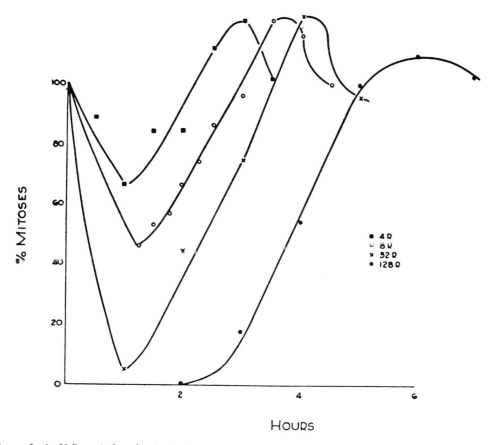

Figure 3–4. X-Ray–induced mitotic depression and "overshooting" in cells of rat corneal epithelium. (From Friedenwald and Sigelman, 1953.)

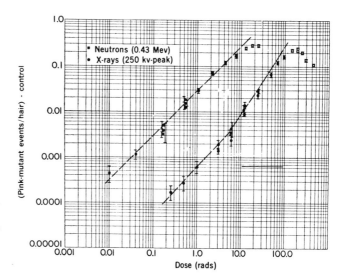

Figure 3–5. Yield of pink-mutant events in stamen hairs of treadescantia clone 02 as a function of dose of neutrons or X rays. (From Sparrow et al., 1972.)

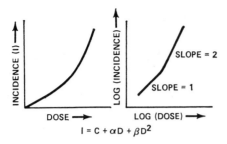

Figure 3–6. Graphic illustration of linear quadratic dose–effect relationship. (From J. M. Brown, 1977.)

observed in peripheral blood lymphocytes cultured from patients many years after irradiation. The combined frequency of dicentric and ring aberrations in human lymphocytes cultured shortly after whole-body irradiation in vivo has been observed to approximate 0.002 per cell per rem, from which it may be inferred that the dose required to double the frequency of such ab-

errations is only a few rem (UN, 1972, 1977; Lloyd et al., 1980).

DNA damage, expressed in the form of *mutations*, has been investigated in somatic cells (Puck, 1979) as well as germ cells (UN, 1977). In mouse spermatogonia and oocytes, the most extensively studied mammalian cells, the dose–effect relationship for specific-locus mutations resembles that for induction of chromosome aberrations, discussed above. With high-LET radiations, the curve rises steeply as a function of dose and is relatively independent of the dose rate, whereas with low-LET radiations the curve rises less steeply and is highly dependent on the dose rate (Figures 3-7 and 3-8). At high dose rates, the curves for both high-LET and low-LET radiations pass through a maximum and turn downward because of excessive cell injury (Figure 3-7). On appropriate protraction or fractionation of low-LET irradiation in this dose range, turning over of the curves is not observed, presumably be-

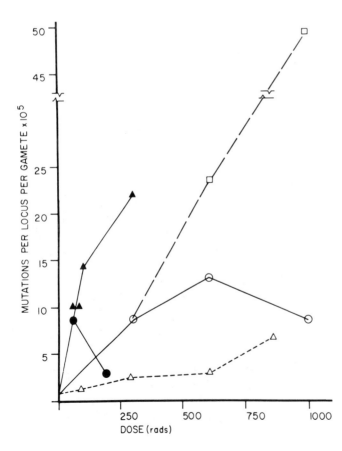

Figure 3–7. Frequency of specific-locus mutations in mouse spermatogonia as a function of the dose and dose rate of irradiation. Shaded symbols denote data for neutrons; open symbols denote data for X rays and γ rays. Circles denote data for acute exposures; squares denote data for fractionated exposures; and triangles denote data for chronic, daily exposures. (From Upton, 1974, based on data of W. L. Russell et al.)

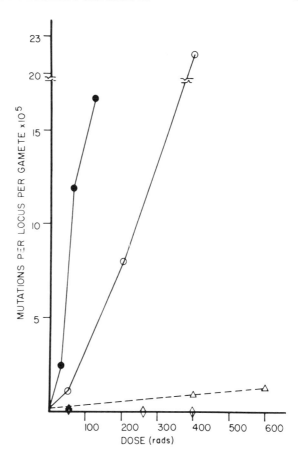

Figure 3–8. Frequency of specific-locus mutations in mouse oocytes as a function of the dose and dose rate of irradiation. Symbols are the same as in Figure 3–7, with the addition that the diamonds denote data for matings more than 7 weeks after irradiation. (From Upton, 1974, based on data of W. L. Russell et al.)

cause injury that would otherwise interfere with expression of the mutational damage is repaired (Figure 3-9).

Another complicating feature of the dose–effect curves is the absence of a detectable increase in mutations in offspring born to irradiated female mice mated more than 7 weeks after irradiation (Figure 3-8). The absence of mutations in these animals implies the existence of differentiation-dependent variations in the radiation sensitivity of successive oocyte maturation stages. Because of these variations, one must be cautious in extrapolating from one germ cell stage or system to another, especially across species (Figure 3-9).

The *killing of cells* by irradiation may occur through interference with mitosis (mitotic, or reproductive death), or it may be independent of cell division (interphase death, or apoptosis) (Berdjis, 1971; Kerr and Searle, 1980; Casarett, 1981). In general,

the susceptibility of cells to killing by irradiation varies in proportion to their rate of proliferation and inversely in relation to their degree of differentiation, as noted early in this century by Bergonie and Tribondeau (Rubin and Casarett, 1968). The survival of dividing cells, as measured by their ability to proliferate and form colonies, tends to decrease exponentially with increasing dose (Figure 3-10).

On irradiation with high-LET radiation, the dose–survival curve is characteristically steeper than it is with low-LET radiation and is relatively independent of the dose rate. With low-LET radiation, the curve usually has an initial shoulder in the low dose region, beyond which survival decreases exponentially with increasing dose (Figure 3-10). Moreover, on fractionation of low-LET radiation into two exposures (D_2) the shoulder reappears between successive exposures, owing presumably to repair of

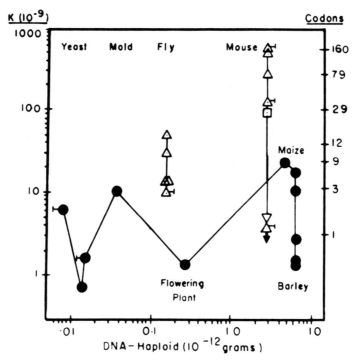

Figure 3–9. Mutations per gene per rad *(K)* and equivalent codons (estimated per target gene) plotted against test organism haploid DNA for various X-irradiated genes and groups of genes. In the case of the mouse, three sets of genes were used: the seven-locus test, represented by triangles (plain, spermatogonia; hooked, mature oocytes; arrow and hooked immature oocytes); the six-locus test by a square (spermatogonia); the H test by an inverted triangle (spermatogonia). The upper and lower points for mature oocytes were for 400 and 500 rad, respectively. The upper and lower spermatogonial points were for 1000 rad (split, 1 day apart) and 300 rad, respectively. (From Kohn, 1980.)

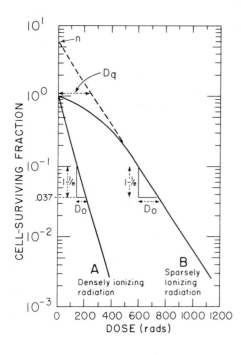

Figure 3–10. Characteristic survival curves for clonogenic mammalian cells exposed to ionizing radiation, as scored by ability to proliferate and form macroscopic colonies. The two parameters characterizing the curve are the slope (D_0) of the straight portion of the curve and the extrapolation number *(n)*, which is a measure of the "width" of the initial shoulder; the width of the shoulder may also be expressed in terms of the quasi-threshold dose (D_q). (From Hall, 1978.)

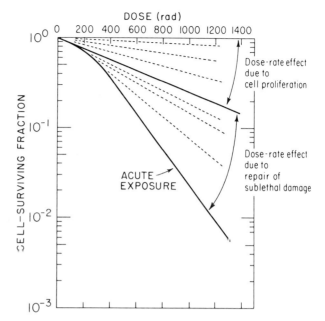

Figure 3–11. Illustration of how decrease in dose rate increases population survival through (a) repair of sublethal damage within cells and (b) replacement of dead or damaged cells by proliferation of survivors. (From Hall, 1978.)

sublethal damage during the interval (Figure 3-11). On protraction of low-LET radiation the slope of the curve likewise decreases, presumably because the accumulation of potentially lethal damage is offset by concomitant repair.

The slope of the exponential part of the survival curve is customarily expressed in terms of the dose that is required to reduce the number of clonogenic cells to 37% of their control value, the so-called D_{37} or D_0. In mathematical terms, it represents the tangent of the angle between the slope and the horizontal axis, that is,

$$\frac{\log(1-0.37)}{D_0}$$

For most clonogenic mammalian cells, including cancer cells, the D_0 has a value of 100 to 200 rem. Under hypoxia, however, the D_0 of low-LET radiation may be two to three times higher, which has important implications in terms of the resistance of poorly vascularized cancer tissue in radiotherapy (Denekamp et al., 1977; Hall, 1978).

The mechanisms of cell killing remain a subject of conjecture, although most current theories invoke incomplete repair or misrepair of damage to DNA (Cole et al., 1980; Elkind, 1980; Painter, 1980); Tobias

et al., 1980). Degenerative changes (cloudy swelling, pyknosis, karyorrhexis, etc.) are detectable within minutes after intensive irradiation (>100 rad) in the cells of lymphoid follicles and other radiosensitive tissues, followed within hours by frank necrosis and other evidence of cellular injury (Warren et al., 1942, 1943; Rubin and Casarett, 1968; Upton and Lushbaugh, 1969). The entire, complex sequence of reactions, including interactions among the damaged cells and homeostatic responses elicited in response to injury, is incompletely understood.

Neoplastic transformation of cells in culture is increased in frequency by irradiation (Borek, 1979, 1980; Kennedy and Little, 1980). The yield of transformants rises more steeply with dose in the case of neutron irradiation than in the case of X irradiation, passes through a maximum at intermediate dose levels, and then decreases with further increase in the dose (Figure 3-12). Fractionation of low-LET irradiation into two exposures, separated by an interval of 5 hours, has been observed to enhance the yield of transformants at doses below 300 rem, for reasons that are still to be determined. It can be postulated, however, that the enhancement may result from greater misre-

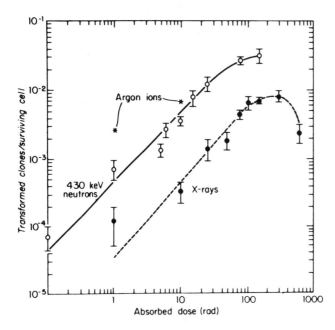

Figure 3–12. Rate of hamster embryo cell transformation in relation to dose of argon ions, neutron, or X rays. (From Borek et al., 1978.)

pair of DNA damage following appropriately fractionated exposures than following a single exposure alone, owing to induction of error-prone repair systems by the first exposure that accentuate the damaging effects of the second (Borek, 1979). Unrepaired or misrepaired damage to DNA bases, as opposed to DNA strand breaks, has been interpreted to be the most likely molecular mechanism of X-ray–induced neoplastic transformation (Little, 1978).

The transforming effects of ionizing radiation on cells in vitro, which can be elicited in human as well as animal cells (Borek, 1980), are consistent with the carcinogenic effects of radiation in vivo, discussed below. Although studies of radiation-induced neoplastic transformation in vitro are still limited in number and scope, they are useful for quantifying effects on cells in the low to intermediate-dose range, for exploring interactions between radiation and other factors influencing neoplasia, and for investigating directly mechanisms of carcinogenesis at the cellular level.

Non-Neoplastic Effects on Tissues

The effects of radiation on tissues comprise a spectrum of responses, reflecting both direct injury to cells and indirect reactions, some of which may evolve slowly. Although mitotic inhibition and cytologic abnormalities may be evident within minutes after intensive irradiation in radiosensitive tissues, some forms of degeneration and reactive fibrosis may not become manifest until months or years later. In general, tissues in which there is a high rate of cell turnover tend to exhibit injury sooner than others, as noted above; however, tolerance to long-term damage is not consistently correlated with mitotic rate (Rubin and Casarett, 1968).

Because damage to tissues is a function of the number of cells injured, the severity of damage is generally greater when an entire organ or the whole body is irradiated than when exposure is limited to only a part of an organ or a part of the body. Similarly, a given dose is generally less damaging when accumulated gradually in small increments over an extended period of time than when received in a single brief exposure, owing both to repair of damage at the intracellular level and to partial replacement of damaged cells by the compensatory proliferation of uninjured cells (Figure 3-11).

The pathologic effects of radiation are generally mimicked to varying degrees by other physical and chemical agents. Hence they are not strictly pathognomonic. Nevertheless, the changes in tissue parenchyma, stroma, and vasculature are often sufficiently characteristic to implicate radiation in the differential diagnosis. In general, most radiation reactions evolve through the following phases: (1) *acute* phase, with mitotic abnormalities, cytologic degeneration, necrosis, and acute inflammation, (2) *subacute* phase, with evidence of regenerative hyperplasia, phagocytosis, and other reparative phenomena, and (3) *chronic* phase, with progressive atrophy, fibrovascular sclerosis, and secondary complications (Rubin and Casarett, 1968; Berdjis, 1971; Casarett, 1981). Because the response of tissue to radiation varies somewhat from one organ to another, the reaction cannot be characterized in detail without considering each organ individually.

It is beyond the scope of this chapter to review the reaction of each tissue or organ. Suffice it to say that radiosensitivity varies appreciably from one organ to another and that few mature organs are known to exhibit severe or lasting degenerative changes at dose levels below 1000 rem absorbed within hours or days (Table 3-2). Notable exceptions, however, are the bone marrow, gonads, and lens of the eye (Table 3-2). The reactions of these organs are discussed briefly below.

BONE MARROW AND HEMOPOIETIC TISSUES

Hemopoietic cells are among the most radiosensitive in the body. The D_0 of hemopoietic stem cells has been estimated at 65 to 70 rem (Lajtha, 1965). Cytologic changes are demonstrable in the bone marrow and lymphoid follicles within minutes after acute whole-body irradiation at doses in excess of 100 rad (Bond et al., 1965; Berdjis, 1971). Changes in peripheral blood counts also become manifest soon after comparable whole-body irradiation, with almost immediate decline in the lymphocyte count (Figure 3-13). The changes reflect the high radiosensitivity of rapidly dividing hemo-

poietic cells—which undergo reproductive death as they attempt to divide, thus interfering with normal blood cell replacement—and of lymphocytes, which are unusual in undergoing interphase death within minutes after exposure (Bond et al., 1965; Maisin et al., 1971; Proukakis and Lindop, 1971). In general, granulocytes, erythrocytes, platelets, and their nondividing precursor cells are radioresistant.

After an initial granulocytosis, which results from the mobilization of leukocytes from extravascular spaces in response to stress, the granulocyte count falls, at a rate related to the normal granulocyte turnover time; that is, the maximum depression in humans is reached in the third to fifth week after acute whole-body irradiation (Figure 3-13), while in rats and mice it is reached in 5 to 10 days (Bond et al., 1965). The platelet count falls slightly less rapidly (Figure 3-13). The erythrocyte count falls much less rapidly, in the absence of hemorrhage (Figure 3-13).

The magnitude and duration of pancytopenia depend on the volume of hemopoietic tissue irradiated, the dose and quality (LET) of radiation, and the distribution of the dose in time. Granulocytopenia (complicated by infection) and thrombocytopenia (complicated by hemorrhage) are the main causes of death after acute whole-body irradiation in the midlethal dose range (Bond et al., 1965; Upton, 1969). The dose required to cause death in 50% of exposed individuals varies among species, from 200 to 300 rem in humans and other large mammals to more than 1000 rem in small rodents (Table 3-3). While doses below 50 to 100 rem produce too little depletion of hemopoietic cells to affect survival in humans, doses above 500 to 1000 rem are invariably lethal (Figure 3-14).

In contrast to the doses shown in Table 3-3, which cause hemopoietic death when delivered to the whole body in a single brief exposure, far larger doses can be tolerated when only a small fraction of hemopoietic tissue is exposed, or when the dose is spread out over a long period of time. Under continuous, whole-body irradiation at a dose

Table 3–2. Estimated Doses Required to Cause Various Types of Tissue Damage (TD) within 5 Years after Irradiation[a]

| Organ | Injury at 5 years | Percentage affected | | Fraction of organ irradiated (cm^3) |
		1–5% TD$_{5/5}$(rad)	25–50% TD$_{50/5}$(rad)	
Skin	Ulcer, severe fibrosis	5,500	7,500	100
Oral mucosa	Ulcer, severe fibrosis	6,000	7,500	50
Esophagus	Ulcer, stricture	6,000	7,500	75
Stomach	Ulcer, perforation	4,500	5,000	100
Intestine	Ulcer, stricture	4,500	6,500	100
Colon	Ulcer, stricture	4,500	6,500	100
Rectum	Ulcer, stricture	5,500	8,000	100
Salivary glands	Xerostomia	5,000	7,000	50
Liver	Liver failure, ascites	3,500	4,500	Whole
Kidney	Nephrosclerosis	2,300	2,800	Whole
Bladder	Ulcer, contracture	6,000	8,000	Whole
Ureters	Stricture, obstruction	7,500	10,000	5–10 cm
Testes	Permanent sterilization	200–600	2,000	Whole
Ovary	Permanent sterilization	200–300	625–1,200	Whole
Uterus	Necrosis, perforation	<10,000	<20,000	Whole
Vagina	Ulcer, fistula	9,000	<10,000	5 cm
Breast				
Child	No development	1,000	1,500	5
Adult	Atrophy + necrosis	<5,000	<10,000	Whole
Lung	Pneumonitis, fibrosis	4,000	6,000	Lobe
Capillaries	Telangiectasia, sclerosis	5,000–6,000	7,000–10,000	
Heart	Pericarditis, pancarditis	4,000	<10,000	Whole
Bone				
Child	Arrested growth	2,000	3,000	10
Adult	Necrosis, fracture	6,000	15,000	10
Cartilage				
Child	Arrested growth	1,000	3,000	Whole
Adult	Necrosis	6,000	10,000	Whole
CNS (brain)	Necrosis	5,000	<6,000	Whole
Spinal cord	Necrosis, transection	5,000	<6,000	5
Eye	Panophthalmitis, hemorrhage	5,500	10,000	Whole
Cornea	Keratitis	5,000	<6,000	Whole
Lens	Cataract	500	1,200	Whole
Ear (inner)	Deafness	<6,000	—	Whole
Vestibular	Meniere's disease	6,000	10,000	Whole
Thyroid	Hypothyroidism	4,500	15,000	Whole
Adrenal	Hypoadrenalism	<6,000	—	Whole
Pituitary	Hypopituitarism	4,500	20,000–30,000	Whole
Muscle				
Child	No development	2,000–3,000	4,000–5,000	Whole
Adult	Atrophy	<10,000	—	Whole
Bone marrow	Hypoplastic	200	550	Whole
		2,000	4,000–5,000	Localized
Lymph nodes	Atrophy	3,500–4,500	<7,000	Localized
Lymphatics	Sclerosis	5,000	<8,000	Localized

[a]Tabulated levels are estimates of dose required to cause an incidence of 5% (TD$_{5/5}$) or 50% (TD$_{50/5}$), respectively, of effects, with the following radiation conditions: supervoltage therapy (1–6 MeV); 1000 rad/week in five daily fractions with a 2-day rest; and treatment completed in 2 to 8 weeks, depending on the total dose.

Source: Modified from Rubin and Casarett (1972).

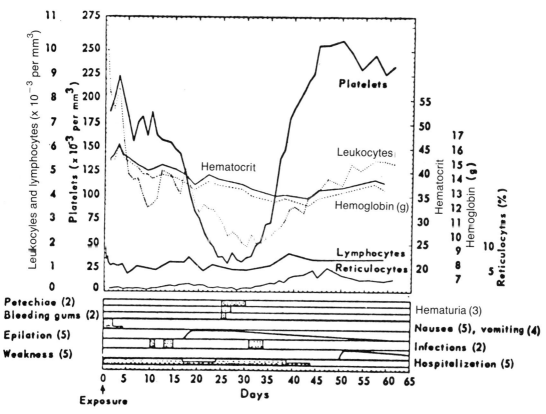

Figure 3–13. Hematologic values, symptoms, and clinical signs in five men exposed to whole-body irradiation in a criticality accident. The blood counts are average values for the five men; the figures in parentheses denote the number showing the symptoms and signs indicated. (From Andrews et al., 1961.)

Figure 3–14. Probability of death after acute whole-body irradiation in humans as a function of dose. (Modified from Langham et al., 1965. Overlapping range estimates are those of NAS, 1960; and UN, 1962.)

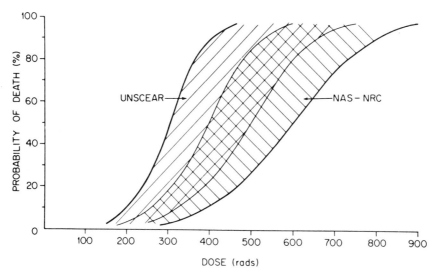

Table 3–3. Species Differences in Dose of Whole-Body Radiation Required to Cause Fatally Severe Hemopoietic Injury in 50% of Exposed Individuals (LD_{50})

Species	LD_{50} (rads)
Laboratory mouse	600–900
Desert mouse	1500
Gerbil	1000–1100
Hamster	600–900
Rat	700–900
Guinea pig	250–500
Marmoset	200
Rabbit	700–900
Monkey	400–600
Dog	200–300
Sheep	150–250
Goat	200–300
Swine	200–300
Burro	250
Human	250–550

Sources: From Bond et al. (1965); Hall (1978).

rate of up to 50 rad/day, compensatory proliferation of hemopoietic cells enables rodents to survive for weeks (Porteus and Lajtha, 1966). If the volume of marrow irradiated is small, relatively few effects are observed even after a dose of 2000 to 10,000 rem, apart from localized necrosis, atrophy, and fibrosis (Knospe et al., 1966).

Among the physiologic changes complicating damage to lymphoid tissues, is depression of the immune response. Following whole-body irradiation in the mid-lethal dose range, the depression is profound enough to enable transplantation of allogeneic bone marrow (Micklem and Loutit, 1966). Early stages in the immunologic response, including the process of antigen recognition, appear to be more sensitive than later stages, including antibody synthesis itself (UN, 1972; Anderson and Warner, 1976).

GONADS

The high radiosensitivity of type A spermatogonia makes the testis one of the most radiosensitive organs of the body. Late spermatogenic maturation stages, sperma-

tozoa, and other components of the testis are relatively radioresistant (Casarett, 1981). A single dose as low as 15 rem has been observed to cause a temporary reduction in the sperm count after a latent period of several weeks, followed by gradual recovery of normal sperm numbers and fertility. Permanent sterility has been reported to result from a dose of 200 rem or more (Sandeman, 1966; Lushbaugh and Ricks, 1972). The testis is unusual in that fractionated irradiation may cause even greater damage than acute exposure (Lushbaugh and Ricks, 1972); however, as much as 0.3 rem/week may be tolerated indefinitely without impairment of fertility in dogs (Rubin and Casarett, 1968).

Like the testis, the ovary is also highly radiosensitive. In this case, however, mature germ cell stages are radiosensitive and are killed in interphase. Moreover, in contrast to spermatozoa, which are formed throughout reproductive life by the proliferation of precursor cells, the ovary's entire supply of oocytes is present at puberty and is not replenished thereafter. To the extent, therefore, that the number of oocytes is reduced by irradiation, the reproductive potential of the ovary is diminished irreparably. Temporary sterility has been observed to result from a dose of 150 to 200 rem and permanent sterility from a dose as low as 200 to 300 rem (Lacassagne et al., 1962; Lushbaugh and Ricks, 1972).

LENS OF THE EYE

Opacification of the lens, or cataract, is a well-known complication of radiation exposure. Because cells of the anterior lens epithelium continue to divide throughout life, mitotic inhibition and cytologic abnormalities are detectable microscopically in such cells soon after exposure. Opacities observable with the slit lamp do not become evident, however, until after months or years, depending on the species and conditions of irradiation (Upton et al., 1956).

In humans, minimal subcapsular opacities at the posterior pole of the lens have been observed after a dose of 100 to 200 rem received in a single, bried exposure, but a larger dose is required to cause opacification severe enough to impair vision. The threshold for a vision-impairing cataract is estimated to vary from about 200 to 300 rem received in a single exposure to 550 to 1400 rem received over a period of months (Merriam et al., 1972). The occurrence of radiation cataracts in pioneer cyclotron physicists and heavily irradiated atomic bomb survivors is consistent with the high relative biologic effectiveness of fast neutrons for cataractogenesis in animals (Upton et al., 1956).

Carcinogenic Effects

The first cancer attributed to X rays, reported in 1902, arose as a complication of long-standing radiation dermatitis on the hand of a radiologist (Frieben, 1902). During the ensuing decade, scores of similar cases were reported in pioneer radiation workers, along with results of experiments confirming the carcinogenicity of X rays in laboratory animals (Furth and Lorenz, 1954; Upton, 1975).

Because the earliest cases of radiation-induced cancer occurred in heavily irradiated tissues, typically as a late complication of gross radiation injury, it was generally assumed that carcinogenesis required doses large enough to cause severe damage and disorganization of tissue (Furth and Lorenz, 1954). With further study, however, carcinogenic effects have been detected at lower and lower dose levels in human and animal populations. In some instances, moreover, the dose–effect data have been interpreted to imply that the incidence of a given type of cancer increases as a linear, nonthreshold function of the dose (Upton, 1975, 1981). Concern about the possible existence of a linear, nonthreshold dose–incidence relationship for radiation carcinogenesis, with its obvious implications of risks attributable to low-level irradiation, has thus had a major influence on the direction of relevant radiation research and on the development of radiologic protection poli-

cies (ICRP, 1977; UN, 1977; Upton, 1977, 1981; NAS, 1980).

From the wealth of information that is now available from observations in humans (Table 3-4) and laboratory animals, it can be inferred that neoplasms of most types may be induced by radiation under appropriate conditions of exposure, and that all forms of ionizing radiation possess carcinogenic activity to varying degrees (Upton, 1975; UN, 1977).

Because the neoplasms induced by irradiation do not differ individually in any known respect from those resulting from other causes, their induction by radiation can be inferred only on statistical gounds, that is, on the basis of an increase in frequency following exposure to radiation. It is noteworthy that the magnitude of the increase varies with (1) the susceptibility of the exposed tissue (which, in turn, depends on species, strain, sex, age at irradiation, and other factors), (2) the time after irradiation, and (3) the conditions of exposure (dose, dose rate, quality of radiation, and anatomic distribution of dose). The relationship among these variables can be characterized only to a limited degree on the basis of existing knowledge (UN, 1977). Hence, attempts to assess the carcinogenic risks of low-level irradiation must depend largely on extrapolation from limited observations at higher doses and dose rates, based on unproven assumptions about the dose–incidence relationship and the relevant mechanisms of carcinogenesis.

The hypothesis that the cumulative incidence of cancer might increase as a linear, nonthreshold function of radiation dose rests on several lines of evidence, which have been reviewed extensively elsewhere (UN, 1977; NAS, 1980). Cogent empirical data on cancer in humans include the incidence of leukemia in various irradiated populations, especially atomic bomb survivors of Hiroshima, in whom the cumulative excess appears to increase linearly with dose, even at the lowest dose levels that can be analyzed (Figure 3-15), and the incidence of breast cancer in women who received repeated fluoroscopic examinations of the chest for

Table 3–4. Various Types of Cancer Associated with Radiation in Different Populations[a]

Type of cancer	Atom bomb radiation			Medical radiation											Occupational radiation			
	Japanese atom bomb survivors	Marshall Islanders	Nuclear test participants	Ankylosing spondylitis (X ray)	Ankylosing spondylitis (radium)	Benign pelvic disease	Benign breast disease	Multiple chest fluoroscopy	Tinea capitis (children)	Enlarged thymus (infants)	Thorotrast	Thyroid cancer (I-131)	In utero X ray	Diagnostic X ray	Radium dial painters	Radiologists	Uranium and other miners	Nuclear workers
Leukemia	***		*	***		**			**	***	*	***	**	**		***		*
Thyroid	***	**		**					***	***		***	*	*				
Female breast	***			**			***	**		**								*
Lung	***			**						**							***	
Bone					***										***			
Stomach	**			**														
Esophagus	**			**														
Bladder	**			*														
Lymphoma (including multiple myeloma)	**			**						*	*							*
Brain																**		
Uterus						*												
Cervix						*										**		
Liver											*							
Skin									**	***						***	**	
Salivary gland									**									
Kidney										*								
Pancreas															*			
Colon	*					**												
Small intestine						*												
Rectum						**												

[a]Strong associations are indicated by ***, meaningful associations by **, and suggestive but unconfirmed associations by *.
Source: From U.S. Dept. of HEW (1979).

72

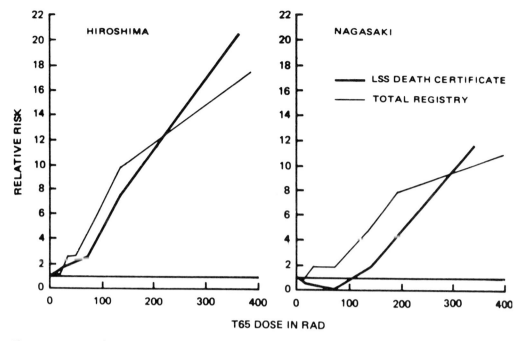

Figure 3–15. Leukemia mortality in atomic bomb survivors of Hiroshima and Nagasaki as a function of radiation dose. Data based on LSS sample and death certificates, 1950–1974, are compared with those based on atomic bomb survivors' survey and total leukemia registry, 1946–1974. (From Beebe et al., 1978.)

treatment of pulmonary tuberculosis with artificial pneumothorax, in whom the cumulative excess per unit dose is comparable to that resulting in other women from a single intensive radiation exposure (Figure 3-16). While the dose–incidence data for these two types of cancer are more extensive than those for other cancers, they are not the only dose–incidence data consistent with a linear, nonthreshold relationship (UN, 1977; NAS, 1980). In animals, a variety of dose–incidence patterns has been observed, which presumably reflect differences among different types of neoplasms in the mechanisms of carcinogenesis (UN, 1977).

Radiation at high dose levels causes such a diversity of effects on cells and tissues that it would be fortuitous if the dose–incidence relation for a given neoplasm were actually linear over a broad range of doses and dose rates. Nevertheless, if the carcinogenic effects of low-level radiation on a tissue are postulated to result from the neoplastic transformation of one of its cells by damage to the cell's genome, then a function of

the following form can be predicted on radiobiologic grounds:

$$I_D = (C + aD + bD^2)e^{-(pD + qD2)}$$

where I_D is the incidence of neoplasms at dose D, and a, b, p, and q are constants (Upton, 1977). The ratio of the coefficients a and b for low-LET radiation is such that the linear term (aD) predominates at low doses and low dose rates, and the quadratic term (bD^2), at high doses and high dose rates. With high-LET radiation, on the other hand, the ratio is such that the linear term predominates at all doses and dose rates. The values of the coefficients p and q are such as to account for the saturation of the dose–incidence curve at high doses.

Although this expression must be assumed to be a gross oversimplification of the dose–incidence relationship, for the reasons stated, it is more consistent with many of the existing dose–incidence data than a simple linear or simple quadratic model (Robinson and Upton, 1978; NAS, 1980). However, there are neoplasms in

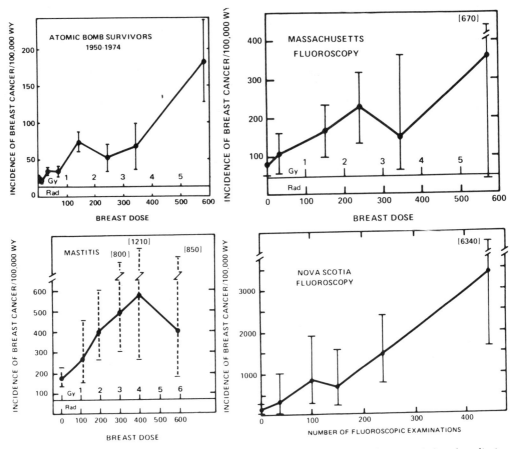

Figure 3–16. Dose–incidence curves for breast cancer in women exposed to atomic bomb radiation, multiple fluoroscopic examinations of the chest in the treatment of pulmonary tuberculosis, and X-ray therapy to the breast for postpartum mastitis. (From Boice et al., 1979.)

which the killing of cells is thought to play an important role in promoting carcinogenesis, in which the model must be modified accordingly (UN, 1977; Marshall and Groer, 1977).

While existing evidence is insufficient to define unambiguously the dose–incidence relationship for low-level carcinogenesis, or even to exclude the possibility of a threshold, the following generalizations can be made: (1) High-LET radiations (α particles, protons, fast neutrons) are more carcinogenic per unit dose than low-LET radiations (X rays, γ rays, β radiations), at least in the low to intermediate-dose range; (2) the excess of many, if not most, types of neoplasms per unit dose decreases with decreasing dose and dose rate of low-LET ra-

diation, but decreases less, if at all (or may even increase), with decreasing dose and dose rate of high-LET radiations; (3) at high dose rates, the dose–incidence curve for most neoplasms passes through a maximum at intermediate to high doses and decreases with further increase in the dose; (4) although radiation is carcinogenic in essentially all tissues, susceptibility to radiation carcinogenesis varies widely among species, strains, organs, tissues, and cells, for reasons that are poorly known; (5) the induction of neoplasms may be enhanced or inhibited after irradiation by hormonal, immunologic, or other factors modifying the expression of radiation-induced carcinogenic changes; (6) the neoplasms induced by irradiation are indistinguishable from

Table 3–5. Parameters and Values Assumed in Estimating Cancer Risks

Age at irradiation	Type of cancer	Duration of latent period (years)	Duration of plateau region[a] (years)	Risk estimate	
				Absolute risk[b] (deaths/10^6/ year/rem)	Absolute risk (% increment in deaths/rem)
In utero	Leukemia	0	10	25	50
	All other cancers	0	10	25	50
0–9 Years	Leukemia	2	25–30	2.0	5.0
	All other cancers	15	Life	1.0	2.0
10+ Years	Leukemia	2	25–30	1.0	2.0
	All other cancers	15	Life	5.0	0.2

Source: From NAS (1972).

[a] Plateau region, interval following latent period during which risk remains elevated.

[b] The absolute risk for those aged 10 or more at the time of irradiation for all cancer excluding leukemia can be broken down into the respective sites as follows:

Type of cancer	Deaths/10^6/year/rem
Breast	1.5 *
Lung	1.3
GI including stomach	1.0
Bone	0.2
All other cancers	1.0
Total	5.0

* Derived from the value of 6.0 for women, corrected for a 50% cure rate and the inclusion of men as well as women in the population.

those arising through other causes (UN, 1977; NAS, 1980).

The evidence at hand allows one to estimate the carcinogenic risks of low-level irradiation only by extrapolating from observations at higher doses and dose rates, through the use of an appropriate dose–incidence model. The model most widely used to date is the linear nonthreshold model, which is generally considered to provide conservatively high estimates of risks at low doses, in the case of low-LET radiation, in that it makes no allowance for biologic repair at low doses and low dose rates. Some of the assumptions used in applying this model, and estimates of the lifetime risks of radiation-induced cancer in various tissues derived with the model, are shown in Tables 3-5 and 3-6. According to such estimates, it has been calculated that no more than 1–3% of all cancers in the general population are attributable to natural background radiation (Table 3-7).

Table 3–6. Estimated Cumulative Lifetime Cancer Risks of Low-Level Radiation

Site of cancer	Risk per million person-rem	
	Fatal cancers	Incident cancers
Breast (women only)	50	50–200
Thyroid	10	20–150
Lung	25–50	25–100
Bone marrow (leukemia)	15–40	20–60
Brain		
Stomach		
Liver	10–15	15–25
Colon	(each)	
Salivary glands		
Bone		
Esophagus		
Small intestine	2–5	5–10
Urinary bladder	(each)	
Pancreas		
Lymphatic tissue		
Skin	1	15–20
Total (both sexes)	100–250	300–400

Sources: From NAS (1972, 1980); UN (1977); Jablon and Bailer (1980); Upton (1981).

Table 3–7. Estimates of the Contribution of Radiation Exposure to Overall Cancer Mortality in the United States

Source of radiation	Annual dose (person-rem)	Cumulative lifetime cancer mortality commitment (number of fatal cancers)
Natural background	20,000,000	5,000
Healing arts	17,000,000	4,250
	(14,800,000)[a]	(3,670)[a]
Nuclear weapons fallout	1,300,000	375
Technologically enhanced natural radiation (mining + milling, etc.)	1,000,000	250
Nuclear energy	30,000	9
Consumer products	6,000	1.5
Total	39,345,000	<10,000[b]

Source: From Jablon and Bailar (1980).
[a]Proportion of healing arts made up of diagnostic X-rays.
[b]Value = 2.5% of total natural cancer mortality per year (i.e., 400,000).

Heritable Effects

Radiation-induced genetic changes in germ cells are transmissible to offspring in the form of (1) gene mutations, (2) chromosome aberrations, and (3) changes in chromosome number (aneuploidy). These effects can express themselves in an increase in the frequency of traits and diseases of types attributable to naturally occurring mutations and chromosome changes (UN, 1977; NAS, 1980).

Among the categories of such genetic diseases are disorders caused by dominant gene mutations, which appear in the first generation (e.g., polydactyly, Huntington's chorea, and achondroplasia). Such diseases, of which there are thought to be hundreds, are estimated to affect, collectively, about 1% of the population (McKusick, 1974).

Another category of genetic damage is attributable to autosomal recessive mutations and, hence, may not express itself for many generations. It includes hundreds of other diseases, most of which are rare (e.g., Tay-Sachs disease, phenylketonuria, cystic fibrosis, and sickle cell anemia). Diseases resulting from recessive genes located on the X chromosomes can, of course, express themselves as dominants and affect males exclusively (e.g., hemophilia) (McKusick, 1974).

Alterations in chromosome number are generally lethal to the embryo but may give rise to disturbances in sexual development, systemic disorders such as Down's disease, or other abnormalities. Similarly, chromosome aberrations (deletions, translocations, inversions, and other structural alterations) vary in their consequences, depending on the severity of genetic imbalance they cause (UN, 1977; NAS, 1980).

Additional categories of heritable detriment include traits and diseases influenced in a more complicated way by gene variation. Although difficult to assess, the effects of elevation in the mutation rate might include an increase in the frequency of these diseases, leading to impairment of the overall mental and physical vigor of the population (UN, 1977; NAS, 1980).

Although inherited effects of radiation have been studied extensively in species other than humans, such effects have yet to be documented unequivocally in humans. The largest human investigation thus far, on the children of atomic bomb survivors, has been negative to date (UN, 1977; NAS, 1980). Assessment of genetic risks to humans must thus be based primarily on extrapolation from observations in experimental animals. For this purpose, our best information comes from large-scale studies with the mouse.

From experiments on the induction of

specific locus mutations in mice, which have provided data on recessive mutations at 12 loci affecting external features observable in weanlings, a number of conclusions may be drawn. First, the yield of mutations per rad varies with dose, dose rate, dose fractionation, LET, sex, age, and time after irradiation, in a manner that cannot be fully explained at present (UN, 1977). Second, the yield after a dose of 100–600 rad of low-LET radiation is several times smaller at low dose rates (<0.1 rad/minute) than at high dose rates (>50 rad/minute). Third, no such influence of dose rate—which is tentatively ascribed to repair of premutational injury—is observed with high-LET radiation. Fourth, the frequency of mutations in spermatogonia increases as a linear function of the dose at low dose rates, with a slope corresponding to roughly 0.5×10^{-7} mutations/locus/rem/gamete; from this, in comparison with the spontaneous rate of roughly 8.1×10^{-6} mutations/locus/gamete, the mutation rate-doubling dose may be estimated at about 160 rem. Fifth, comparison of the sexes is complicated by the fact that mutations attributable to irradiation of females have been detectable only in offspring conceived within 7 weeks after exposure, pointing to variations in radiosensitivity among oocyte maturation stages that remain to be explained (UN, 1977; NAS, 1980).

Information on dominant mutations is more limited than that on recessive mutations. The yield of dominant visible mutations induced by acute X irradiation in mouse spermatogonia approximates 5×10^{-7} mutations/locus/rad/gamete (UN, 1977). The corresponding rate for mutation affecting the skeleton is about 1.1×10^{-5}, as compared with a spontaneous rate of 2.9×10^{-4} per gamete (UN, 1972, 1977).

Data are available on the yield of chromosomal abnormalities induced by irradiation in various germ cell stages of the mouse, based on cytologic examinations and on genetic analysis of affected offspring for semisterility. The yield of translocations from acute X irradiation has been estimated to be about 3×10^{-5} per gamete per rem (UN, 1972).

Although translocations constitute a minority of all of the chromosome aberrations observed in newborns, they may be expected to represent the bulk of chromosome abnormalities transmitted to the next generation in irradiated male germ cells, in that reproductive cells carrying other abnormalities are nonviable in the mouse (UN, 1972). This may be less true of female germ cells, however, in view of evidence that offspring lacking an X chromosome are produced at a rate of about $5-15 \times 10^{-6}$ per rem by appropriate irradiation of inseminated female mice (UN, 1972).

Direct empirical observation has failed to demonstrate the accumulation of injury in populations of laboratory animals irradiated serially through successive generations. The negative findings, however, may simply be attributable to the relatively small number of animals examined and the insensitivity of the methods for detecting small genetic differences in the presence of substantial nongenetic variability (UN, 1972, 1977; NAS, 1980).

From the evidence that is now available, it has been estimated that the dose required to double the mutation rate in humans lies between 20 and 250 rem (UN, 1977; NAS, 1980). On the basis of this estimate, the effects of radiation on the incidence of various types of genetically related diseases have been assessed. Although it is difficult to relate the amount of genetic disease in a population to the mutation rate, the results of the assessment (Table 3-8) imply that only a small percentage of naturally occurring, genetically determined diseases is attributable to natural background radiation.

Effects on Growth and Development of the Embryo (Teratogenesis)

The high radiosensitivity of embryonal, fetal, and juvenile animals is well recognized. Acute exposure of the embryo to doses as low as 25 rem during critical stages in organogenesis have been observed to cause disturbances in growth and development (UN, 1977). Similarly, atomic bomb survivors who were irradiated under 16 weeks of gestational age in Hiroshima have shown

Table 3–8. Estimates of Genetic Detriment per Million Offspring Attributable to a Gonadal Dose of 3 rem to the Parental Generation

Type of genetic detriment	Natural incidence	Effects of 3 rem per generation[a]	
		First generation	Equilibrium generations
Dominant traits + diseases	10,000	3–30	150–3,000
Chromosomal + recessive traits + diseases	10,000	<30	<120
Recognized abortions			
Aneuploidy + polyploidy	35,000	33	33
XO	9,000	9	9
Unbalanced rearrangements	11,000	216	276
Congenital anomalies	15,000		
Anomalies expressed after birth	10,000	3–300	30–3,000
Constitutional + degenerative diseases	15,000		
Total (rounded)	115,000	300–900	500–6,000

Sources: Modified from reports of the National Academy of Sciences (1972, 1980) and the United Nations (1977), based on an assumed doubling dose of 20 to 250 rem.

[a] Equivalent to 0.1 rem/year, or average dose from natural background.

an increased incidence of microcephaly at doses as low as 25 rad (UN, 1977).

During the preimplantation stage, the embryo is more susceptible to killing than at any other time during life, but is not susceptible to induction of malformations by irradiation. Susceptibility to a given malformation is characteristically confined to a sharply circumscribed "critical" period during organogenesis, which may not coincide with the critical period for any other malformation. The complexity of these effects, in which cell killing may play an important role, complicates estimation of dose–response relationships in the low-dose range, because at low dose rates the amount of radiation accumulated during the stage of maximal sensitivity for any one effect is relatively small. It is not astonishing, therefore, that teratogenic effects have not been detected in laboratory animals at dose rates below 1 rem/day (NAS, 1972; UN, 1980).

Although numerical risk estimates for teratogenic effects in humans have yet to be derived, the evidence at hand implies that the risks of teratogenic effects of low-level radiation are appreciably smaller per unit dose than the risks of carcinogenic and mutagenic effects (UN, 1977; NAS, 1980).

Acknowledgment

Support for the preparation of this report was provided by Grant ES00260 from the National Institute of Environmental Health Sciences and Grant CA 13343 from the National Cancer Institute.

The author is grateful to G. Cook, K. Griffin, D. Natalizio, J. Smith, and L. Witte for their assistance in the preparation of this manuscript.

REFERENCES

Anderson, R. E., and Warner, N. L. 1976. Ionizing radiation and the immune response. *Adv. Immunol.* 24:216–335.

Andrews, G. A. 1957. A few notions involved in the clinical use of radioisotopes. *Ann. Intern. Med.* 47:922–938.

Andrews, G. A., Sitterson, B. W., Kretchmar, A. L., and Brucer, M. 1961. Criticality accidents at the Y-12 plant. In *Diagnosis and treatment of acute radiation injury,* pp. 27–48. Geneva: World Health Organization.

Beebe, G. W., Kato, H., and Land, C. E. 1978. Studies of mortality of the A-bomb survivors. 6. Mortality and radiation dose, 1950–1974. *Radiat. Res.* 75:138–201.

Berdjis, C. C. 1971. *The pathology of irradiation.* Baltimore: Williams and Wilkins.

Boice, J. D., Jr., Land, C. E., Shore, R. E., Norman, J. E., and Tokunaga, M. 1979. Risk of breast cancer following low-dose exposure. *Radiology* 131:589–597.

Bond, V. P., Fliedner, T. M., and Archambeau, J. O. 1965. *Mammalian radiation lethality*. New York: Academic Press.

Borek, C. 1979. Neoplastic transformation following split doses of X-rays. *Br. J. Radiol.* 50:845–846.

Borek, C. 1980. X-ray induced *in vitro* neoplastic transformation of human diploid cells. *Nature* 283:776–778.

Borek, C., Hall, E. J., and Rossi, H. H. 1978. Malignant transformation in cultured hamster embryo cells produced by X-rays, 430-kev monoenergetic neutrons, and heavy ions. *Cancer Res.* 38:2997–3005.

Brown, J. M. 1977. The shape of the dose–response curve for radiation carcinogenesis: Extrapolation to low doses. *Radiat. Res.* 71:34–50.

Brown, P. 1936. *American martyrs to science through the roentgen rays*. Springfield, Ill.: Charles C Thomas.

Casarett, G. 1981. *Radiation histopathology*. West Palm Beach, Fla.: CRC Press.

Cerutti, P. A. 1974. Effects of ionizing radiation on mammalian cells. *Naturwissenschaften* 61:51–59.

Cole, A., Meyn, R. E., Chen, R., Corry, P. M., and Hittelman, W. 1980. Mechanisms of cell injury. In *Radiation biology in cancer research*, eds. R. E. Meyn and H. R. Withers, pp. 33–58. New York: Raven Press.

Denekamp, J., Fowler, J. F., and Dische, S. 1977. The proportion of hypoxic cells in a human tumor. *Int. J. Radiat. Oncol. Biol. Phys.* 2:1227–1228.

Elkind, M. M. 1980. Cells, targets and molecules in radiation biology. The Ernst W. Bertner Memorial Award Lecture. In *Radiation biology in cancer research*, eds. R. E. Meyn and H. R. Withers, pp. 71–93. New York: Raven Press.

Frieben, A. 1902. Demonstration eines Cancroids des rechten Handruckens, das sich nach langdauernder Einwirkung fon Röntgenstrahlen entwickelt hatte. *Fortschr. Geb. Röntgenstr.* 6:106.

Friedenwald, J. S., and Sigelman, S. 1953. The influence of ionizing radiation on mitotic activity in the rat's corneal epithelium. *Exp. Cell Res.* 4:1–31.

Furth, J., and Lorenz, E. 1954. Carcinogenesis by ionizing radiations. In *Radiation biol-ogy*, vol. 1, ed. A. Hollaender, pp. 1145–1201. New York: McGraw-Hill.

Gaulden, M. E. 1973. Genetic effects of radiation. In *Medical radiation biology*, eds. G. V. Dalrymple, M. E. Gaulden, G. M. Kollmorgen, and H. H. Vogel, Jr., 1933. pp. 52–83. Philadelphia: W. B. Saunders.

Glasser, O. 1933. *The science of radiology*. Springfield, Ill.: Charles C Thomas.

Hall, E. J. 1978. *Radiobiology for the radiologist*, 2nd Ed. New York: Harper and Row.

International Commission on Radiation Units. 1980. *Radiation quantities and units*. ICRU Report No. 33, April. Washington, D.C.: ICRU.

International Commission on Radiological Protection. 1977. *Recommendations of the International Commission on Radiological Protection*. ICRP Publication 26, Annals of the ICRP, vol. 1, no. 3. Oxford: Pergamon Press.

Jablon, S., and Bailar, J. 1980. The contribution of ionizing radiation to cancer mortality in the United States. *Prev. Med.* 9:219–226.

Kennedy, A. R., and Little, J. B. 1980. Radiation transformation *in vitro*: Modification by exposure to tumor promoters and protease inhibitors. In *Radiation biology in cancer research*, eds. R. E. Mayn and H. R. Withers, pp. 295–307. New York: Raven Press.

Kerr, J. F. R., and Searle, J. 1980. Apoptosis: Its nature and kinetic role. In *Radiation biology in cancer research*, eds. R. E. Mayn and H. R. Withers, pp. 367–384. New York: Raven Press.

Knospe, W. H., Blom, J., and Crosby, W. H. 1966. Regeneration of locally irradiated bone marrow. I. Dose-dependent, long-term changes in the rat, with particular emphasis upon vascular and stromal reaction. *Blood* 28:398–415.

Kohn, H. I. 1980. X-ray induced mutation rates: A target-theory estimate of their reduction *in vivo* owing to selection and repair. In *Radiation biology in cancer research*, eds. R. E. Mayn and H. R. Withers, pp. 327–330. New York: Raven Press.

Lacassagne, A., Duplan, B. M., and Marcovitch, J. F. 1962. The action of ionizing radiations on the mammalian ovary. In *The ovary*, eds. S. Luckerman, A. M. Mandel, and P. Eckstein, pp. 498–501. New York: Academic Press.

Lajtha, L. G. 1965. Response of bone marrow stem cells to ionizing radiations. In *Current topics in radiation research*, eds. M. Ebert and A. Howard, pp. 139–162. Amsterdam: Elsevier-North Holland.

Langham, W. H., ed. 1967. *Radiobiological factors in manned space flight.* Washington, D.C.: National Academy of Sciences.

Langham, W. H., Brooks, P. M., Grahn, D., Adams, D. A., Holly, F. E., Curtis, H. J., Lambersten, C. J., Campbell, D. P., Galbraith, T. C., Gibbons, L. V., Kloster, R. L., Rudman, S. W., Spear, V. D., and Warneke, C. H. 1965. Radiation biology and space environmental parameters in manned spacecraft design and operations. *Aerospace Med.* 36:1–55.

Little, J. B. 1970. Biological consequences of X-ray induced DNA damage and repair processes in relation to cell killing and carcinogenesis. In *DNA repair mechanisms*, eds. P. C. Hanawalt, E. C. Friedberg, and C. F. Fox, pp. 701–711. New York: Academic Press.

Lloyd, D. C., Purrott, R. J., and Reeder, E. J. 1980. The incidence of unstable chromosome aberrations in peripheral blood lymphocytes from unirradiated and occupationally exposed people. *Mutat. Res.* 72:523–532.

Lushbaugh, C. C., and Ricks, R. C. 1972. Some cytokinetic and histopathologic considerations of irradiated male and female gonadal tissues. *Front. Radiat. Ther. Oncol.* 6:228–248.

Maisin, J., Dunjic A., and Maisin, J. R. 1971. Radiation pathology of lymphatic system and thymus. In *The pathology of irradiation*, ed. C. C. Berdjis, pp. 496–541. Baltimore: Williams and Wilkins.

Marshall, J. M., and Groer, P. G. 1977. A theory of the induction of bone cancer by alpha radiation. *Radiat. Res.* 71:149–192.

McKusick, V. A. 1974. *Mendelian inheritance in man. Catalogs of autosomal dominant, autosomal recessive, and X-linked phenotypes*, 4th Ed. Baltimore: The Johns Hopkins Press.

Merriam, G. R., Schechter, A., and Focht, E. F. 1972. The effects of ionizing radiation on the eye. *Front. Radiat. Ther. Oncol.* 6:346–385.

Micklem, H. S., and Loutit, J. F. 1966. *Tissue grafting and radiation.* New York: Academic Press.

National Academy of Sciences (NAS), National Research Council (NRC). 1960. *The biological effects of atomic radiation. Summary reports.* Washington, D.C.: National Academy of Sciences.

National Academy of Sciences (NAS), Advisory Committee on the Biological Effects of Ionizing Radiation (BEIR). 1972, 1980. *The effects on populations of exposure to low levels of ionizing radiation.* Washington, D.C.: National Academy of Sciences, National Research Council.

Painter, R. B. 1980. The role of DNA damage and repair in cell killing induced by ionizing radiation. In *Radiation biology in cancer research*, eds. R. E. Meyn and H. R. Withers pp. 59–68. New York: Raven Press.

Porteus, D. D., and Lajtha, L. J. 1966. On stem-cell recovery after irradiation. *Br. J. Haematol.* 12:177–188.

Proukakis, C., and Lindop, P. J. 1971. Hematological changes following irradiation. In *Pathology of irradiation*, ed. C. C. Berdjis, pp. 447–495. Baltimore: Williams and Wilkins.

Puck, T. T. 1979. Histological perspective on mutation studies with somatic mammalian cells. In *Mammalian cell mutagenesis: The maturation of test systems*, eds. A. W. Hsie, J. P. O'Neill, and V. K. McElheny, pp. 3–14. Cold Spring Harbor, N.Y.: Cold Spring Harbor Laboratory.

Robinson, C. V., and Upton, A. C. 1978. Competing-risk analysis of leukemia and non-leukemia mortality in X-irradiated male RF mice. *J. Natl. Cancer Inst.* 60:995–1007.

Rubin, P., and Casarett, G. W. 1968. *Clinical radiation pathology*, vols. 1 and 2. Philadelphia: W. B. Saunders.

Rubin, P., and Casarett, G. W. 1972. A direction for clinical radiation pathology: The tolerance dose. *Front. Rad. Ther. Oncol.* 6:1–16.

Sandemann, T. F. 1966. The effects of X-irradiation on male human fertility. *Br. J. Radiol.* 39:901–907.

Sparrow, A. H., Underbrink, A. G., and Rossi, H. H. 1972. Mutations induced in *Tradescantia* by small doses of x-rays and neutrons: Analyis of dose-response curves. *Science* 176:916–918.

Tobias, C. A., Blakely, E. A., Ngo, F. Q. H., and Yang, T. C. H. 1980. The repair-misrepair model of cell survival. In *Radiation biology in cancer research*, eds. R. E. Meyn and H. R. Withers, pp. 195–230. New York: Raven Press.

Report of the United Nations Scientific Committee on the Effects of Atomic Radiation. 1962. *Report to the General Assembly*. Official Records, 17th Sess., Suppl. No. 16 (A/5216). New York: United Nations.

United Nations Scientific Committee on the Effects of Atomic Radiation. 1972. *Ionizing radiation: Levels and effects*. Report ot the Gerneral Assembly. Official Records, 27th Sess., Suppl. No. 25 (A/8725). New York: United Nations.

United Nations Scientific Committee on the Effects of Atomic Radiation. 1977. *Sources and effects of ionizing radiation*. Report to the General Assembly, with annexes. New York: United Nations.

Upton, A. C. 1969. *Radiation injury. Effects, principles and perspectives*. Chicago: University of Chicago Press.

Upton, A. C. 1974. Somatic and genetic effects of low-level radiation. In *Recent advances in nuclear medicine*, vol. 4, ed. J. H. Lawrence, pp. 1–40. New York: Grune and Stratton.

Upton, A. C. 1975. Physical carcinogenesis: Radiation-history and sources. In *Cancer, a comprehensive treates*, vol. 1, ed. F. F. Becker, pp. 387–403. New York: Plenum Press.

Upton, A. C. 1977. Radiobiological effects of low doses: Implications for radiological protection. *Radiat. res.* 71:51–74.

Upton, A. C. 1981. Radiation hazards. In *International symposium on cancer research*.

Upton, A. C., Christenberry, K. W., Melville, G. S., Furth, J., and Hurst, G. S. 1956. The relative biological effectiveness of neutrons, x-rays and gamma rays for the production of lens opacities. Observations on mice, rats, guinea pigs and rabbits. *Radiology* 67:686–696.

Upton, A. C., and Lushbaugh, C. C. 1969. The pathological anatomy of total-body irradiation. In *Atomic medicine*, 5th Ed. eds. C. F. Behrens, E. R. King, and J. W. J. Carpender, pp. 154–188. Baltimore: Williams and Wilkins.

U.S., Dept. of Health, Education and Welfare. 1977. *Human health and the environment—some research needs*. Report of the Second Task Force for Research Planning in Environmental Health Science. Washington, D.C.: Dept. of Health, Education and Welfare, DHEW Publication No. (NIH) 77-1277.

U.S., Dept. of Health, Education and Welfare, Interagency Task Force on the Health Effects of Ionizing Radiation. 1979. *Report of the Work Group on Science*. Washington, D.C.: Dept. of Health, Education and Welfare.

Warren, S. 1942. Effects of radiation on normal tissues. *Arch. Pathol.* 34:443–450, 917–1084; (with C. E. Dunlap) 562–608; (with N. B. Friedman) 749–788.

Warren, S. 1943. Effects of radiation on normal tissues. *Arch. Pathol.* 35:121–139, 304–323, 340–353; (with O. Gates) 323–340.

Yamagiwa, K., and Ichikawa, K. 1918. Experimental Study of the pathogenesis of carcinoma. *J. Cancer Res.* 3:1–29.

4

Morphogenic Injury by Chemical Agents

N. Karle Mottet

Teratology

The period in a person's lifespan of greatest susceptibility to exogenous injury is during the early stages of morphogenesis. This occurs despite the protective adventages of the developing mammal, residing in the uterus of the maternal organism during this sensitive period rather than being directly exposed to the external environment. The fertilized eggs and embryos of oviparous animals, being directly exposed to changes in temperature, pressure (trauma), pH, and chemicals in the surrounding medium, have an extremely high mortality rate. Not only does the uterine environment of viviparous animals provide protection from the drastic changes of temperature and pressure and pH, but also the maternal organism and placenta can block, metabolize, or sequester toxic chemicals, thus limiting their access to the developing organisms. An environmental chemical must be able to traverse cell membranes at the pulmonary, gastrointestinal, or epidermal portals of entry of the maternal organism, and be able to traverse epithelial cell layers before gaining entry into blood vascular or lymphatic circulation. Once within the circulatory system, it must be present in sufficient quantity to overcome the dilution effect of body fluid and come the dilution effect of body fluid and

exceed the capacity of the body to sequester, biotransform, or eliminate the agent or its metabolic products. Further, it must be able to traverse the placental barrier. Despite the protective mechanisms, many exogenous agents, both physical and chemical, cause frequent fetal loss or damage in mammals by altering the genetic or epigenetic controls of morphogenesis.

In its broadest sense, environmental teratology is a study of the adverse effects of environmental etiologic agents on the developing system. It refers to all influences external to the developing individual, that is, amniotic fluid, placenta, uterus, maternal metabolism, and the external physical and chemical surrounding environment. Thus, the broadest view would hold that all abnormal development is due to some external influence acting either on the morphogenic controls exercised through the genome, or through indirect (maternal) or direct (fetoplacental) action on the cells of the new developing individual. Temporally viewed, the environmental etiologic agent can affect the gonads of the paternal or maternal organism, resuting in genetic injury to the germ cells prior to fertilization; second, the injurious interaction can occur during the interval between fertilization and the implantation of the zygote in the uterine wall. Third, following implantation the injurious agent, by transport through the maternal bloodstream, can enter the developing embryo or fetus by passage through the placenta, resulting in injury at any time during fetal development.

Common usage limits environmental teratology to nonbiotic etiologic agents. To attempt to describe all the physical and chemical environmental agents that may exert their effects on the developing individual is beyond the scope of this chapter. A catalog of teratogens (Shepard, 1980) alphabetically lists known teratogens and provides selected references thereto. To illustrate mechanisms of injury, this chapter will be limited to consideration of some of the most important exogenous environmental chemicals and radiation.

The mechanisms by which these environmental agents produce abnormal development are the same cellular and molecular mechanisms associated with diseases in the adult: necrosis, cell differentiation, migration, inflammation, proliferation. Therefore, the study of teratogenic mechanisms is an integral part of pathology. Its unique features are related to the fact that the pathologic processes are superimposed on cells during a period of unusually rapid proliferation and differentiation, rather than on the more stationary tissues in the adult organism. Also, protective and reparative processes are not fully developed. There are no strict borders between anomalous development and diseases. Common usage has limited the term "malformations" to deal with anatomic abnormalities, whereas the word "anomaly" refers to any gross anatomic, histopathologic, or molecular changes occurring in organs, tissues, cells, or subcellular molecules.

Assessment of the risk of environmentally induced congenital anomalies can be viewed by two approaches: the opportunity for exposure or the incidence of congenital anomalies. The risk of exposure to radiation has been discussed in Chapter 3. The general risk of exposure to chemical etiologic agents in an industrial society is great, but a definitive estimate is elusive. One

Table 4–1. Number of Chemicals in Different Categories in Use, November 1977

Total chemicals listed in ACS registry	4,039,907
New chemicals per week	6,000
Chemicals in common use	50,000
Pesticides	1,500
Food additives	5,500
Drugs	6,000
Total in common use	63,000

measure is provided by the American Chemical Society (ACS) Abstracts Service, which has a unique computer registry of reports on all chemicals synthesized or isolated. The number of chemicals reported in several categories as of 1977 is given in Table 4-1 (Maugh, 1978).

Not only is the number of different chemicals dramatically increasing, but the quantity of production of some of them is also increasing. *Chemical Engineering News* recorded six chemicals (sulfuric acid, ethylene, sodium hydroxide, chlorine, phosphoric acid, and nitric acid) are produced at a rate of 8500 to 40 million tons/year. Fifteen other organic agents, many of them known toxins, are produced at the annual rate of 650 million to 13 billion pounds (Anonymous, 1981).

Incidence of Anomalies

It is commonly estimated that approximately 3% of all livebirths in the United States have significant birth defects discovered during the neonatal period (Kalter and Warkany, 1983). This represents 100,000 congenital anomalies in a total of 3 million livebirths annually. These figures are approximations because of several sources of error:

1. *Definition.* The boundary between normal variation in a human population and birth defects is indefinable objectively. If one were to include in the above data abnormalities that have no significant threat to the survival of the individual, then the figure would be much higher.

2. *Detection rate.* Most congenital defect statistics are based on observations made soon after birth, usually in a hospital nursery. Such surveys overlook the congenital defects that are undetectable during the early days of extrauterine life, but that in later years become apparent. Included among the latter are mental retardation, abnormal sexual differentiation, and polycystic kidneys. If one were to include anomalies that appear later in life, the percentage of congenital defects would be much higher, probably twice the figure given above. Another variable in the detection rate is how carefully one looks for the malformation at the time of birth. Comparative studies in which the incidence of malformations at the time of birth in two western European countries and the United States and Canada, based on birth certificate records, reveals a rate of less than 1%. However, if one searches hospital and clinic records, this increases to almost 2%. If intensive and careful examination were carried out at the time of birth, the study reveals an incidence of approximately 4.5%.

About 7.5% of livebirth congenital anomalies have a monogenic mechanism, and another 6% of the liveborn anomalies have chromosomal abnormalities. Excluding maternal causes (diabetes, thyrotoxicosis, infections, etc.), a very rough estimate would indicate that approximately half of the liveborn congenital anomalies are due to exogenous (environmental) causes.

The above data are based on livebirths. If one were to include lost cases—that is, those fetuses with congenital defects that die before birth—the figures would be markedly higher. The incidence of preimplantation deaths has been difficult to establish but is suspected to be frequent. Some estimates indicate that 30% of fertilized ova are lost by early (usually undetected) miscarriage. Clinically apparent abortions during early pregnancy and stillbirths resulting from congenital defects have been estimated to increase the number of congenital anomalies to about 2.5 times the percentage given, to approximately 560,000 per year. Furthermore, the effects of exogenous agents on growth retardation (fetal and newborn size) are not included in these data. One of the most definitive studies on lost cases was done by Semba (1976), who painstakingly dissected the hearts of more than 1200 human embryos from induced abortions and found double the rate (2.1%) of congenital heart lesions in Japan as compared with the newborn congenital heart incidence (0.5–1.2%). He observed that the most severe types of heart anomalies were scarce in liveborn infants but were very common in the early embryos, suggesting that those with the severe anomalies are not able to survive to birth.

Maceration of stillborns due to autolysis severely limits the opportunity to determine precisely the incidence of congenital anomalies in stillbirths. However, eight independent studies revealed an incidence of defects in stillbirths to be between 13 and 25%.

Numerous studies have established the relative population frequency of common types of human developmental anomalies (Tables 4-2 and 4-3).

Exposure and Site of Injury

To characterize fully a teratogenic etiologic agent, one must consider the period of development at which the exposure occurs, the dose, and the site of action of the agent. Has the chemical acted on the genome of previous generations, on the sperm, ovum, or zygote, on the process of implantation, or directly on the developing embryo? The etiologic agents can be broadly classified into two groups: those that alter the genetic control mechanisms and those that act on the developing phenotype of the new individual. Many agents affect both control mechanisms of morphogenesis.

Critical Periods

Both in human and in experimental animals, it is apparent that the susceptibility of an individual to a teratogenic agent varies with the developmental stage at which the exposure occurs. The thalidomide problem, described in a later section, is an example

Table 4–2. Frequency of Some Common Anomalies

System	Anomaly	Population frequency (%)
Central nervous	Anencephaly	0.2
	Spina bifida	0.3
	Mental retardation	0.4+
Cardiovascular	Congenital heart defect	1.2
Gastrointestinal	Hypertrophic pyloric stenosis	0.3
	Congenital megacolon	0.02
	Inguinal hernia	1.0
Musculoskeletal	Kyphoscoliosis	0.2
	Clubfoot, syndactyly	0.12
	Congenital hip dislocation	0.1
Oral	Cleft lip and/or palate	0.15

of the importance of critical periods of exposure. Anotia occurred when the developing fetus was exposed to thalidomide between 34 and 38 days of gestation, whereas arm anomalies tended to predominate between 40 and 44 days; leg anomalies predominated toward the latter part of this period through 50 days of gestation. Throughout the period of organiogenesis the many internal organs were subject to malformation. Exposure to thalidomide after 50 days of gestation did not produce any anomalies.

Table 4–3. Human Gross Malformations by Site

Malformation	Percentage of total
Central nervous system (anencephaly, meningomyelocele)	17
Face (cleft lip and/or palate)	9
Cardiovascular system (septal defects, transposition, tetralogy of Fallot)	4
Gastrointestinal system (hypertrophic pyloric stenosis, imperforate anus, bile duct atresia, tracheoesophageal fistula)	8
Limbs (clubfoot, syndactyly, polydactyly)	26
Genitourinary system (hypospadias, renal agenesis)	14
"Polymorphous" and miscellaneous	22
Total	100

Although relatively little is known about preimplantation stages of development, there is accumulating evidence that a variety of teratogenic agents can concentrate in the ovarian follicular fluid or testis and semen, causing death of germ cells. Similarly, the preimplantation zygote can be exposed. It is difficult to establish the incidence of these types of early injury because of the minimal physiologic change in this early stage of pregnancy. In later preimplantation stages during the blastula stage, Fabro and Seiber found that many chemicals and drugs accumulate in the blastocyst fluid in rabbits (Fabro and Seiber, 1968). The period of organogenesis following implantation is a period generally very sensitive to many teratogens. In laboratory rodents this usually extends from 5 to 14 days of gestation. In the human it is the first trimester. Some agents such as X radiation have different embryopathic effects depending on the stage of development when exposure occurs.

The *site of injury* by chemical teratogens (maternal, placental, or fetal) is often unknown. Important features of the metabolism of teratogenic agents are related to such maternal processes as rate of absorption, distribution within the body, biotransformation, and excretion.

PLACENTA

The significance of the placenta as a site of injury has extensive experimental evidence to substantiate it (Juchau, 1981; Waddell and Marlow, 1981). Many teratogenic agents appear to be producing their effect on the fetus indirectly by altering maternal metabolism or the maternal–fetal exchange of metabolic substances. Development of our knowledge in this important area of teratology has been delayed, because the placentas of most readily available experimental animals are not structurally or functionally comparable to the human placenta. Of the species that have chorioallantoic placentas, the structural features are markedly different from the human. For example, in laboratory rats and mice, a yolk sac placenta is a structure that persists throughout most of the early stages of gestation, and is at least as important during organogenesis as the subsequent chorioallantoic placenta. A large inverted yolk sac surrounds the fetus and provides direct contact with the uterine tissue. The cells lining the yolk sac are continuous with those that form the fetal gut. The yolk sac may be viewed as an outpouching from the mid gut. The epithelial surface of the yolk sac closely resembles the epithelium of the intestine and kidney, and thus apparently is well adapted for both absorption and excretory function. Study of the chorioallantoic placenta at term can yield erroneous teratogenic information, because the yolk sac placenta is the important one during the early phases of gestation when the fetus is most susceptible to injury by many agents. Whereas the transport of materials from the mother to the fetus in the human and subhuman primates involves its movement across the vascular endothelium, connective tissue, and trophoblastic epithelium of the fetal cell layers, the laboratory rodents generally have only the endothelium and connective tissue layers in their placental villi. The guinea pig has only the endothelial layer. These laboratory species have hemoendothelial placentas, whereas the humans and monkeys have hemochorial placentas. Although these anatomic boundaries differ, this does not fully represent the functional differences between these different types of placentas.

Furthermore, one must keep in mind that not only the structural but also the functional capacities of these placentas vary with the period of gestation. During early gestation the yolk sac placenta is usually the predominant organ for transfer of material between mother and fetus in the rodents and rabbits.

The importance of the placental histologic features can be readily seen as one examines the significant features of fetal and placental development in laboratory animals compared with the human (Mossman, 1937; Stevens, 1975). In the rat, implantation occurs at 5.5 days following fertilization, which is 3 days before the beginning of gastrulation. Throughout this period the nutrition of the developing embryo is largely histiotrophic. By the stage of gastrulation the yolk sac placenta develops, and at this stage the embryonic nutrition is largely associated with the ability of the extraembryonic endoderm of the yolk sac to degrade macromolecules. The histiotrophic nutrition appears to come from maternal blood serum, secretion of uterine glands, and the destruction of endometrial cells by the trophoblastic layer of the developing blastocyst. At about the 20-somite stage, the chorioallantoic placenta begins to develop as a result of the fusion of the allantois with the chorion. A third phase of nutrition in the rat begins at 11 days of gestation. However, the yolk sac endoderm and yolk sac placenta continue to be active until full term. For example, the yolk sac placenta is able to take up radioactive iodine-labeled bovine serum albumin and digest it, and is able to ingest and degrade horseradish peroxidase at 17 to 18 days gestation.

The human and primate placental systems differ markedly from that of the rat. Implantation begins at about 7.5 days, and a small hillock of trophoblasts is formed at the point of penetration. Histiotrophic nutrition begins by digestion of endometrial tissue and endometrial secretions, and within 4 to 5 days thereafter the blastocyst becomes completely buried in the compact layers of the endometrium. Circulation through these evolving placental structures begins at about 13 days of gestation, and within 3 days gastrulation begins. Nutrition of the developing embryo is still principally histiotrophic. About a week after the beginning of gastrulation, circulation is established through the chorionic villi and the embryonic nutrition becomes hemotrophic. In contrast to the rodents, the human chorionic vesicle begins to develop rapidly following a brief period of histiotrophic nutrition, and soon the precocious development of the circulatory system results in hemotrophic nutrition through a hemochorial placenta at the five-somite stage.

Old World monkeys follow a similar course of placental differentiation. As with the human, the cardiovascular system develops rapidly within 2 days of gastrulation, and the hemotrophic nutrition is established early at about the five-somite stage of development. Thus, the subhuman primates most nearly approximate the human in placental development and functions, and represent the best available model for the study of placental function and the effects of noxious agents.

The placenta, being an organ derived from fetal cells, has the same genome as the fetus. The various cell layers of the placenta are derived from the developing embryo. The trophoblastic layer of cells is derived from the inner cell mass, and evidence strongly supports the idea that the connective tissue cells of the villous blood vessels, yolk sac, and so on, are all derived from cells emanating from the embryo. The decidual layer that surrounds the placenta is derived from the endometrial stroma of the mother.

Primary disease conditions of the placenta are rare and seldom are associated with fetal abnormalities. Gross anatomic lesions of the placenta usually reflect pathologic processes of the mother, which in turn may affect the development of the fetus. There is no evidence relating environmental chemical and physical agents to such commonly recognized gross placental abnormalities as amniotic bands, circumvallation, marginal insertion of the cord, or

abnormalities in the positioning of the placenta. A review of the gross pathology of the placenta has been written by Benirschke (1977).

The transfer of teratogens across the placenta and the functional role of placenta in transforming teratogens remain poorly understood. Reviews of our current state of knowledge on the subject have been written by Waddell and Marlowe (1981) and by Juchau (1981). In most instances the specific chemical that is transferred across the placenta to produce the teratogenic effect is not known. Chemicals that are transported through the placenta by various species of animals have been catalogued by Schultz (1970).

For many years the placenta was considered an organ for the passive transfer of all molecules of low molecular weight (less than 1000), and that it excluded virtually all larger molecules. Evidence now indicates that there is no specific separation of this type, but rather that there is a gradation of molecular sizes that traverse the placenta to the fetus. One must consider the same features that are associated with selective accumulation of compounds in other organs and tissues. Features such as lipid solubility, ionic exchange, molecular size, structural configuration, all appear to contribute to the transfer of molecules between the mother and the fetus. Placental transfer of water and small molecules occurs by diffusion and is regulated by placental blood flow and lipid solubility. Hydrostatic pressure contributes to the transfer of water and solutes from the mother to the fetus in most types of palcentas.

Active transfer of chemicals into the fetus as an energy-dependent mechanism has been established for some nutritional and pharmaceutical agents. Several amino acids are actively transported through the placenta; thus, one could hypothesize that a teratogen could produce defective embryonic development by interfering with the active transport of essential nutrients to the placenta, diminishing their availability to the metabolism of the fetus. Olson and Massaro (1975) have suggested this as the mechanism of action of methylmercury on the amino acid uptake of the developing fetus. Carrier-mediated transfer of some essential nutrients has been established, and the demonstration of carriers has been achieved in human placentas. This transport does not appear to require energy.

Passive transfer, as alluded to above, is the mechanism for the transport of most substances across the placenta. Lipid-soluble molecules cross more readily than do hydrophilic molecules. Crossing of the latter is dependent on the size and structure of the molecule, as well as the specific stage of gestation of the animal.

Waddell and Marlowe (1981) extensively reported the transfer of elements between the mother and fetus, using radioaudiographic methods that enabled the identification of the distribution in each of the tissues of the mother, fetus, and placenta. For example, elemental mercury administered by injection or inhalation caused a much higher accumulation of mercury in the fetal tissues than had previously been suspected. Methyl mercury chloride administered to pregnant rats in mid- and late gestation demonstrated accumulaion in the fetal brain of much more mercury than appeared in the brain of the pregnant animal. These observations suggest a greater opportunity for mercury damage of the fetal nervous system than the maternal, particularly when the mercury is methylated. The distribution of mercury among the maternal and fetal tissues is dependent on the chemical state of the mercury.

EMBRYONIC MORPHOGENESIS AS A SITE OF INJURY

Normal development depends on two mechanisms of control: the genetic instructions for morphogenesis, and the unaltered metabolism of cells established to carry out the genetic instructions (epigenetic or morphogenic mechanisms). The effects of environmental agents on the genetic controls are dealt with in Chapter 1. Environmental teratogenic chemical and physical agents may

Table 4–4. Cellular Mechanisms of Teratogenesis

Morphogenic cellular alteration	Cellular Mechanism
1. Cell proliferation	Mitotic rate Dividing fraction
2. Cell location	Migration Aggregation Delamination (Decreased adhesion)
3. Cell loss	Necrosis Exfoliation
4. Cell size	Hypertrophy Hypotrophy
5. Cell differentiation	Neoplasia Metaplasia Biosynthesis alterations
6. Tissue interaction	Induction

injure both the genome and the cell metabolism to produce anomalies. In the processes of genetic replication, transcription, translation, and biosynthesis, any step in the chain of responses may be attacked by the agents. Irrespective of whether the injury is to the genome or the cells' capacity to respond to the genetic instruction, the fundamental result is a biochemical change affecting the structural and ultrastructural integrity of the cell, which is reflected in altered cell activity, which in turn may lead to anomalous morphogenesis. There are at least six major cellular responses that can be altered (see Table 4-4).

Morphogenic Mechanisms

CELL PROLIFERATION

Following fertilization, the initial and main activity of the zygote is proliferation. A fertilized egg is approximately 0.14 mm in diameter. By 2 months of gestation in the human, the volume of the fetus increases about 27,000 times. Proliferation is the dominant main feature of early morphogenesis. Cell differentiation and biosynthetic activity are present in early morphogenesis, but become increasingly important as gestation progresses.

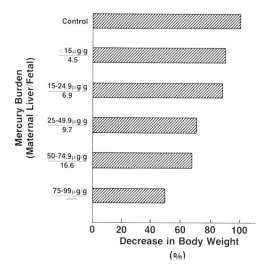

Figure 4–1. The effect of maternal methyl mercury burden on the body weight of offspring. Maternal exposure was continuous at low doses throughout gestation.

An example of how an environmental chemical agent may affect cell proliferation is the effect of methyl mercury on microtubules. It has been shown that methyl mercury decreases the size of the offspring (Figure 4-1) in many species of animals in a dose-related way (Mottet, 1974; Chen et al., 1979). It has been shown in vitro that methyl mercury impedes the assembly of microtubules, a major element of the mitotic spindle, in a comparable way (Schlaepfer, 1971; Schliwa, 1976). Some presumptive evidence indicates that the mercury binds to the sulfhydryl groups in the microtubule protein, tubulin. This alteration in the cell organelle interferes with the assembly of the microtubules into tubulin, a principal component of the mitotic spindle (Sager et al., 1982). This in turn may be associated with a decrease in cellular proliferative rate, and thus may alter the development of individual organs or, as in this case, the total weight of the offspring (Sager et al., 1983).

Although the above illustrates an in vitro mechanism whereby an environmental agent may alter the size of the fetus, it does not preclude other possible mechanisms or alterations of cells by mercury, such as membrane transport and mitochondrial energy turnover. Because of the complexity of the problem, the normal control mechanisms of embryonic cell proliferation are poorly understood (Troup, 1971). During the early phases of embryogenesis, the cells are dividing at a maximal rate, that is, about 8 to 9 hours for each cell cycle. Thus, the pool of cells from which each organ differentiates is increased rapidly. One can reason a priori that the controls of the rate of proliferation involved extracellular as well as intracellular mechanisms. For example, Rutter and co-workers (1973) have isolated a protein from connective tissues capable of stimulating the proliferation of epithelial cells, such as the glandular exocrine portion of the pancreas, by acting on the cell surfaces. Also, thyroxin produced by the mother's thyroid gland may have an overall stimulatory effect on fetal development as it does in oviparous embryos.

Intrauterine growth retardation can be caused by many etiologic agents, including X irradiation, pharmaceuticals, environmental chemicals, maternal endocrine and nutritional factors, and hypoxia. An additional growth-controlling factor is self-inhibition. As a population of cells enlarges, the density of the population may within itself diminish proliferation, due in part to the decreased availability of nutritional substances. Numerous growth factors are currently under investigation. Among these are the epithelial factor, the fibroblast growth factor, and the nerve growth factor, all of which apparently affect the surface membrane receptors as a signal to alter rates of self-proliferation.

The proliferative rate in embryonic tissues is extremely rapid. For example, Kohler et al. (1972) studied the growth kinetics in mammalian embryos in the early stages of differentiation, and calculated that between days 8 and 10 of pregnancy the rat embryo has a minimum of 10 mitotic divisions. This allowed for an average of 5 hours per cell cycle if one assumes that all cells are proliferating at the same rate. Even the most rapidly growing neoplasms or the intestinal crypt epithelium do not proliferate at this rate.

In assessing the effects of a teratogenic agent on proliferating cells, one must consider not only the proportion of cells that are undergoing mitosis at a given time (i.e., the mitotic index), but also the rate at which cells that are dividing proceed through the various stages of the cell cycle. The features of the cell cycle have recently been reviewed (Baserga, 1981).

CELL LOCATION

Throughout the period of embryonic development, many types of cells undergo carefully coordinated active and passive movement from one region of the embryo to another. The developmental events assoicated with cell movements are migration, aggregation, cavitation, delamination, and folding of tissues. Many cells in the developing embryo undergo active ameboid movement from one site to another. Major examples of these are the migration of germ cells from their original location in the yolk sac to the developing gonad. Similarly, the epithelial-derived neural crest cells adjacent to the neural tube of early embryos migrate to many distant sites in the body. They give rise to pigment-forming cells (the melanoblasts) and autonomic nerve ganglia. Similarly, portions of cells such as the developing axons of neurons migrate and pursue a path within the central nervous system or through the connective tissues of the body extending to the distal sites, where they establish contact with muscle fibers or sensory end organs. Cells may migrate singly or in groups.

Two types of subcellular structures, the microfilaments and microtubules, appear to be essential for cell movement. Intermediate filaments such as neurofilaments and tonofilaments may also be involved. The microfilaments appear similar in size and function to actin found in muscles, and appear to have a similar function within the cells. Using energy provided by ATP, the microfilaments react with myosin to produce a contractile activity in the cell analogous to that seen in muscle cells. However, the way in which these contractile proteins interact to produce directional cell movement is still unknown. It appears that the cytoplasmic actin and myosin are inserted into regions of the plasma membrane, and that contraction by a sliding-filament mechanism similar to that in muscle pulls selective portions of the cell membrane together, resulting in the production of a pseudopod much as is seen in ameboid movement. Microtubules are larger than microfilaments and intermediate filaments, and appear hollow when seen in cross section. Microtubular protein, tubulin, appears to provide structural support for cellular shapes other than simple globular shape. Cell migration has been most extensively studied using fibroblasts. As the cell undergoes ameboid movement in vitro, one can see bundles of microfilaments parallel to the lower surface of the cell, and immediately under the plasma membrane. There microfilaments are most prominent in the portions of the cell periphery most active in forming pseudopodia for movement and in the leading ruffled membranes. The rays of parallel microfilament form a sheath along the bottom of the cell and on the dorsal surface. Some of these microfilaments appear to insert on the plasma membrane where the cell is adhering to the substratum or to other cells. Disruption of the microfilaments by chemical agents such as cytochalasin B causes a cessation of movement.

Not only the migratory movement of cells, but also the ability of the internal skeleton of the cells to maintain diverse rearrangements, is important in embryogenesis. Cavitation appears to involve similar activities of the filamentous and tubular subskeleton of the cell. For example, epithelium may give rise to an organ rudiment by infoldings or outpouchings. With electron microscopy, bands of microfilaments can be seen in the regions of the folds, suggesting that they may be involved in the folding process. This has been shown to be true in lower forms of marine life. In mammalian species, for example, the pancreatic and lung buds arise as outpouchings from the primitive gut. The pancreatic rudiment formation is the product of changes in the shape and relative position of a few cells in the epithelium of the duct. Microfilament bundles are abundant at the apical end of such cells and appear to be involved in shape changes. The controls of morphogenetic movement are poorly understood. During early embryogenesis, migratory activity is much more extensive than it is in late embryogenesis, and it is much less active in adult mature cells.

There is some evidence that the control of migration may in part reside in the matrix surrounding the cells (Tool, 1973). Although many human congenital defects appear to be due to impeded morphogenic movements, a clear association with specific environmental agent changes has not been shown. Cytochalasin effects on neural tube closure represent an experimental model. Similarly, Zimmerman et al. (1981) have shown that the absence of neural crest-derived cells (presumably impeded migration) in the palatine shelves results in cleft palate formation. The cells normally respond to a neurotransmitter to rotate the palatine shelves into their proper position.

One important aspect of cell movement is cell aggregation. Once cells have migrated to a new site, they must in some way recognize the new environment and establish relationships there with similar or stromal cell types. The organization of the human embryo into tissue and organs depends on the ability of individual cells to be linked in very specific orientation to other appropriate cells. These multicellular patterns arise in the course of embryonic development and differentiation. The mechanisms that direct the assembly of cells into tissues are dependent on genetic as well as environmental factors that control embryonic development. As we have seen, many cells leave their place of origin and move individually or in groups to new sites by migrating through tissues, between tissue layers and cells, or by the bloodstream, and arrive at specific new sites distant from their origin. The cells reassemble and reassociate with each other and with local cells to form new structural entities within which differentiation, histogenesis, and organogenesis occur.

Much of our knowledge of how cells associate following the migratory pattern has been developed by Moscona (1973). He reasoned that following the process of migration, the cells must have an affinity for similar types of cells (contact selectivity) that enables them to select and establish their new site of residence. The surface of embryonic cells undergoes various changes in structure, composition, and function in the course of embryonic development and differentiation. These changes are reflected in changes of selective adhesiveness of cells, their movements and migrations, and changes in metabolism, intercellular communication, and so on. Among the properties of the cell surface that appear to be very important in the process of cell migration and the subsequent assembly of like cells into tissues and organs, is the development of mutual adhesiveness of cells, and the major characteristic of this enveloping adhesiveness is its selectivity. Thus, the cells have a capacity to recognize and identify other cells of similar nature, and accordingly to adhere and interact developmentally.

The recognition process involves not only self-recognition but also recognition between different but functionally matching or complementary types. Detailed examination of the process of cell aggregation reveals the initial clustering to be more attributable to random collisions between the cells than to active cell movements or contractions of protoplasmic filaments between cells resulting in fusion of clusters of cells of like type. Unlike cells would not adhere. Gently swirling the suspension of cells resulted in a more rapid formation of the aggregation of cells from each separate organ. Cells dissociated from different tissues of the same embryo show the same striking differences in their ability to aggregate when tested under identical conditions. Dissociated cells from older embryos aggregate less effectively than cells from the same tissues of younger embryos. Cells that have been fully committed to specialized biosynthesis are less capable or are incapable of effectively regenerating the histologic association. Following reaggregation, the cells undergo an internal reorganization and formation of tissues similar to those found in the original embryo. There appears to be a progressive sorting out of cells, resulting in a grouping according to type or functional relationships and into a histologic organization. Not only do the different types of cells sort themselves out, they also tend to be grouped in a predictable region of the aggregate; thus, in combinations of cartilage cells with liver and kidney cells, the cartilage cells almost always are found in the center of the aggregate and the other cells form external zones. When cells from different species of animals are suspended, one finds there is a greater organ specificity than there is a species specificity. Thus, if kidney and liver cells from two species such as chicken and mouse are mixed in suspension, the liver cells from the two species will have a greater affinity for one another than will liver and kidney cells of the same species.

The specific details of the mechanism of cell recognition remain to be discovered. It appears to be associated with the glycoprotein coat of cell surface that links adjacent cells by interaction of complementary receptor sites.

CELL LOSS

Cell death is another mechanism for diminution of the pool of cells available for the development of an organ. Necrosis is a normal developmental event that occurs in many sites in the body and appears to have a role in the shaping of organs. For example, the sternum in some species of animals originates as a pair of structures on each side of the midline; between these paired structures extensive necrosis ensues, and with the dissolution of the tissues the paired structures move and join at the midline to produce the ultimate sternum (Fell, 1939). Individual necrotic cells or small patches of cell necrosis can be seen throughout the developing embryo, and the significance of these changes remains to be determined. They may represent spurious cell development that is nonviable, or they may represent a programmed type of cell destruction

that enables the shaping and formation of the pool of cells that gives rise to a particular organ (Glucksmann, 1951).

The accompanying electron micrographs (Fig. 4-2) reveal the presence of selective cell necrosis within the developing limb buds of chick embryos (Hammar and Mottet, 1971; Mottet and Hammar, 1972). Necrosis occurs in the interdigital space as well as in an anterior and posterior zone at the attachment of the bud to the body wall. The latter necrosis has many interesting features. Several stages prior to necrotic changes, long before there is ultrastructural evidence of degeneration and necrosis, the cells appear to be destined to die (Saunders, 1966). For example, transplanting this region at stage 17 to a different region of the body of the embryo results in cell death in the usual manner. However, if transplanted at a prior stage the cells do not undergo necrosis.

Many cyotoxic agents have been shown to produce necrosis in the developing embryo. Some have a selective effect, inducing necrosis in some cells but not harming adjacent cells. Why this should happen is unknown. Some have speculated that the difference in cytotoxic effet may be due to the amount of the agent transported to the cell. Factors such as the differential distribution, permeability of the cell membrane to the agent, the amount of intracellular or extracellular binding, and different levels of metabolic activity might result in variation of the sensitivity and resistance of cells.

Although decreased proliferation and necrosis are associated with malformations, the precise mechanism is not as yet understood. Most human malformations are reductionist in nature. The diminished pool of cells necessary for the formation of an organ may have a critical mass. A certain minimal number of cells may be necessary to produce a smaller but functional organ, whereas excessive diminution of the pool may result in hypoplasia, agenesis, or malformation. In other instances, the diminution of a cellular activity, such as the inductive interaction between different cell types, may occur. The effect of arsenic in renal agenesis is an example to be discussed later.

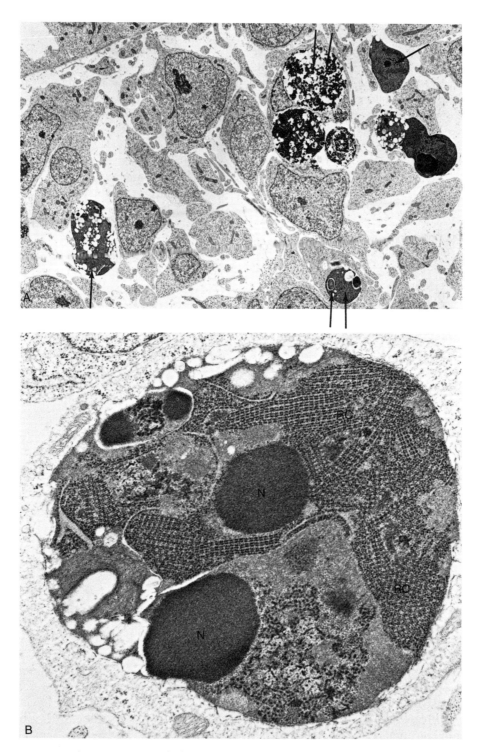

Figure 4–2. (A) Electron micrograph showing necrotic cells in the posterior zone of the chick embryo limb bud mesenchyme. Some are interstitial (↑), whereas others have been phagocytosed (↑ ↑) (× 5500). (B) Electron micrograph showing a phagocytosed cell. Fragments of a pyknotic nucleus (N) and ribosomal crystals (RC) are prominent features. The latter are unique to this type of programmed necrosis (× 12,000).

Radiation, as well as virtually every class of chemical in sufficient dose, has been shown to produce cytotoxicity in the developing embryo. Many of the anticancer agents such as vincristine, 6-aminonicotinamide, 5-fluorouracil, and nitrogen mustards as well as many other agents (ethyl alcohol, vitamin deficiencies, hormones, rubella virus, cytomegalovirus, etc.) have been shown to be cytotoxic. Diminution of the oxygen supply to the embryo and hyperthermia have a similar effect, as do ultraviolet radiation and X radiation.

Cell Size

Alteration in cell size is another mechanism associated with teratogenesis. An increase in size of cells (hypertrophy) or a decreased size of cells (hypotrophy) are produced by altered biosynthetic rates of the cells. Biosynthesis is the central activity of all living cells, and the extent of its activity is carefully regulated. Inhibition may decrease the synthesis of DNA and/or RNA and the production of proteins in the cell. Thus, any step along the replication, transcription, or translation of the genetic code may be inhibited by cytotoxic agents. In contrast, many inhibitors of protein synthesis have little or no teratogenic effect unless the inhibition is extreme. Some cytotoxic agents may induce teratogenesis by inhibiting the energy storage mechanism. Cellular energy is stored in organic compounds such as glucose, which is ultilized by a process of glycolysis and in the terminal electron transport system to make ATP. ATP in turn provides the energy for the biosynthesis of macromolecules in membrane integrity, energy for cell movement, osmotic regulation, and so on. Thus, anything that impedes or reduces the ATP level can be expected to alter markedly the development of an embryo. Decreased ATP levels can be produced by nutritional deficiencies and some chemical agents and some metals.

Cell Differentiation

Cell differentiation is an increasingly dominant feature as morphogenesis progresses.

Most types of defective differentation are the result of heritable mutations of the genome. Resultant enzyme defects cause aberrant cell differentiation by blocking the synthesis of a cellular product, producing a defective product, or the accumulating or storing a product that is useless to the cells or tissue. One type of aberrant cell differentiation is its misdirection by transplacental carcinogens. The concept that exposure of pregnant women to carcinogens can lead to the development of neoplasia in the offspring has existed for many years (Peller, 1960; Tomatis and Mohr, 1973). The concept received new impetus in the mid-1960s when it was demonstrated that a relatively rare type of neoplasm of the human vagina, clear cell adenocarcinoma, began to occur frequently. Between 1966 and 1969 eight cases of clear cell adenocarcinoma of the vagina were seen in women between the ages of 14 and 22 years (Herbst et al., 1974). A retrospective case–control epidemiologic investigation revealed an association with the ingestion of diethylstilbestrol (DES) during pregnancy by mothers of the patients. The use of DES to support high-risk pregnancies in habitually aborting women began in the mid-1940s. Over the next two decades hundreds of thousands of women received this drug or a chemically related but nonsteroidal estrogen during pregnancy. The effectiveness of the drug has never been satisfactorily proven for this purpose. By 1975 over 250 cases had been accessioned by the clear cell adenocarcinoma registry, and many thousands more were encountered in hospital pathology services throughout the country (Herbst et al., 1977). The dose of DES administered during pregnancy to these mothers range from 1.5 to 225 mg daily. The duration of treatment also varied from 1 week to the entire length of pregnancy. Three congenital anomalies are associated with this pattern of exposure to DES in the human. First, persistent mucous glandular epithelium in the vagina and cervix (vaginal adenosis) occurs in about 95% of the cases in which clear cell adenocarcinoma occurs. Second, glycogen-free metaplastic squamous epithelium is seen in association with the vaginal adenosis. Third, a transverse fibrous ridge in the upper third of the vagina and cervix creates the appearance that has given rise to the descriptive terms cockscomb cervix, cervical hood, or cervical pseudopolyp, which is seen in about 25% of the exposed subjects.

Most clear cell adenocarcinomas develop in the adenoses of the vagina and cervix. They are usually grossly nodular, polypoid, or papillary in appearance, but a few may be flat or ulcerated. They usually are between 1 and 3 cm in diameter when found. The microscopic appearance of the neoplastic glandular tissue reveals cells that have a clear cytoplasm, are hobnailed shaped, may be of flattened or indifferent epithelial cell appearance, and may resemble endometrial epithelium.

Prospective studies have revealed that vaginal adenosis occurs in as many as 90% of DES-exposed females; fortunately, only a small percentage develop clear cell adenocarcinomatous change, estimated to be 1.4 per 1000 exposed population through age 24. In all cases of clear cell adenocarcinoma the maternal therapy had been initiated before the eighteenth week of getation. The mortality rate among women who develop the neoplasm is approximately 25%.

The pathogenic mechanism for the effects of DES on the developing female reproductive tract and the consequent development of carcinoma is not known. The evidence suggests that the hormones administered increase the transformation zone between the squamous and columnar junction of the cervix, and it eventually becomes transformed into squamous epithelium by metaplasia. This zone extends into the vagina to produce a large area of vulnerable glandular tissue on which some as yet unidentified carcinogenic initiator or promoter can act in late childhood or early adult life. Conversely, one may hypothesize that premalignant changes (initiation) may have occurred in the embryonic period during the development of the glandular epithelium producing the vaginal adenosis during early fetal life, but that cancer does not develop until many years later after exposure to an additional, as yet unidentified,

promoter. Because these tumors occur after puberty, the role of the offsprings' ovarian estrogens may be a significant factor. During early fetal development, it appears that the DES acts either on the Müllerian duct or urogenital sinus at a time when portions of these structures are being transformed into the lower female reproductive tract, thus causing persistence of abnormal glandular epithelium in the vagina and ectocervix where ordinarily these glands would not occur. Normally an upgrowth of squamous epithelium from the urogenital sinus occurs, replacing the Müllerian epithelium. The development of the vaginal–cervical ridge is further evidence of a disturbance in the early vaginal morphogenesis.

More recent investigations have shown that intrauterine exposure to DES also affects the development of the human male genital tract (Gill et al., 1976). Both anatomic and functional abnormalities have been identified. These consist of epididymal cysts, hypotrophic testes, and in about 25% of the exposed males a decrease in spermatogenesis. In another 25% of the exposed males there are abnormalities in sperm morphology. Malignancies in the males have not been identified. However, an increase in cryptorchidism occurs, which in itself is associated with a higher than normal incidence of testicular neoplasms. It should also be parenthetically added that the mothers to whom DES was administered have an incidence of breast cancer above normal.

With the impetus provided by DES-induced transplacental carcinogenesis, numerous other agents have been studied for their transplacental carcinogenicity in experimental animals. Of particular interest is a group of nitrosourea compounds that have been shown to produce neoplasms in laboratory animals. The neoplasms may be located in a variety of organs including the lung, nervous system, liver, kidneys, and intestine (see Table 4–5). The significance of nitrosourea compounds in human transplacental carcinogenesis has not been established. Benzo[a]pyrene is another compound that has been of concern as a transplacental carcinogen. However, its effect in the human has not been established

Table 4–5. Some Transplacental Carcinogens

Compound	Species	Target organ
Ethyl carbamate (urethane)	Mouse	Lung
Methylnitrosourea	Rat	Nervous system
	Mouse	Lung, liver
	Mouse	Nervous system
n-Propylnitrosourea	Rat	Nervous system
Methylnitrosourethane	Rat	Multiple
Dimethylnitrosamine	Rat	Kidney
Diethylnitrosamine	Rat	Kidney
	Hamster	Trachea
	Mouse	Lung
Cycasin (methylazoxymethyl-β-D-glucoside	Rat	Jejunum; multiple
1,2-Diethylhydrazine, azoethane, azoxyethane	Rat	Nervous system
Methyl methanesulfonate	Rat	Nervous system
7,12-Dimethylbenz[a]anthracene	Mouse	Multiple
Benz[a]pyrene	Mouse	Lung, skin
Diethylstilbestrol	Human	Vagina

Source: Modified from Rice (1973).

(see placental biotransformation). Evidence for radiation as a congenital carcinogen has been presented in Chapter 3.

TISSUE INTERACTION

There is a large body of information showing that inductive tissue interactions are of utmost importance in controlling the differentiation and morphogenesis throughout gestation. Since the early work of Spemann (1938), these interactions have been known as embryonic induction. Most, if not all, of the tissues of embryonic and later stages of development are engaged in these interactions, functioning as inducers, as reactors, or in both capacities in some instances. Some of the better known examples of these interactions have been more extensively investigated, such as the epithelial mesenchyme interaction identified by Fell (1953), the influence of the peripheral innervated field on neuron differentiation (Mottet, 1952, 1954), and more recently by Young et al. (1975) and Warren et al. (1980), salivary gland epithelium and mesenchyme interaction (Borghese, 1958), the pancreas (Wessels and Evans, 1968), and the kidney (Grobstein, 1955, 1957, 1967).

The interaction between the ureteric bud and kidney differentiation is an example of how environmental chemicals can alter morphogenesis by interfering with an inductive interaction. Grobstein (1957) has shown that the differentiation of the metanephric blastema into the definitive kidney in higher mammals does not ensue unless an interaction occurs with the developing ureteric bud derived from the mesonephric duct. In his elegant experiments, when the analogs of these two structures were cultured in vitro in contact with one another, the differentiation of the blastema ensued. However, if they were cultured a short distance from one another in the same vessel, no differentiation resulted. If the two primordia are separated by a thin impermeable membrane, then again no differentiation is seen. However, if the two primordia are separated by a thin permeable membrane, then differentiation ensues, implying that there is a transfer of a stimulus from the ureteric bud to the blastema leading to tubule and nephron formation.

Recently Ferm et al. (Ferm and Carpenter, 1968a,b; Ferm et al., 1972; Ferm and Kilham, 1977) have shown that administration of relatively high doses of sodium arsenate at a critical period during renal organogenesis in rats resulted in defective renal formation or complete renal agenesis. Beaudoin (1975) confirmed Ferm's observation, and Burk and Beaudoin (1978) have shown that the renal agenesis is due to a failure of ureteric bud formation; thus, arsenic interferes with the inductive interaction by impeding or destroying the ureteric bud formation. When the ureteric bud is partially formed, the resultant kidney is also partially formed, or if the ureteric bud formed unilaterally, the nephrogenesis was unilateral as well.

Another potentially significant aspect of this demonstration of environmental agents interfering with the inductive interaction was the observation by Ferm and Kilham (1977) that if the dose of sodium arsenate was decreased by one-half, normal renal morphogenesis ensued. However, at this dose level, if the animals were also exposed to hyperthermia during the sensitive period, the renal agenesis would result. Hyperhthermia alone did not cause renal agenesis. This may be a model of how two or more agents could act synergistically to produce an anomaly when each individual agent was unable alone to produce anomalies.

Teratogenic Agents

RADIATION

Many of the features of radiation teratogenesis were presented in Chapter 3. Dose—response relationships and the effects on the developing young have been discussed. It remains to amplify further some details of the morphologic effects. Radiation is one of the more extensively studied teratogenic agents, and reviews of the subject have been written (Brent, 1977, 1980).

Before the blastocyst stage, the embryo is a multicellular organism with a low sensitivity to the teratogenic and growth-retarding effects of radiation. However, the developing organism is highly sensitive to the lethal effects of radiation at this time. During early organogenesis the embryo is very sensitive to the growth-retarding, ter-

atogenic, and lethal effects of radiation, but may overcome the growth-retarding effect in the postpartum period. During the early period the fetal visceral organs have a diminished sensitivity to radiation; however, the central nervous system remains very sensitive throughout the latter part of gestation and cannot overcome the growth-retarded brain development postnatally. During the later fetal stages the embryo is not grossly deformed by radiation, but may have a permanent cell depletion of various organs and tissues if the radiation dose is high enough.

Of the pathogenic mechanisms, cell death, mitotic delay, disturbance of cell migration, and alteration of macromolecular structure are potentially involved, although these mechanisms have not been established experimentally.

Necrosis may be an important factor in a later phase of gestation, because the embryo is not able to replace the killed cells, whereas at an earlier stage it may still have the proliferative capacity to replace them. Also, the cell necrosis must be sufficiently extensive to deplete the pool of cells available for organ development.

These embryopathic effects have been observed in human fetal development as well as extensively investigated in experimental animals. Each of these responses, during different stages of gestation, has a specific dose relationship and a threshold exposure below which there is no detectable difference between the irradiated and control populations as revealed by available methods of investigation. Growth retardation and central nervous system defects, microcephaly, and eye malformations are the major intrauterine effects in the human. Microcephaly is the commonest malformation observed in humans randomly exposed to high doses of radiation during pregnancy. At 100 rad or more, microcephaly was accompanied by mental retardation. A variety of other malformations may accompany this effect, such as cleft palate or genital tract anomalies. Intrauterine growth retardation is present in most.

Growth retardation, microcephaly, and

mental retardation are predominant observable effects following acute exposures greater than 50 rad. The opportunity to study human embryos soon after the radiation exposure is rare. The acute effects on two human fetuses exposed to radiation from radium with which women were being treated for cancer of the cervix has been reported. The fetuses were 15 and 21 cm in crown–rump length and were examined 2 and 10 days after the beginning of radiation. They received about 800 and 1600 rad of radiation. In both, the destruction of primitive, proliferative, and migratory cells in the brains and granulopoietic cells in the hematopoietic tissue occurred, and there was evidence of necrosis in lymphoid and hemopoietic cells throughout. Irradiation of human fetuses from diagnostic exposures below 5 rad have not been observed to cause congenital malformation or growth retardation.

Recently Schull et al. (1981) reviewed the frequency of untoward pregnancy outcomes (stillbirths, major congenital defects, death during first postnatal week) and the occurrence of death in liveborn children over an average span of the first 17 years of life. The frequency of sex chromosome aneuploidy and children with mutations born to survivors of the atomic bombings of Hiroshima and Nagasaki was also studied. There was no evidence of a statistically significant effect of parental exposure on these parameters of development. However, for all the indicators, the observed effect is in the direction suggested by the hypothesis that genetic damage may result from the exposure.

TRACE ELEMENT TERATOGENESIS

Mercury

Metallic and ionic forms of mercury occur in fossil fuels. At the present rate of burning coal in the United States, about 3000 tons of mercury are added to our environment per year. Petroleum combustion adds a similar amount (U.S. Geologic Survey, 1970). Inorganic mercury released into our environment can be inhaled as a vapor, consumed with foods (Clarkson, 1971, 1976), or absorbed through the skin. Metallic and inorganic mercury liberated into the environment are converted to methyl mercury by bacterial action. Methyl mercury is of special biologic significance because, unlike its inorganic counterparts, it is widely distributed in the mammalian body, it gains ready access to the brain and spinal cord, and it is eliminated from the human body much more slowly. Methyl mercury readily passes through the human placenta, and thus the unborn human is at risk. The average daily intake of mercury by the adult human is estimated at 0.35 µg/kg/day. The maximum allowable intake is 1.4 µg/kg/day (Berlin, 1969). These estimates are currently under revision.

Knowledge that methyl mercury can pass through the placenta has stimulated investigation of its effects on fetal development (Tejning, 1969). The majority of the investigations have administered one or two doses of the agent at a sensitive period during organogenesis (Gale and Ferm, 1971; Inouye et al., 1972). The doses used are usually very high. Table 4–6 shows the pattern of anomalies experimentally produced in a variety of laboratory animals receiving acute high doses (Nonaka, 1969). The pattern of genital defects is not uniform. This can be explained by differences in animal species, mercury compound, dose, and dosage schedule.

Recent major human population exposures in Japan (Kutsuna, 1968) and Iraq Bakir et al., 1973; Amin-Zaki et al., 1974) were apparently relatively continous high-dose exposures throughout pregnancy. Although these poisonings clearly establish organic mercurials to be human teratogens, the dose and duration of exposure during gestation and nursing can only be estimated retrospectively. Other variables such as general nutrition and specificity of mercurial were poorly defined. Experiments to correlate mechanisms of methyl mercury teratogenesis with dose and duration of exposure in rats and nonhuman primates have been in progress for more than a decade (Mottet, 1974; Chen et al., 1979).

Table 4–6. Teratogenic Effects of Acute High Doses of Organomercurials

Species	Hg compound	Dose	Day of gestation	Congenital defects
Rats	Methyl mercury chloride	0.2–2.0 mg/100 g	9 or 11	Retarded cerebellum development
Hamsters	Phenyl mercuric acetate	2–4 mg/kg	8	Syndactyly, rib fusion, cleft lip and palate, anophthalmia, exencephaly
Hamsters	Methyl mercury perchloride	8 mg/kg	5, 8, or 9	Clubfoot, hydrocephalus, fetal death
ddM mice	Methyl mercury chloride	30 mg/kg	6–13	Vaulted cranium, cleft palate, micrognathia, microglossia, general edema
Rats	Methyl mercury chloride	5 mg/kg	6–13	Possible brain damage
Mice	Methyl mercury chloride	30 mg/kg	6–13	Cleft palate, retarded growth
Mice (A strain)	Methyl mercury dicyandiamide	2, 4, 8 mg/kg	6–13	No malformation
Mice (strain 129)	Methyl mercury dicyandiamide	2, 4, 8 mg/kg	6–13	Palate and jaw malformations
Mice and rats	Methyl mercury chloride	5 mg/kg	6–17	Cerebellar defects, exencephaly, syndactyly, absent tail

Continuous low-dose exposure of pregnant rats to methyl mercury did not increase the rate of anatomic malformation as did acute high doses, but rather the fetuses were smaller (Mottet, 1974). The extent of the decrease in fetal weight was dose related. At higher doses, fetal deaths increased, and the number of fetuses per litter was decreased (Figure 4-1). Experiments using animals that develop free from the maternal influence—the nonplacentates such as fish, amphibia, and fowl—reveal that their offspring are also smaller than normal following continuous exposure to methylmercury during embryogenesis (Dial, 1974, 1978; Weis and Weis, 1977). Birthweights of human congenitally exposed newborns (although tending to be smaller than the mean) are mostly within two standard deviations of the mean. In no instances were the exact dose and duration of human exposure known. Very often the mercury was incorporated either in seafood or in bread from seed grain treated with mercury compounds. The amount ingested can only be estimated from general dietary habits.

Alteration of three morphogenic mechanisms could explain the decreased fetal size. These involve a decreased number of cells (hypoplasia) resulting from (1) reduced proliferation because of lengthened cell cycle or decreased dividing fraction, (2) increased rate of necrosis, or (3) decreased size of cells (hypotrophy) or interstitium (collagen, elastin, proteoglycans) because of diminished biosynthesis.

Currently available evidence suggests that mercury decreases the proliferative rate (Mottet, 1974; Chen et al., 1979). We have measured the organ content of DNA and protein in experimental and control animals. Because each diploid cell in a given species has a constant amount of DNA, the DNA assay can be used as an index of the number of cells in a given organ or quantity of tissue. Organ weights (kidney, liver, cerebellum) were significantly subnormal. The total DNA per kidney and liver was also lower in the experimentals than in the controls. The total protein per kidney and liver was similarly decreased. The DNA and protein per unit weight (gram) of tissue were normal. This confirmed that the cells in the kidneys and liver were of normal size but were fewer in total number.

The incorporation of tritiated thymidine into nuclear DNA as an indicator of cell-proliferative activity was also used to confirm the above (Chen et al., 1979). [³H]Thymidine (0.5 μCi/mg body weight) was intraperitoneally injected on day 20 of gestation of methyl mercury–exposed and control pregnant rats 2 hours before sacrifice. The data show that less [³H]thymidine is incorporated in the fetal organs of experimental animals than in controls. One can deduce from this that fewer kidney and liver cells were synthesizing DNA at the time of sacrifice. This is consistent with the DNA data on cell proliferation described above. Biochemical mechanisms for the decreased proliferation induced by methyl mercury have not been defined.

Much remains to be learned about the biologic and biochemical effects of mercury compounds. Biochemical evidence suggests that the toxic action of mercurials is due to specific actions on certain groups, primarily sulfhydryl (SH) groups of enzymes, rather than on specific denaturation. The inhibition may be competitive, noncompetitive, or mixed. In vitro studies have shown mercurials to inhibit heart lactic dehydrogenase and liver cytochrome C reductase by blocking SH groups. They also inhibit enzymes of the electron transport chain, and oxidative phosphorylation at concentrations of 1 to 100 ppm. Southard and Nitisewojo (1974) confirmed these findings. Some organic mercurials have been shown to inhibit NADH dehydrogenase—flavoprotein complex and the respiratory chain (Murakami, 1971; Southard and Nitisewojo, 1974; Lucier et al., 1973). Mitochondrial changes induced by both inorganic and organic mercurials have been reviewed by Goyer and Rhyne (1975) and Fowler (1974). They emphasize that organic mercurials are more easily transported across cell membranes than are inorganic mercurials, and are firmly bound to organelles.

Other mechanisms cannot as yet be ruled out. Cell necrosis may be a factor in some organs, especially at higher doses. Its effect on biosynthesis of extracellular matrix represents a largely unstudied possibility. Methyl mercury's multiple effects on cellular metabolism in vitro illustrate the complexity and importance of establishing the biochemical mechanism operative during in vivo development. Methyl mercury has been shown to produce chromosomal damage under some human exposure situations (Skerfuing et al., 1970, 1974; Khera and Tabacova, 1973). Also, Sirover and Loeb (1976) have shown mercury to induce infidelity in DNA synthesis in vitro.

Arsenic

Like mercury, arsenic is a contaminant of fossil fuels and many ores, and is also found in artesian water in some regions. Excessive intake of arsenic has been associated with a variety of disease processes in the human. Chronic exposure has been associated with neoplastic changes in the skin and other organs. That arsenic compounds in the pregnant woman can be transported to the developing fetus has also long been known, because organic arsenicals were used as antisyphilitic agents long before the development of antibiotics (Underhill and Amatruda, 1923). The organic arsenicals are stored within the fetus and placenta, and are slowly released into the fetal circulation (Eastman, 1931). At the clinical doses used to treat syphilis, there was no knowledge of causing arsenic congenital malformations. A case of maternal human inorganic arsenic poisoning during pregnancy with subsequent fetal death has been reported by Lugo et al. (1969). However, no unusual pathologic changes were seen in the fetus other than hyaline membrane disease.

Teratogenic effects of arsenic compounds in experimental animals have been recognized only recently. Ridgeway and Karnofsky (1952) and Amcel (1946) injected sodium arsenate into chick embryos at 4 days of incubation and observed relatively nonspecific anomalies in the embryos at hatching. Growth retardation, impaired feather growth, and abdominal swelling were present. However, more recently sodium arsenate has been shown to be teratogenic to hamsters (Ferm and Carpenter, 1968a), mice (Hood and Bishop, 1972), and rats (Beaudoin, 1975). Ferm and co-workers (Ferm and Carpenter, 1968a; Ferm and Kilham, 1977) were the first to show in hamsters that sodium arsenate, administered 20 mg/kg intravenously as a single dose on day 8 or 9 of gestation, was critical in producing a high incidence of anencephaly and increased fetal mortality. Of the fetuses that died during gestation, there was a markedly increased incidence of anencephaly, exencephaly, and genitourinary anomalies. This period of administration corresponds to the period of very rapid differentiation of the organs affected. The spectrum of defects produced by arsenate in the hamster included exencephaly, encephaloceles, skeletal defects, and renal agenesis. Administration of selenium simultaneously significantly reduced the incidence of defects (Ferm, 1977).

Hood and Bishop (1972) administered single doses of 24 to 25 mg/kg of sodium arsenate in mice intraperitoneally on days 6–12 of gestation and observed a variety of consequent malformations. There were many dead and resorbed fetuses, in addition to defects including exencephaly, micrognathia, cleft lip, fused vertebrae, and forked ribs. Similar results have been reported by Beaudoin (1975) for rats. He administered varying doses of ranging from 20 to 50 mg/kg to pregnant Wistar rats during days 7–12 of gestation. The most common malformations included eye defects, exencephaly, and renal and gonadal dysgenesis. The morphologic changes in the neural tube associated with exencephaly were investigated by Morrissey and Mottet (1983). They showed that the basic lesion was a failure of the anterior neuropore to close as a result of an increased number of necrotic neuroepithelial cells at the site of closure. More recently, Denckar et al. (1983), using whole-body autoradiographs, have shown a higher than usual concentration of arsenic in these cells.

Extensive investigations have been done on the subcellular and biochemical mechanisms of action of arsenate compounds on mammalian tissues. Unfortunately, there are no experiments to relate these biochemical reactions directly to the aforementioned anomalies. The mechanisms of action of arsenicals on the cellular metabolic processes have been well reviewed by Klevay (1976) and Fowler (1977). The reader is referred to these reviews for further reference to details of the metabolic effects of arsenicals.

Arsenic metabolism appears to involve several diverse aspects of general cellular metabolism, and in part this diversity of effects may reflect the fact that arsenic has a strong affinity for SH groups. Oxidative phosphorylation effects of arsenicals are an important site of action on the inner mitochondrial membrane. Arsenicals appear to be involved in the formation of cytochromes and of several cofactors in the oxidative process, nicotinamide adenine dinucleotide (NAD), flavin adenine dinucleotide (FAD), and coenzyme Q. During the process of oxidation of substrates and the transfer of electrons from these substrates to molecular oxygen, about 40% of the free energy is stored in the form of ATP, so it can be released as needed to perform work.

The toxicity of an arsenic compound is highly dependent on its chemical form and oxidation state. Thus arsenite (As^{3+}), arsenate (As^{5+}), arsine gas (AsH_3), and organic arsenicals vary in their degree of toxicity. Generally, trivalent arsenite is more toxic than arsenate, although arsenate is the form most commonly encountered in the environment. All these forms of arsenicals inhibit cellular respiration and the cell's energy-producing system. Arsenate has long been known as an uncoupler of mitochondrial oxidative phosphorylation. The mechanism by which this occurs is thought to be related to competitive substitution of arsenate for inorganic phosphate, with subsequent formation of an unstable arsenate ester. The inhibitory effect of arsenate has been observed in vivo and in vitro. Associated with these metabolic effects is the induction of mitochondrial swelling by arsenate, which has been shown both in vivo and in vitro in several organs, including kidney and liver.

In addition to these metabolic effects, arsenate has been shown to substitute for phosphate in the DNA chain, causing chromosomal abnormalities. Arsenate is also known to inhibit DNA repair following UV irradiation (Rossman et al., 1975). Jung et al. (1969) reported autoradiographic studies demonstrating a decrease in enzymatic DNA repair following UV irradiation and incubation of skin samples in an arsenate solution. Trivalent arsenite compounds are primarily sulfhydryl reagents. These arsenicals cause enzymic inhibition of the tricarboxylic acid cycle as well as inhibition of a number of other enzyme systems.

Lead

Excessive exposure to lead salts has important effects on the reproductive processes. Specific toxic effects on embryonic tissues were reported as early as 1915 (Weller, 1915). Subsequently, a teratogenic effect of lead salts on chick embryos that induced malformations of the brain has been reported (Ridgeway and Karnofsky, 1952; Butt et al., 1952).

In addition to direct effects on the fetus, there is evidence that lead may induce a necrosis and hemorrhage within placental tissues, involving the trophoblasts and resulting in defective development of surviving fetuses (Baker, 1960). More recently, Ferm and Carpenter (1967) and Ferm (1972) demonstrated teratogenic activity of lead salts in mammalian embryos. When injected intravenously in pregnant hamsters on day 8 of gestation, maldevelopment of the tail bud and stunting of the sacral vertebra were identified. Lead, in a dose of about 25 ppm, results in the loss of the strain of mice or rats in two generations (Schroeder and Mitchener, 1971) when the lead is administered in the drinking water, reinforcing the evidence for a reproductive failure.

Lead effects on human reproduction also have been reported. Exposure of pregnant females to high levels of lead has resulted in abortion (Wilson, 1977). Lead has been shown by Barltrop (1968) to cross the human placenta readily. Following excessive industrial exposure of women with no neurologic symptoms, the offspring frequently have both an intrauterine and postnatal growth retardation.

In adult animals the principal effect of lead toxicity within the cells is on mitochondrial function as reported by Goyer (1971). Barltrop et al. (1971) also established a time-dependent distribution of radioactive lead within various tissues after intraperitoneal injection in rats. The most rapid decrease in lead content occurred in the microsomal and the slowest in the lysosomal fraction, suggesting that the latter might have a high affinity for lead. However, only a minor portion of the lead in the tissue was present in this subfraction. The extent of accumulation of renal lead in subcellular fractions 48 hours after injection was in the following order; beginning with the largest: supernatant, microsomal, mitochondrial, and nuclear. When the rats had been pretreated daily with lead, mitochondrial uptake was reduced by 30% to 40%, implying some saturation of its binding capacity.

Mitochondrial accumulation of lead in kidneys is potentially damaging to normal renal function. ADP-stimulated respiration in mitochondria is completely inhibited on incubation with lead, as revealed by Goyer et al. (1968; Goyer, 1971) and by Rhyne and Goyer (1971). Mitochondria from the proximal convoluted tubules of lead-loaded rats generally showed a reduced rate of respiration and partial uncoupling of oxidative phosphorylation, possibly as a result of altered membrane structure. The respiratory abnormalities of these mitochondria could have resulted from reduced cytochrome content (Labbe and Hubbard, 1961). The cells studied, although functionally impaired, were still viable at cellular lead concentrations that would have been lethal to mitochondria in in vitro studies. This protection of mitochondria from exposure to lead uptake in vivo may be the result of the intranuclear inclusion bodies, which may serve to trap and sequester lead. As the concentration of the lead and the cells increases, much of the additional lead is found in the nuclear fraction with over 50% in the inclusion bodies. These workers have suggested that the metal is thus maintained in a nondiffusible, nontoxic form until the cell in which the inclusion body exists is itself excreted in the urine. In this way the kidney can secrete large amounts of lead without excessive damage to the tubular lining of the cells.

The lead in the intranuclear inclusion bodies occurs as a lead–protein complex (Choie and Richter, 1972). The protein appears to be derived from preexisting intranuclear nonhistone protein. These effects appear rapidly after administration of lead.

Ridgeway and Karnofsky (1952) reported brain hemorrhage and damage followed by hydrocephalus in chick embryos exposed to 1.1 mg of lead nitrate on day 4 of incubation. Byers and Lord (1943) recorded the late effects of lead poisoning congenitally in the human. They observed 20 schoolchildren who had been hospitalized in infancy or early childhood because lead poisoning was identified. In all but one of the children there was a failure in the normal process of growth and mental development of the cerebral cortex that prevented their satisfactory functioning in school. Subsequent to this early report, there have been many reports of similar behavioral changes in children who suffered congenital or early childhood exposures to lead. The median blood level of lead in the United States is 16–21 μg/100 ml of blood.

In the adult guinea pig, acute lead encephalopathy was induced by administering oral doses of lead carbonate daily (Baudin et al., 1975). During the process of development of the lesion, the structural and functional integrity of the blood–brain barrier was evaluated by electron microscopy and tracer probes. There was no evidence of blood–brain barrier dysfunction. However, there was a progressive rise in lead concentration in the cerebral tissues and evidence that the encephalopathic effects of lead were mediated directly at the neuronal level.

Wide and Nilsson (1977) studied the effects of lead administration on the preimplantation period of embryonic development in the mouse. All stages of implantation were adversely affected by lead, resulting in a decrease in frequency of normal offspring.

Administration of lead in the diet to pregnant female mice resulted in a reduction in litter size in a number of pregnancies. The blastocyst formed normally, although it was reduced in size. The formation of the decidua was impaired, and estrogen and progesterone secretion had diminished (Wide and Nilsson, 1977).

In the Carpenter and Ferm (1977) study, the pregnant golden hamsters were given intravenous injections of lead nitrate at a dose of 15 mg/kg on day 8 of gestation. The earliest morphologic change was the presence of edema in the developing tail region. This occurred consistently about 30 hours after treatment. Later, grossly visible blisters and hematomas developed in the tail region. Following this there was a disruption in morphogenic tissue interaction between the tissues just described, with extensive dysgenesis or agenesis of caudal structures. Accompanying these changes was a sharp increase in embryonic death and resorption. Death was observed in approximately 70% of the embryos by day 13 of a 16-day gestation period. Those surviving to birth displayed varying degrees of caudal malformation.

Press (1977) studied the development of the cerebellum of neonatal rats with lead encephalopathy produced by administering daily doses of lead by esophageal catheter. During this early postnatal period, matrix cells and neuroblasts of the external granular layer were minimally altered prior to day 8, but thereafter the number of mitotic figures per folium decreased moderately and the number of pyknotic cells increased markedly. The thickness of the molecular layer in lead-poisoned animals persistently lagged behind that of control animals after 3 days. Purkinje cells survived the cerebellar alterations of lead encephalopathy very well for the first 5–8 days. However, the rate of Purkinje cell maturation decreased after 10 days. The processes of the Purkinje cells maintained synaptic contact with climbing fibers, whereas the climbing fibers of control animals formed asymmetric synapses in the lower dendritic field, and the cell soma had symmetric basket-fiber synapses.

It is difficult to correlate the gross pathologic changes in embryonic development in the several species with subcellular biochemical mechanisms. However, there are many studies on the effects of lead at the cellular and subcellular biochemical levels that, to a certain extent, seem to correlate with the pathology just described.

Kusell and co-workers (1978) studied the growth of cultured cells in the presence of lead. A rat liver cell line was cultured in chemically defined medium in the presence of lead nitrate. Lead reversibly inhibited the growth of these cells even after 6 days of exposure to the heavy metal. Glioma and neuroblastoma cell lines were similarly affected, with comparable LD_{50} values. Gerber and Maes (1978) have shown that heme synthesis is depressed in liver cells of lead-intoxicated mouse embryos.

Brunn and Brunk (1974) studied in vitro–cultured embryonic rat fibroblasts to test the concentration that would cause widespread cellular injury but not cell death. Doses between 1 and 100 μ and 25 mg of lead nitrate/ml culture medium were used for the study of the mechanism of cell injury. The lead was present in those lysosomes having a decreased stability of the lysosomal membrane.

Decreased heme biosynthesis in lead-poisoned rats and a depression of the microsomal P-450 and b_5 is found. The rate-limiting enzyme for heme biosynthesis, δ-aminolevulinic acid synthetase, was inhibited, as was the activity of other heme-biosynthetic enzymes, including δ-aminolevulinic acid dehydratase and ferrochelatase. Inorganic lead inhibits the cellular respiration and ADP-dependent (stage 3) respiration. These observations were made in isolated mitochondria from rat brain.

Copper

Chronic exposure to excessive copper has not been proven to be a major toxicologic problem in human medicine, although occasionally it may occur in infants as a result of excessive intake. Copper is an essential trace element. Women with Wilson's disease (a genetically determined trait characterized by massive accumulation of copper in tissues, especially the liver and brain) give birth to children without evidence of copper-induced anomalies. (There is some evidence that they have increased fetal death.)

The effects of exogenous excessive copper exposure on the developing embryo are less well defined than the effects of deficiency. Intravenous or subcutaneous injection of copper salts during pregnancy has a major effect in rats, resulting in interruption in pregnancy in about 50% of the cases (Oster and Salgo, 1976). However, intravenous injections of similar salts in pregnant rabbits have no effect even when doses are very high. Copper salts injected into pregnant hamsters are teratogenic (Ferm and Hanlon, 1974). The intraperitoneal injection of copper salts into pregnant hamsters on day 5 of gestation caused an increase in embryonic resorption. Malformations of the heart appeared to be a specific result of the toxicity of these copper compounds (Di-Carlo, 1980). The types of defects were those commonly associated with decreased endocardial cushion development. Copper in a chelated form was only slightly embryocidal but considerably more embryopathic than that of the uncomplexed form, copper sulfate. Carnes (1971) reviewed the role of copper in connective tissue metabolism. The congenital heart lesions observed by Di-Carlo are principally due to a deficiency in the connective tissue development of the endocardial cushion. Additional studies on the permeability of the early hamster placenta during the critical stage of organogenesis revealed that the placenta was permeable to radioactive copper, indicating that this metal may have a direct teratologic effect on the developing embryo. Injection of copper salt in the chick egg is teratologic and embryocidal (Ridgeway and Karnofsky, 1952).

Experiments on the use of copper intrauterine devices (IUDs) revealed no effect on fertilization in the rat (Webb, 1973). Progressively fewer embryos survived, however. The later the device was removed during pregnancy, the progressively fewer embryos survived. The presence of a copper IUD during the first few hours of embryonic life completely suppressed implantation and caused the death of the embryos. It is suspected that the copper IUD interferes with pregnancy by liberating copper ions that are toxic to the early fetus. Copper wire wound around plastic IUDs gives increased effectiveness (Brinster and Cross, 1972). In vitro studies show that two-cell embryos placed in a medium containing 10^{-4}–10^{-5} M copper chloride have markedly decreased survival. Lower concentrations did not interfere with the development of the blastocyst.

Recent clinical investigation by WHO suggests the possibility that deficiency of copper and/or zinc may be associated with an increased incidence of congenital malformations, especially in diabetic mothers. In one study of 243 births, five of the eight malformed infants were born to women with the lowest serum zinc. Diabetics may be particularly liable to zinc deficiency.

Cadmium

In a classic study of cadmium-induced teratogenesis by Ferm and co-workers (Ferm and Carpenter, 1968b), golden hamsters were given 2–4 mg/kg cadmium salts intravenously on day 8 of gestation. There were subsequent facial developmental malformations and some resorptions of the embryos. This was first seen on day 9 of gestation (24 hours after intravenous cadmium administration). Many of the embryos showed obvious disparity in the size of the first brachial arch. Within a given litter, there was sometimes a range of severity (from normal configuration to unilateral cleft of

the lip, to bilateral cleft, to complete or incomplete palatal cleft), or the degree of malformation could be fairly consistent within the litter. In conjunction with the gross facial malformations were defects of the eye, neural tube anomalies of microphthalmia, anophthalmia, encephalocele, and exencephaly. Infrequently observed were defects of the developing heart and limb buds.

Barr (1972) conducted a similar study in rats, administering intraperitoneally teratogenic doses of cadmium on days 9, 10, or 11 of gestation (doses given subcutaneously did not produce developmental anomalies). Embryos treated on day 9 frequently had anophthalmia, dysplastic or absent ears, and attenuated abdominal wall, whereas those treated on day 10 were observed to have eye and forelimb malformations. Day 11 treatment showed individuals with hydrocephaly and absence of the left leaf of the diaphragm.

In those fetuses with attenuated abdominal walls, the walls were paper-thin and ballooned out, but there was no evidence of increased intraabdominal pressure or visceromegaly. No distinction could be made between cutaneous and musculofascial layers. Those fetuses with deficient abdominal musculature had a higher general malformation rate than did fetuses with normal muscle from the same litter. At day 21, 43% of fetuses had the musculature syndrome with a high degree of correlation with hydronephrosis, hydroureter, undescended testes, and limb malformation. The occurrence of this anomaly was more frequent among the male than among the female fetuses. Fetal mortality and malformation were dose related.

In addition to the immediate repercussions of orally administered cadmium salts on resorption of embryos, fetal mortality, runting, and congenital malformations, Schroeder and Mitchener (1971) noted a long-term effect on the reproductive capacity of experimental animals. Mice and rats exposed to trace elements in drinking water (10 ppm) resulted in the loss of the strains within two generations, with many abnormalities occurring in the offspring before the cessation of mating (Gunn et al., 1967).

Sublethal (to the mother) concentrations of cadmium were administered, resulting in 51% of the embryos being malformed and 73% being either malformed or resorbed. The wide range of developmental anomalies has already been alluded to, but most often they were confined to the craniofacial region and with especially high frequency of cleft palate and lip. Malformations were focused in the cranial regions, where rapid morphogenesis occurs during day 8 of gestation.

When pregnant hamsters were injected intravenously with radioactive cadmium on day 8 of gestation, significant amounts could be detected in the embryo within 24 hours (Ferm et al., 1969; Berlin and Ullberg, 1963). This interval corresponds to the period during which cadmium is teratogenic for hamster fetuses. At 96 hours after injection, there was a relative decrease in embryonic concentration of radioactive cadmium. This may be accounted for on the basis of (1) dilution effect (increase in size of the conceptus relative to a constant initial amount of cadmium), (2) an active block in placental transport of cadmium, perhaps in the developing yolk sac placenta, or (3) a fetal excretion mechanism.

It is unknown if the action of cadmium is directly on the fetus, or if cadmium acts secondarily through maternal or placental effects, or if there is a combination of these factors. The placenta can act as a barrier against small amounts of cadmium, but administration of large amounts can result in significant amounts detectable in the fetus.

Zinc alone produces mild teratogenic effects and, as already remarked, cadmium alone produces marked embryocidal and teratogenic effects affecting up to 73% of the concepti. Simultaneous injection of zinc sulfate almost completely inhibits the deleterious developmental effects of cadmium on the embryo, sometimes to such a degree that teratogenesis in cadmium- and zinc-treated animals is no higher than that in controls (Chaube, 1973). Interestingly, zinc does not prevent placental transfer of cad-

mium, so rather it must inhibit the effects of cadmium at specific sites. There is a remarkable increase in zinc concentrations between days 31–35 and 39–79, suggesting that during these early stages of development, morphogenic events are occurring that require zinc for local happenings such as palatal fusion, unless both processes represent two different expressions of derangement of embryonic mesenchymal cell activity.

Thallium

The toxic effects of thallium on children and adults is well established in the medical literature. Numerous instances of thallotoxicosis due to the misuse of thallium compounds, usually thallium sulfate, a rodenticide or medicinal (for the removal of hair or the treatment of syphilis or gonorrhea, gout, or dysentery), have been recorded (Munch, 1934; Reed et al., 1963). The biochemical mechanism of action of thallium remains poorly understood. Human fetal cases of thallium poisoning reveal that much of the thallium accumulates in the kidneys, intestinal mucosa, thyroid, testes, pancreas, skin, and bone. Postmortem examination in fatal cases revealed the presence of punctate hemorrhages in the gastrointestinal mucosa, fatty changes in the liver and kidneys, and small hemorrhages and degeneration in the adrenal gland. Varying degrees of cerebral edema have been identified, as well as congestion of the cerebral vessels. A very large percentage of the children poisoned by thallium die in acute episodes (Stevens and Barbier, 1976).

Despite the rather common occurrence of acute thallium intoxication in adults, relatively little is recorded in the medical literature regarding human congenital exposure. One report from Germany (Stevens and Barbier, 1976) identified six cases of human thallium intoxication during the first trimester of pregnancy. No congenital anomalies were found in these cases. When the intoxication occurred after the first trimester, some of the features of the adult acute syndrome were observed in the newborn. Those exposed had alopecia, skin rash, low birth rate, and premature birth.

Experimental studies of the effects of thallium on the developing embryo have been conducted with chick embryos (Ford et al., 1968). Injection of thallium sulfate into the yolk sac of the developing chick embryo at any time from 4 to 12 days of incubation causes abnormal skeletal development. The most consistent finding is a bowing and shortening of the long bones of the extremities. The changes appear to be dose related. In the developing chick skeleton the thallium salts appear to alter the metabolic pathways of glycosaminoglycan synthesis with an increased necrosis and defective differentiation of the chondrocytes, whereas no alteration in hydroxyproline synthesis was demonstrable (Hall, 1972). In the experimental group there was approximately a 17% decrease in glycosaminoglycan synthesis. One hour after injecting radioactive ^{204}thallium sulfate into the yolk of 11-day-old chick embryos, the label localized mainly in the narrow, vascular spaces of the bone, and on the surface of the bone trabeculae. The thallium appeared to be cytotoxic for chondrocytes, even though no marked intracellular concentration of thallium could be demonstrated.

The congenital effects of thallium have been studied in rodents (Gibson and Becker, 1970) when administered intraperitoneally to rats on days 8, 9, and 10 or on days 12, 13, and 14 of gestation. The studies revealed that thallium sulfate administration at each dose during appropriate stages of gestation significantly reduced the fetal body weight and produced a hydronephrosis and a failure of ossification of vertebral bodies. However, it did not increase the fetal resorption rate. Low potassium did not alter the severity of the teratogenic effects. These investigators further studied the placental transfer of thallium and found that the maternal blood level of thallium was much higher that that which passed through the placenta. The diminished teratogenic effect of thallium on the rat as compared with the chick was due to the limited placental passage of thallium.

The biochemical mechanism of action of thallium is not well established. The cellular injury to the chondrocyte appears to be associated principally with changes in the mitochondria.

Nickel

Although there are no reports of embryotoxicity of nickel in the human, its toxicity to embryos and fetuses in experimental animals is well established (Sunderman, 1977; Sunderman et al., 1978). Administration of nickel chloride and nickel subsulfide in rats on day 8 reduced the number of live pups per dam and resulted in a diminished body weight of the fetuses on day 20 when the examinations were carried out. Similarly, the weights of the offspring were diminished 8 weeks postnatally. There were no specific congenital malformations found in these fetuses. The distribution of nickel in the fetal tissues was studied extensively, and the investigations showed that nickel injected into the pregnant female early in gestation can cross the placental barrier to the fetus. Doses that do not produce mortality in the pregnant female cause extensive embryonic mortality. Other investigations (Schroeder and Mitchener, 1971) have shown that continuous administration of nickel in the drinking water through three generations of rats also produced a diminution of the size of the offspring and increased neonatal mortality in each of the three generations tested. Administration of nickel acetate to pregnant hamsters by intravenous injection on day 8 of gestation at doses from 0.07 to 0.10 mg/kg resulted in a few congenital malformations that did not follow a consistent pattern (Ferm, 1972). Similarly, increased fetal resorption was noted in investigations with hamsters.

All these animal experiments on the embryotoxicity of nickel indicate that the administration to pregnant rodents produces fetal mortality and impairs intrauterine growth. Although the growth defects are well established, there are virtually no data to explain the biochemical mechanisms of the effects of nickel on fetal metabolism.

Cobalt

The effects of cobalt deficiency or excess in the developing young are minimal. Vitamin B_{12} deficiency, induced by a variety of techniques, has caused congenital anomalies in rats and pigs (Ross et al., 1944). Although cobalt can cause a polycythemia in several species, there is little evidence that it is significantly toxic to the developing fetus. Cobalt itself is not a teratogen, as revealed in its effect on the golden hamster by Ferm and Carpenter (1968a). Others have injected chick embryos on day 4 of development of an anemia in the embryos that survive to 20 days, and observed some thyroid epithelial hyperplasia in a small percentage of their embryos.

Fluorine

Congenital exposure to excessive amounts of fluorine as fluoride can lead to alterations in the development of the teeth and bone (Smith and Smith, 1935). Mottled enamel has been observed in the deciduous teeth of children whose mothers used well water containing 12–18 ppm of fluorine (Schour and Smith, 1935). This fluorine level is over 20 times higher than that usually found in water, and that which is added to water in the fluoridation process. Attempts to link fluoridation with other specific human developmental malformations have been unsuccessful. In explanted chick embryos, a differential inhibition of cardiac development has been reported. Sporadic case reports of increased bone density without alteration of the overall bone structure have been reported from areas of high fluorine intake. Calcification often extends into the ligaments. The biochemical mechanisms for the effects of this trace element have not been elucidated.

Chaube and Murphy (1969) produced defects in the offspring of rats receiving 700–1000 mg/kg of fluorine on day 11 or 12 of gestation. These defects included cleft lip and palate, micrognathia, and other skeletal defects. They observed that fluorine per se was considerably less effective than the ter-

atogen 5-fluorodeoxycytidine, a fluorinated compound that has been studied as a cancer chemotherapeutic agent. Fleming and coworkers (Fleming and Greenfield, 1954) produced similar results in fetal mice by administering fluorides to the pregnant mother.

Iodine

Although the association of maternal iodine deficiency and the occurrence of cretinism have been recognized for more than 100 years, relatively little is known about the biochemical mechanisms involved (Warkany, 1971). Epidemiologic studies have shown in Switzerland and parts of Austria that endemic cretinism can be eradicated by the addition of iodine to the maternal diets in these iodine-deficient areas. The elimination of cretinism did not occur immediately following the introduction of iodine in maternal diets but rather often required a second generation. Although the association of endemic cretinism with iodine as a principal causative factor has been established, evidence suggests that other trace elements may play a part. Calcium, cobalt, and fluorine are elements that have been associated with increased demand for iodine. These elements appear to alter the capacity of the thyroid to bind iodine. A hereditary predisposition to cretinism appears to exist. Although a genetic predisposition may play a role in the etiology of endemic goiter and cretinism, it probably is the result of pathologic manifestation only in the presence of iodine deficiency (Stanbury and Querido, 1957). Mothers of cretins usually have goiters. The increased risk of cretinism with increasing birth order and the increasing risk of abortion and stillbirth are probably due to the depletion of iodine in the maternal organism and the progressive malfunction of the thyroid gland. Similarly, chronic infection appears to enhance the occurrence of cretinism. It has been demonstrated that fever is associated with a marked increase in the need for iodine ingestion, because urinary excretion of iodine is enhanced by fever.

Cretinism is not merely the deficiency of

hormone and thyroid gland function in the newborn, but rather of alteration in morphogenesis of the fetus during gestation. Tissues other than the thyroid are congenitally damaged, suggesting developmental disturbances between the second and third trimesters of pregnancy.

Newborn cretins are somnolent, hypothermic, tend to feed poorly, have a hoarse cry, are constipated, and may have umbilical hernias and an excessive amount of neonatal jaundice. Physical growth and mental retardation become apparent within the first few months of life. Skeletal development is slow. The head appears unusually large for the size of the body, the nose tends to be flat and broad, and the tongue is enlarged. The neck is usually short and thick and the abdomen protuberant. The skin is rough and dry with sparse hair. The infants often are deaf and cannot speak. Serum levels of thyroid hormone are usually very low. However, in rare instances maternal antithyroid hormone antibodies block the function of the infant thyroid gland (Blizzard et al., 1960). Usually however, the thyroid hormone deficiency (which is usually present) reduces the feedback inhibition of the pituitary; thyroid-stimulating hormone levels are typically elevated, and the thyroid gland is enlarged.

The cause of endemic cretinism clearly is associated with deficient maternal ingestion of iodine (Hamilton, 1976). However, there are other causes of cretinism (occurring sporadically) that are not associated with the ingestion of this trace element. Maternal ingestion of drugs such as thiourea and other chemical goitrogens can be associated with cretinism.

Although much is known about the biochemical mechanism of the synthesis of the hormone thyroxin by the thyroid gland, relatively little is known about the effects of the deficiency of this hormone on the developing fetus. The biochemical mechanism of this interaction is virtually unknown. Perhaps this deficit in our understanding can be attributed to the absence of an animal model that closely simulates cretinism in the human. In rats, prenatal iodine deficiency

produces fetal thyroid hyperplasia but not cretinism. Even if iodine deficiency continues in postnatal life, the animals develop normally. Even when the rats are raised through several generations, cretinism does not result. The same is true for mice. Smith and co-workers (1951) induced hypothyroidism in puppies by administering radioactive iodine to pregnant dogs. Although some of the puppies had some of the features of cretinism, the overall pattern of deficits did not mimic cretinism as seen in the human.

Several of the medications that can induce hypothyroid cretinism in the developing fetus and the features of cretinism, including growth impairment and mental retardation, have been detailed by Hassan and co-workers (1968). Congenital goiter and hypothyroidism in the offspring can result when the pregnant woman uses iodine-containing drugs. These drugs are often used for the relief of asthma or as expectorants in respiratory infections. Over-the-counter and prescription use of potassium iodide and other iodine-containing drugs provide the equivalent of 25,000 to 350,000 μg of iodine in a single dose. The levels at which iodine intake can cause goiter in the fetus or in children are not known. Some people appear to be especially susceptible to the goitrogenic effects (Murray and Stewart, 1967). Iodides do not produce malformation of the fetus when administered during the first trimester of pregnancy, although it is known that the iodine is easily transferred across the placenta, and after 12 weeks of gestation the iodine administered is taken up by the fetal thyroid. Administration of iodides to the mother can induce fetal goiter by inhibiting the synthesis and release of thyroid hormone, thereby stimulating pituitary thyrotropic hormone. This, in turn, leads to hypertrophy and hyperplasia of the thyroid gland. The enlarged thyroid can cause respiratory distress and asphyxia in the newborn due to its compression of the trachea. In many instances the goiter can be associated with hypothyroidism and its consequence—impaired growth and development. Similarly, cobalt antianemic medication should be avoided during pregnancy because of its goitrogenic effect. In rare instances, lithium used in the treatment of depression may also cause goiter by its synergistic effect.

Lithium

Since Cade (1949) introduced the use of lithium as a treatment for psychiatric disturbances in 1948, it has gained wide acceptance as an antidepressive drug. Since his discovery, over 100 studies on the use of lithium in major psychiatric syndromes were published. These investigations generally supported the contention that lithium salts are of marked value in the treatment of manic and certain other depressive disorders. Because the depressive disorders are most likely to become manifest in women during the childbearing decades, the question has arisen whether lithium might have teratogenic effects in humans. This concern about lithium exposure during pregnancy was heightened by a century of accumulation of evidence that lithium was teratogenic in a variety of animal forms including rodents (Wright et al., 1967). Concern about this risk led to the development of an international registry of lithium babies to develop data on its possible effects on humans (Weinstein, 1976). By 1966 the registry had accumulated 166 instances of the use of lithium during pregnancies from which 18 malformed children were born. Thirteen of the 18 malformations involved the cardiovascular system, 2 the central nervous system, and 1 each the external ears, endocrine system, and ureters (Weinstein and Goldfield, 1975). One infant had multiple defects associated with intrauterine infection with toxoplasmosis. Of the 13 who had cardiovascular abnormalities, 12 had changes in the heart and great vessels and 1 had a single umbilical artery. Six of the 166 pregnancies resulted in stillbirths for a rate of 3.6%. One stillbirth was malformed, with a congenital heart anomaly. Two children of the group had Down's syndrome. Thus, it appears that the cardiovascular anomalies are of significantly higher incidence in

the lithium-treated group than in a control population. The other anomalies are questionable as to their statistical significance.

Recently, Wright and co-workers (1967) studied the teratogenic effects of lithium in rats. Intraperitoneal administration of lithium chloride to pregnant rats resulted in malformation almost exclusively in the cephalic region, primarily affecting the eyes, ears, and palate. In addition, the fetal resorption rate was increased. Lithium has been shown to be teratogenic in a variety of invertebrates, as well as in fish and amphibians, chicks, and mice. In mice, lithium induced a decrease in litter size. In Wright et al.'s investigation (1967), lithium was administered intraperitoneally, beginning on days 4, 7, and 9 and continuing through day 16. A dose of 50 mg/kg of lithium chloride was injected initially into each rat, followed by a maintenance dose of 20 mg/kg for the subsequent injections. This dose is quite large in comparison with that used in the human. In mice of the strain Ha M/Icr, which are known to have a low incidence of spontaneous malformations, the administration of lithium has resulted in a statistically significant increase in the rate of cleft palate. Johansen (1971), using a different strain of rat than that used by Wright, found only one defect in 42 animals injected with 212 mg/kg of lithium chloride on days 4, 7, and 9.

These studies are fragmentary at best. There is little concordance between the cardiovascular defects found in the human and the cephalic defects found in experimental rodents. Virtually nothing is known about the biochemical mechanism of action of lithium either in the human or in experimental animals. Lithium decreases the cell proliferative rate (Timson and Price, 1971).

Drugs

Almost 50 years ago it was discovered that a deficiency of vitamin A resulted in maldevelopment of the eyes in weanling pigs; relatively little systematic investigation of the effects of pharmaceutical agents on the developing fetus was made in ensuing years until the thalidomide disaster in the late 1950s. Even today, relatively few well-documented epidemiologic studies are available to establish strong presumptive evidence of the effects of a given pharmaceutical agent as a teratogen (Nelson and Forfar, 1971). The average pregnant human receives four prescription drugs during pregnancy, and self-administers many more nonprescription remedies. Therefore, the association of a deformed offspring with a particular agent is difficult in the human. Also, the relevance of animal studies to the human have many causes for doubt. The dose, time of application, and duration of exposure to the agent, coupled with the dif-

fering responses of various laboratory animals to the agent, often leaves the relevance of animal experiments questionable. This topic has been reviewed by Tuchmann-Duplessis (1975) and in a monograph by Presaud (1979).

Table 4-7 lists some of the suspected teratogens, taken either from experimental animal investigations or from reported human cases. Except for thalidomide, ethanol, and diethylstilbestrol, the human cases represent sporadic case reports or small collections, which generally are insufficient to make a presumptive causal association. The cancer therapeutic agents in the human represent the rare circumstance where the

Table 4–7. Drugs and Developmental Defects: Some Suspected Teratogens in Experimental Animals (A) and Humans (H)

Drugs	Abortion, fetal death (resorptions)	Growth retardation	Malformations
Cancer chemotherapeutic agents			
Nitrogen mustard	A		A
Cyclophosphamide	A	A	AH
Chlorambucil	A	A	AH
Busulphan	A	AH	AH
Colchicine	A		
Vinblastine			A
Actinomycin-D	A	A	A
Mitomycin-C	A		A
6-Mercaptopurine	A	A	A
Azathioprine (Imuran)	A (mouse)		A (rabbit)
Aminopterin	AH	AH	AH
Methotrexate	AH	AH	AH
Antibacterial/antiprotozoal			
Tetracyclines			H
Rifampicin			A
Quinine	AH	A	
Anticoagulant			
Warfarin (Dicumarol)	A		
CNS-Active			
Barbiturates			?H
Thalidomide	A		AH
Lysergic acid diethylamide (LSD)	AH	A	AH
Cannabis		A	A
Diphenylhydantoin	A	A	A
Amphetamines	A	A	AH
Ethanol	AH	AH	AH
Endocrine			
Diethylstilbestrol	AH	AH	AH

Source: From Wilson (1977).

woman has both cancer and a pregnancy, and the clinical decision was to treat the cancer and not interrupt the pregnancy; thus, the number of human cases is extremely sparse in this group. Aminopterin was tried as abortifacient. Although it does produce a high incidence of abortions, it also produces malformation in offspring that survive the abortion attempt, and therefore it has been discarded. The maldevelopment associated with tetracycline is defective tooth formation with some deposition of the tetracycline in bone, and thus is of limited significance.

Of the central nervous system–active pharmaceuticals, thalidomide is the one that has been studied most thoroughly and is most clearly associated with maldevelopment in the human and experimental animals. In the mid-1950s, the agent thalidomide was developed as one of the least toxic hypnotics and was extensively prescribed in many countries as a hypnotic and as an antiemetic for women during pregnancy. It was immensely successful in this respect and was licensed in many countries between 1956 and 1961. Shortly after its general use an extremely rare form of congenital anomaly, namely phocomelia (seal flipper-like extremities) became much more frequent. Independently, Von Lenz (1961; Von Lenz and Knapp, 1962) in Germany, and McBride (1961) in Australia made careful clinical observations and began to incriminate thalidomide as the cause of the increased frequency of phocomelia. As more cases were accumulated, a large constellation of internal and external anomalies were identified including phocomelia, amelia (shortening of the extremities on one or both sides), defective ear development, and a wide distribution of internal anomalies involving virtually any organ system. An extensive study of these cases showed that about 5% of the children had total amelia, and 65% had aplasia of the humerus and/or radius and digits; 15% of the cases had only malformation of the thumb associated with some synostosis of the radius and ulna. Following these reports the agent was removed from the market, and the incidence of these anomalies returned to their original background level. Thalidomide was not licensed in the United States, and therefore the occasional sporadic case that occurred was the result of illicit transport of the drug into the United States.

The thalidomide disaster illustrates many important features of teratogenesis and its discovery in the human. Because of the diversity of exposures of pregnant humans to chemicals in the environment, current methods dictate that a marked increase in frequency of a relatively rare anomaly is necessary to develop evidence for a causal relationship by statistical methods. Because of multiple exposures to chemical agents, a slight increase of a particular anomaly in a population due to exposure to a particular agent may not be detectable by present methods of study. Further, the thalidomide disaster changed the general attitudes of medical scientists toward drug-induced malformation. Previously, virtually all new pharmaceutical agents were tested on laboratory animals, and the results of this were the basis for predicting what would happen in the pregnant human if she were to consume this drug. Common laboratory rodents are minimally affected by thalidomide. Rabbits and primates are the two common laboratory species that do respond to thalidomide exposure during gestation, producing offspring with anomalies of a pattern similar to the human. Thus, increasing doubt exists as to the relevance of many animal studies to the human for testing pharmaceutical agents.

Thalidomide also illustrates the importance of periods of sensitivity to an agent during gestation. Women who received thalidomide before day 34 of gestation or after 50 days of gestation produced offspring without anomalies. Between 34 and 50 days the pattern of anomalies varied depending on the day or days of exposure. Thus, failure for the ear to develop properly (anotia) occurred when exposure was between 34 and 38 days, whereas defective thumb development occurred when exposure was between 46 and 50 days of gestation. Upper extremity malformations tended to occur in the period earlier than the lower extremities, because the upper extremities embryologically develop slightly in advance of the lower extremities. Seldom does one encounter such a highly specific pattern of anomalies associated with specific days of exposure during a sensitive period. Despite intensive investigation during the last two decades it has not been possible to identify another teratogen similar to thalidomide. Thalidomide appears to be a chemical of unique effects in human and some experimental animal development, in that it possesses toxicologic properties not shared by any other substance as yet tested. The compound is of very low toxicity in adult animals and humans, and has an exclusive sensitivity in the embryos. The species difference in responses and sensitivity to this teratogen is also unexplained.

Although it is well established that thalidomide and its metabolites readily penetrate the placenta and are distributed throughout the embryo, relatively little is known about the biochemical mechanisms by which it produces malformations. Numerous hypotheses have been advanced including interaction with folic and glutamic acid metabolism, interference with nucleic acid metabolism, immunosuppression, uncoupling of oxidative phosphorylation, and acylation effects. This latter hypothesis is based on the observation that thalidomide reacts with a number of polyamines. According to this hypothesis, thalidomide may be a biologic acylating agent, and by forming stable reaction products with polyamines it may deprive the embryo of the necessary biogenic amines, resulting in the anomalies identified. However, a clear understanding of the mechanism by which thalidomide exerts its teratogenic effects remains elusive after almost two decades of intensive research. The reader is referred to Fabro (1981) for a more detailed description of the biochemical reactions of thalidomide and an inclusive list of references.

Organic Solvents

The embryotoxicity and teratogenicity of aliphatic hydrocarbons are not well established for the human, and relatively few studies have been done on experimental an-

imals. The effects of gasoline and kerosene are largely unknown except for the effects of tetraethyl lead additives to gasolines. The effects of methylene chloride on pregnant mice and rats exposed to this vapor in concentrations that were twice the maximum allowable limit for human industrial exposure (1225 ppm) for 7 hours per day on day 6 through 15 of gestation revealed no fetal toxicity or teratogenicity. Carbon tetrachloride exposure of pregnant rats on day 2 or 3 of gestation caused no congenital defects in the offspring. However, some degeneration of the embryonic disk of rabbits was noted. Trichloroethylene does not produce fetal toxicity or teratogenicity in mice or rats exposed to concentrations of the vapor at twice the maximum allowable limit for human industrial exposure (300 ppm).

Aliphatic alcohols can have major embryotoxic effects. The prime example of this group is the *fetal alcohol syndrome* induced by ethanol ingestion. A group of anatomic and functional changes occur in some offspring of women who consumed alcoholic beverages during pregnancy, ranging from severe growth deficiency, mental retardation, and abnormal facial features to mild mental changes (Table 4-8). This may be the foremost public health problem in our society today, and the major cause of birth defects, including mental retardation. Despite references to the adverse effects of alcohol on prenatal development dating from biblical times, and four reports in the medical literature during this century, the interest and detailed investigation of this syndrome occurred following the report of Jones and Smith (1973). The original and subsequent observations included children born to severely alcoholic mothers from three races, all having pre- and postnatal growth deficiency. At 1 year of age, all continued to be small and failed to thrive. The children averaged 65% of normal height, their weight gain was 38% of normal, and their head circumference remained below the third percentile for their height and chronologic age. Similarly, all were below average in performance on standard intelligence tests, motor dysfunction tests, grasp, and tremulousness, and had poor hand-to-eye coor-

Table 4–8. Malformations Associated with Fetal Alcohol Syndrome

Frequent (80% of patients)	Occasional (26–50% of patients)	Uncommon (1–25% of patients)
Microcephaly	Ptosis	Blepharophimosis
Short palpebral fissures	Strabismus	Auricular conchal mal-
Short upturned nose	Epicanthal folds	development
Hypoplastic filtrum	Posterior auricular rotation	Cleft lip or palate
Hypoplastic maxilla	Prominent lateral palatine	Small teeth
Thin upper vermillion	ridges	Pulmonary artery stenosis
Infantile micrognathia	Atrial septal defect	Ventricular septal defect
Prenatal and postnatal	Genitolabial hypoplasia	Atrioventricular canal
growth deficiency	Cutaneous hemangiomas	Right aortic arch
	Abnormal palmar creases	Tetralogy of fallot
	Pectus excavatum	Horseshoe kidney
		Hydronephrosis
		Renal crossed ectopia
		Renal dysplasia
		Renal pelvicalyectasis
		Ureteropelvic obstruction
		Joint contractures
		Nail hypoplasia
		Polydactyly
		Klippel-Feil anomaly
		Scoliosis
		Hernias
		Diastasis recti

Source: Modified from Clarren and Smith (1978).

dination. Physical abnormalities included limitation of joint motion, increased congenital heart malformation rate, short palpebral fissures, and maxillary hypoplasia with relative prognathism. Morphologic abnormalities in the structure of the brain were found in the patient that died and was autopsied (Clarren et al., 1978). The brain was small, the corpus callosum was absent, and heterotopias resulting from abnormal neuronal migrations were found. Similar reports from three countries of Western Europe now confirm these findings (Krous, 1981).

The frequency of adverse outcome of pregnancies of chronic alcoholic women is very high. There is an eightfold increase in perinatal mortality, and the frequency of the fetal alcohol syndrome in the surviving children is common. Almost half of the offspring had IQs below 80, and a smaller percentage had the dysmorphic features noted above. The grouping of abnormal facial features is sufficiently characteristic to alert physicians to possible unrecognized alco-

holism in the mother, and to enable the diagnosis of the syndrome during the neonatal period. When occurring together, the features produce a rather characteristic appearance. However, when seen individually, they may not be distinguishable from normal variations (Streissguth et al., 1980).

It now is becoming increasingly apparent that although the complete fetal alcohol syndrome is seen in children born to severely alcoholic mothers, lesser degrees of change can be found in some offspring of women who consume lesser amounts of alcoholic beverage (Streissguth, 1976). Is there a threshold dose of alcohol consumption during pregnancy below which no fetal injury results? The answer to this question is not completely established at this time.

A recent surgeon general advisory recommends that women who are pregnant or considering pregnancy should not drink alcoholic beverages. The deleterious effects include a significant decrease in birthweight in children of some women who average 1 ounce of absolute alcohol per day during pregnancy, a significant increase in spontaneous abortions at 1 ounce twice a week, and some or all of the features of the fetal alcohol syndrome in the offspring of heavy drinkers.

Laboratory animal studies reveal that lesser amounts of alcohol during pregnancy may also be deleterious to the developing fetus. The current status of extensive epidemiologic studies on humans suggests a similar result. In one investigation, infants born to mothers who reported an average consumption of 2 or more ounces of hard liquor per day, or who reported being intoxicated during pregnancy (e.g., ingestion of five or more drinks per occasion), were studied. Of 163 infants reported in this study, 11 had the fetal alcohol syndrome with nearly all of its manifestations. The mothers of 9 of these 11 infants reported consuming alcoholic beverages to the above degree, whereas two of the mothers of infants who had a few of the fetal alcohol syndrome facial features reported consuming less than 3 ounces of alcohol daily before recognition of pregnancy. Of 16 women who consumed as much as four or more drinks of hard liquor per day before the recognition of pregnancy, three were delivered of infants with partial fetal alcohol syndrome. These data suggest that there is a dose–response curve for maternal alcohol intake relative to the well-being of the fetus. It suggests that the risk of the fetal alcohol syndrome increases proportionately with the increase in average daily alcohol consumption. The severity of the dysmorphic features (Streissguth et al., 1980) appears to correlate with the extent of mental retardation. There are not, as yet, sufficient data to determine whether there is a safe level of alcohol consumption during pregnancy. There do not appear to be major fetal defects at a maternal alcohol intake level of less than four drinks per day. However, even at a level of two drinks per day, infants average about 60 to 160 g below the expected birthweight for gestational age. Fertilization of the ovum in women occurs about 2 weeks before the "first missed period," and implantation and embryogenesis have already begun. Whether

small amounts of alcoholic beverages produce injury or death of the embryo during these early stages of development remains to be established. The existing evidence suggests that early in pregnancy even moderate amounts of alcohol can have adverse effects.

The pathogenic mechanism by which ethanol produces these changes in the developing fetus is not known. Some experimental evidence suggests that ethanol is degraded to acetaldehyde by the normal liver but is not so degraded in the chronic alcoholic person. The suspicion is strong that the acetaldehyde may directly affect the proliferation of fetal cells. However, there is other evidence to suggest that ethanol itself can produce the changes noted. Whether the concurrent use of alcohol and tobacco or the commonly associated nutritional deficiencies associated with alcoholism have a potentiating role, remains to be determined. Similar morphologic disorders, including the impairment of growth and development and cognitive functions, have been observed following the maternal use of a number of central nervous system–active agents. Thus, the syndrome described may be the product of a variety of agents, or may be the result of a common mechanism induced by a variety of agents.

Methanol effects on the developing fetus are poorly established for both the human and experimental animals.

Glycol groups of organic solvents can produce developmental defects. Ethylene glycol is the most widely used glycol, and it has been shown to produce some fetal skeletal defects in rats with doses of over 100 μl/kg/day, but no defects were caused in mice or rabbits.

Aromatic hydrocarbon solvents such as benzene and toluene, although toxic to the adult human, have not been shown to be toxic to the developing embryo or to produce developmental anomalies.

Pesticides

Pesticides are useful in our society because of their increased toxicity to pests and insects, but lesser toxicity to humans and domesticated animals. Some of the rodenti-cides, insecticides, and fungicides are particularly toxic to mammals. This is true of those containing trace metals (mercury, arsenic, chromate), which are discussed in another section. Almost every person in our society is exposed to pesticides in some form or another. Data from the American Chemical Society referred to earlier in this chapter indicate more than 1500 pesticides are currently manufactured in the United States. The people most likely to be exposed are the workers in the fields and food-preparing industries, the manufacturers of pesticides, and those who formulate the product. Commonly these operators are men; however, women are an increasing percentage of the work force, and thus the unborn may be increasingly exposed. Cases of pesticide intoxication have occurred in such people as the result of neglect of safety precautions. However, there are no reports of toxic effects other than acute intoxica-tion followed by death or complete recov-ery, or occasionally a delayed neurotoxicity and dermatitis. Thousands have been ex-posed to organophosphorus insecticides, and there have been many intentional fatal poi-sonings especially with parathion. How-ever, the literature does not reveal reports of abortion, miscarriage, stillbirths, or live-births with malformations associated with these exposures, whether toxic or nontoxic.

The lack of proven cases of embryopathy associated with ingestion of pesticides has not removed the basis for concern. Exten-sive animal studies have been carried out and embryotoxic effects have been demon-strated. The most extensive and up-to-date review of this subject is the one by Wilson (1977). Tables 4-9, 4-10, and 4-11 are from that chapter, and the reader who seeks fur-ther details should refer to it. As one can see from the tables, even though the dosage in many instances was remarkably high, even to the level of maternal toxicity, many had no embryopathic effects—malformations, intrauterine death and resorption, or intra-uterine growth retardation. In fact, the in-secticides as a group have a remarkably low embryotoxic potential, even though they may cause general toxicity in the adults at a relatively low dose. It is further notewor-thy that DDT has not been found to cause embryotoxic changes in mammals, al-though some of the other organochlorine insecticides do reveal teratogenic effects (Zavon, 1969). Numerous investigations of the embryonic effects of herbicides such as 2,4,5-T and 2,4-D reveal them to be non-teratogenic to several rodent species except when large doses are given. The claims that human birth defects occurred in pregnant women exposed to 2,4,5-T when used as a defoliant in the Vietnam War has not been validated. Attempts to demonstrate that there was an increase in birth defects in areas of its usage have not been borne out by the data.

Fungicides are also not very toxic to the embryos. Relatively high doses in experi-mental animals are necessary to produce evidence of embryopathic effects.

Dioxin

Chlorophenols and products produced from them, such as the herbicide 2,4,5-trichlo-rophenoxyacetic acid (2,4,5-T), contain dioxins such as 2,3,7,8-tetrachlorodibenzo-p-dioxin (TCDD). TCDD and other chlo-rodibenzo-p-dioxins are among the most toxic compounds known, and have been implicated in human outbreaks of chlor-acne and other toxic manifestations among chemical workers. Experimental animal studies have shown guinea pigs to be the most sensitive to the lethal effects of TCDD, with 90% dying from a single 3-μg/kg dose. A 100-μg/kg dose was lethal to approxi-mately 50% of rats treated. Administration of daily or weekly sublethal doses does not raise the threshold level of TCDD toxicity (Harris et al., 1973).

The major sites of toxic effects of TCDD are the hematopoietic system, liver, and thymus. Mice, guinea pigs, and monkeys given TCDD became leukopenic with an associated decreased cell-mediated immune response. Rats and guinea pigs also became thrombocytopenic. Liver damage was evi-denced by increased SGOT and SGPT, hy-

Table 4–9. Insecticides Reported To Be Embryotoxic When Given during Pregnancy in Mammals

Agent	Species	Treatment (dose; route; gestational days)	Embryonic effects[a]
Aldrin	Hamster	50 mg/kg; oral; 7, 8, or 9	MAL, IDR, IGR
	Mouse	25 mg/kg; oral; 9	MAL
	Rat	12.5 ppm; diet; 3 generations	Reduced pregnancies
Carbaryl	Guinea pig	300 mg/kg; oral; var. 11–20	MAL, IDR, IGR
	Rabbit	50–200 mg/kg; oral; 5–15	None
	Hamster	125–250 mg/kg; oral; 6–8	IDR
	Rat	200 mg/kg; diet; 3 generations	None
	Guinea pig	300 mg/kg; diet; 0–35	None
	Rat	2000–100,000 ppm; diet; 3 generations	Reduced fertility, 2nd generation
	Gerbil	2000–100,000 ppm; diet; 3 generations	Reduced fertility, 3rd generation
	Dog	3–50 mg/kg; diet; throughout	MAL, IDR, PGR
	Pig	4–32 mg/kg; diet; various	±MAL, IDR
	Monkey	2–20 mg/kg; oral; throughout	IDR
Carbofuran	Dog	10 ppm; diet; throughout	None
	Rat	50 ppm; diet; throughout	None
	Rabbit	50 ppm; diet; throughout	None
DDT	Rat	20 ppm; diet; throughout	None
	Rat	25 ppm; diet; 3 generations	None
Demeton	Mouse	7–10 mg/kg; ip; var. 7–10	MAL IDR, IGR
Diazinon	Rat	100–200 mg/kg; ip; 11	±MAL, IDR, IGR
	Rat	9–95 mg/kg; oral; var. 8–15	±MAL, IDR
	Dog	1–5 mg/kg; oral; throughout	SB
	Pig	5–10 mg/kg; oral; throughout	±MAL
	Hamster	0.125–0.25 mg/kg; oral; 6–8	None
	Rabbit	7–30 mg/kg; oral; 5–15	None
Dichlorvos	Rat	15 mg/kg; ip; 11	MAL
Dieldrin	Hamster	30 mg/kg; oral; 7, 8, or 9	MAL, IDR, IGR
	Mouse	15 mg/kg; oral; 9	MAL
	Mouse	5 ppm; diet; 1 generation	±IDR
	Mouse	1.5–6.0 mg/kg/days; oral; 7–16	None
	Rat	1.5–6.0 mg/kg/day; oral; 7–16	None
	Rat	2.5 ppm; diet; 3 generations	Reduced pregnancies
Endrin	Hamster	5 mg/kg; oral; 7, 8, or 9	MAL, IDR, IGR
	Mouse	2.5 mg/kg; oral; 9	MAL
	Mouse	5 ppm; diet; 1 generation	±IDR
Fenthion	Mouse	40–80 mg/kg; ip; var. 7–10	MAL, IDR, IGR
Imidan	Rabbit	35 mg/kg; oral; 7–12	None
Isoflurophate	Rat	1–4 mg/kg; ip; 8, 9, or 12	IGR
Kelthane	Mouse	7 ppm; diet; 3 generations	MAL, PGR 3rd generation
Lindane	Dog	7.5–15.0 mg/kg; oral; throughout	SB
Malathion	Rat	240 μg/day; diet; 2 generations	Reduced fertility, 2nd generation
	Rat	600–900 mg/kg; ip; 11	None
	Rat	105–355 mg/kg; oral; var. 8–15	±MAL, IDR
Methylparathion	Rat	5–10 mg/kg; ip; 12	IGR
	Mouse	20–60 mg/kg; ip; 10	MAL, IDR, IGR
Parathion	Rat	3.5 mg/kg; ip; 11	IDR, IGR
	Rat	0.5–5.0 mg/kg; ip; var. 8–16	SB, PGR
Photodieldrin	Mouse	0.15–0.6 mg/kg/day; oral; 7–16	None
	Rat	0.15–0.6 mg/kg/day; oral; 7–16	None
Tsumacide	Rat	80–4000 ppm; diet; 8–15	None

[a] MAL, Malformations; IDR, intrauterine death and resorption or abortion; IGR, intrauterine growth retardation; SB, stillbirth or perinatal death; PGR, postnatal growth retardation.
Source: From Wilson (1977).

Table 4–10. Fungicides Studied for Embryotoxicity in Pregnant Mammals

Agent	Species	Treatment (dose; route; gestational days)	Embryonic effects[a]
Alkyldithiocarbamate salts	Rat	5–50% LD_{50}; oral; various	MAL
Benomyl	Rat	0.01–0.5% LD_{50}; diet; 6–15	None
Captan	Hamster	125–1000 mg/kg; oral; throughout	IGR, IDR
	Rat	500–2000 mg/kg; oral; 8–10	±MAL
	Rabbit	19–75 mg/kg; oral; 6–18	IDR, IGR
	Rabbit	80 mg/kg; oral; 7–12	None
	Rabbit	37.5–75.0 mg/kg; oral; 6–16	MAL
	Dog	15–60 mg/kg; oral; throughout	MAL, IDR
	Dog	30–60 mg/kg; diet; throughout	None
	Monkey	10–75 mg/kg; oral; 21–34	None
Difolatan	Hamster	200–1000 mg/kg; oral; 7 or 8	MAL, IDR
	Rat	100–500 mg/kg; oral; 8–10	None
	Rabbit	37–150 mg/kg; oral; 6–18	±IDR, IGR
	Monkey	6.25–25.0 mg/kg; oral; 6–18	None
Disulfiram	Hamster	125–500 mg/kg; oral; 7 or 8	±IDR
Folpet	Hamster	500–1000 mg/kg; oral; 7 or 8	MAL, IDR
	Rat	100–500 mg/kg; oral; 8–10	None
	Rabbit	19–75 mg/kg; oral; 6–18	IGR, IDR
	Rabbit	75–150 mg/kg; oral; 6–16	None
	Rabbit	80 mg/kg; oral; 7–12	None
	Monkey	10–75 mg/kg; oral; 21–34	None
Griseofulvin	Rat	500 mg/kg; oral; 7–10, 11–14	MAL, IDR
	Rat	125–1500 mg/kg; oral; 6–15	MAL, IDR, IGR
	Cat	500–1000 mg/kg; oral; various	MAL, ?IDR
Pentachlorophenol	Rat	10–30 mg/kg; oral; 6–15	IDR
Pyrithione	Rabbit	20–50 mg/kg; dermal; 7–18	None
	Pig	100–330 mg/kg; dermal; 12–36	None
Tetrachlorophenol	Rat	5–50 mg/kg; oral; 6–15	MAL, IDR, IGR
Thiram	Hamster	125–500 mg/kg; oral; 7 or 8	MAL, IDR, IGR

[a]MAL, Malformations; IDR, intrauterine death and resorption or abortion; IGR, intrauterine growth retardation.
Source: From Wilson (1977).

perbilirubinemia, and hypoproteinemia. Hepatocellular necrosis is the main toxic action of TCDD in the rat, but the platelet effect is also important.

The main target organs of TCDD appear to be the liver of rats and the thymus of rats, guinea pigs, and mice. TCDD causes thymic atrophy in all three species. The liver lesions were extensive enough to account for death only in the rats. Degenerative changes in kidneys and thyroid, lymphoid depletion of the spleen and lymph nodes, hyperplasia of the bladder mucosa, and atrophy of the adrenal zona glomerulosa (in guinea pigs) were also seen. The hepatotoxic changes were characterized by hepatocyte swelling, fatty change, and necrosis. Large multinucleate giant hepatocytes were also found.

Ultrastructurally, proliferation of both the rough and smooth endoplasmic reticulum was seen in rat hepatocytes.

Lymphoid organs (especially thymus) were consistently affected over a wide dose range in all species examined. Decreased thymic weight and cortical thymocytes was a sensitive indicator of TCDD exposure.

After explosion of a chemical plant in Seveso, Italy, toxic compounds, particularly dioxin (TCDD), were released. Epidemiologic investigations of pregnant humans exposed indicate that abortion and malformation rates were not increased. Thus far, postnatal development has been normal. Whether these findings are due to inadequate sample, low-dose exposure (actual dose unknown), or a human embryo

Table 4–11. Herbicides Reported To Be Embryotoxic When Given during Mammalian Pregnancy

Agent	Species	Treatment (dose; route; gestational days)	Embryonic effects[a]
2,4-D	Rat	87.5 mg/kg; oral; 6–15	IGR
	Rat	100–150 mg/kg; oral; 6–15	±MAL
Diquat	Rat	7–14 mg/kg; diet; 8–15	MAL, IGR, IDR
MCPA (ethylester)	Rat	60–100 mg/kg; diet; 8–15	MAL, IGR, IDR
Norea	Hamster	2000 mg/kg; oral; 6–8	IDR
Paraquat	Rat	6.5–13.0 mg/kg; ip; 6–14	±MAL, IDR
Silvex	Rat	100 mg/kg; sc; 6–15	None
2,4,5-T	Mouse	46–103 mg/kg; oral; 6–14	MAL, IDR
	Mouse	15–120 mg/kg; oral; 6–14	MAL, IGR, IDR
	Hamster	400–100 mg/kg; oral; 6–10	MAL, IGR, IDR
	Rat	10–46 mg/kg; oral; 10–15	MAL, IDR
	Rat	60–120 mg/kg; oral; 12–16	None
	Rat	1–50 mg/kg; oral; 6–15	None
	Rat	100–150 mg/kg; oral; 6–15	±MAL, ±IGR
	Rabbit	10–40 mg/kg; oral; 6–18	None
	Sheep	100–113 mg/kg; oral; 14–36	None
	Monkey	5–40 mg/kg × 12; oral; 20–48	None

[a] MAL, Malformations; IDR, Intrauterine death and resorption or abortion; IGR, intrauterine growth retardation.
Source: From Wilson (1977).

response to dioxin that is different from laboratory animals, is unknown (Emerson et al., 1970; Neubert et al., 1973; Dougherty et al., 1973; Harris et al., 1978; Tuchmann-Duplessis, 1978).

Polycyclic Aromatic Hydrocarbons

Products of incomplete combustion of coal, wood, petroleum, and tobacco have been extensively studied as mutagens and carcinogens, but relatively little is known about their teratogenic potential. Virtually no controlled epidemiologic studies on human pregnancy outcome have been done, and there have been remarkably few experimental animal studies. One experiment on pregnant rats fed 1 mg benzo[a]pyrene per gram of diet resulted in many resorptions, fetal deaths, and only one malformed offspring in seven litters (Rigdon and Rennels, 1964). Mice exposed to benzo[a] pyrene had increased infertility (Mackenzie et al., 1979).

In a more extensive study, Mattison (1979) exposed three strains of rats and mice to 3-methylcholanthrene (MC), benz[a] pyrene (BAP), and 7,12-dimethylbenz[a] anthracene (DMBA). In mice almost all pri-

mordial oocytes were destroyed after 6 days of 80 mg/kg of DMBA. Rats were less affected at 100 mg/kg. Mice were also more susceptible to MC with 100% destruction of oocytes after 6 days exposure. BAP was slightly less toxic than MC and DMBA. The rate of primary oocyte destruction was proportional to the activity of ovarian microsomal *P*-450–dependent monooxygenase. No evidence of toxicity to the granulosa or ovarian stroma cells was found. DMBA also destroyed large follicules and oocytes.

REFERENCES

Amcel, P. 1946. Recherche experimentale sur le spina bifida. *Arch. Anat. Microsc. Morphol. Exp.* 36:45–68.

Amin-Zaki, L., Elhassani, S., Majeed, M., Clarkson, T. W., Doherty, R. A., and Greenwood, M. 1974. Intrauterine methylmercury poisoning in Iraq. *Pediatrics* 54:587–595.

Anonymous. 1981. Top 50 chemicals. *Chem. Engineering News* 49:33–38.

Baker, J. B. E. 1969. The effects of drugs on the fetus. *Pharmacol. Rev.* 12:37–90.

Bakir, F., Damluji, S. F., Amin-Zaki, L., Murtadha, M., Khaliki, A., Al-Rawi, N. Y.,

Tikriti, S., Dhahir, H. I., Clarkson, T. W., Smith, J. C., and Doherty, R. A. 1973. Methylmercury poisoning in Iraq. *Science* 181:230–241.

Barltrop, D. 1968. The transfer of lead to the human fetus. In *Mineral metabolism in pediatrics*, eds. D. Barltrop and W. L. Burland, pp. 93–124. Oxford: Blackwell.

Barltrop, D. S., Barret, A. J., and Dingle, J. T. 1971. Subcellular distribution of lead in the rat. *J. Lab. Clin. Invest.* 77:705–712.

Barr, M. J. 1972. The teratogenicity of cadmium chloride in two stocks of Wistar rats. *Teratology* 7:237–242.

Baserga, R. 1981. The cell cycle. *N. Engl. J. Med.* 304:453–459.

Baudin, T. W., Mushak, P., O'Tuama, L. A., and Krigman, M. R. 1975. Blood–brain barrier dysfunction in acute lead encephalopathy. *Environ. Health Perspect.* 12:81–88.

Beaudoin, A. R. 1975. Teratogenicity of sodium arsenate in rats. *Teratology* 10:153–158.

Benirschke, K. 1977. Effects of placental pathology on the embryo and fetus. In *Handbook of teratology*, eds. J. G. Wilson and F. C. Fraser. New York: Plenum Press.

Berlin, M. 1969. Maximum allowable concentrations of mercury compounds. *Arch. Environ. Health* 19:891–905.

Berlin, M., and Ullberg, S. 1963. The fate of Cd 109 in the mouse. *Arch. Environ. Health* 7:686–693.

Blizzard, R. M., Chandler, W. R., Landing, B. H., and Pettit, D. M. 1960. Maternal autoimmunization to thyroid as a probable cause of athyroidic cretinism. *N. Engl. J. Med.* 263:327–336.

Borghese, E. 1958. Organ differentiation in culture. In *The chemical basis of development*, eds. W. McElroy and B. Glass. Baltimore: The Johns Hopkins University Press.

Brent, R. L. 1977. Radiation and other physical agents. In *Handbook of teratology*, vol. 1, eds. J. G. Wilson and F. C. Fraser, pp. 153–223. New York: Plenum Press.

Brent, R. L. 1980. Radiation teratogenesis. *Teratology* 21:281–298.

Brinster, R. L., and Cross, P. C. 1972. Effect of copper on the preimplantation mouse embryo. *Nature* 238:398–399.

Brunn, A., and Brunk, U. 1974. Lead induced injury of in vitro cultured fibroblasts. *Acta Pathol. Microbiol. Scand.* A.82:311–318.

Burk, D., and Beaudoin, A. R. 1978. Arsenate-induced renal agenesis in rats. *Teratology* 16:247–260.

Butt, E. M., Pearson, H. E., and Simonsen, D. G. 1952. The production of meningoceles and cranioschisis in chick embryos with lead nitrate. *Proc. Soc. Exp. Biol. Med.* 79:247–249.

Byers, R. K., and Lord, E. E. 1943. Late effects of lead poisoning on mental development. *Am. J. Dis. Child* 66:471–494.

Cade, J. F. J. 1949. Lithium salts in the treatment of psychotic excitement. *Med. J. Aust.* 2:349–352.

Carnes, W. H. 1971. Role of copper in connective tissue metabolism. *Fed. Proc.* 30:995–1000.

Carpenter, S. J., and Ferm, V. H. 1977. Embryopathic effects of lead in the hamster. *Lab. Invest.* 37:369–385.

Chaube, S. 1973. Zinc and cadmium in normal human embryos and fetuses: Analysis by atomic absorption spectrophotometry. *Arch. Environ. Health* 26:237–240.

Chaube, S., and Murphy, M. L. 1969. The teratogenic effects of 5-fluorocytosine in the rat. *Cancer Res.* 29:534–557.

Chen, W. -J., Body, R. L., and Mottet, N. K. 1979. Some effects of continuous low dose congenital exposure to methylmercury on organ growth in the rat fetus. *Teratology* 20:31–36.

Choie, D. D., and Richter, G. W. 1972. Lead poisoning: Rapid formation of intranuclear inclusions. *Science* 177:1194–1195.

Clarkson, T. W. 1971. Epidemiological and experimental aspects of lead and mercury contamination of food. *Food Cosmet. Toxicol.* 9:229–243.

Clarkson, T. W. 1976. Quantitative measure of the toxicity of mercury in man. In *Essential and toxic elements*, ed. A. S. Prasad, pp. 274–296. New York: Academic Press.

Clarren, S., Alvord, E. C., Sumi, M., Streissguth, A. P., and Smith, D. W. 1978. Brain malformations related to prenatal exposure to alcohol. *Pediatrics* 92:64–67.

Clarren, S., and Smith, D. W. 1978. Fetal alcohol syndrome. *N. Engl. J. Med.* 298:1063–1067.

Denckar, L., Danielsson, B., Khayat, A., and Lindgren, A. 1983. Disposition of metals in the embryo and fetus, pp. 607–633. In *Reproductive and developmental toxicity of metals*, eds. T. W. Clarkson, G. Nordberg, and P. R. Sager. New York: Plenum Press.

Dial, N. A. 1974. Methylmercury: Teratogenic and lethal effects on frog embryos. *Teratology* 13:327–334.

Dial, N. A. 1978. Methylmercury: Some effects on embryogenesis in the Japanese Medaka, *Oryzias latipes. Teratology* 17:83–92.

Di Carlo, F. J. 1980. Syndromes of cardiovascular malformations induced by copper citrate in hamsters. *Teratology* 21:89–101.

Dougherty, W. H., Coulston, F., and Goldberg, L. 1973. Non-teratogenicity of 2,4,5-trichlorophenoxyacetic acid in monkeys. *Toxicologist* 12:7.

Eastman, N. J. 1931. The arsenic content of the human placenta following arsphenamine therapy. *Am. J. Obstet. Gynecol.* 21:60–64.

Emerson, J. L., Thompson, D. J., Gerbig, C. G., and Robinson, V. B. 1970. Teratogenic study of 2,4,5-trichlorophenoxyacetic acid in the rat. *Toxicol. Appl. Pharmacol.* 17:317–323.

Fabro, S. 1981. Biochemical basis of thalidomide teratogenicity. In *The biochemical basis of chemical teratogenesis*, ed. M. R. Juchau, pp. 159–173. New York: Elsevier-North Holland.

Fabro, S., and Seiber, S. M. 1968. Penetration of drugs into the rabbit blastocyst before implantation. In *International Symposium on the Fetal Placental Unit*, eds. A. Pecile and I. C. Phinz, pps. 313–320. Amsterdam: Excerpta Medica International Congress Series 183.

Fell, H. B. 1939. The origin and developmental mechanics of the avian sternum. *Philos. Trans. R. Soc. Lond. (Biol.)* 229:407–459.

Fell, H. B. 1953. Metaplasia produced in cultures of chick extoderm by high vitamin A. *J. Physiol.* 119:470–488.

Ferm, V. H. 1972. The teratogenic effects of metals on mammalian embryos. *Adv. Teratol.* 5:51–76.

Ferm, V. H. 1977. Arsenic as a teratogenic agent. *Environ. Health Perspect.* 19:215–217.

Ferm, V. H., and Carpenter, S. J. 1967. Developmental malformations resulting from administration of lead salts. *J. Exp. Molec. Pathol.* 7:208–213.

Ferm, V. H., and Carpenter, S. J. 1968a. Malformation induced by sodium arsenate. *J. Reprod. Fertil.* 17:199–201.

Ferm, V. H., and Carpenter, S. J. 1968b. The relationship of cadmium and zinc in experimental mammalian teratogenesis. *Lab Invest.* 18:429–432.

Ferm, V. H., and Hanlon, D. P. 1974. Toxicity of copper salts in hamster embryonic development. *Biol. Reprod.* 11:97–101.

Ferm, V. H., Hanlon, D. P., and Urban, J. 1969. The permeability of hamster placenta to radioactive cadmium. *J. Embryol. Exp. Morphol.* 22:102–133.

Ferm, V. H., and Kilham, L. 1977. Synergistic teratogenic effects of arsenic and hyperthermia in hamsters. *Environ. Res.* 14:483–486.

Ferm, V. H., Saxon, A., and Smith, B. M. 1972. The teratogenic profile of sodium arsenate in the Golden hamster. *Arch. Environ. Health* 22:557–560.

Fleming, H. S., and Greenfield, V. S. 1954. Changes in the teeth and jaws of neonatal mice after administration of NaF and CaF_2 to the female parent during gestation. *J. Dent. Res.* 33:780–788.

Ford, J. K., Eyring, E. J., and Anderson, C. E. 1968. Thallium chondrodystrophy in chick embryos. *J. Bone Joint Surg.* 50:687–700.

Fowler, B. A. 1974. Lysosomal uptake of mercury in renal proximal tubule cells of rats given methylmercury. *Fed. Proc.* 33:257.

Fowler, B. A. 1977. Cellular mechanisms of arsenical toxicity. In *Advances in modern toxicology*, vol. 2, eds. R. A. Goyer and M. A. Mehlman, pp. 96–108. New York: John Wiley & Sons.

Gale, T. F., and Ferm, V. H. 1971. Embryopathic effects of mercuric salts. *Life Sci.* 10:1341–1347.

Gerber, G. B., and Maes, J. 1978. Heme synthesis in the lead intoxicated mouse embryo. *Toxicology* 9:173–179.

Gibson, J. E., and Becker, B. A. 1970. Placental transfer, embryotoxicity, and teratogenicity of thallium sulfate in normal and potassium-deficient rats. *Toxicol. Appl. Pharmacol.* 16:120–132.

Gill, W. B., Gebhard, F. B., Schumacker, M. D., and Bibbo, M. 1976. Structural and functional abnormalities in the sex organs of male offspring of mothers treated with diethylstilbestrol (DES). *J. Reprod. Med.* 16:147–153.

Glucksmann, A. 1951. Cell deaths in normal vertebrate ontogeny. *Biol. Rev.* 26:59–86.

Goyer, R. A. 1971. Lead toxicity: A problem in environmental pathology. *Am. J. Pathol.* 64:167–179.

Goyer, R. A., Krall, A., and Kimball, J. P. 1968. The renal tubule in lead poisoning. *Lab. Invest.* 29:78–83.

Goyer, R. A., and Rhyne, B. C. 1975. Toxic changes in mitochondrial membranes and mitochondrial function. *Pathobiol. Cell Membranes* 1:383–413.

Grobstein, C. 1955. Inductive interaction in the

development of the mouse Metanephros. *J. Exp. Zool.* 130:319–339.

Grobstein, C. 1957. Some transmission characteristics of the tubule induction influence on mouse metanephrogenic mesenchyme. *Exp. Cell Res.* 13:575–587.

Grobstein, C. 1967. Mechanisms of organogenetic tissue interaction, Monograph No. 26. *J. Natl. Cancer Inst.*, pp. 279–295.

Gunn, S. A., Gould, T. C., and Anderson, W. A. D. 1967. Specific response of mesenchymal tissue to carcinogenesis by cadmium. *Arch. Pathol.* 83:493–499.

Hall, B. K. 1972. Thallium induced achondroplasia in the embryonic chick. *Dev. Biol.* 28:47–60.

Hamilton, W. 1976. Endemic cretinism. *Dev. Med. Child. Neurol.* 18:386–391.

Hammar, S., and Mottet, N. K. 1971. Tetrazolium salt and electron microscopic studies of cellular degeneration and necrosis in the interdigital areas of the developing chick limb. *J. Cell Sci.* 8:229–251.

Harada, Y. 1968. Congenital (or fetal) minamata disease. In *Minamata disease,* ed. M. Kutsuna, pp. 87–96. Kumamoto, Japan: Kumamoto University Press.

Harris, M. W., Moore, J. A., Vos, J. G., and Gupta, B. N. 1973. General biologic effects of TCDD in laboratory animals. *Environ. Health Perspect.* 5:101–162.

Harris, S. J., Cecil, H. C., and Bittman, J. 1978. Embryotoxic effects of polybrominated biphenyls (PBB) in rats. *Environ. Health Perspect.* 23:295–300.

Hassan, A. I., Aref, G. H, and Kassem, A. S. 1968. Congenital iodide induced goiter with hypothyroidism. *Arch. Dis. Child.* 43:702–710.

Herbst, A. L., Scully, R. E., Robboy, S. J., Welch, W. R., and Cole, P. 1977. Abnormal development of the female genital tract following prenatal exposure to diethylstilbestrol. *Cold Springs Harbor Symp. Quant. Biol.* 4:399–412.

Hood, R. D., and Bishop, S. L., 1972. Teratogenic effects of sodium arsenate in mice. *Arch. Env. Health.* 24:62–65.

Hunter, C. G. 1965. Embryopathies associated with exposure to pesticides. In *Embryopathic activity of drugs,* ed. J. M. Robson. Boston: Little, Brown.

Inouye, M., Hoshino, K., and Murakami, U. 1972. Effects of methylmercury chloride on embryonic and fetal development in rats and mice. *Annu. Rep. Res. Inst. Environ. Med. (Nagoya Univ.)* 19:69–74.

Johansen, K. T. 1971. Lithium teratogenicity. *Lancet* 1:1026–1027.

Jones, K., and Smith, D. W. 1973. Recognition of the fetal alcohol syndrome in early infancy. *Lancet* 2:999–1001.

Juchau, M. R. 1981. Enzymatic bioactivation and inactivation of chemical teratogens and transplacental carcinogenesis/mutagenesis. In *Biochemical basis of chemical teratogenesis,* ed. M. R. Juchau, Chapter 2. New York: Elsevier-North Holland.

Jung, E. G., Trachsel, B., and Immich, H. 1969. Arsenic as an inhibitor of the enzymes concerned in the cellular recovery (dark repair). *Germ. Med. Monthly* 14:614–616.

Kalter, H., and Warkany, J. 1983. Congenital malformations. Etiologic factors and their role in prevention. *N. Engl. J. Med.* 308:424–431.

Khera, K. S., and Tabacova, S. A. 1973. Effects of methylmercury chloride on the progeny of mice and rats treated before and during gestation. *Food Cosmet. Toxicol.* 11:245–254.

Klevay, L. M. 1976. Pharmacology and toxicology of heavy metals: Arsenic. *Pharmacol. Ther.* 1:189–209.

Kohler, E., Merker, H. J., Ehmke, W., and Wojnorwica, F. 1972. Growth kinetics of mammalian embryos during the stage of differentiation. *Naunyn-Schmiedebergs Arch. Pharmacol.* 272:169–181.

Krous, H. F. 1981. Fetal alcohol syndrome: A dilemma of maternal alcoholism. In *Pathology annual,* part 1, eds. S. C. Sommers and P. P. Rosen, pp. 295–313. New York: Appleton-Century-Crofts.

Kusell, M., O'Cheskey, S., and Gerschenson, L. E. 1978. Cellular and molecular toxicology of lead. Effects of lead on cultured cell proliferation. *J. Toxicol. Environ. Health* 4:503–513.

Kutsuna, M., ed. 1968. *Minamata disease.* Kumamoto, Japan: Kumamoto University Press.

Labbe, R., and Hubbard, N. 1961. Metal specificity of the iron-protoporphyrin chelating enzymes from rat liver. *Biochim. Biophys. Acta* 52:130–135.

Lucier, G. W., Fowler, B. A., and Folsom, M. D. 1973. Methylmercury-induced changes in rat liver microsomes. *Environ. Health Perspect.* 4:102–106.

Lugo, G., Cassady, G., and Palmiseno, P. 1969.

Acute maternal arsenic intoxication with neonatal death. *Am. J. Dis. Child.* 117:328–330.

MacKenzie, K. M., Lucier, E. W., and McLachian, J. A. 1979. Infertility in mice exposed prenatally to benzo[a]pyrene. *Teratology* 19:37A.

Mattison, D. R. 1979. Difference in sensitivity in rat and mouse primordial oocytes to destruction by polycyclic aromatic hydrocarbons. *Chem. Biol. Interact.* 28:133–137.

Maugh, T. H. 1978. Chemicals: How many are there? *Science* 199:162.

McBride, W. G. 1961. Teratogenic action of thalidomide. *Lancet* 2:1358.

Morrissey, R. E., and Mottet, N. K. 1983. Arsenic-induced exencephaly in the mouse and associated lesions occurring during neurulation. *Teratology* 28:399–411.

Moscona, A. A. 1973. Cell aggregation. In *Cell biology in medicine*, ed. E. E. Bittar, Chapter 17. New York: John Wiley & Sons.

Mossman, H. W. 1937. Comparative morphogenesis of the fetal membranes and accessory uterine structures. *Contrib. Embryol.* 26:129–246.

Mottet, N. K. 1952. The effects of the removal of the somatopleure on the development of motor and sensory neurons in the spinal cord and ganglia. *J. Comp. Neurol.* 96:519–553.

Mottet, K. and Barron, D. H. 1954. Some effects of the peripheral field on the cytochemical differentiation of neurons. Yale J. Biol. Med. 26:275–284.

Mottet, N. K. 1974. Effects of chronic low-dose exposure of rat fetuses to methylmercury hydroxide. *Teratology* 10:173–189.

Mottet, N. K. 1981. Biochemical basis of trace metal teratogenesis. In *Biochemical basis of teratogenesis*, ed. M. R. Juchau. New York: Elsevier-North Holland.

Mottet, N. K., and Hammar, S. P. 1972. Ribosome crystals in necrotizing cells from the posterior necrotizing zone of the developing chick limb. *J. Cell Sci.* 11:403–414.

Mulvihill, J. E., Ganam, S. H., and Ferm, V. H. 1970. Facial formation in normal and cadmium-treated golden hamster. *J. Embryol. Exp. Morphol.* 24:393–403.

Munch, J. C. 1934. Human thallotoxicosis. *J.A.M.A.* 102:1929–1934.

Murakami, U. 1971. Embryo-fetotoxic effect of some organic mercury compounds. *Annu. Rep. Res. Inst. Environ. Med. (Nagoya Univ.)* 18:33–43.

Murray, I. P. C., and Steward, D. H. 1967. Iodide goitre. *Lancet* 1:922–925.

Nelson, M. N., and Forfar, J. O. 1971. Association between drugs administered during pregnancy and congenital abnormalities of the fetus. *Br. J. Med.* 1:523–527.

Neubert, D., Zens, P., and Rothenwallner, A. 1973. Survey of the teratogenic effects of TCDD in mammalian species. *Environ. Health Perspect.* 5(18):67–71.

Nonaka, I. 1969. An electron microscopical study on the experimental congenital Minamata disease in the rat. *Kumamoto Med. J.* 22:27–40.

Olson, C. F., and Massaro, J. E. 1975. Methylmercury induced cleft palate and alterations in palatine C-AMP levels. *Fed. Proc.* 35:1758.

Olson, F. C., and Massaro, E. J. 1977. Effects of methylmercury on murine fetal amino acid uptake, protein synthesis and palate closures. *Teratology* 16:187–194.

Oster, G., and Salgo, M. P. 1976. Copper in mammalian reproduction. *Adv. Pharmacol. Chemother.* 14:327–382.

Peller, S. 1969. *Cancer in childhood and youth.* London: J. Wright & Sons, Ltd.

Presaud, T. V. N. 1979. *Perinatal pathology.* Springfield, Ill.: Charles C Thomas.

Press, M. F. 1977. Neuronal development in the cerebellum of lead poisoned neonatal rats. *Acta Neuropathol. (Berl.)* 40:259–268.

Reed, D., Drawley, J., Faro, S. N., Pierper, S. J., and Kurland, L. T. 1963. Thallotoxicosis. J.A.M.A. 183:96–102.

Rhyne, B. C., and Goyer, R. A. 1971. Cytochrome content of kidney mitochondria in experimental lead poisoning. *Exp. Mol. Pathol.* 14:386–391.

Rice, J. M., ed. 1979. *Perinatal carcinogenesis.* National Cancer Institute Monograph No. 51. Washington, D.C.: U.S. Government Printing Office.

Rice, J. R. 1973. An overview of transplacental carcinogenesis. *Teratology* 8:113–126.

Ridgeway, L. P., and Karnofsky, D. A. 1952. The effects of metals on chick embryos. *Ann. N.Y. Acad. Sci.* 55:203–215.

Rigdon, R. H., and Rennels, E. G. 1964. The effect of feeding benzo[a]pyrene on reproduction in the rat. *Experimentia* 20:224–226.

Ross, O. B., Philips, P. H., Bohstedt, G., and Cunha, T. J. 1944. Congenital malformation, syndactylism, talipes and paralysis agitans of nutritional origin in the swine. *J. Anim. Sci.* 3:405–414.

Rossman, T., Meyn, M. A., and Troll, W. 1975. Effects of sodium arsenate on the survival of UV-irradiated *Escherichia coli. Mutat. Res.* 30:157–162.

Rutter, W. J., Pictet, R. L., and Morris, T. W. 1973. Toward molecular mechanisms of developmental practices. *Ann. Rev. Biochem.* 42:601–618.

Sager, P. R., Doherty, R. A., and Rodier, P.M. 1982. Effects of Methylmercury on developing mouse cerebellar cortex. *Exp. Neurol.* 77:179–193.

Sager, P. A., Doherty, R. A,., and Olmstead, J. B. 1983. Interactions of methylmercury with microtubules in cultured cells in vitro. *Exp. Cell Res.* 146:127–138.

Saunders, J. W. 1966. Death in embryonic systems. *Science* 154:1–9.

Schlaepfer, W. W. 1971. Experimental alteration of neurofilaments and neurotubules by calcium and other ions. *Exp. Cell Res.* 67:73–80.

Schliwa, M. 1976. The role of divalent cations in the regulation of microtubule assembly. *J. Cell Biol.* 70:527–540.

Schour, I., and Smith, M. C. 1935. Mottled teeth: An experimental and histologic analysis. *J. Am. Dent. Assoc.* 22:798–813.

Schroeder, H. A., and Mitchener, M. 1971. Toxic effects of trace elements on the reproduction of mice and rats. *Arch. Environ. Health* 23:102–106.

Schull, W. J., Otake, M., and Neel, J. V. 1981. Genetic effects of the atomic bomb: A reappraisal. *Science* 213:1220–1227.

Schultz, R. L. 1970. Placental transport. *Obstet. Gynecol. Surv.* 25:979–1019.

Semba, R. 1976. Cardiovascular malformations found in 1286 externally normal human embryos alive in utero. *Teratology* 13:341–344.

Shepard, T. H. 1980. *Catalog of teratogenic agents*, 3rd Ed. Baltimore: The Johns Hopkins University Press.

Sirover, M. A., and Loeb, L. A. 1976. Infidelity of DNA synthesis in vitro: Screening for potential metal mutagens or carcinogens. *Science* 194:1434–1436.

Skerfving, S., Hansson, K., and Lindsten, J. 1970. Chromosome breakage in humans exposed to methylmercury through fish consumption. *Arch. Environ. Health* 21:133–139.

Skerfving, S., Hansson, K., Mangs, C., Lindsten,

J., and Ryman, N. 1974. Methylmercury induced chromosome damage in man. *Environ. Res.* 7:83–98.

Smith, C. M., and Smith, H. V. 1935. The occurrence of mottled enamel on the temporary teeth. *J. Am. Dent. Assoc.* 22:814–817.

Southard, J. H., and Nitisewojo, P. 1974. Mercurial toxicity and the pertubation of the mitochondrial control system. *Fed. Proc.* 33:2147–2154.

Spemann, H. 1938. *Embryonic development and induction.* New Haven, Conn.: Yale University Press.

Stanbury, J. B., and Querido, A. 1957. On the nature of endemic cretinism. *J. Clin. Endocrinol.* 17:803–904.

Stevens, D. H. 1975. *Comparative placentation.* New York: Academic Press.

Stevens W. J., and Barbier, F. 1976. Thalliumintoxicatic gedurende de zgangerschap. *Acta Clin. Belg.* 31:188–192.

Streissguth, A. P., 1976. Psychological handicaps in children with fetal alcohol syndrome. *Ann. N.Y. Acad. Sci.* 273:140–145.

Streissguth, A. P., Landesman-Dwyer, S., Martin, J., and Smith, D. W. 1980. Teratongenic effects of alcohol in humans and laboratory animals. *Science* 209:353–361.

Sunderman, F. W., Jr. 1977. A review of the metabolism and toxicity of nickel. *Ann. Clin. Lab. Sci.* 7:377–398.

Sunderman, F. W., Jr., Shen, S. K., Mitchell, J. M., Allpass, P. R., and Danjanov, I. 1978. Embryotoxicity and fetal toxicity of nickel in rats. *Toxicol. Appl. Pharmacol.* 43:381–390.

Tejning, S. 1969. Accumulation of mercury in the human fetus. In *Methylmercury*, Bulletin No. 4, ed. G. Lofroth, pp. 203–218. Stockholm: Swedish National Research Council.

Timson, J., and Price, D. J. 1971. Lithium and mitosis. *Lancet* 2:93–95.

Tomatis, L., and Mohr, U. 1973. *Transplacental carcinogenesis*, IARC Scientific Publication No. 4. Lyons, France: International Agency for Research on Cancer.

Toole, B. P. 1973. Hyaluronate and hyaluronidase in morphogenesis and differentiation. *Am. Zool.* 13:1061–1065.

Troupe, G. M. 1971. II. Growth and development. *Hum. Pathol.* 2:493–499.

Tuchmann-Duplessis, H. 1975. *Drug effects on the fetus.* Sydney, Australia: Adis Press.

Tuchmann-Duplessis, H. 1978. The Seveso accident: Present data on the human pre- and postnatal development. *Bull. Acad. Natl. Med.* 162:389–394.

Underhill, F. R., and Amatruda, F. G. 1923. The transmission of arsenic from mother to fetus. *J.A.M.A* 81:2009–2012.

U.S., Dept. of Health and Human Services, Public Health Service. 1981. *FDA drug bulletin*, HFI-22. Rockville, Md.: Food and Drug Administration.

U.S., Geological Survey. 1970. *Mercury in the environment*, professional paper No. 713. Washington, D.C.: U.S. Government Printing Office.

Von Lenz, W. Die Thalidomid Embryopathie. *Dtsch. Med. Wochenschr.* 86:2555–2556.

Von Lenz, W. and Knapp, K 1962. Die Thalidomid Embryopathie. *Dtsch. Med. Wochensch.* 87:1232–1242.

Waddell, W. J., and Marlowe, C. 1981. Biochemical regulation of the accessibility of teratogens to the developing embryo. In *Biochemical basis of chemical teratogenesis*, ed., M. R. Juchau, Chapter 1. New York: Elsevier-North Holland.

Warkany, J. F. 1971. Endemic goiter and cretinism. *Congenital malformations*, pp. 102–124, Chapter 12. Chicago: Year Book Medical Publishers.

Warren, S., Fanger, M., and Neet, K. E. 1980. Inhibition of biological activity of mouse B-nerve growth factor by monoclonal antibody. *Science* 210:910–912.

Webb, F. T. G. 1973. The contraceptive action of the copper I.U.D. in the rat. *J. Reprod. Fertil.* 32:429–439.

Weinstein, M R. 1976. The international register of lithium babies. *Drug Info. J.* April/Sept. pp. 94–100.

Weinstein, M. R., and Goldfield, M D. 1975. Cardiovascular malformations with lithium use during pregnancy. *Am. J. Psychiatry* 132:529–531.

Weis, P., and Weis, J. S. 1977. Methylmercury teratogenesis in the killifish, *Fundulus heteroclitus. Teratology* 16:317–326.

Weller, C. V. 1915. The blastophthoric effect of chronic lead poisoning. *J. Med. Res.* 33:271–293.

Wessels, N. K., and Evans, J. 1968. Ultrastructural studies of early morphogenesis and cytodifferentiation in the embryonic mammalian pancreas. *Dev. Biol.* 17:413–446.

Wide, M., and Nilsson, O. 1977. Differential susceptibility of the embryo to inorganic lead during peri-implantation in the mouse. *Teratology* 16:272–276.

Wilson, J. G. 1977. Environmental chemicals. In *Handbook of teratology*, Vol. 1, eds. J. G. Wilson and F. C. Fraser, pp. 357–366. New York: Plenum Press.

Wright, T. L., Hoffman, L. H., and Davies, J. 1967. Teratogenic effects of lithium in rats. *Teratology* 4:151–156.

Young, M., Ogen, J., Blanchard, M. H., Asdourian, H., Amos, H., and Arnason, B. G. W. 1975. Secretion of a nerve growth factor by primary chick fibroblast cultures. *Science* 187:361–362.

Zavon, M. R., Tye, R., and Laton, L. 1969. Chlorinated hydrocarbon insecticide content of the neonate. *Ann. N.Y. Acad. Sci.* 160:196–200.

Zimmerman, E. F., Wee, E. L., Phillips, N., and Roberts, N. 1981. The presence of serotonin in the palate just prior to shelf elevation. *J. Embryol. Exp. Morphol.* 64:233–250.

II
Systemic Reactions to Injury by Environmental Agents

5

Reproductive Toxicity

Robert A. Ettlin and Robert L. Dixon

The complicated biologic interactions on which successful mammalian reproduction depends presents many targets for toxic chemicals (Figure 5-1). During the past decade, laboratory and clinical efforts have intensified considerably to identify and describe more readily those chemicals in our environment that, by perturbing essential molecular and cellular processes, result in morphologic and functional alterations. Our understanding of the underlying biologic mechanisms of reproductive toxicity remains incomplete, however, as does the predictability of our current test approaches. Yet advances have been made. As this chapter shows, we now have a clearer understanding of the biologic properties of the various cells and tissues that comprise the male and female reproductive systems. We also have a greater appreciation of their unique developmental and chemical susceptibilities. Likewise, our understanding of the events involved in fertilization and implantation continues to increase. We know more about the pharmacokinetic (toxicokinetic) factors that determine the amount of active chemical that reaches its site of toxicity, and we know more about how the organism adapts to chemicals and recovers from damage. We are even beginning to understand the molecular dynamics of the toxic event and its direct and indirect consequences.

Experimental pathology plays an important role in all of these activities. Improved fixation and embedding procedures allow better preservation of the tissue and thinner sectioning. These methods aid the investigator in recognizing more clearly the subtle morphologic changes that occur. Newer techniques of microscopy, including scanning electron microscopes, also provide new opportunities. Modern pathology is no longer a descriptive science. Rather, it represents a multidisciplinary effort not only to describe alterations in biologic structure, but also to understand the etiology of chemically induced disease. In the near future, sensitive "markers" should allow the identification of toxic effects before the expression of serious and often irreversible clinical endpoints.

This chapter first outlines the components of the male and female reproductive systems and the events of fertilization. After mentioning those factors that modulate toxicity and differential tissue susceptibility, we summarize approaches for detecting gonadal and accessory sex organ toxicity. The text emphasizes the manner in which environmental agents affect reproduction and attempts to describe those agents af-

129

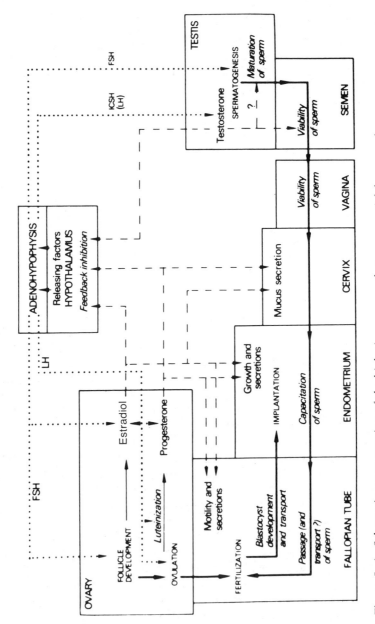

Figure 5–1. Schematic representation of the biologic processes that are essential for normal reproduction. (From Bowman and Rand, 1980.)

fecting humans and to define their mechanisms of action. Wherever possible, we indicate the relationship of biochemical and morphologic effects induced by chemicals and the functional consequences of such interactions. Finally, we discuss the sensitivity and specificity of both laboratory and clinical approaches for defining hazards and analyzing risk to human health. For our purposes here, we define reproduction to include those events from earliest gametogenesis through implantation.

Structure, Function, and Targets for Toxicity

Hypothalamo-Pituitary-Gonadal Axis

Hypothalamic neuroendocrine neurons secrete a specific gonadotropin-releasing hormone (LHRH) into the hypophyseal portal system, which carries it to the adenohypophysis where it acts to stimulate the release of anterior pituitary gonadotropins. These neurons have terminals containing monoamines (norepinephrine, dopamine, serotonin). If the hypophyseal–pituitary control system is excessively stimulated, the following abnormalities may occur: delayed puberty, hypogonadism, crypt orchidism, and functional amenorrhea. If these control systems are inhibited, precocious puberty, infertility (anovulation, arrest of spermatogenesis), luteolysis, endometriosis, premature menopause, benign prostatic hypertrophy, and hormone-dependent tumors may develop. The effects of reserpine or chlorpromazine and other agents that alter the influence of brain monoamines on reproductive function will be discussed later in this chapter.

Follicle-stimulating hormone (FSH) probably acts primarily on the Sertoli's cells of the testis, but it also appears to stimulate the mitotic activity of spermatogonia. Luteinizing hormone (LH) stimulates steroidogenesis. A testicular defect leading to decreased production of sperm or testosterone will tend to be reflected in increased levels of FSH and LH in serum because of the lack of the "negative feedback" effect.

The same cell type in the pituitary produces and secretes LH and FSH. In infancy and prepuberty their concentrations in plasma are measurable but quite low. At puberty, gonadotropin secretion increases, probably as a result of diminished feedback inhibition of secretion by sex steroids. In men, gonadotropin concentrations are relatively constant, while rates of secretion in women are somewhat higher and vary according to the phases of the menstrual cycle. In some gonadal disorders, in postmenopausal women, and to some extent in elderly men, concentrations of gonadotropins increase because of diminished concentrations of sex steroids and resultant loss of their feedback inhibition on the pituitary and brain.

Prolactin promotes mammary development during pregnancy in humans followed by lactogenesis during lactation. This is the only recognized function for prolactin. Whereas the identification of prolactin receptors in mammary tissue corresponds with the necessary lactogenic function of prolactin, the finding of prolactin receptors in other tissues has not been associated with a complementary physiologic role for prolactin. A role for prolactin in steroid biosynthesis has been suggested. Hyperprolactinemia may result from the loss of inhibitory control due to disrupted dopamine synthesis or activity in the hypothalamus. The number of drugs associated with hyperprolactinemia continues to grow.

The sensitive and complex hypothalamo–pituitary—gonadal system presents several targets for environmental and industrial chemicals, and there are many drugs thought to alter the normal functional state. It is well established that the effects of toxic agents on neuroendocrine processes in the brain or pituitary gland may indirectly inhibit spermatogenesis, alter steroidogenesis, cause abnormal sexual development, and result in sterility. Possible sites where chemicals may interfere with the hypothalamo–pituitary–gonadal axis are shown in Figure 5-2.

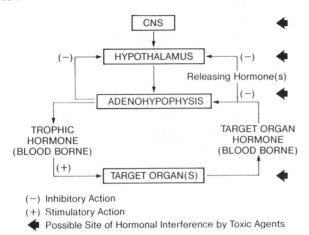

Figure 5–2. Hypothalamo–pituitary–gonadal interrelationships. The heavy arrow indicates possible targets for toxicity. (From Thomas and Bell, 1982.)

MALE

The male component of an effective reproductive system functions to produce adequate quantities of viable sperm with normal chromosomes in an appropriate fluid milieu and to ejaculate this semen into the female vagina. Human male infertility is usually associated with faulty semen, a varicocele, or an obstruction of the vas deferens.

Testis

The two testes can each be divided into major compartments: the seminiferous tubules, which produce sperm, and the interstitium (interstitial space), which produces steroids (Figure 5-3). Kerr and de Kretser (1981) have recently reviewed the cytology of the human testis.

SEMINIFEROUS TUBULES. The seminiferous tubules contain germ cells at different stages of differentiation, as well as Sertoli's cells. In a cyclic fashion, spermatogonia A of certain areas of a tubule become committed to divide synchronously, and the cohorts of the resulting cells differentiate in unison. Thus, a synchronous population of developing germ cells occupies a defined area within a seminiferous tubule. Cells within each cohort are connected by intercellular bridges.

In many laboratory species, a cross section through a seminiferous tubule contains a single cellular association. However, this

is not true for humans, where different associations are intermingled in a mosaic-like fashion. Depending on the species and the observer, from 6 to 14 cellular associations have been discerned. Each cellular association contains four or five types of germ cells organized in a specific layered pattern. Each

Figure 5–3. Cross section of seminiferous tubules and interstitial spaces. ① basement membrane. ② Sertoli's cell (nucleus often perpendicular to 1). ③ spermatogonium (ovoid nucleus parallel to 1). ④ spermatocyte (large nucleus with condensed chromosomes). ⑤ young spermatid (aligned mitochondria clearly mark cell boundary). ⑥ late spermatid (elongated and dark nucleus). ⑦ tubular lumen (with tails of 6). ⑧ blood vessel (empty because of fixation by perfusion). ⑨ interstitial cell (Leydig's cell). ⑩ lymphatic space.

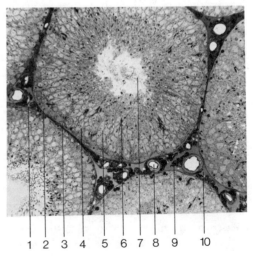

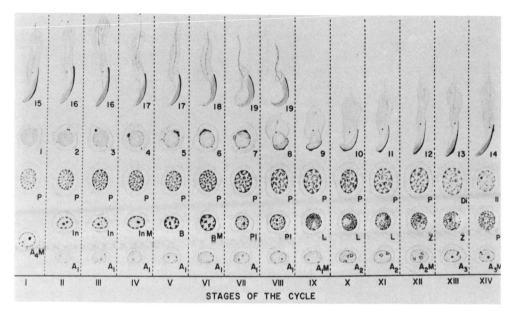

Figure 5–4. Schematic representation of spermatogenesis (horizontally from bottom left to top right) and of the 14 cellular associations stages I–XIV) observed in the seminiferous epithelium of the rat, which are represented vertically. The figure represents a composite of the different cross sections found in the seminiferous spermatogenic cycle. If the same point in a tubule could be observed during a full cycle, the 14 different patterns of cellular associations would be observed in the sequence indicated.

layer represents one cellular generation. The 14 cellular associations observed in seminiferous epithelium in the rat are presented in Figure 5-4 (Clermont, 1972).

If a fixed point within a seminiferous tubule could be viewed as the germ cells develop, it would sequentially acquire the appearance of each of the cellular associations characteristic of that species. This progression through the series of cellular associations would continue to repeat itself in a predictable fashion. The interval required for one complete series of cellular associations to appear at one point within a tubule is termed the *duration* of the cycle of the seminiferous epithelium. The duration of one cycle of the seminiferous epithelium depends on, and is thus equal to, the cell turnover rate of spermatogonia. It takes approximately 13 days to complete one cycle in the rat, approximately 16 days in man. Spermatids, originating from spermatogonia committed to differentiate approximately 4.5 cycles earlier, are continuously released from the germinal epithelium. Ta-

ble 5-1 compares the duration of the seminiferous epithelial cycle and other aspects of seminiferous tubule function for various species (Galbraith et al., 1982).

The spermatogenic process offers unique stages of susceptibility to toxic chemicals. The replication of spermatogonia necessitates intensive DNA, RNA, and protein synthesis and considerable DNA synthesis also takes place in early spermatocytes preparing for meiosis. Protein synthesis is high in preleptotene and pachytene primary spermatocytes as well as in elongated spermatids; RNA synthesis is particularly high in late primary spermatocytes, secondary spermatocytes, and early spermatids. Finally, morphogenesis of spermatids is a complex process which, when disturbed, may result in spermatid malformation or degeneration.

Adjoining Sertoli's cells form a biologic barrier (the blood–testis barrier), which partitions the seminiferous epithelium into two compartments: a basal compartment containing spermatogonia and early sper-

Table 5–1. Criteria for Spermatogenesis in Laboratory Animals and Man

Criterion	Mouse	Rat	Rabbit (New Zealand White)	Dog (beagle)	Monkey (rhesus)	Man
Duration of cycle of seminiferous epithelium (days)	8.6	12.9	10.7	13.6	9.5	16.0
Life span (days) of:						
B-Type spermatogonia	1.5	2.0	1.3	4.0	2.9	6.3
L + Z spermatocytes[a]	4.7	7.8	7.3	5.2	6.0	9.2
P + D spermatocytes[a]	8.3	12.2	10.7	13.5	9.5	15.6
Golgi spermatids	1.7	2.9	2.1	6.9	1.8	7.9
Cap spermatids	3.5	5.0	5.2	3.0	3.7	1.6
Fraction of a life span as:						
B-Type spermatogonia	0.11	0.10	0.08	0.19	0.19	0.25
Primary spermatocyte	1.00	1.00	1.00	1.00	1.00	1.00
Round spermatid	0.41	0.40	0.43	0.48	0.35	0.38
Testes weight (g)	0.2	3.7	6.4	12.0	49	34
Daily sperm production						
Per gram testis (10^6/g)	28	24	25	20	23	4.4
Per male (10^6)	5	86	160	300	1100	125
Sperm reserves in cauda (at sexual rest; 10^6)	49	440	1600	?[b]	5700	420
Transit time (days) through (at sexual rest)						
Caput + corpus epididymids	3.1	3.0	3.0	?	4.9	1.8
Cauda epididymids	5.6	5.1	9.7	?	5.6	3.7

[a] D, diplotene; L, leptotene; P, pachytene; Z, zygotene.
[b] Data are unclear or inadequate.
Source: From Galbraith et al. (1982).

matocytes, and an adluminal compartment containing the more developed spermatogenic cells. A third compartment, the intermediate one, is represented by the passage of leptotene to zygotene primary spermatocytes through the occluding cellular junctions. An ionic gradient is maintained between the two tubular compartments, and a unique chemical milieu exists. Nutrients, hormones, and other chemicals must pass either between or through Sertoli's cells in order to diffuse from one compartment to another. Germinal cells are either situated between adjacent pairs of Sertoli's cells or embedded in their luminal margins. The release of sperm from the germinal epithelium into the lumen of the seminiferous tubule is termed *spermiation.* Before release the germ cells are called *spermatids;* after spermination they are called *sperm.* The differentiation of spermatids from spherical cells with considerable cytoplasm to characteristically shaped cells with a highly condensed nucleus and scant cytoplasm is termed *spermiogenesis.*

Some germ cells normally degenerate during certain stages of their development. It is possible that genetically defective germ cells are eliminated or that the number of germ cells is limited by nutritive or growth factors. Because of the interrelationship between germ cells of the same age, germ cells may tend to degenerate in clusters.

In the absence of gonadotropic hormones, the loss of germinal cells during spermatogenesis in the rat is considerably enhanced; very few cells reach step 7 of spermiogenesis. The administration of gonadotropins or testosterone to hypophysectomized animals prevents to variable degrees the massive regression of the seminiferous tubules. Some central and local mechanisms that regulate seminiferous epithelial function have been reviewed by Parvinen (1982).

Aging is sometimes accompanied by reduced testicular weight and by unilateral or bilateral testicular atrophy. More subtle histologic alterations include thickening of the basal membrane of the seminiferous tubules, progressive fibrosis, and thinning or desquamation of the spermatogenic epithelium. Focal degeneration or calcification may obliterate the lumen of the tubule. The prevalence of malformed sperm increases with age. Multinucleated Sertoli's cells are observed in testes of older animals and men.

Sertoli's cells secrete several products including androgen-binding protein (ABP), inhibin, müllerian-inhibiting hormone (MIH), and proteases. In some rodents, ABP is thought to be a carrier of testosterone (or dihydrotestosterone) transporting androgens from the testis to the epididymis.

Inhibin appears to inhibit the release of FSH by the anterior pituitary. MIH suppresses the formation of the female internal genitalia during fetal development. Proteases may facilitate the passage of germ cells through the inter-Sertoli's cell junctions during maturation. The Sertoli's cells also phagocytize degenerating germ cells and the residual cytoplasm of spermatids.

The Sertoli's cells are essential to normal spermatogenesis. Chemicals affecting spermatogenesis may act indirectly via an effect on the Sertoli's cells rather than directly on the germ cells. Too little attention has been directed to the role of Sertoli's cell function in normal spermatogenesis and to its potential as a target for drugs and other environmental chemicals.

INTERSTITIUM. The Leydig's cells within the interstitium are the main site of testosterone synthesis. Their close association with the testicular blood vessels and lymphatic space facilitates androgen transport. The spermatic arteries to the testes are tortuous, and their blood flows parallel but in the opposite direction of blood in the pampiniform plexus of spermatic veins. This anatomic arrangement seems to facilitate a countercurrent exchange of heat, androgens, and other chemicals.

LH stimulates testicular steroidogenesis. Androgens, the dominant steroids secreted by the testis, are essential to spermatogenesis, epididymal sperm maturation, growth and secretory activity of accessory sex organs, somatic masculinization, male behavior, and various metabolic processes.

Men with disorders of testicular function may consult their physician because of infertility, impotency, or gynecomastia. Abnormalities of virility, genitalia, and breasts receive particular attention in the assessment of men with testicular disorders.

Efferent Ducts

The fluid produced in the seminiferous tubules moves into a system of spaces called rete testis that is confluent with the efferent ducts. The chemical composition of the rete testis fluid is unique and has a total protein concentration much lower than that of the plasma. The efferent ducts open into the caput epididymidis. The concentration of chemicals in the rete testis fluid relative to unbound plasma concentration has been used to estimate the permeability of the blood–testis barrier for selected chemicals (Okumura et al., 1975).

Epididymis

The epididymis is conventionally and macroscopically divided into the head (caput), body (corpus), and tail (cauda). In most species from 1.8 (man) to 5.4 days (boar) are required for sperm to move through the caput and corpus epididymi, where maturation takes place (Table 5-1). In contrast, the transit time for sperm through the cauda epididymi, regarded as the site for sperm storage, in sexually rested males, differs greatly among species. Average transit time for 21- to 30-year-old man is about 3.7 days. The number of sperm in the caput and corpus epididymi is similar in sexually rested males and in males ejaculating daily. However, the number of sperm in the cauda epididymis is more variable, being lower in males ejaculating regularly.

The important functions of the epididymis are reabsorption of tubular fluid, metabolism, epithelial cell secretions, sperm maturation, and sperm storage. It is likely that the chemical composition of the epididymal plasma plays an important role in both the sperm maturation process and sperm storage, and that environmental chemicals may affect it to produce dysfunction. However, even considering the potential for interference with numerous physiological functions, few examples of chemical effects on epididymal function are known.

Progressive motility is acquired gradually by the sperm during epididymal passage. From the epididymi, sperm move into the vas deferens, where glandular secretions are added to the seminal plasma.

Accessory Organs

The seminal plasma functions as a vehicle for conveying the ejaculated sperm from the male to the female reproductive tract (Mann and Lutwak-Mann, 1981). The seminal plasma is produced by the secretory organs of the male reproductive system, which, along with the epididymides, include the prostate, seminal vesicles, ampullary glands, bulbourethral (Cowper's) glands, and urethral (Littré's) glands. Seminal plasma is normally an isotonic, neutral medium that, in many species, contains sources of energy such as fructose and sorbitol that are directly available to sperm. Similar secretory processes exist in a number of other organs, of which the renal proximal tubule is the most familiar. Thus, diuretic drugs might be expected to have an effect also on fluid production in reproductive accessory organs.

Because all of the accessory organs are androgen dependent, they serve as indicators of Leydig's cell function and androgen action. The weights of the accessory sex glands are an indirect measure of circulating testosterone levels. The ventral prostate of rats has been used as a model to study the actions of testosterone and to investigate the molecular basis of androgen-regulated gene function.

Although all male mammals have a prostate, the organ differs anatomically, physiologically, and chemically among species. The rat prostate is notable for its complex structure and its prompt response to castration and androgen stimulation. The human prostate is a tubuloalveolar gland made up of two prominent lateral lobes that contribute about one third of the ejaculate.

As with the prostate, the structure of the seminal vesicle varies across animal species. There are two seminal vesicles, one on each side of the lower dorsal part of the urinary bladder. Each gland is made up of an elongated, convoluted tube coiled upon itself and held together by connective tissue. Neither the dog nor cat has a seminal vesicle. In humans, the seminal vesicle contributes about two thirds of the seminal fluid.

Semen

The human male ejaculates 2.5 to 3.5 ml of semen after several days of continence. Semen volume and sperm count decrease rapidly with repeated ejaculations. Although there are normally about 100 million sperm per milliliter of semen, the count varies widely within a single individual (Belsey et al., 1980). There are those who feel that sperm count and semen quality have been decreasing during the past decade (James, 1980, 1982; Dougherty et al., 1981). James examined evidence related to changes in sperm count during the past 45 years and concluded that it seems likely that a secular decline has occurred. It is, however, very difficult to correlate sperm counts with fertility directly. Nevertheless, about 50% of men whose sperm count is between 20 and 40 million per milliliter and nearly all of those with counts below 20 million per milliliter are sterile. Sperm morphology and motility are other indicators of sperm quality. Human sperm move at a speed of about 30 mm/minute through the female genital tract and reach the oviducts 30–60 minutes after copulation. Few chemicals are known that have an in vivo effect on sperm motility.

Erection and Ejaculation

Parasympathetic nerve activity results in dilatation of the arterioles of the penis, which initiates the erection. Ejaculation is a two-part spinal reflex that involves emission and ejaculation. Emission is the movement of the semen into the urethra; ejaculation is the propulsion of the semen out of the urethra at the time of orgasm. Afferent pathways involve fibers from receptors in the glans penis that reach the spinal cord through the internal pudendal nerves. Emission is a sympathetic response effected by contraction of the smooth muscles of the vas deferens and accessory sex organs. Semen is ejaculated out of the urethra by contraction of the bulbocavernosus muscle.

Since few laboratory and clinical studies are available, relatively little is known concerning the effects of chemicals on erection or ejaculation. However, many drugs, which will be discussed later, appear to act on the autonomic nervous system to affect potency (Woods, 1984).

Sperm Capacitation

Ejaculated sperm are not yet functional; they must undergo capacitation. This biochemical process prepares the sperm for morphologic changes that the acrosome undergoes when the sperm makes contact with the egg. Capacitation destabilizes the sperm membrane and may also involve the removal of blocking agents (or decapacitation factors) and the activation of receptor sites.

Sperm Enzymes

Sperm possess two major enzyme systems. One is associated with the midpiece and tail, and includes the enzymes involved in the membrane transport of chemicals, glycolysis, the citric acid cycle, oxidative phosphorylation, and other metabolic activities. Numerous compounds can inhibit these glycolytic and respiratory enzymes and thus immobilize sperm. However, most of these compounds are nonspecific and generally toxic.

The second enzyme system is associated with the acrosome and includes mucolytic enzymes such as hyaluronidase, proteolytic enzymes such as acrosin, and various other enzymes. Hyaluronidase facilitates sperm passage through the follicular cell layers. Acrosin, a proteinase, is apparently also involved in several aspects of the fertilization process, including the breakdown of the acrosomal membranes and the penetration of the egg investments. A naturally occurring acrosin inhibitor seems to be present in seminal plasma.

Acrosome Reaction

The acrosome reaction is a membrane fusion and vesiculation that releases the acrosome contents and exposes the inner acrosomal membrane. These processes are also targets for chemical intervention. A number of naturally occurring and synthetic sperm enzyme inhibitors have been shown to prevent fertilization, but only a few have been investigated in detail. The greatest attention has been directed to inhibitors of hyaluronidase and acrosin. However, no contraceptive product that affects these enzymes is available clinically. The only spermicides currently on the market are employed in vaginal contraceptives. The primary agent is nonoxynol-9, which immobilizes sperm by its surfactant action. Immunologic research is aimed at developing antibodies that would result in the agglutination of sperm. The development and clinical success of sperm enzyme inhibitors for contraception has been reviewed by Zaneveld (1982).

FEMALE

Oogenesis and Ovulation

Oogenesis, in contrast to spermatogenesis, is a prenatal (or perinatal) event in most eutherian mammals. Ovulation is a complex cellular process that involves the oogonium, the primary oocytes, the fully grown primary oocyte in the graafian follicle, and the ovulated secondary oocyte. The ova of the mouse and rat achieve fertilizability during the last 6–8 hours before ovulation. The size and morphology of ova vary greatly among species. The approximate diameter of the rabbit ovum is 120–140 μm, of primates 110–140 μm, and of rodents from 75 to 85 μm. While women (and other primates) ovulate 1–2 eggs at a time, rodents ovulate 12–20. Some mammals ovulate more than 500 (Chang and Austin, 1976).

The morphology of the ovum is intricate. A plasma membrane, often with microvilli, surrounds its cytoplasmic body. Just below the surface of the unpenetrated ovum lie the cortical granules, which are surrounded by membranes. Cytoplasmic organelles include mitochondria, multivesicular bodies, the endoplasmic reticulum, and Golgi bodies. At the time of fertilization, the ovum is surrounded by several investments.

In humans, between 300,000 and 400,000 follicles are present at birth in each ovary. Under normal conditions, there is a continual reduction in the number of viable ovarian follicles. Any agent that damages the follicles or oocytes may accelerate the depletion of the pool, perhaps resulting in reduced female fertility. About one half of the number of oocytes present at birth remain at puberty, and this number is further reduced to about 25,000 by the age of 30. On an average, only 400 primary follicles will yield mature ova during the reproductive life span of a woman. Spontaneous alterations in the ovary include hypoplasia of the theca cells or stroma, cysts, and a wide variety of neoplasms.

Postovarian Processes

The female accessory sex organs function to bring together the ovulated ovum and the ejaculated sperm. Chemical composition and viscosity of reproductive tract fluids, as well as the epithelial morphology of these organs, are controlled by ovarian (and trophoblastic) hormones.

OVIDUCTS. The oviducts perform specialized functions including the taxis of the fimbria, which are under chemical and muscular control. The involvement of the autonomic nervous system in this process, as well as in oviductal transport of both ova and sperm, raises the possibility that pharmacologic agents that affect the autonomic nervous system may alter function and therefore fertility. Since oviductal fluid provides the environment for the gametes during fertilization, the accumulation of xenobiotics in the fluid may be deleterious.

ENDOMETRIUM. In primates, at the end of menstruation, all but the deep layers of the endometrium have sloughed. From the point of view of endometrial function, the proliferative phase represents the restoration of the epithelium from the preceding menstruation; the secretory phase defines the preparation of the uterus for the implantation of the fertilized ovum.

Secretion of specialized products is an important differentiated function of endometrial cells. Disorders of differentiation (including neoplasia) and disruption of the cellular cycle can be assessed by a variety of tests. Currently, the most common is histology of the tissue (in humans, timed endometrial biopsies). Other tests that merit development and validation include determination of the number of steroid receptors and their binding affinities in specific cell types, and quantitative cytochemistry. Xenobiotics may also accumulate in the uterine fluid that bathes the early conceptus.

MYOMETRIUM. The major role of the myometrium is contractile. This process may be vulnerable to chemicals that stimulate or disrupt neuromuscular function. The role of such dysfunction in premature labor should be considered. Current tests (tocography) include mechanical and electrophysiologic determination of uterine smooth muscle function.

CERVIX. The mucosa of the uterine cervix does not undergo cyclic desquamation, but there are regular changes in the cervical mucus. Estrogen, which makes the mucus thinner and more alkaline, promotes the survival and transport of sperm. Progesterone makes the mucus thick, tenacious, and cellular. The mucus is thinnest at the time of ovulation and dries in an arborizing, fernlike pattern on a slide. After ovulation and during pregnancy, the mucus becomes thick and fails to form the fern pattern. Major functional disruptions of the cervix may be expressed as disorders of differentiation (including neoplasia), disturbed secretion, and incompetence. Exfoliative cytologic (Papanicolaou's stain) and histologic techniques are currently used to assess disorders of differentiation. Studies of the cervical mucus are clinically routine.

VAGINA. Under the influence of estrogens, the vaginal epithelium becomes cornified, and cornified cells can be identified in the vaginal smear. Under the influence of progesterone, the epithelium proliferates, becoming infiltrated with leukocytes. The cyclic changes in the vaginal smear in rats are particularly clearly identifiable. The changes in humans and other species are similar but unfortunately not so apparent. Cervical fluid analysis and cytologic studies of desquamated vaginal cells (quantitative cytochemistry) are generally quite predictive of ovarian function. Alteration in vaginal flora is a possible toxicologic problem that was highlighted by the association of the toxic shock syndrome with the use of vaginal tampons.

Infertility in women is often associated with a failure to ovulate, endometriosis, or oviductal blockage. About 20% of female infertility comes from anovulation, which is usually due to hormonal imbalance. Endometriosis involves the ectopic growth of the endometrium which can block the reproductive tract. Endometriosis or infection can cause blockage of the oviducts. Even so, more than one half of the cases of female infertility have no known cause.

FERTILIZATION

In the human, fertilization of the ovum by sperm normally occurs in the distal part of the oviduct. Cell division and cleavage continue during the transit through the oviduct. Oviductal transit takes approximately 4 days, a period considered essential for the developing conceptus to prepare for implantation. Progestins administered before ovulation accelerate the passage of the ovum from the oviduct to the uterus and thus decrease the chance of fertilization.

The biologic steps involved in fertilization are intricate, and the process is likely to be perturbed by chemicals. Yet little is known of the toxic effects of drugs and other environmental chemicals. Fertilization seems to be a neglected area of toxicologic study, which would most likely reveal not only subtle mechanisms of toxicity but new approaches to contraception as well.

IMPLANTATION

Normal implantation in women occurs about 7 days after ovulation (twenty-first day of the menstrual cycle), when the endometrium is at its peak of secretory activity. During the initial stages of attachment between the endometrium and the embryonic trophoblast, it is possible that drugs and other environmental agents could disrupt the biochemical interactions that must occur. About one half of human conceptuses fail to implant successfully and complete their gestation (Wilcox, 1983).

SEXUAL BEHAVIOR AND FECUNDITY

One of the first questions to be dealt with in any reproductive study is whether or not the animals actually mate. In rodents, this can be determined by inspecting females each day for vaginal plugs. If the male is not copulating, then the emphasis of further investigation must be on neuromuscular or behavioral defects. In humans, loss of libido may occur as a result of either psychologic or somatic factors. The loss may be complete in individuals with serious organic diseases or advanced age.

A variety of drugs have been associated with impotence. The list includes narcotics (morphine), ethanol, psychotropic drugs [chlorpromazine, diazepam, tricyclic anti-depressants, and monoamine oxidase (MAO) inhibitors], hypotensive agents (methyldopa, clonidine, reserpine, and gu-anethidine), and estrogenic hormone ago-nists and androgen hormone antagonists. These drugs are discussed further later in this chapter.

In men under 45 years of age, 95% of impotence is traceable to psychologic roots. However, once past 45 years of age, one half of male impotence has a physical cause. Arteriosclerosis to the penis is the major cause. Diabetes, alcoholism, nerve disease, kidney disease, traumatic injury to the spinal cord, and blood pressure medications can contribute, as can surgery for the prostate, colon, or bladder.

All ovarian functions decline in aged fe-male mammals, and reproductive capacity is lost well before the end of an average life span. In humans, the ultimate loss of fertil-ity is caused primarily by the exhaustion of normal oocytes. In other mammalian spe-cies, reproduction ceases because of age-related changes in other areas of the repro-ductive system. In mice, reproductive fail-ure is due almost exclusively to age-related changes in the uterus, whereas in hamsters and rabbits degenerative changes take place in both the uterus and ova.

Modulating Factors

The ultimate objective of all toxicological studies is to assess the toxic effects of a chemical in laboratory animals and to ex-trapolate the experimental data relevant to humans. To accomplish this, one must con-sider the main factors that may influence and modulate the toxic effects of chemicals in an organ. These include the pharmacoki-netic factors that determine the amount of the chemical (or its metabolites) that reaches its target as well as adaptive, repair, and homeostatic processes. Although these pro-cesses are equally important in both the male and female gonads, much more informa-tion is available regarding the testis than the ovary (Dixon and Lee, 1980; Mattison, Shiromizu, and Nightingale, 1983b).

THE BLOOD–TESTIS BARRIER

The blood–testis barrier (BTB) retards the passage of chemicals from the blood to the lumen of the seminiferous tubule. Setchell and co-workers (1969) first demonstrated that immunoglobulins and iodinated albu-min, inulin, and a number of small mole-cules were excluded from the seminiferous tubules by the BTB. Dym and Fawcett (1970) suggested that the primary permeability barrier for the seminiferous tubules was composed of the surrounding layers of myoid cells, whereas specialized Sertoli's cell–Ser-toli's cell junctions within the seminiferous epithelium constituted a secondary cellular barrier. Okumura and co-workers (1975) quantified permeability rates for nonelec-trolytes and selected drugs. Small molecules such as water and urea were transported readily across the BTB, while larger mole-cules such as galactose and inulin moved much more slowly.

A positive correlation between the lipid solubilities of chemicals and their mem-brane penetrabilities was demonstrated. The rate-determining factors for transport of compounds across the BTB are molecular size, ionization, and lipid solubility at phys-iologic pH. The permeability characteris-tics of the BTB are similar to those of the membrane barriers that limit penetration of foreign chemicals to the central nervous system and aqueous humor of the eye. The ability of the BTB to control the entry of chemicals to the seminiferous tubules is af-fected by a number of physiologic, chemi-cal, and pathologic factors (Dixon, 1981).

BIOTRANSFORMATION OF EXOGENOUS CHEMICALS

A number of investigators have reported on the capability of the testis to biotransform exogenous chemicals. Mukhtar, Bend, and Lee and their co-workers (1978a, b) found appreciable activities of both mixed-function oxidases and epoxide-degrading enzymes, as well as cytochrome P-450, in testicular tissues.

Although aryl hydrocarbon hydroxylase

(AHH) activity in testicular microsomes was only 5% of that of hepatic microsomes, the close proximity of activating enzymes to the germ cells may be important for enzyme-activated chemicals. Factors that affect enzyme activity and cytochrome P-450 levels are likely to play a significant role in germ cell toxicity. 2,3,7,8-Tetrachlorodibenzo-p-dioxin (TCDD) significantly induces testicular and prostate AHH activity and cytochrome P-448 (Lee et al., 1981). The metabolism of benzo[a]pyrene by the isolated perfused testis has been contrasted to cell-free testicular systems such as homogenates (Nagayama and Lee, 1982). Qualitative and quantitative differences in the metabolites that were observed suggest that the perfused organ system is a better model for extrapolating data to the whole animal.

UNSCHEDULED DNA SYNTHESIS

Our laboratory and others have also been interested in the capacity of spermatogenic cells to repair DNA damage as a consequence of exposure to environmental chemicals (Lee, 1983). It has been shown that both physical (ultraviolet and X-ray radiation) and chemical agents can cause damage to DNA molecules. Damage inflicted on the DNA templates, unless repaired, may interfere with transcription or cellular replication. Lethal mutations (cell death) and mutations that result in transformed cells, or altered gene function may also occur. Testes of various mouse strains have been found to differ in their abilities to repair DNA damage.

The velocity sedimentation cell separation technique has been used to identify spermatogenic cells capable of unscheduled DNA synthesis (Dixon and Lee, 1980). To study unscheduled DNA synthesis after methyl methane-sulfonate (MMS) treatment, male mice were first treated with varying doses of MMS followed 2 hours later by the intratesticular administration of [³H]thymidine 1 hour before sacrifice. Spermatogenic cell types were then isolated. Control mice receiving saline followed by intratesticular injection of [³H]thymidine showed a single peak of radioactivity that identified spermatogonial cells passing through S phase. In contrast, the radioactive profiles obtained after MMS treatment demonstrated that thymidine incorporation now occurred not only in the spermatogonia but also in the leptotene, zygotene, pachytene, and diplotene cells in decreasing order. Normally no DNA synthesis occurs in these premeiotic cells; therefore, the thymidine incorporation in untreated cells is very low. These studies suggest that non–S phase spermatogonial cells were also induced to undergo unscheduled DNA synthesis. In contrast, no thymidine radioactivity was present in spermatids or sperm (spermiogenic cells). However, other investigators have demonstrated DNA repair in postmeiotic stages (Sega, 1982; Warking and Butterworth, 1984.) Therefore, spermiogenic cells appear less able to repair DNA damage and thus may be more vulnerable to the effects of monofunctional alkylating agents such as MMS.

Because unscheduled DNA repair in spermatogenic cells appears to be dose and time dependent, the DNA repair systems might be saturated at high test doses or with repeated exposures to toxic chemicals. Overwhelming the repair system could result in a larger number of affected cells and increased toxicity. Thus, the DNA repair system is another protective mechanism with regard to toxic effects of environmental chemicals, as well as a sensitive indicator of chromosome damage. Sega and colleagues at Oak Ridge National Laboratory have reviewed DNA repair in spermatocytes and spermatids and have commented on the potential of unscheduled DNA synthesis in testing for mutagens (Sega, 1982; Sega and Sotomayor, 1982). Working and Butterworth (1984) have also reported an assay for DNA repair in spermatocytes.

Pedersen and Brandriff (1980) have reviewed studies showing that ultraviolet light or drug-induced unscheduled DNA synthesis in mammalian oocytes and embryos indicate that the female gamete has an excision repair capacity from the earliest stages of oocyte growth. In contrast to the mature sperm, the fully mature oocyte maintains a repair capacity and contributes this to the zygote. However, the oocyte's demonstrable excision repair capacity decreases at the time of meiotic maturation for unknown reasons.

Differential Tissue Susceptibility

An appreciation of the unique susceptibility of the reproductive system components during their different stages of development or adult function will aid hazard identification and human risk analysis.

GAMETOGENESIS

The human primordial germ cells first become discernible at about 21 days of gestation. They migrate to and invade the germinal ridge, which provides the supporting cells of the gonad. Until about the end of the sixth week, the human embryonic gonad remains undifferentiated, having the same morphologic appearance in both sexes.

Spermatogenesis

Testicular development, because it involves both the prenatal and postnatal periods and includes the differentiation of various tissues, offers a number of possible targets for chemicals capable of perturbing biologic processes. Gonocytes are present in the sex cords of rats from birth until about 4 days of age, when they begin mitotic division to form type A spermatogonia. By 6 days of age, type A cells are common, and some type B and intermediate-type spermatogonia can be identified, a few of which actively divide. At 9 days of age, gonocytes disappear and a few primary spermatocytes develop. Three successive stages of the cycle of the seminiferous epithelium can be identified in 18-day-old animals, with the most mature spermatocytes progressing to the pachytene stage of meiotic prophase. By 26 days, primary spermatocytes complete meiosis to form secondary spermatocytes, and a few of these go on to form spermatids, thus finishing the second meiotic division. Following the first appearance of spermatids, spermiogenesis progresses with the formation and release of mature sperm by 45 days of age. Cellular division during spermatogenesis and oogenesis are summarized in Figure 5-5.

In normal adult rats there are several vulnerable stages of spermatogenesis during which germinal cells spontaneously degenerate, resulting in less sperm than theoretically expected. It has been shown that some type A spermatogonia degenerate during some of their mitotic peaks, spermatocytes degenerate as mid-pachytene spermatocytes during their meiotic divisions, and steps 9–11 spermatids degenerate during the acrosome phase of spermiogenesis. Some later spermatids undergo regressive changes and are eventually phagocytized by Sertol's cells.

Sertoli's Cells

Sertoli's cells divide only during the early postnatal period. In laboratory rodents this is from birth until approximately 15 days of age; structural maturation and the formation of tight inter-Sertoli's cell junctions occur approximately between days 16 and 18. These junctional complexes play a critical role in the formation of the blood–testis barrier, which becomes functional at this time. The seminiferous tubular lumen appears concurrently with the development of these tight intercellular junctions and is thought to result from fluid production initiated by the Sertoli's cells. Sertoli's cells continue to mature until about 45 days of age, when they attain their adult structural and functional characteristics. In the adult, the Sertoli's cell population is stable with no evidence of further cellular replication.

Leydig's Cells

Leydig's cells undergo biphasic development in rodents. A fetal phase lasts from the seventeenth day of gestation to the second postnatal week, and an adult phase begins at the third postnatal week. Fetal androgens are critical to the development of the male phenotype. Following the fetal

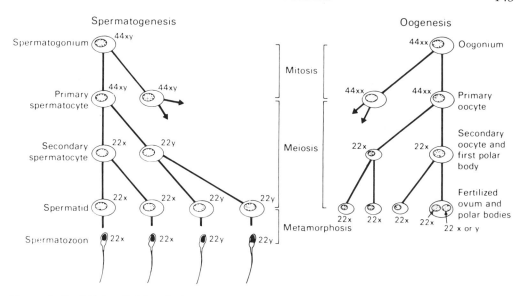

Figure 5–5. Cellular division during spermatogenesis and oogenesis.

phase, testosterone levels remain relatively low until they rise rapidly to adult levels at approximately 60 days of age.

Because during development, critical molecular and cellular processes must respond with integrity to a variety of hormones and other growth factors to ensure normal postnatal function, there is real potential for environmental chemicals to affect these processes. The development of normal reproductive capacity may offer particularly susceptible targets for toxins. Environmental factors might alter the genetic determinants of gonadal sex, the hormonal determinants of phenotypic sex, fetal gametogenesis, reproductive tract differentiation, as well as postnatal integration of endocrine functions and other processes essential for the propagation of the species. While the effects of environmental agents on sexual differentiation and the development of reproductive capacity are largely unstudied, a number of chemicals with diverse structures and actions have been shown to exert dramatic effects, especially on hormone synthesis and function (Dixon, 1982).

The prenatal testis is much more resistant to toxic effects than the prenatal ovary (McLachlan, Newbold, Korach, et al., 1981). Only a few chemicals have been identified

as having effects on the developing male offspring. The male germ cell–damaging effects of prenatal exposure to benzo[a]pyrene have been described (MacKenzie and Angevine, 1981). Certain chemicals may interfere with the normal hormonal function regulating spermatogenesis. For example, studies on male offspring of women treated with diethylstilbestrol (DES) during pregnancy indicate that the average values for sperm density and total motile spermatozoa ejaculated are less than half those of controls. Furthermore, the number of abnormal sperm in the DES-exposed offspring was significantly greater than in the control group (Bibbo et al., 1977). Gonadal abnormalities in the mouse include cryptorchid testes and a reduction in number of spermatogonia in more than half of the males (McLachlan, Newbold, and Bullock, 1975). The gonadal toxicity of chemotherapeutic agents administered to children is discussed in a later section.

A thorough understanding of any differences in the effects of a chemical on the immature as compared to the mature gonad is critically important to hazard identification and human risk analysis. Unique tissue and cellular susceptibility of developing testes has been observed when anticancer agents were administered to rats at selected postnatal periods (Bechter et al., 1982; Ettlin et al., 1982; Matter et al., 1983). Vincristine, cyclophosphamide, cytosine arabinoside, procarbazine, and doxorubicin were studied. Histologic evaluations suggested an association between damage to a particular developing cell type and an observed reproductive dysfunction. By selecting the drug, the dose, and the treatment schedule, these investigators were able to target Sertoli's, Leydig's, or spermatogenic cells. The possibility exists that laboratory animals could be produced in which one of these cell types is absent. Such animals would be valuable models, especially to explore further the physiologic role of the Sertoli's cells.

Oogenesis

During the early differentiation of the ovary, the primordial germ cells become oogonia (the ovarian stem cells), which undergo repeated mitotic divisions and increase greatly in number. Once this period of intense mitotic activity is completed, the oogonia enter meiotic prophase and then proceed to the diplotene stage. Meiosis is only resumed after puberty in oocytes that have sustained normal follicular growth to become graafian follicles. LH induces the oocyte to progress to metaphase II, just before ovulation. The great majority of oocytes never progress beyond the diplotene stage and are eliminated from the ovary by atresia. Events of oogenesis are presented in Figure 5-5.

Female primordial germ cells are highly sensitive to damage induced by chemicals (or radiation) capable of altering cell replication. For example, in embryonic rats exposed to X rays on day 10 of gestation, the germ cell population is reduced by two thirds within 5 days of treatment. Depending on the time of exposure and the severity of the cytotoxicity, the total population may be partially restored owing to the mitotic proliferation of surviving primordial germ cells. The high sensitivity of the embryonic gonad may involve a failure of the stem cells to reach the developing gonadal ridges, or a reduction or elimination of the stem cell population.

Thus, since oogenesis occurs prenatally (or perinatally) and no new germ cells are formed later in life, the female fetus of most mammals is particularly vulnerable to germ cell toxicity during gametogenesis. When mouse fetuses were exposed to procarbazine (a potent antineoplastic agent that interferes with DNA, RNA, and protein synthesis) either before, during, or after peak oocyte DNA synthesis, the fertility of the female offspring was significantly affected. Male offspring were relatively unaffected at the dose levels tested (MacLachlan, Newbold, Shah, et al., 1982).

Additional chemicals that, when administered prenatally, affect reproductive capacity in the offspring at puberty include those presented in Table 5-2. Antineoplastic agents, pesticides, synthetic nonsteroidal estrogen, pyrolysis products, and various environmental pollutants are included (McLachlan et al., 1981).

PUBERTY

Subtle mechanisms are responsible for the onset of puberty, and aberrations of puberty can be produced in laboratory animals with chemical treatment.

After birth, the androgen-secreting Leydig's cells in the fetal testes become quiescent. In all mammals, there follows a period in which the gonads of both sexes remain inactive until activated by gonadotropins from the pituitary to bring about the final maturation of the reproductive system. Puberty, strictly defined, is the period when the endocrine and gametogenic functions of the gonads have first developed to the point where reproduction is possible. Although the nature of the pituitary-inhibiting gonadal secretion is uncertain, it is obvious that a complex triggering of the hypothalamo–pituitary–gonadal axis is involved. Puberty is initiated when the brain starts secreting a hormone, LHRH, in periodic bursts. LHRH stimulates the pituitary to release gonadotropins; these, in turn, stimulate steroidogenesis in the gonads, which accounts for sexual maturation. The rate at which the brain releases LHRH is crucial to sexual development. Aberrations

Table 5–2. Some Compounds Reported to Alter Fertility after Prenatal Exposure

Compound given to mother	Major effects in offspring	Species
Methoxychlor	Reduced fertility in males and females	Rat
Dimethylbenzanthracene (DMBA)	Gonadal dysplasia and reduced fertility in males and females	Mouse
Benzo[a]pyrene	Gonadal dysplasia and reduced fertility in males and females	Mouse
Diethylstilbestrol (DES)	Genital tract abnormalities and reduced fertility in females	Mouse
Diethylstilbestrol (DES)	Genital tract abnormalities and reduced fertility in females	Human
Diethylstilbestrol (DES)	Genital tract abnormalities and reduced fertility in males	Mouse
Diethylstilbestrol (DES)	Genital tract abnormalities including sperm	Human
Methyl methanesulfonate (MMS)	Sterility in males	Rat
Procarbazine	Reduced fertility in females	Mouse
Cyclophosphamide	Reduced fertility in males and females	Mouse
Clomid	Reproductive tract	Rat
Busulfan	Gonadal dysplasia in males and females	Rat
Cyanoketone	Altered estrous cycles	Rat

Source: From McLachlan et al. (1981).

of puberty can be produced in laboratory animals following chemical treatment, and they also are observed clinically.

Assessment of Reproductive Toxicity

A histopathologic approach using light microscopy (LM) and electron microscopy (EM) for detecting gonadal and accessory sex organ toxicity is essential to a better understanding of chemical toxicity. Because human data are relatively rare and often difficult to interpret because of multiple chemical exposures and advanced pathologic changes, laboratory studies using experimental animals play an essential role in reproductive toxicology.

Morphologic methods are often focused on the assessment of rather obvious cytotoxic phenomena. Additional methods to detect more subtle effects are necessary to understand mechanisms of reproductive toxicity more fully and to interpret the etiology of chemically induced disease. The

proceedings of a symposium organized by Niswender, which focused on cellular and molecular approaches to the study of reproduction were published by the Society for the Study of Reproduction (Ewing, 1983).

Methods complementary to morphologic investigations are summarized in Table 5-3 for assessing male reproductive toxicity and in Table 5-4 for assessing female reproductive toxicity. Table 5-3 is taken from a recent EPA workshop (Galbraith et al., 1982) and Table 5-4 was compiled by the authors. However, scientific consensus regarding either list is lacking.

MALE

Testis

The number of sperm produced per day by a normal male is largely determined by testicular size. In a scrotal mammal, testicular size can be measured easily and precisely.

Table 5–3. Potentially Useful Tests of Male Reproductive Toxicity for Laboratory Animals and Man

Test target	Tests accepted	Tests considered and rejected
Whole body	Body weight	

Testis	Size in situ
	Weight
	Spermatid reserves
	Gross histology
	Nonfunctional tubules (%)
	Tubules with lumen sperm (%)
	Tubule diameter
	Counts of leptotene spermatocytes
		Tonometric measurement of testicular consistency
		Qualitative testicular histology
		Stage of cycle at which spermiation occurs
		Quantitative testicular histology
		  Counts of degenerating germ cells
		  Complete germ cell counts
		  Stem cell counts
		  Relative frequency of stages of cycle

Epididymis	Weight of distal half Number of sperm in distal half Motility of sperm, distal end (%) Gross sperm morphology, distal end (%) Detailed sperm morphology, distal end (%) Gross histology	Histology Biochemistry of epididymal fluids
Accessory sex glands	Weight of vesicular glands Weight of total accessory sex glands	Histology
Semen	Total volume Gel-free volume Sperm concentration Total sperm/ejaculate Total sperm/day of abstinence Sperm motility, visual (%) Sperm motility, videotape (% and velocity) Gross sperm morphology Detailed sperm morphology Concentration of agent in sperm Concentration of agent in seminal plasma Concentration of agent in blood Biochemical analyses of sperm/seminal plasma	Biochemical analysis of sperm Sperm membrane characteristics Biochemical analysis of seminal plasma Evaluation of sperm metabolism Fluorescent Y bodies in spermatozoa Flow cytometry of spermatozoa Karyotyping human sperm pronuclei Cervical mucus penetration test
Prepubertal animals		Studies
Endocrine	Luteinizing hormone Follicle-stimulating hormone Testosterone Gonadotropin-releasing hormone	
Fertility	Ratio of exposed:pregnant females Number of embryos or young/pregnant female Ratio of viable embryos:corpora lutea Ratio of implantations:corpora lutea	

Test target	Tests accepted	Tests considered and rejected
Fertility	Number of 2- to 8-cell eggs Number of unfertilized eggs Number of abnormal eggs Sperm per ovum Number of corpora lutea	
In vitro	Incubation of sperm in agent Hamster egg penetration test	

[a] See Galbraith et al. (1982) for complete table and discussion of the relative usefulness of these tests.

Table 5–4. Potentially Useful Tests of Female Reproductive Toxicity for Laboratory Animals and Women

Test target	Nature of test
Whole body	Body weight
Ovary	Organ weight Histology Number of oocytes Rate of follicular atresia Follicular steroidogenesis Follicular maturation Oocyte maturation Ovulation Luteal function
Hypothalamus	Histology Altered synthesis and release of neurotransmitters, neuromodulators, and neurohormones
Pituitary	Histology Altered synthesis and release of trophic hormones
Endocrine	Gonadotropin-releasing hormone levels LH, FSH, prolactin levels Chorionic gonadotropin levels Estrogen levels Progesterone levels Cyclicity of steroid hormone levels
Oviduct	Histology Gamete transport Fertilization Transport of early embryo
Uterus	Cytology Histology Luminal fluid analysis (xenobiotics, proteins) Decidual response Dysfunctional bleeding
Cervix	Cytology Histology Mucus production Mucus quality (sperm penetration test)
Vulva/vagina	Cytology Histology Virilization Adenosis

Table 5–4. (Continued)

Test target	Nature of test
Fertility	Ratio of exposed:pregnant females
	Number of embryos or young/pregnant female
	Ratio of viable embryos:corpora lutea
	Ratio of implantations:corpora lutea
	Number of 2- to 8-cell eggs
	Number of unfertilized eggs
	Number of abnormal eggs
	Number of corpora lutea
In vitro	In vitro fertilization of superovulated eggs, either exposed to chemical in culture or from treated females

At autopsy, the testis should be freed from the epididymis, spermatic cord, and fat, and then weighed. Because testes weight and body weight are largely independent variables, absolute testis weight should be reported rather than weight relative to body weight. Testicular degeneration correlates well with a reduction in testis size and weight.

The preparation of testicular tissue involves problems that generally are not thoroughly discussed in technical handbooks. Good tissue preservation and high resolution are essential for the early detection of subtle and specific cellular changes. The testis presents special challenges. Fixatives slowly penetrate the seminiferous tubules, because the germ cells are protected by a complex system of membrane barriers. In addition, the connective tissue and tubules are too fragile to allow unfixed testicular tissue to be cut into thin sections to facilitate penetration by fixatives.

TISSUE FIXATION. Basic methods for histologic preparation of the testis are summarized in Table 5-5. In the past, formalin fixation and paraffin embedding were the most widely used methods. However, there is considerably less shrinkage and therefore improved preservation of the testicular architecture when Bouin's fluid, Zenker-formol (Helly's fluid), or other fixatives containing picric acid are used. Special care must be taken to remove all of the picric acid from the tissue to ensure long-lasting staining. Immersion of the testis in such a fixative for approximately 15 to 20 minutes hardens the tissue enough to allow cutting of 2- to 3-mm slices, which facilitates further fixation. Glutaraldehyde is a particu-

Table 5–5. Basic Methods for Histologic Preparation of Testicular Tissue

Fixative		Embedding material	Characteristics of sections				Field of application
Application	Type		Thickness (μm)	Field	Quality	Staining	
Immersion	Formalin	Paraffin	5–7	cs[d]	(+)	Normal stains	(Routine)
Immersion	Bouin's[a]	Paraffin	5–7	cs	+	Normal stains	Routine
Immersion	Bouin's[a]	GMA[c]	2	cs	+ +	Normal stains	Special cases
Perfusion	Bouin's[b]	GMA	2	cs	+ + +	Normal stains	Research
Perfusion	Glutaraldehyde	Epon, Araldite	1	15 tubules	+ + + +	Toluidine blue	Research

[a] Or Zenker-Formol.
[b] Or mixture of formalin and glutaraldehyde.
[c] Glycol methacrylate.
[d] Cross section.

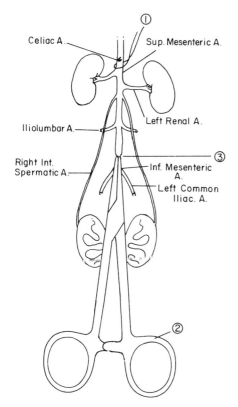

Celiac A.

Sup. Mesenteric A.

Left Renal A.

Iliolumbar A.

Right Int.
Spermatic A.

Inf. Mesenteric
A.

Left Common
Iliac. A.

Figure 5–6. Diagrammatic representation of the technique for perfusing testes with fixative. This is a modified version of the procedure originally described by Vitale et al., 1973. ① ligature prepared blindly around big subdiaphragmatic vessels and tightened at the beginning of the perfusion. ② curved hemostat which slightly lifts the aorta cleaned from surrounding connective tissue. ③ point where aorta is incised for collection of blood and insertion of a 19-gauge needle connected to an infusion set.

larly efficient and rapid fixative, but it penetrates the tissues very slowly.

ORGAN PERFUSION. Because no fixative will penetrate more than a few millimeters of whole testis in a 24-hour period, optimal fixation is achieved only by delivering the fixative directly into the organ's vascular system. A retrograde perfusion method (diagrammed in Figure 5-6) that delivers the fixative to the gonads via the lower abdominal aorta can be used (Vitale et al., 1973).

EMBEDDING. The principal disadvantages of paraffin embedding are the effects of exposing the tissue to the heat of melted paraffin (~60°C) and the difficulty involved in cutting sections thinner than a few microns. The exposure of the tissue to heat can be reduced by the use of celloidin. However, this embedding procedure is time-consuming, more complicated, and less rewarding than paraffin.

A breakthrough regarding higher resolution for light microscopy was achieved by embedding samples of well-preserved perfused tissue in plastic materials. These materials polymerize and harden, thus providing thinner sections with less superposition of cellular details. Glycol methacrylate (GMA)-embedded section bind stains in much the same manner as tissue embedded in paraffin and are preferable to epoxy. Epoxy resins react with some of the dye-binding sites, thus reducing the number of stains that can be used. Furthermore, because GMA does not become as hard as epoxy (with certain precautions), tissue blocks as large as 1 cm^2 can be cut (Bennett et al., 1976). Figure 5-7 demonstrates degree of cellular resolution obtained using these techniques.

Russell (1983) has recently described the morphological evaluation of chemically induced testicular toxicity. Short-term (mechanistic) and long-term (end-stage maturation deletion) effects are described along with methods to quantify the toxicological response.

However, if staining properties and the size of the sections are not crucial, tissue samples of 1 to 2 mm in diameter can be embedded in an epoxy resin such as Epon 812 or Araldite. Before embedding, postfixation with osmium tetroxide will enhance contrast, particularly for electron microscopy. Thick sections of 0.5 to 1 μm (also called semithin sections) can be stained, for instance, with toluidine blue and evaluated with the light microscope. Very high resolution is obtained even at 1500× magnification. Such a section usually contains 15–20 tubules. The same block can be trimmed down to focus on one or two particularly

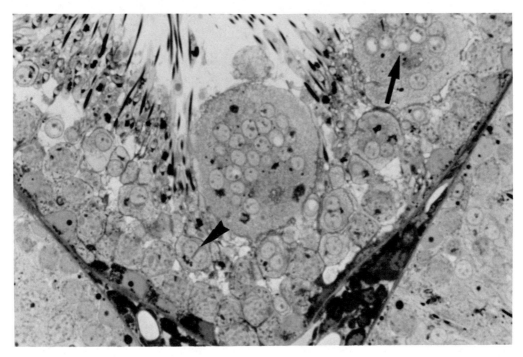

Figure 5–7. Example of cellular resolution obtained with glutaraldehyde perfusion, osmium tetroxide postfixation, Araldite embedding, toluidine blue staining, and 1 μm sectioning. Testicular tissue from a rat 1 week after treatment with a single 200 mg/kg dose of procarbazine is shown. Note multinucleated cells of different size, among them giant cells, with subcellular structures characteristic of early spermatids (acrosomes and chromatoid bodies). An arrowhead indicates that some of the spermatid nuclei have a common acrosome. Margination of chromatin in certain spermatid nuclei is probably an early sign of degeneration (marked with arrow). Also apparent is the pronounced reduction of early spermatids and the absence of late spermatogonia or early primary spermatocytes.

interesting tubules, and thin sections can then be studied using transmission electron microscopy (TEM).

To take full advantage of this technique, special microtomes such as the Sorval JB-4 must be used. Sections considerably thinner that 0.5 μm obtained using ultramicrotomes generally do not have enough contrast for light microscopy.

STAINING. Testicular tissues routinely are stained with hematoxylin–eosin (H&E), and with periodic acid Schiff's (PAS); the latter better identifies the acrosomal system. Stains for connective tissue such as Masson's trichrome or van Gieson also may be useful. However, they do not stain epon-embedded tissues.

Histochemical investigations of gonadal tissue allow a visualization of biochemical processes such as steroidogenesis. Some of the substrates and enzymes that can be detected histochemically are listed in Table 5-6. Adenosine triphosphate and alkaline phosphatase are involved in energy production. Thiamine pyrophosphatase catalyzes the decarboxylation of α ketoacids and is considered a marker of the Golgi apparatus. Acid phosphatase is involved in degradation processes and therefore associated with phagocytosis. Glucose-6-phosphate dehydrogenase and α-glycerophosphate dehydrogenase are involved in steroid biosynthesis, lipogenesis, and carbohydrate metabolism. 3-β-Hydroxysteroid dehydrogenase is a key enzyme for steroidogenesis. Several isoenzymes of lactic dehydrogenase are involved in carbohydrate metabolism. LDH-X, determined by using D,L-α-hydroxyvalerate as a substrate, is con-

Table 5–6. Histochemical Localization of Carbohydrates, Fats, and Enzymes in Rat Testis[a]

	Connective cells	Basement membrane	Seminiferous tubule	Sertoli's cells	Leydig's cells
Carbohydrate (PAS)	+ +	+	+ + + (sperm)	−	+
Neutral fat (Oil red O)	−	−	+ + + (sperm)	+ +	−
Alkaline phosphatase	+ +	+ +	+ +	−	−
Acid phosphatase	−	−	+	+	+
Adenosine triphosphatase	+ + +	−	+ + + (sperm)	−	−
Thiamine pyrophosphatase	−	−	+ + +	+ +	−
α-Glycerophosphate dehydrogenase	−	−	+ + + (sperm)	−	−
Glucose 6-phosphate dehydrogenase	−	−	+	+	+ + +
3-β-Hydroxysteroid dehydrogenase	−	−	−	−	+ + +
Lactic dehydrogenase	−	−	−	−	+ + +
Lactic dehydrogenase-X	−	−	+ + +	−	−

[a]Intensity of reaction is graded from no visible reaction (−) to a maximal reaction (+ + +).
Source: Adapted from Livni and Yaffe (1974).

sidered a specific marker for primary spermatocytes and more advanced spermatogenic cells. Further details concerning histochemical techniques for the testis are available in a review by Hodgen (1977) and for the ovary in a review by Bjersing (1977).

Immunohistochemical and immunofluorescence techniques are available, and both methods show promise for basic research and toxicologic investigations, especially with regard to hormones and their cytoplasmic receptors. Immunofluorescence detection of LDH-X variants in sperm populations has been proposed as a measure of mutagenicity.

ELECTRON MICROSCOPY (EM). Electron-microscopic investigations have broadened considerably our understanding of gonadal morphology and response to toxic chemicals. Tissues from perfused organs that are then embedded in plastic can be used for both light microscopy and electron microscopy. After LM evaluation of semithin sections, interesting blocks can be trimmed down to focus on special features and then cut into ultrathin sections for EM study. Thus, these newer techniques allow a careful selection of specimens for EM, saving both time and money, and improve the correlation between light and electron microscopy.

Lanthanum, an electron-opaque substance, added to the perfusate, can be used to demonstrate the integrity of Sertoli's cell–Sertoli's cell junctions of the blood–testis barrier.

OTHER MORPHOLOGIC APPROACHES. Freshly prepared, living, unstained seminiferous tubules can be studied using a phase-contrast light microscope (Parvinen and Vanha-Petulta, 1972). The various stages of spermatogenesis as well as degenerating cells can be identified by observing differences in light absorption. Following such evaluation, segments of the tubules can be studied in greater morphologic detail or used for biochemical investigations.

QUANTIFYING TOXICITY. To quantify changes more effectively, one or more germ cell types can be counted in a fixed number of tubular cross sections of one cellular association (Galbraith et al., 1982). A more convenient approach is to count the number of leptotene spermatocytes. They are readily discernible and are present in only about 8% of the tubules because of the short duration of the leptotene stage. This procedure establishes the number of primary spermatocytes formed, it samples a finite cell population, and it avoids the need to establish cellular associations. Expression of the data in terms of the number of leptotene spermatocytes per Sertoli's cell nucleolus corrects for differences due to tissue shrinkage during histologic processing and variations in the thickness of histologic sections. Thus, variation is minimized. This approach provides a sensitive test for detecting chemicals that affect mitosis or otherwise decrease the production of leptotene spermatocytes (Amann, 1981).

The percentage of tubules with spermatids lining the lumen and the percentage of nonfunctional tubules can be determined by scoring a few hundred tubular cross sections. For normal rats, these values are approximately 30% and less than 5%, respectively (Amann, 1981). Germ cell, Leydig's cell, Sertoli's cell nuclei can also be quantified in the homogenates prepared from glutaraldehyde-fixed tissues (Johnson et al., 1981). A simple measurement of morphologic change is that of tubular diameter.

ANALYSIS OF SPERMATOGENESIS. To study early and subtle alterations in spermatogenesis as well as to follow the development of cellular damage and repair, in vivo studies using laboratory animals are indispensable. The test animal, usually a rodent, is treated once with different doses of the test chemical. Doses are selected to produce toxic effects ranging from slight to severe, to define a dose–response relationship, and to establish the threshold for toxicity. Necropsies are conducted serially at various times following exposure. The exposure period usually covers at least the time necessary for early spermatogonia to become sperm. Because cellular regeneration may require a much longer period, additional investigations at later time points may be necessary to define recovery. Using this approach, it is possible to determine which stages of germ cell differentiation have been altered morphologically, and then to extrapolate back to determine which cells were the primary target. Serial necropsies also

permit an analysis of both the extent of stem cell killing and the time necessary to reestablish the normal cell population. This reasoning assumes that the chemical has a reasonably short biologic half-life and that specific toxic effects are produced.

Such an analysis is possible because of the regularity of the spermatogenic process. No chemical treatment is known that accelerates or decelerates the spermatogenic cycle. However, researchers have observed effects on certain cell stages that desynchronize the development of germ cells (Ettlin et al., 1982). By knowing the time of each stage of spermatogenesis, the stage when a cell was first damaged can be identified (Figure 5-8; Ettlin et al., 1984).

Multiple-exposure regimens are necessary if the toxic effect of the chemical is schedule dependent and does not display its usual toxicity after a single treatment, or if effects of low exposure over prolonged periods are to be assessed. Because spermatogenesis requires about 4.5 cycles of the seminiferous epithelium, it is generally necessary to follow chemical effects on spermatogenesis over 6.0 cycles of the seminiferous epithelium for the test species. To assess recovery, 12 cycles without treatment should allow normal spermatogenesis to be re-established (Amann, 1981). Although an interval of 12 cycles probably is sufficient to allow regeneration of the germinal epithelium in test animals, a longer recovery time has been demonstrated for men exposed to dichlorobromopropane (DBCP) (Whorton and Milby, 1980).

Any experiment to evaluate the effect of an agent on male reproductive function must include sufficient males per treatment group to detect a treatment effect. Amann (1981) presents the following analysis: For normal rabbits, a 25% decrease in testicular weight, in spermatid reserves per gram of testis, in the percentage of seminiferous tubules with sperm lining the tubule lumen, or in seminiferous tubule diameter would have an 80% chance of being detected at the 5% level if 12–15 rabbits per test group were used. Variance associated with the evaluation of seminal characteristics is larger. A reduc-

Figure 5–8. Plot relating time of observed effect after treatment to the cell type damaged following acute exposure to a reproductive toxin. The same time scale is used for the ordinate (weeks after treatment) and abscissa (spermatogenesis). Thus, damaged cells observed can be related to the cell injured initially, which accounts for the observed delayed effect. For instance, step 1 spermatids observed to be abnormal 3 weeks after treatment can be traced back to a toxic effect during the last mitotic cell division.

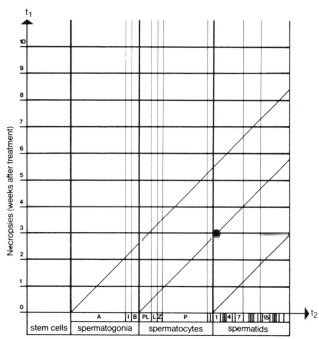

tion in daily sperm output of nearly one half would have to occur to ensure an 80% chance of detection using 15 rabbits per group. Measurements of motile or morphologically normal sperm seem to be more sensitive indicators of effect and thus would require fewer animals (Wyrobek, 1983).

Epididymis

Weighing of the cauda epididymidis provides a rough estimate of stored sperm. However, the epididymis must not be squeezed, as partial loss of fluid and tissue damage may result. Histologic examination of epididymal lumina can reveal alterations in sperm number that reflect changes in the germinal epithelium. The number of sperm within the epididymis can be determined by homogenizing the tissue (Robb et al., 1978). In sexually rested animals, the number of sperm in the distal epididymis is a function of the daily sperm produced by the associated testis and the rate of movement of sperm through the epididymal duct. The motility and morphology of sperm in a small drop of fluid expressed from the cauda epididymis also can be evaluated. An increased

incidence of immotile sperm is clear evidence of abnormal testicular or epididymal function. Fluorescence-conjugated lectins and monoclonal antibodies that can be quantified visually have been employed at the National Institute of Environmental Health Sciences and other laboratories to determine modifications in rat sperm surface proteins during testicular and epididymal maturation (Vernon et al., 1982).

Male Accessory Sex Organs

The male accessory sex organs do not require any special techniques to obtain good-quality preparations for histopathology. Their size and weight are useful indicators of circulating levels of androgens.

Gross and microscopic evaluation of selected endocrine organs will aid in detecting indirect effects. To exclude reproductive side effects secondary to general organ toxicity, organs such as the kidney, liver, and bone marrow should be examined as well. Examination of other organs with rapid cell turnover rates, such as the intestinal epithelium and bone marrow, may define the specificity of the agent's toxic effect on the germinal epithelium. The diagnostic and predictive power of morphologic investigations consists mainly in providing detailed information regarding the type, severity, location, and outcome of cytotoxic effects. Genotoxic and functional alterations may go undetected. Therefore, additional methods must supplement histologic observations.

Semen Analysis

Semen analysis does not play a major role in the assessment of reproductive toxicity using laboratory animals, although advances are being made in this area. In the human, the preliminary semen examination concerns volume (usually about 3.5 ml), sperm count, motility, and analysis of sperm morphology. Chemical analysis of semen focuses on pH and viscosity (coagulated semen usually liquefies in 20 minutes), as well as prostatic and seminal vesicle secretions. Prostatic secretions are rich in acid phosphatase, lysozymes, citric acid, aminotransferase, dehydrogenases, zinc, and magnesium. Seminal vesicle secretions are rich in fructose and prostaglandins. The extended semen analysis includes estimates of nuclear maturation, metabolic patterns, survival and motility patterns, and intracellular constituents, as well as sperm penetration of cervical mucus (Eliasson, 1983). For guidelines regarding semen evaluation, an excellent reference is the WHO handbook (Belsey et al., 1980).

The clinical detection (semen analysis) of human reproductive capacity is generally unreliable. Therefore, a number of investigators have sought to develop a heterologous (interspecies) in vitro fertilization test system that utilizes human sperm and ova of laboratory animals (Hall, 1981).

Fertility Testing

Mating of rodents or rabbits is a useful but rather insensitive predictor of human toxic effects. The number of sperm available for ejaculation can be reduced by nearly 90% in rats before a decreased number of off-spring is consistently observed. A 50% reduction in either the daily sperm production or in the functionality of the ejaculated sperm is unlikely to alter fecundity. However, serial mating studies are a good approach to assess genotoxic effects, which are generally not identified morphologically. Malformed germ cells may be associated with genotoxic effects of reactive chemicals such as procarbazine, and of agents such as vincristine that disrupt spermatogenesis by affecting microtubules (Ettlin et al., 1983).

FERTILITY PROFILES. The serial mating technique using rodents can be used to test both dominant lethal mutations and male reproductive capacity (Epstein et al., 1972; Lee and Dixon, 1972).

HORMONAL STATUS. Hormonal deficiencies induce characteristic changes particularly in the testes. In such cases, it is useful to measure hormone levels in the serum and in the target organ. Repeated estimations are often necessary as normal individual levels show a relatively high variability. The influence of circadian rhythms and other variables is minimized by sampling during the same hour of the day. Hormonal levels can also be affected by stress. Hormone measurements in men include FSH, LH, testosterone, estradiol (measured in men with gynecomastia of sudden onset), and prolactin. Hyperprolactinemia has been associated with oligospermia and impotence.

PROTEIN MARKERS. "Marker proteins" indicative of normal or abnormal cellular differentiation or function have been sought by many investigators. Shen and Lee (1977) have used testicular enzymes in an attempt to predict testicular development and chemically induced toxicity. Androgen-binding protein (ABP) may be a useful indicator of Sertoli's cell function in some rodents. The isoenzyme LDH-X is specific for pachytene primary spermatocytes and older germ cells, and might be used to quantify the effect of chemicals affecting these cell types.

FEMALE

As with the male, female animals should be inspected to assess the general appearance of their external genitalia. This is particularly important when studying the postnatal effects of gestational chemical exposure. The genito–anal distance can be measured to determine the sex of newborn animals, the distance in females being shorter than in males. After sacrifice, the animals can be examined internally for conformity of anatomic relationships, cystic ovaries, and other gross abnormalities. Organ weights, especially of the ovaries and adrenals, are important indicators of toxicity.

Using light microscopy, all organs important to reproduction should be examined. These include the ovaries, oviducts, uterus, cervix, adrenals, and pituitary. PAS stain can be used to identify mucus-secreting cells in the vagina and uterus. Transmission electron microscopy (TEM) sometimes provides additional information, particularly with regard to the ovary and pituitary. Scanning electron microscopy (SEM) of luminal surfaces of the vagina, cervix, and uterus may reveal early anatomic changes (Newbold and McLachlan, 1982).

Ovary

TISSUE FIXATION. In routine procedures for light microscopy, ovaries are fixed in Bouin's solution, and serial sections are prepared. Elaborate systems have been proposed for classifying oocytes and follicles. The following types of follicles are typically classified: primordial, primary, secondary, tertiary or vesicular, and graafian or mature. It is difficult at times to distinguish between the primordial and early primary follicles using light microscopy, and some investigators lump them together. Primary, secondary, and tertiary follicles are sometimes referred to as growing follicles. Oocyte counts are made generally on every fifth section, and stages of follicular development are quantified and compared. This provides information on the mean number of follicles, on the percentage of atretic follicles, and on the relative percentage of primordial, growing, and graafian follicles (Mattison, Nightingale, and Shiromizu, 1983a; Vouk and Sheehan, 1983).

For evaluating toxic effects on the ovary, it is useful to distinguish the three types of atresia. The first type is characterized by fresh degenerative changes including karyorrhexis, pyknosis, cytoplasmic eosinophilia, and distortion of the cell membranes of oocytes and follicular cells, as well as leukocytic infiltration of the whole follicle. After oocyte degeneration, a second type of atresia is observed characterized by amorphous eosinophilic material in a cavity surrounded by flattened epithelial cells. This type of degeneration might be associated in particular with secondary follicles. In the third type of atresia, the oocyte degenerates while the surrounding follicles appear normal.

To prepare samples for electron microscopy, the ovary can be cut easily into small blocks and fixed rapidly with glutaraldehyde.

Ovarian Cyclicity

Estrous cycles can be determined by vaginal smears in laboratory animals. Vaginal smears are obtained by inserting a spatula, a smooth rod, or a cotton swab into the vagina, or by washing the vagina with a small amount of saline. The cells are then smeared onto a microscope slide and air-dried; they may be stained, cleared, and permanently preserved under a cover glass (Champlin et al., 1973).

Estrogen Responsiveness

Tissue and organ responses to estrogens include time of vaginal opening in immature rats, onset of reproductive capacity, age of reproductive senescence, total reproductive capacity, uterine weight, endometrial morphology, and serum levels of FSH and LH (Mattison et al., 1983a).

The study of nuclear and cytoplasmic hormone receptors in target tissues is a rapidly developing field with important toxicologic applications. The cellular content and affinity of receptors for natural hormones may be modified by exposure to foreign chemicals. Quantification of cytoplasmic estrogen receptors in human breast cancer is a useful adjunct to the therapy of this disease, and such measurements have helped to predict those mammary neoplasms that respond best to estrogen therapy.

Female Accessory Sex Organs

The female accessory sex organs do not require any special fixation or embedding techniques to obtain quality specimens. Attention should be directed to the vulva, vagina, cervix, uterus, and oviduct to assess congenital malformations, disorders in sexual differentiation, hypertrophy, hyperplasia, and malignant tumors. Cyclic changes in body temperature and the cytology of the cervix and vagina are convenient endpoints that reflect the complex hormonal regulation of the female reproductive system.

Biochemical analysis, including electrophoresis, of vaginal and uterine luminal fluid, is in many ways analogous to semen analysis in the male. In larger laboratory species like the rabbit, monkey, or dog, follicular fluid from the ovary can be analyzed for changes in certain components that indicate altered function. The text, *Pathology of the Female Genital Tract*, edited by Blaustein (1977), is an excellent reference for the basic or clinical scientist concerned with the details of this general area.

Reproductive Capacity

Although less extensive than for the male, a number of functional, morphologic, and biochemical parameters are available to assess toxic effects on female reproductive function (Table 5-4). Essential aspects of reproductive capacity include gametogenesis, conception, implantation, and successful pregnancy. Total reproductive capacity is a useful approach for studying chronic reproductive toxicity in rodents (Dixon and Hall, 1982). The effects of gestational ex-

posure to DES have been studied using this technique (McLachlan et al., 1982). Lamb et al. (1984) designed a continuous breeding test protocol. Relatively simple procedures exist for studying sperm and ovum transport, fertilization success, the rate of tubal transport of the zygote, early embryonic development, implantation, and the spacing of conceptuses along the uterine horns (West et al., 1977).

Multigenerational Tests

Multigenerational studies are intended to provide data on gonadal function, estrous cycle, mating behavior, conception, implantation, abortion, fetal and embryonic development, parturition, postnatal survival, lactation, maternal behavior, and postpartum growth. The classical three-generation reproduction study requires continuous exposure of the parental generation (F_0) and the offspring of each succeeding generation to the test chemical (Collins, 1978). The advantages of multigenerational tests include the wide range of reproductive processes that are assessed and the possibility of observing genetic and behavioral effects (Vouk and Sheehan, 1983). The multigenerational study involves only gross observations; histopathology is rare. There are several variations on this classic scheme, and recent analyses suggest that no more than two generations are required or scientifically justified (Dixon and Hall, 1982). The Environmental Protection Agency design for multigeneration reproductive study is presented in Figure 5-9.

Agents Affecting Reproduction

Most humans are exposed to a vast number of chemicals that may be hazardous to their reproductive capacity. Many chemicals have been identified as reproductive hazards in laboratory studies (Dixon and Hall, 1982). Although the extrapolation of data from laboratory animals to humans is inexact, a number of these chemicals have also been shown to exert detrimental effects on human reproductive performance. The list in-

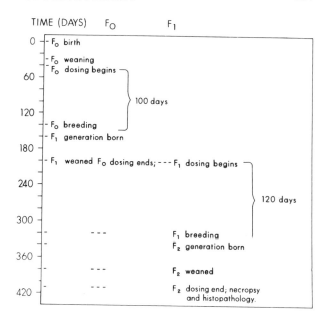

Figure 5–9. Approximate breeding and dosing schedule for EPA Reproduction Study. F_0, parents; F_1, first filial generation produced by crossing two individuals; F_2, second filial generation produced by mating two members of the F_1 generation. (From Dixon and Hall, 1982.)

cludes drugs (especially steroid hormones and chemotherapeutic agents), metals and trace elements, pesticides, food additives and contaminants, industrial chemicals, and consumer products. Cause-and-effect relationships are particularly difficult to establish in the human population, which probably accounts for the fact that fewer than a dozen nontherapeutic environmental chemicals have been linked with effects on men; fewer still have been shown to alter reproductive performance in women.

It is not the purpose of this section to present a complete account of all chemicals that have been implicated as affecting reproduction or to discuss dose–response relationships or species differences in detail. Reviews and textbooks are available concerning both male and female reproductive toxicity (Gomes, 1970, 1977; Bingham, 1977; Lucier et al., 1977; Hunt, 1979; Davies, 1980; Walsh and Egdahl, 1980;). Sieber and Adamson (1975) and Shalet (1980) have focused on the effects of cancer chemotherapeutic agents on reproduction. Spira and Jouannet (1982) have recently edited *Human Fertility Factors*. The Council on Environmental Quality (1981) and Barlow and Sullivan (1982) treat the subject more broadly.

Four primary references were used to prepare this section (Davies, 1980; Gilman et al., 1980; CEQ, 1981; Barlow and Sullivan, 1982). The reader is referred to these sources for more details and for the specific references to the studies summarized below. In addition, one of us (R.L.D.) maintains a reproductive toxicity information file at the E.P.A. and is willing to receive inquiries.

Gonadal (and accessory sex organ) toxicity depends on not only the level of exposure (or dose) but also the frequency and duration of exposure. Findings are also influenced by the time of observation after exposure was initiated or ceased, the quality of the histologic preparations, and the experience and training of the investigator. Very few systematic attempts have been made to define the potential of therapeutic or environmental chemicals to induce biochemical, morphologic, and functional changes associated with reproduction. Clinical assessment of reproductive effects is even more difficult. Thus, both the laboratory and clinical data bases need to be qualitatively and quantitatively strengthened.

The basic types of morphologic reactions of reproductive tissues to chemicals and other environmental agents can be classified as follows: (1) regressive changes, which include various degrees of degeneration, hypoplasia, and atrophy, (2) progressive changes involving hypertrophy and hyperplasia, and (3) neoplastic transformations. The pattern of morphologic response of the reproductive system can provide clues to the mode of action of toxic chemicals.

In the male, reproductive dysfunction may be related to altered hypothalamo–pituitary–gonadal interactions, spermatogenesis, Sertoli's cell function, hormone synthesis and action, accessory sex organ function, gene integrity, libido, potency, or ejaculation. Likewise, female reproduction may be perturbed by altered hypothalamo–pituitary–gonadal interactions, oogenesis, steroidogenesis and ovulation, or accessory sex organ function. As the sperm and egg come together in the oviduct, fertilization occurs and the embryonic tissues start to differentiate. Extraembryonic tissues are involved with implantation and the production of hormones that help maintain the pregnancy. These processes are likewise targets for toxicity.

THERAPEUTIC AGENTS

In our efforts to understand more fully the underlying mechanisms of reproductive toxicity and to identify more accurately chemicals that might pose a reproductive hazard, side effects and toxicity associated with therapeutic agents have provided valuable insights. For this reason, a number of drugs that affect reproduction will be mentioned and an attempt made to link the altered biologic process with a toxic reproductive effect.

Drugs Acting on the Central Nervous System

The effect of a drug is considered to be specific when it affects an identifiable molecular mechanism unique to target cells that bear receptors for the drug. Conversely, a drug is regarded as nonspecific when it produces effects on many different target cells and acts by diverse molecular mechanisms.

Mechanisms of toxicity fall into similar categories. This separation is often a function of the dose–response relationship of the drug and the cell or mechanisms under scrutiny. A drug (or chemical) that is highly selective when tested at a low concentration may exhibit nonspecific actions at substantially higher doses. The general or nonspecific CNS depressants include the anesthetic gases and vapors, alcohols, and some hypnotic-sedative drugs. These agents share the ability to depress excitable tissue at all levels of the CNS. Drugs that selectively modify CNS function include the anticonvulsants, antiparkinsonism drugs, narcotic and nonnarcotic analgesics, appetite suppressants, antiemetics, analgesic antipyretics, certain stimulants, neuroleptics (antidepressants, antimanic, and antipsychotic agents), hypnotics, sedatives, and tranquilizers. Many of the individual agents in these drug categories are capable of altering reproductive performance.

GENERAL ANESTHETICS. Laboratory animal studies do not reveal any consistent adverse effect on mating or fertility induced by anesthetic agents. Rates of implantations, resorptions, viable fetuses, and congenital malformations are similar in experimental and control groups. The effects of acute exposure to anesthetic gases do not appear to be long-lasting in humans. Within days, decreased LH and testosterone levels have returned to normal ranges.

However, chronic occupational exposure to waste anesthetic gases does appear to affect human reproduction. Women working in operating rooms apparently have an increased rate of spontaneous abortions and a higher incidence of birth defects. It has also been suggested that wives of male oral surgeons chronically exposed to unspecified concentrations of anesthetics before their wives' pregnancies had an increased rate of spontaneous abortions. However, other studies fail to confirm the higher incidence of abortions in the wives of men working in operating rooms. It is likely that these effects are linked to the halogenated anesthetic agents, such as halothane, enflurane, and methoxyflurane, which undergo biotransformation. Trichlorethylene and chloroform represent older halogenated compounds that are no longer employed for anesthesia. However, both of these agents are used in industrial processes, and each has been associated with embryolethal and fetotoxic effects in laboratory animals (Marshall and Wollman, 1980).

HYPNOTICS AND SEDATIVES. Incidences of reduction of libido have been associated with the benzodiazepine antianxiety agents.

ALCOHOLS. Alcoholic beverages have been used since the dawn of history, and the opinions and traditions of the past often cloud the discussion of toxic effects. It is a popular notion that alcohol is an aphrodisiac, but this is not the case. Laboratory and clinical experiments have confirmed the observations of the gatekeeper in *Macbeth* that drink "provokes the desire, but taketh away the performance." Although aggressive sexual behavior is often seen after alcohol ingestion, it is usually as a result of a loss of inhibition and restraint. Furthermore, objective measurements of penile tumescence and vaginal pressure show that ethanol significantly decreases sexual responsiveness in both men and women (Ritchie, 1980).

In men, chronic ingestion of alcohol may lead to impotency, sterility, and gynecomastia. This feminization has a dual origin. First, alcohol-induced hepatic injury leads to a hyperestrogenization and a reduced rate of production of testosterone; second, by increasing the activity of the enzymes of the hepatic endoplasmic reticulum, ethanol markedly increases the rate of metabolic inactivation of testosterone.

Although teratogenic effects of alcohol have been suspected for a long time, the fetal alcohol syndrome has only recently been fully described.

Disulfiram, used in the treatment of chronic alcoholism because it alters the intermediate metabolism of ethanol, affects spermatogenesis, and reduces sexual potency.

Drugs Used in Psychiatric Disorders

PHENOTHIAZINES. Chlorpromazine is the prototype of the phenothiazine class of antipsychotic agents. Most neuroleptic drugs have the ability to increase the rate of prolactin secretion in humans. This effect is likely responsible for the breast engorgement and galactorrhea that is sometimes associated with their use, even in male patients. Chlorpromazine can also reduce urinary concentrations of gonadotropins, estrogens, and progestins. In female animals, chlorpromazine can block ovulation, suppress the estrous cycle, cause infertility and pseudopregnancy, as well as maintain an endometrial decidual reaction. In males, inhibition of secretion of gonadotropins can result in decreased testicular weight. Nonreproductive endocrinologic functions are also affected (Baldessarini, 1980).

TRICYCLIC ANTIDEPRESSANTS. Therapeutic use of tricyclic antidepressants such as imipramine and amitriptyline has been associated with delay of orgasm and orgasmic impotence in both men and women. The safety of using antidepressants during pregnancy and lactation is not clearly established.

BENZODIAZEPINE DERIVATIVES. The benzodiazepine derivatives, presently used for the treatment of anxiety, have been associated with menstrual irregularities and failure to ovulate.

MISCELLANEOUS ANTIDEPRESSANTS. A number of nonsteroidal drugs and chemicals used as antidepressants impair fertility in the male by reducing gonadotropin production. It appears that the effect is on the hypothalamus. Reserpine, serotonin, and MAO inhibitors such as iproniazid have been reported to depress spermatogenesis.

Antiepileptic Drugs

Phenytoin, a primary drug for all types of epilepsy, has been associated with hirsutism in young women. Anticonvulsant therapy with aminoglutethimide has been reported to cause virilization due to an effect on adrenocortical steroid biosynthesis. Menstrual disorders and ovarian dysfunction have been observed in patients receiving aminoglutethimide, which is also used for the treatment of breast cancer.

Drugs for Parkinson's Disease

Levodopa, the prototype of central dopaminergic drugs, has been associated with endocrine and reproductive side effects. Central dopaminergic systems play an important role in the modulation of hypothalamic–pituitary function which modulates FSH and LH secretion. Dopamine also inhibits the secretion of prolactin in humans. Thus, levodopa and other dopaminergic agonists decrease the secretion of prolactin, while dopaminergic antagonists have the opposite effect.

Opioids

Among their effects in humans, opioids and opioid-like peptides suppress the secretion of LH and enhance the release of prolactin. LH suppression leads to a substantial decrease in concentrations of testosterone in the plasma. Depending on the dose and the degree of tolerance, males maintained on methadone exhibit decreased sexual drive, as well as decreased motility of sperm and volume of ejaculate. Heroin addicts had lower total and free plasma testosterone levels and higher levels of sex steroid-binding globulin than age-matched controls. Inhibition of the action of LH on the testis may be involved in the reduction of plasma testosterone levels. Heroin addicts may have decreased libido, ejaculation difficulties, or be impotent (Jaffe and Martin, 1980).

Histamine and Serotonin (and Their Antagonists)

Depending on what responses to histamine are prevented, antagonists that act at receptors for histamine are classified as H_1- or H_2-receptor blocking agents (Douglas,

1980). Chlorcyclizine, a representative of the H_1-receptor blocking drugs, caused severe testicular damage affecting germinal, Sertoli's, and Leydig's cells in rats fed the drug in their diet for 6 weeks or longer.

The H_2-receptor blocking agents have provided a new and effective therapeutic approach to the treatment of gastric hypersecretory states. Cimetidine, an H_2-blocking agent, has a weak antiandrogenic effect that has been demonstrated in rats and dogs given high doses of the drug. In men, cimetidine has been reported to impair sexual function by exerting an antiandrogenic action. In treated patients the plasma testosterone level was normal, but the levels of LH, FSH, and prolactin were elevated though not in all cases. Gynecomastia has been noted in men and galactorrhea in women who have taken the drug for long periods of time. A reduction of sperm count by 40% has also been noted in human males receiving cimetidine. The reduction was associated with a reduced response of LH to the administration of gonadotropin-releasing hormone and elevated concentrations of testosterone in plasma (Van Thiel et al., 1979). Because of its weak antiandrogenic activity, cimetidine reduced the rates of growth of the prostate and seminal vesicles in treated rats.

Drugs Affecting the Autonomic Nervous System

The muscular movements of the accessory sex organs are under the control of the autonomic nervous system, as are the processes of penile erection and ejaculation. Willis (1981) has reviewed the drugs that take the joy out of sex. Sexual side effects have been demonstrated for drugs in the following categories: antihypertensives, antiarrhythmics, cholesterol- and lipid-lowering agents, antipsychotics, antidepressants, anxiolytics (antianxiety), and weight control agents. Thus, drugs (or other chemicals) that interrupt the nervous system can have adverse effects on reproductive performance and capacity (Mayer, 1980; Woods, 1984).

ANTICHOLINESTERASE AGENTS. Anticholinesterase agents inhibit acetylcholinesterase by terminating the action of acetylcholine at the junctions of the various cholinergic nerve endings. In addition to their uses in medicine, anticholinesterase agents are used as agricultural insecticides and potential chemical warfare "nerve gases." Impotency and decreased libido have been associated with exposure to anticholinesterase agents.

ANTIMUSCARINIC DRUGS. These drugs antagonize the muscarinic actions of acetylcholine an autonomic effectors innervated by postganglionic cholinergic nerves as well as on smooth muscles that lack cholinergic innervation. Atropine and related belladonna alkaloids are antimuscarinic drugs that may affect reproduction by altering potency.

ANTIADRENERGIC DRUGS. Many substances of diverse structure and mechanism of action interfere with the function of the sympathetic nervous system. Several drugs, such as α- and β-blocking agents, clonidine, methyldopa, guanethidine, bretylium, and reserpine, are used in clinical medicine, particularly for the control of hypertension and cardiac disorders. Adrenergic neuron-blocking agents interfere with the release of norepinephrine consequent to nerve stimulation. They may produce this effect by inhibiting the synthesis, storage, or release of the neurotransmitter. The consequence of these effects is a reduction in the amount of norepinephrine released by each nerve impulse. Other drugs, adrenergic receptor-blocking agents, inhibit the ability of the neurotransmitter or other sympathomimetic amines to interact effectively with their receptors. Their reproductive side effect could be expected to be due to an interruption of adrenergic function, especially with regard to smooth muscle function and penile erection and ejaculation.

Although there are several reports of impotence related to β-adrenergic receptor-blocking agents such as atenolol and propranolol, the α-adrenergic receptor-blocking agents are more often associated with sexual dysfunction. Phenoxybenzamine and prazosin affect ejaculation. All adrenergic neuron-blocking agents are capable of causing ejaculation failure and impotence. Some patients receiving clonidine have reported impotence. Methyldopa also causes impotence in varying degrees. About one half of the patients receiving either bethamidine or guanethidine fail to ejaculate; other patients taking either of these drugs are impotent. The failure of ejaculation is attributed to the loss of sympathetic activity necessary for erection and ejaculation. The use of reserpine also causes reduced libido and impotence. This effect has been related to both CNS depression and to increased serum prolactin levels.

Hypnotics and Sedatives

The principal use of sedative-hypnotic drugs such as the benzodiazepines, barbiturates, chloral derivatives, and glutethimide is to produce drowsiness and promote sleep. In humans, barbiturates may induce a deficiency of steroid delta 4-5-α-reductase. Reduction of libido has been associated with the benzodiazepine antianxiety agents.

Anti-inflammatory, Analgesic, and Antipyretic Drugs

Aspirin is the prototype of drugs whose therapeutic activity appears to depend to a large extent on the inhibition of a defined biochemical pathway. Aspirin and aspirin-like drugs inhibit the biosynthesis of prostaglandins. Most of the common aspirin-like drugs are "irreversible" inhibitors of cyclooxygenase. These aspirin-like drugs may have undesirable effects on male fertility. Human seminal fluid is probably the richest natural source of prostaglandins, and in some subfertile males decreased concentrations of prostaglandins in seminal fluid correlate well with infertility. Indomethacin, another prostaglandin inhibitor, inhibits hyaluronidase in the testis. Colchicine is used for the treatment of gout. Azoospermia might be produced by colchicine as a result of an inhibition of mitotic and meiotic spindles necessary for cell division. The impairment of spindle activity may also result in aneuploidy caused by nondisjunction of chromosomes. Similar effects are associated with the vinca alkaloids used to treat cancer.

Antiparasitic Drugs

Hycanthone, an anthelmintic drug useful to treat schistosomiasis, has been shown to be both mutagenic and carcinogenic in several experimental systems. The antimalarial drugs, quinine, quinacrine, and chloroquine, are thought to have an antifertility effect perhaps due to an action on sperm motility. These drugs are also capable of inhibiting steroidogenesis in Leydig's (and ovarian) cell cultures, and may also inhibit prostaglandin synthesis.

Antimicrobial Agents

Antibiotics are chemical substances produced naturally by various species of microorganisms that suppress the growth of other microorganisms and may eventually kill them. Many antimicrobial agents are also the product of chemical synthesis. Most of the antimicrobial antibiotics have a high degree of microbial specificity and low mammalian toxicity. Thus, few of the agents in this category are associated with reproductive side effects. However, the nitrofurans (furacin, furadoxyl, and furadantin) arrest spermatogenesis in rats at the primary spermatocyte stage. Spermatogenesis returned to normal on the cessation of treatment. Furacin was the most potent of the nitrofurans tested. It has been reported that the nitrofurans might affect Sertoli's cell function in addition to acting on germ cells (Davies, 1980). A number of recent reports have also suggested that male patients treated with sulfasalazine developed oligospermia and became infertile. Semen quality improved on withdrawal of the drug, and subsequent pregnancies were normal.

Antineoplastic Drugs

In contrast to antimicrobial agents, antineoplastic agents are generally nonspecific in their action and have a low therapeutic index. It is now generally accepted that the entire population of neoplastic cells must be eradicated in order to obtain a cure (Skipper, 1983). The concept of "total cell kill" applies to chemotherapy as it does to toxicity, especially that associated with spermatogonia replication. An understanding of cell cycle kinetics is essential to use the current generation of antineoplastic agents properly and to predict the tissues they will affect. Because most antineoplastic agents act specifically on processes such as DNA synthesis, transcription, or mitotic spindle formation, they are regarded as cell cycle-specific. Many of the most potent cytotoxic agents are only effective against cells that are in the process of division. Likewise, reproductive tissues, depending on their stage of differentiation and degree of cellular replication, are uniquely susceptible to drugs acting by various mechanisms of action.

Some antineoplastic agents, particularly certain antimetabolites, that were originally developed for cancer treatment have earned important roles in the management of non-neoplastic disorders. Examples include the application of allopurinol in controlling hyperuricemia in gout, the use of methotrexate in psoriasis, and the inhibitory actions of analogs of pyrimidine and purine nucleosides on the proliferation of certain DNA viruses. Cytotoxic agents such as azathioprine are used to suppress the immune response, which plays an essential role in organ transplantation and in the treatment of diseases characterized by altered immunologic reactivity and autoimmunity. Azathioprine does not affect sperm counts or sperm motilty but does increase the proportion of abnormal forms present in the semen of some men being treated for chronic hepatitis (Calabresi and Parks, 1980).

Almost all classes of antineoplastic agents have been associated with reproductive toxicity, especially in males. Because anticancer agents are administered at cytotoxic doses, their effects on the gonads are generally apparent and have been relatively well studied. An additional insight is provided by the fact that the different classes of anticancer drugs generally represent unique mechanisms of action. These classes include alkylating agents, antimetabolites, mitotic inhibitors, and antitumor antibiotics (Sieber and Adamson, 1975; Lu and Meistrich, 1979; Davies, 1980).

ALKYLATING AGENTS. This class includes the nitrogen mustards (e.g., cyclophosphamide), ethylenimine derivatives (e.g., Thiotepa), alkyl sulfonates (e.g., busulfan), nitrosoureas (e.g., BCNU), and the triazenes (e.g., Dacarbazine). These agents cross-link DNA and prevent normal cell replication. Germ cell damage is known to result from the administration of busulfan, chlorambucil, and cyclophosphamide. Cyclophosphamide has also been reported to cause oligospermia and azoospermia in young men treated for nephrotic syndrome. Treatment with cytotoxic drugs can also impair the function of Leydig's cells. The deleterious effect of antitumor drugs on Leydig's cell function is more evident in prepubertal boys than in adult men.

Busulfan arrests the development of spermatogonia by affecting those cells that are dividing actively (Hodel et al., 1984). Ionizing radiation has a similar selective action on spermatogonia. Exposure of rodents in utero to busulfan eradicates germ cells, so that the tubules of the male offspring contain only Sertoli's cells.

Procarbazine, a methylhydrazine derivative, has been shown to cause sterility in rats, mice, monkeys, and man. It is a carcinogen that disrupts the chromosomes of zygotene and mid-pachytene cells. Procarbazine also has a mutagenic action on all spermatogenic cell types (Bechter et al., 1982). Spermatogonia and spermatids were most heavily affected by the genotoxic action of procarbazine, the first probably because they are the least protected, the latter because they lack the ability to repair damage to DNA by unscheduled DNA synthesis. Development of early spermatids is retarded in a unique fashion, and spermiation is inhibited (Ettlin et al., 1982).

ANTIMETABOLITES. Members of this class include the folic acid analogs (e.g., methotrexate), pyrimidine analogs (e.g., 5-fluorouracil, cytosine arabinoside), and the purine analogs (e.g., 6-mercaptopurine). These drugs act by a variety of mechanisms to prevent the synthesis of ribonucleotides and deoxyribonucleotides essential for gametogenesis. Generally they are less toxic for the gonads than alkylating agents, but cytosine arabinoside has also been reported to reduce the proportion of tubules containing spermatids in boys being treated for acute lymphoblastic leukemia.

VINCA ALKALOIDS. The vinca alkaloids include vinblastine and vincristine, which inhibit the function of microtubules. Parvinen et al. (1978) examined the effects of vinblastine and vincristine on spermatogenesis in adult rats after intratesticular application and reported there was arrest of mitotic and meiotic divisions at metaphase similar to that produced by colchicine. There was also a premature loss of spermatids from Sertoli's cells. Early spermatids were damaged, acrosomes had vacuoles, and cytoplasmic bridges were disrupted, which resulted in the formation of multinucleated giant cells. Sertoli's cells were also damaged by these vinca alkaloids. These drugs bind to tubulin and prevent microtubule assembly. Effects after single ip injection of 0.6 mg/kg into rats were more subtle. In particular, meiosis was less affected than mitosis, possibly because spermatocytes—in contrast to spermatogonia—lie inside the protective Sertoli–Sertoli cell tight junctions (Ettlin, 1983).

NATURAL PRODUCTS (ANTIBIOTICS). This class includes drugs such as actinomycin D, daunomycin, bleomycin, mithramycin, and mitomycin which affect macromolecular synthesis. Prominent among the mechanisms of action of these agents is the ability to interacalate with DNA and prevent cell division. Other members of the class inhibit RNA synthesis. Morphological, biochemical, and functional effects of daunomycin on the testis have been described by Matter and co-workers (1983).

The drug combination responsible for the cure of Hodgkin's disease causes sterility in 95% of men and about 50% of women treated. This drug-induced infertility has persisted in patients followed for as long as 12 years. Men generally are more susceptible to gonadal damage from chemotherapy than women. In men, spermatogonia are primarily affected; in women, the drugs destroy a certain number of oocytes in the ovary. Because the number of oocytes decreases with age, sterility risk is higher for older women. Therefore, women over 35 often become sterile while women under 35 usually continue to ovulate. There is a concern that the onset of menopause will be premature in young women who have received chemotherapy. Age plays a critical role in the susceptibility of patients to gonadal toxicity.

Diuretics

Most diuretics act by inhibiting sodium and chloride reabsorption. Treating rats with the carbonic anhydrase inhibitor diuretics, acetazolamide and ethoxyzolamide, reduced the rate of flow of rete testis fluid, thus suggesting that the secretion of testicular fluid is an active process. Acetazolamide has also been shown to decrease fluid production and the pressure in the aqueous humor of the eye and the cerebrospinal fluid of the brain.

Hormones and Hormone Antagonists

The essential role of the hypothalamo–pituitary–gonadal axis in reproduction is well appreciated. As already mentioned, it can be perturbed by a variety of drugs (and other environmental chemicals). Those agents used therapeutically are usually synthetic analogs of the natural hormone but differ in some important aspect. The design of synthetic products seeks to escape enzyme degradation while retaining an affinity for the specific hormone receptor. The first nonsteroid estrogen, diethylstilbestrol (DES), was synthesized nearly 50 years ago. A wide variety of hormone agonists and antagonists has been developed in more recent years.

ORAL CONTRACEPTIVES. The oral contraceptives offer a good example of the reproductive effects of estrogens and progestins; the most common type of oral contraceptive contains both. Their contraceptive efficacy is nearly 100%. Other modifications of steroidal contraception include sequential preparations where estrogen is taken initially followed by combined estrogen and progestin for the last 5–6 days of the dosage regimen. A wide variety of estrogen and progesterone analogs are used in these preparations.

Ovulation is prevented by suppressing the synthesis of pituitary gonadotropins and possibly also by reducing the ovarian response to gonadotropins. The most widely used preparations today owe their effectiveness in inhibiting ovulation to the estrogenic component. The progestin serves the major purpose of ensuring that withdrawal bleeding will be prompt, brief, and essentially physiologic. The oral contraceptives also could interfere with implantation by their direct actions on the endometrium. The coordinated contractions of the cervix, uterus, and oviducts also appear essential for the transport of sperm to the egg and the precisely timed movement of the blastocyst to the uterine lumen.

Many natural and synthetic hormones, such as methyltestosterone, can disrupt the hormonal regulation of spermatogenesis. This area has been investigated quite intensively, mainly in an effort to develop effective male contraceptives (Neumann et al., 1975; Steinberger, 1980). Treating male dogs with estrogens results in tubules containing Sertoli's cells only (Figure 5-10). (Investigational antispermatogenic drugs are considered later in this section.)

HORMONE ANTAGONISTS. The term antiestrogen has been applied generally to several

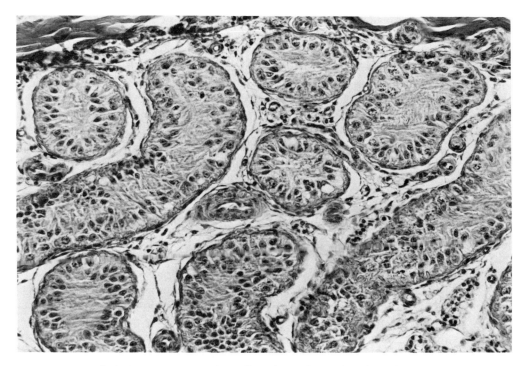

Figure 5–10. Tubules containing Sertoli's cells only, and atrophy of Leydig's cells resulting from chronic exposure of dogs to high doses of estrogens. (Courtesy Dr. G. Zbinden, Institute of Toxicology, Federal Institute of Technology, Schwerzenbach/Zürich, Switzerland.)

different types of compounds that inhibit or modify the action of estrogen. Clomiphene and tamoxifen are clinically available antiestrogens used for treating infertility and carcinoma of the breast. These agents bind to cytoplasmic estrogen receptors, and the modified complex is translocated to the nucleus. Such competition for estrogen-binding sites and the resultant diminished amount of estrogen receptor that is available for endogenous hormone are thought to account for the antiestrogen activity. Cytoplasmic binding affinities are used to predict antiestrogenic activity. Antiestrogens also prevent the normal "feedback inhibition" control of estrogen synthesis in the hypothalamus and pituitary, which results in an increased secretion of LHRH/FSHRH and gonadotropins. Increased concentrations of gonadotropins lead to ovarian stimulation, ovulation, and sustained function of the corpora lutea.

Nonsteroidal antiandrogens have been studied in animals and in in vitro systems. These compounds (e.g., cyproterone, DIMP, flutamide, and cyanoketone) block the action or synthesis of testosterone and include dimethanesulfonate derivatives. Cyproterone acetate, used to treat precocious puberty, is an effective antiandrogen that possesses potent progestational activity and suppresses the secretion of gonadotropins. In androgen-dependent target tissues, cyproterone acetate competes with dihydrotestosterone for its receptor site. Treating pregnant rats with cyproterone acetate causes feminization of their male fetuses. The penis is underdeveloped and resembles a clitoris, the prostate is missing, and the testes are small and undescended (Dixon, 1982).

ENVIRONMENTAL AGENTS

Scientific, regulatory, and public concern continues to increase regarding the potential for chemicals in our environment to affect reproductive capacity. Occupational exposure subjects the worker to the greatest risk because of the regimen and levels of exposure. Other sources of pollutants are the air we breathe, the water we drink, and the food we consume. Even our homes are not without potential reproductive hazards. A very wide variety of chemicals are involved, and exposures are usually multiple.

Metals and Trace Elements

Metals and trace elements are widely distributed in nature. Some metals are essential for life; others have no known biologic function but are not serious toxic hazards. Still others have the potential to produce toxicity. Many metals, both essential and nonessential, are affected by homeostatic mechanisms that determine their physiologic (or toxicologic) action. Tolerance levels in drinking water have been set for the following metals: arsenic, barium, boron, cadmium, chromium, copper, iron, lead, manganese, selenium, silver, uranium (uranyl), and zinc (Hammond and Beliles, 1980). Only a few trace elements have been associated with reproductive toxicity.

ARSENIC. Arsenic has been reported to cause infertility, fetotoxicity, fetolethality, low-birthweight offspring, and congenital malformations in mice and rats. No human reproductive toxicity has been conclusively demonstrated, although arsenic is a suspected mutagen (Beckman et al., 1977).

BORON. Boron is a natural trace element that may be found in ground and well water and that is used medically as boric acid. Laboratory studies confirm that very high doses of boron in the diet of rats for 60 days reduced the number of spermatocytes and spermatids, and eventually caused germinal aplasia that was accompanied by a rise in plasma FSH levels, while LH and testosterone levels were unaffected. Industrial exposure of men to high levels of boron has been associated with oligospermia and loss of libido (Tarasenko et al., 1972). Infertility associated with oligospermia has been reported in workers involved in the pro-

duction of boric acid and in communities where boron concentration in drinking water was high (Krasovskii et al., 1976).

Chronic boron exposure results in testicular atrophy in rats and dogs. Spermatocytes and spermatids seem to be particularly sensitive. Because FSH elevation precedes testicular changes, Sertoli's cells are thought to be affected, thus producing less inhibin. However, the Sertoli's cells are normal under the light microscope. Boron accumulates slowly and persists in the testis for a long time. Thus, recovery may be delayed.

CADMIUM. Cadmium administered parenterally to laboratory animals causes sterility. The mechanisms of action appear to be multiple. Higher doses cause vascular damage, whereas lower doses can be shown to affect the functional capacity of spermiogenic cells and to decrease DNA synthesis by spermatogonial cells. The effects on spermiogenic cells are reversed by zinc (Lee and Dixon, 1973). Chronic cadmium exposure induces metallothionein, a cadmium-binding protein. Reproductive effects in humans have not been associated with cadmium exposure. However, epidemiologic and case studies suggest an association between occupational exposure to cadmium dusts and fumes and prostate cancer (Owen, 1976).

CHROMIUM. Treatment of rats with either the trivalent compound (chromium nitrate) or a hexavalent compound (potassium dichromate) produced seminiferous tubules devoid of spermatocytes. The hexavalent compound was the more toxic and also damaged other types of germ cells. Human data are lacking.

LEAD. Lead, administered orally to rats, causes damage to the seminiferous tubule epithelium, decreased sperm motility, and infertility in males. Treatment of female animals from before breeding until lactation resulted in a reduction in litter size, decreased birthweights, and poor survival. Congenital malformations have been associated with lead exposure of pregnant rats. Lead exposure has also been shown to affect men and women. Occupationally exposed men had morphologically abnormal sperm and decreased libido (Lancranjan et al., 1975); pregnant women had a higher incidence of spontaneous abortions, offspring with lower birthweights, and stillbirths. Lead appears to act directly on the germinal tissues (Nogaki, 1958).

MANGANESE. Manganese is used in steel manufacture, in the chemical industry, and as an additive to gasoline. Large doses of manganese chloride cause loss of testicular germ cells in rats and rabbits. Effects such as decreased libido and impotence have been noted in men occupationally exposed to manganese (Schuler et al., 1957).

MERCURY. Methyl mercury administered parenterally to mice inhibited the early stages of spermatogenesis and reduced fertility. Other laboratory studies suggest that organic mercury increases the incidence of resorptions, decreases fetal weight, and increases fetal death. Teratogenic effects have also been demonstrated. "Fetal Minamata disease" has been documented among the Japanese who consumed fish from Minamata Bay, which contained high concentrations of methyl mercury. Brain damage was reflected as disturbances in motor and mental development, cerebral palsy, and mental retardation (Takeuchi, 1970).

Exposure to inorganic mercury produced fetotoxic and embryolethal effects in laboratory animals. Inorganic mercury has been associated with decreased libido and impotence in male workers (McFarland and Reigel, 1978), and menstrual disorders in exposed female workers (Marinova et al., 1973).

SELENIUM. Selenium has been shown to cause fetotoxicity and embryolethal effects in laboratory animals; human reproductive toxicity has not been reported.

THALLIUM. Thallium alters embryonic development in laboratory animals and can produce fetotoxic and embryolethal effects; human data are lacking.

Pesticides

Reproductive toxicity has been associated with occupational exposure to herbicides and insecticides (Murphy, 1980). Impotence and infertility have been noted in men who are sprayers or applicators of pesticides. Women who worked in vineyards and were exposed to unspecified amounts of various pesticides had detectable levels of DDT in breast milk as well as increased frequency of miscarriages, toxemia, uterine inertia, postpartum hemorrhage, low birthweights, and histopathologic changes in placentas. A number of specific pesticides (discussed below) have been shown to have reproductive effects in laboratory animals. However, only chlordecone and dibromochloropropane (DBCP) have been clearly linked with reproductive toxicity in humans.

CHLORDECONE (KEPONE). Reproductive toxicity produced by chlordecone has been demonstrated in fish, birds, and laboratory rodents (Barlow and Sullivan, 1982). In exposed male mice, rats, and rabbits, depressed spermatogenesis, testicular atrophy, and sterility are seen. In humans, sperm abnormalities including decreased sperm counts, reduced motility, and abnormal morphology have been suggested (Cohn et al., 1978).

Persistent vaginal estrus and anovulation, as well as fetotoxicity, stillbirths, and spontaneous abortions, are seen in female animals treated with chlordecone. Reproduction is completely inhibited in female rats. It is likely that this effect is due to the estrogenicity of chlordecone.

DICHLORODIPHENYLTRICHLOROETHANE (DDT). Reproductive effects have been seen in laboratory animals treated with p,p'-DDT and/or o,p'-DDT. Estrogenic effects are associated with the o,p'-dichlorodiphenyltrichloroethane isomer of DDT. Binding dihydrotestosterone to cytosol receptors is blocked competitively by o,p'-DDT, which also has estrogenic activity. Feeding a diet containing o,p'-DDT to rats for 6 months caused reduced fertility in the treated animals and reduced fecundity in the offspring at the 1000-ppm level. No effects were noted at 20 or 200 ppm. In a multigenerational study there was a marked reduction in fertility and in survival of offspring from the first generation; there were no conceptions in the second generation. In treated mice, in addition to severe adverse effects on reproduction, there was a reduction in lactation and survival of offspring. In dogs, p,p'-DDT caused diminished libido in males; it caused delayed estrus, reduced milk production, infertility, and increased infant and maternal mortality in females. There are no clear-cut reports linking exposure to DDT with reproductive effects in humans, even though it does accumulate in human breast milk.

DIBROMOCHLOROPROPANE (DBCP). Sterility in male workers involved in the manufacture of DBCP is the best quantified and clearest example of human reproductive effects associated with an environmental agent. Before the episode of human toxicity, severe atrophy and degeneration of the testes had been demonstrated in laboratory animals (Torkelson et al., 1961). More recent studies have shown gonadotoxic effects, disturbances of hormonal functions, and altered spermatogenesis in male rats, and altered estrous cycles and low-birthweight offspring in female rats.

Whorton et al. (1977) first reported azoospermia, oligospermia, and elevated FSH levels in men working in the manufacture and formulation of DBCP for more than 3 years. Numerous other reports have been published confirming and expanding on these observations and noting the details of the histopathology. Biopsy of testicular tissue of men reporting decreased libido, impotency, and infertility showed loss of all or most of the germinal cells and a relative increase in the number of Leydig's cells (Biava et al., 1978). An increased frequency of Y chromosome nondisjunction (YFF) has been reported in men exposed to unspeci-

fied levels of DBCP in their workplaces (Kapp et al., 1979), and some men have been rendered permanently azoospermic (Whorton and Milby, 1980).

Fumigants

Fumigants are used in the control of insects, rodents, and soil nematodes. They have in common being in the gaseous form at the time they exert their pesticidal action; furthermore, they have the ability to penetrate to areas otherwise inaccessible to pesticide application. Fumigants may be liquids that vaporize readily, solids that release a gas by chemical reaction, or gases contained in cylinders. Fumigants used in the protection of stored foodstuffs include acrylonitrile, carbon disulfide, carbon tetrachloride, chloropicrin, dibromochloropropane, ethylene dibromide, ethylene oxide, hydrogen cyanide, methyl bromide, and phosphine. These chemicals also have a variety of other applications in industry and agriculture (Murphy, 1980).

CARBON DISULFIDE. Italian factory workers exposed to relatively high concentrations of carbon disulfide had reduced sexual activity and reduced plasma levels of FSH, LH, and prolactin (Cirla et al., 1978). Results of other human studies have been more equivocal. Carbon disulfide appears to have a direct testicular effect, which causes a decreased sperm count and testosterone concentration in rats. Mating behavior is also altered.

ETHYLENE DIBROMIDE (DIBROMOETHANE). In rats, ethylene dibromide (EDB) has been shown to damage spermatids selectively and to induce transient sterility. Testicular weights and serum testosterone levels are both reduced. In bulls, there was decreased sperm motility and a high percentage of sperm abnormalities in the testes, epididymides, ductus deferens, and ejaculate. Decreased fertility in wives of workers in one chemical plant has been reported (Wong et al., 1979).

ETHYLENE OXIDE. Reports have suggested that ethylene oxide exposure is associated with infertility and an increased incidence of spontaneous abortions (Barlow and Sullivan, 1982).

Industrial and Occupational Chemicals

Workers are exposed to a wide variety of chemicals used in industrial processes and manufacture. As more and more women enter the work force, greater attention has been focused on the possible reproductive effects of occupational chemicals. Concern surrounds not only ovarian function and fertility of the women but also the perhaps unique susceptibility of the fertilization and implantation processes as well as the in utero development of the offspring. The books by Barlow and Sullivan (1982) and Hunt (1979) are especially valuable when considering this area, and we refer the reader to those sources for more detail regarding the specific studies cited below.

ANILINE. Treatment of laboratory animals with aniline produces infertility and an increased incidence of abortions; similar effects have been suggested in occupationally exposed women. Women may also experience menstrual and other gynecologic disorders.

BENZENE. Benzene produces testicular damage and reduces fertility in male laboratory animals. There have been suggestions of menstrual and other gynecologic disorders in women occupationally exposed to benzene, and an increased rate of abortions and infertility has also been reported.

BENZO[A]PYRENE. Benzo[a]pyrene is a human carcinogen. Like most other carcinogenic chemicals, it also produces reproductive toxicity when administered to laboratory animals. Benzo[a]pyrene causes testicular damage and reduces fertility in males.

CHLOROPRENE (CHLOROBUTADIENE). Chloroprene induced testicular damage and decreased the sperm counts of mice, rats, and cats. It also induces dominant lethal mutations in mice. Male occupational exposure to chloroprene has been associated with decreased libido, impotence, decreased sperm counts, altered sperm motility, and abnormal sperm morphology. Concern has also been expressed that chloroprene exposure of men might increase the incidence of abortions in their wives.

HEXANE. Testicular lesions have been produced by both hexane and its major metabolite 2,5-hexanedione. Although 2,5-hexanedione induced morphologic changes in the central nervous system that affect both visual and motor function, testicular effects are related to changes in Sertoli's cell biochemistry rather than altered central gonadotropin control systems (Chapin et al., 1982).

FORMALDEHYDE. Formaldehyde has been associated with reproductive toxicity in female workers. Menstrual disorders and increased rates of abortion have been reported, along with decreased fetal growth and low birthweights.

GLYCOL ETHERS. Recent evidence suggests that the glycol ethers may pose severe reproductive hazards to occupationally exposed workers. These hazards include potential sterility or reduced fertility among men, and possible menstrual disorders among women. Testicular toxicity has been reported in rats exposed to ethylene glycol monomethyl and monoethyl ethers, and the potential risk of these chemicals to human reproduction is a growing concern (Lamb et al., 1984).

POLYCHLORINATED BIPHENYLS (PCBS). Treatment of laboratory animals with PCBs produced prolonged estrous cycles in rats and prolonged menstrual cycles in monkeys. Low-birthweight offspring, high perinatal and postnatal mortality, and poor postnatal growth have also been induced in various laboratory species. In women, there have been suggestions of menstrual disorders. Low-birthweight babies, high postnatal mortality, and skin discoloration have also been reported in humans exposed to PCBs.

PHTHALIC ACID ESTERS (PAES). Certain esters of phthalic acid have been found in human and animal tissues as a result of environmental contamination and use in blood transfusion equipment. The phthalic acid esters (PAEs) can adversely affect the rodent testes, but only at high doses. Di(2-ethylhexyl)phthalate (DEHP) and its monomer, monoethylhexyl phthalate (MEHP) appear to have the greatest potency as testicular toxins. Rat gonadal zinc levels can be decreased by the injection of DEHP, and the rat prostate gland seems to be particularly sensitive to PAE-induced zinc depletion. Reproductive effects on humans have not been demonstrated (Thomas et al., 1982).

STYRENE. Styrene exposure disturbed the estrous cycle of rats, and an association between styrene and menstrual disorders in women has been suggested.

TOLUENE. Menstrual disorders in women have been associated with exposure to toluene. There have also been suggestions of decreased fetal growth and low birthweight.

TRIS(2,3-DIBROMOPROPYL)PHOSPHATE (TRIS). TRIS was used as a flame retardant in a variety of fabrics, including acetates and polyesters made into children's sleepwear. The use of TRIS was discontinued after studies indicated numerous toxic effects potentially jeopardizing human health. Dermal exposure of rabbits to TRIS caused testes to shrink and reduced the number of spermatocytes, particularly spermatids. However, neither the extent of toxic effects of TRIS on the organs of the human reproductive system nor its action on fertility are known.

VINYL CHLORIDE. Vinyl chloride is a recognized human carcinogen. It has also been suggested that vinyl chloride affects reproduction by causing decreased libido and impotence in men and decreased fetal growth and low-birthweight babies in exposed women.

Antispermatogenic Drugs (Investigational)

As mentioned, the highly ordered and precise processes that occur during the genesis and maturation of sperm allow many avenues for perturbation or regulation. A variety of compounds can inhibit spermatogenesis. These include antineoplastic agents, antiandrogens, metals, nitrofurans, αchlorohydrin, and dinitropyrrole. However, the irreversible effects of some of these and their toxicity preclude their clinical use. At the present time, the most attractive approach to systemic contraception seems to be the rational administration of androgens, estrogens, and progestins (Nelson and Patanelli, 1965; Murad and Haynes, 1980).

DINITROPYRROLES. Nitrofurans, thiophenes, dinitropyrroles, and bis(dichloroacetyl)diamines have been shown to inhibit gametogenesis without affecting Leydig's cell function. All act directly on the testis and arrest spermatogenesis at the primary spermatocyte stage. However, toxicity and side effects have precluded the use of these chemicals as male contraceptives (Davies, 1980).

BIS(DICHLOROACETYL)DIAMINE (WIN 1446). Bis(dichloroacetyl)diamine is an effective antispermatogenic agent in man. It is relatively nontoxic but causes illness when ethanol is also ingested (Nelson and Patanelli, 1965).

1-P-CHLOROBENZYL-1H-INDAZOLE-3-CARBOXYLIC ACID (AF 1312/TS). 1-*p*-chlorobenzyl-1H-indazole-3-carboxylic acid has an antispermatogenic activity. Diclondazolic acid is a related compound that is 10 times more potent as an antispermatogenic agent.

THIOGLUCOSE. 5-Thio-D-glucose, an analog of glucose, inhibits spermatogenesis in rodents but has no apparent effect on plasma testosterone levels or libido. Because thioglucose inhibits the membrane transport of D-glucose and amino acids, it is felt that this action accounts for its action on germ cells, especially spermatids, which are particularly dependent on glucose for synthetic processes.

CHLORINATED SUGARS. Chlorinated sugars (6-chloroglucose, 6-chlorofructose, and 6-chlorosucrose) administered orally to rats induced infertility. These chlorinated sugars reduced oxygen uptake, ATP, adenine nucleotide, and epididymal sperm motility.

α-CHLOROHYDRIN. α-Chlorohydrin causes readily reversible infertility by damaging sperm in the lower part of the epididymis so that they are incapable of penetrating oocytes. The chemical is active when given orally to rats, guinea pigs, rams, boars, and rhesus monkeys, but is ineffective in mice and rabbits. In rats, irreversible sterility is caused by the formation of spermatoceles. In the epididymis, α-chlorohydrin not only affects metabolism of sperm but also impairs fluid reabsorption. An analog of α-chlorohydrin, 1-amino-3-chloro-2-propanol hydrochloride, causes reversible infertility in male rats, mice, and hamsters at doses that are neither toxic nor affect sexual behavior. The substance appears to abolish the fertilizing ability of epididymal sperm. However, toxicity, including brain damage in monkeys, precluded the clinical trial of this compound as a male contraceptive.

MONOTHIOGLYCEROL. Monothioglycerol affects the fertility of male hamsters. This compound, related chemically to α-chlorohydrin, is thought to affect fertility by causing the seminal vesicles to secrete a substance toxic to sperm.

GOSSYPOL. The collective infertility of a village in China in the 1930s was related to the use of crude cottonseed oil for cooking rather than the traditional soybean oil. Both antispermatogenic effects and menstrual disturbances were reported, as well as not a single childbirth in 10 years. Several groups have demonstrated the male antifertility effect in both laboratory animals and man. Large amounts of work have been done regarding gossypol's antifertility effect and potential as a human contraceptive for men. In clinical trials that lasted longer than 2 years, spermatogenesis was arrested in about 99% of the men tested. This effect was usually reversible. One serious adverse effect is hypokalemia associated with progressive neuromuscular weakness and paralysis.

LHRH ANALOGS. Recent advances in the development of superanalogs of the decapeptide LHRH have increased the efforts to formulate adequate therapeutic regimens which may provide safer and more efficient antifertility methods by taking advantage of the long-term suppressive effects of those peptides on gametogenesis and gonadal function.

Miscellaneous Hazards

The personal habits humans elect are also associated with reproductive hazards. Tobacco smoking and ethanol consumption are the two major contributors to adverse health effects (caffeine, likewise, has raised health-related questions). Agents of abuse such as marijuana and other centrally acting drugs may have reproductive side effects.

SMOKING. Cigarette smokers have been reported to have a significantly higher percentage of morphologically abnormal sperm than nonsmokers. These investigators suggested that the sperm abnormalities in cigarette smokers may reflect genetic damage to those cells as a consequence of exposure to mutagenic products in smoke.

Polycyclic aromatic hydrocarbons produced by smoking tobacco destroy oocytes. A dose-dependent relationship has been found between smoking and the age of menopause (Mattison et al., 1983b).

ETHANOL. Although no clear consensus exists, it appears that ethanol alters the levels of androgens and estrogens in the circulation by mechanisms already discussed. Gonadal dysfunction occurs in alcoholics without liver disease, but the more obvious endocrine features of hypogonadism and feminization are seen in the presence of alcoholic cirrhosis. Testicular biopsies from chronic alcoholics showed severe impairment of spermatogenesis accompanied by raised levels of FSH, prolactin, and sex steroid-binding globulin (Van Thiel and Lester, 1976).

CAFFEINE. Chronically feeding young rats with caffeine, theobromine, or theophylline caused the disappearance of germ cells, and atrophic changes in the epididymis, prostate, and seminal vesicles. However, interstitial cells were hypertrophic, and plasma testosterone levels were elevated. Caffeine has the most marked action on spermatogenesis; theobromine was slightly less potent, and theophylline had a much weaker effect. The methylxanthines appear to act directly on the germ cells. It should be noted that the test concentrations were much higher than the amount of caffeine that would be ingested by heavy drinkers of coffee.

High concentrations of caffeine have also been reported to induce chromosomal abnormalities in both plant and mammalian cells in culture and to have potent mutagenic effects on microorganisms either alone or in combination with other mutagens. These effects seem to be associated with inhibition of DNA repair processes. Concern also surrounds the teratogenicity of caffeine. It has been suggested that women who ingest more than 600 mg of caffeine per day may have an increased incidence of spontaneous abortion, stillbirth, or premature delivery (Davies, 1980).

DRUGS OF ABUSE. Most of the pharmacologic agents commonly used for subjective purposes (excluding caffeine) can be placed into the following major classes: opioids, general CNS depressants, CNS sympathomimetics, nicotine and tobacco, cannabinoids, psychedelics, arylcyclohexylamines (e.g., phencyclidine), and inhalants (including volatile solvents) (Jaffe, 1980). Because the mechanism of action of each of these classes of agents involves the nervous system, it is not surprising that many of them have indirect as well as direct effects on reproductive function and capacity. Drugs acting on the nervous system have been discussed previously.

HALLUCINOGENS. Marijuana and cannabinoids reversibly depress testicular endocrine function in all species studied including man. Marijuana smoking has also been reported to cause significant reductions of sperm counts, yet in other studies this effect was not observed. The timing of the fall in sperm count suggests that marijuana affects spermiogenesis. Cannabinol and delta-1-tetrahydrocannabinol impaired the stimulatory effect of LH on the synthesis of testosterone in vitro. It was suggested that either the conversion of cholesterol to pregnenolone or the availability of cholesterol for steroidogenesis were reduced. Cannabinoids appear to affect corticoid synthesis in a similar manner. Administration of cannabis extract daily to mice reversibly inhibited spermatogenesis by affecting spermatids, spermatocytes, and spermatogonia. Similar histologic changes occurred in dogs treated for 30 days.

Human Risk Analysis

The fertility of humans may be more susceptible to alterations by environmental factors than the reproductive capacity of laboratory animals. One in five couples desiring children are unsuccessful in their attempts to become parents. Yet, only a few chemicals have been conclusively demonstrated to affect human reproductive capacity. One reason for this is that methods to estimate damage to human fertility reliably are not readily available. Also compounding the problem is the difficulty of measuring human exposure to chemicals, identifying situations where an exposure to only a single chemical exists, estimating dose–response relationships for chemicals affecting reproduction, and predicting human risk associated with levels of exposure. These areas have been recently considered by Barlow and Sullivan (1982) and Wilcox (1983). Table 5-7 summarizes those industries that have been associated with reproductive toxicity (Dixon and Schrag, 1984). Suspected chemicals and associated toxic effects are indicated.

FERTILITY ENDPOINTS

Virtually all livebirths are routinely registered. However, many pregnancies end with

Table 5–7. Industries Associated with Reproductive Toxic Effects

Industry	Suspected chemicals	Associated effects
Agriculture (farmers and gardeners)	Pesticides (chlordecone), herbicides, fumigants (DBCP, carbon disulfide, ethylene dibromide, ethylene oxide)	Testicular damage, infertility, abortions
Anesthesia	Anesthetic gases	Infertility, abortions
Construction (builders and painters)	Solvents, glues, tars, building materials (formaldehyde)	Menstrual and gynecologic disorders, infertility, abortions
Degreasing	Glycol ethers	Infertility, menstrual disorders
Drug manufacturing	Oral contraceptives, alkylating agents, hormone agonists and antagonists	Menstrual and gynecologic disorders, infertility, gynecomastia (?)
Dry cleaning	Solvents, glycol ethers	Infertility, menstrual disorders
Electrical power	PCBs	Menstrual and gynecologic disorders
Leather	Solvents, glues, dyes	Menstrual and gynecologic disorders, testicular damage, infertility
Oil and gasoline, refining and retailing	Benzene, organic lead	Menstrual and gynecologic disorders, testicular damage, infertility, abortions, decreased libido, impotency
Painting and dyeing	Aniline, toluene	Menstrual and gynecologic disorders, infertility, abortions
Plastics and polymer manufacturing	Monomers (styrene, toluene diisocyanate, vinyl chloride, PAEs)	Menstrual and gynecologic disorders, decreased libido, impotency
Radio and television	Manganese (?), nonionizing radiation (?)	Decreased libido, impotency
Radiotherapy	Ionizing radiations	Infertility (?)
Rubber manufacturing	Chloroprene	Menstrual and gynecologic disorders, testicular damage, infertility, decreased libido, impotency
Smelting	Lead, mercury, arsenic, other trace metals	Menstrual and gynecologic disorders, infertility, abortions, testicular damage, decreased libido, impotency
Synthetic chemistry	Solvents (hexane, benzene, toluene); mutagenic and carcinogenic chemicals	Menstrual and gynecologic disorders, testicular damage, infertility
Textile manufacturing	Solvents, dyes, flame retardants (TRIS)	Infertility (?)

a miscarriage or stillbirth. More than one third of pregnancies diagnosed by urine assay terminated before becoming clinically apparent (Miller et al., 1980).

INDICATORS OF HUMAN FERTILITY

Although unreliable, semen analysis is commonly used to predict infertility. Endpoints employed include ejaculate volume, sperm number, sperm motility, and sperm morphology. Ejaculate volume and sperm morphology do not correlate well with the length of time required for a couple to achieve pregnancy. Sperm number is related to fertility only when the sperm count is less than 20 million per milliliter. The best predictor of fertility is the fraction of motile sperm and the quality of their activity. However, even this variable was not highly correlated with time to pregnancy (Mann and Lutwak-Mann, 1981). Wyrobek and Bruce (1978) have proposed that abnormal sperm shapes indicate exposure to mutagens. More complex and direct assays of sperm fertilizing capacity have been developed. The heterologous interspecies in vitro fertilization test is such an assay.

In women, the occurrence of anovulatory cycles is commonly observed among about one third of infertile couples but less so in the general population. Ovulation can be monitored easily using daily temperatures or urine assays of female hormones. Understandably, frequency of coitus is clearly related to the probability of conception.

EPIDEMIOLOGIC INVESTIGATIONS

When exposure to a potentially toxic chemical has occurred in a human population, or concern surrounds the use of a certain chemical, epidemiologic approaches may be used to identify effects on reproduction. Epidemiologic investigations are subject to many problems, including low statistical power because of small population size, difficulties in defining exposure, bias in reporting, and the multiple endpoints to be considered. The design of epidemiologic studies may involve either retrospective or prospective gathering of data. Levine and co-workers (1980a, b) have developed a method for monitoring the fertility of workers and have applied it to workers exposed to dibromochloropropane.

ESTIMATION OF RISK

For the relatively few cases where a chemical has produced human reproductive toxicity, correlation between laboratory and human data is good. Particularly strong laboratory and clinical data are available concerning in utero exposure to diethylstilbestrol (DES) on fertility of offspring. Another example is the testicular toxicity produced in men and laboratory animals by exposure to dibromochloropropane (DBCP). Although the data are less extensive, the reproductive effects of both ethylene dibromide and carbon disulfide have been observed in both laboratory animals and man.

Conclusions

Reproductive toxicology is a complex interplay of basic and applied sciences. Today's predictive test methods for toxicity are admittedly inexact, and extrapolation of laboratory data to humans uncertain. The student of this area of toxicology, even more so than others, must remain aware of almost daily research advances in biochemistry and pharmacology, as well as other basic areas, and apply this new information toward a better understanding of the processes by which environmental chemicals and other agents affect the most important of all biologic processes—production of reproductively competent offspring.

Acknowledgments

We acknowledge with appreciation Ms. Susan D. Schrag for her assistance in writing this chapter and Ms. Vickie Englebright for her willingness to prepare numerous drafts as this chapter evolved and for typing the final manuscript. The authors also thank Dr. Chr. Sigg and Dr. C. Genton (Kantonsspital Zürich, Switzerland) as well as Dr. Chr. Hodel and Dr. J. Burckhardt (F.

Hoffmann-La Roche & Co. Ltd., Basel, Switzerland) for critical reading. Thus, this contribution to the scientific literature is a team effort.

REFERENCES

Amann, R. P. 1981. A critical review of methods for evaluation of spermatogenesis from seminal characteristics. *J. Androl.* 2:37–42.

Baldessarini, R. J. 1980. Drugs and the treatment of psychiatric disorders. In *Goodman and Gilman's The pharmacological basis of therapeutics*, 6th Ed., eds. A. G. Gilman, L. G. Goodman, and A. Gilman, pp. 391–447. New York: Macmillan.

Barlow, S. M., and Sullivan, F. M. 1982. *Reproductive hazards of industrial chemicals*. London: Academic Press.

Bechter, R., Ettlin, R.A., and Dixon, R. L. 1982. Assessment of testicular toxicity associated with anticancer agents II. Sperm counts and serial matings. *Proc. West. Pharmacol. Soc.* 25:385–387.

Beckman, G., Beckman, L., and Nordenson, I. 1977. Chromosome aberrations in workers exposed to arsenic. *Environ. Health Perspect.*, 19:145–146.

Belsey, M. A., Eliasson, R., Gallegos, A. J., Moghissi, K. S., Paulsen, C. A., and Prasad, M. R. N. 1980. *Laboratory manual for the examination of human semen and semen cervical mucus interaction*. Singapore: Press Concern.

Bennett, H. S., Wyrick, A. D., Lee, S. W., and McNeil, J. A. 1976. Science and art in preparing tissue embedded in plastic for light microscopy, with special reference to glycol methacrylate, glass knives and simple stains. *Stain Technol.* 51:71–97.

Biava, C. G., Smuckler, E. A., and Whorton, D. 1978. The testicular morphology of individuals exposed to dibromochloropropane. *Exp. Mol. Pathol.* 29:448–458.

Bibbo, M., Gill, W. B., Azizi, F., Blough, R., Fang, V. S., Rosenfield, R. L., Schumacher, G. F. B., Sleeper, K., Sonek, M. G., and Wied, G. L. 1977. Follow-up study of male and female offspring of DES-exposed mothers. *Obstet. Gynecol.* 49:1–8.

Bingham, E., ed. 1977. *Proceedings of the Conference on Women and the Workplace*. Washington, D. C.: Society for Occupational and Environmental Health.

Bjersing, L. 1977. Ovarian histochemistry. In *The Ovary*, 2nd Ed., Vol. 1, eds. L. Zuckerman and B. J. Weir, pp. 303–389. New York: Academic Press.

Blaustein, A., ed. 1977. *Pathology of the female genital tract*, 2nd Ed. New York: Springer-Verlag.

Calabresi, P., and Parks, Jr., R. E. 1980. Antiproliferative agents and drugs used for immunosuppression. In *Goodman and Gilman's The pharmacological basis of therapeutics*, 6th Ed., eds. A. G. Gilman, L. G. Goodman, and A. Gilman, pp. 1256–1313. New York: Macmillan.

Champlin, A. K., Dorr, D. L., and Gates, A. H. 1973. Determining the stage of the estrous cycle in the mouse by the appearance of the vagina. *Biol. Reprod.* 8:491–494.

Chang, M. C., and Austin, C. R. 1976. Mammalian fertilization. *Res. in Reprod.* 8:4.

Chapin, R. E., Norton, R. M., Popp, J. A., and Bus, J. S. 1982. The effects of 2,5-hexanedione on reproductive hormones and testicular enzyme activities in the F-344 rat. *Toxicol. Appl. Pharmacol.* 62:262–272.

Cirla, A. M., Bertazzi, P. A., Tomasini, M., Villa, A., and Graziano, C. 1978. Study of endocrinological functions and sexual behavior in carbon disulphide workers. *Med. Lav.* 69:118–129.

Clermont, Y. 1972. Kinetics of spermatogenesis in mammals: Seminiferous epithelium cycles and spermatogonial renewal. *Physiol. Rev.* 52:198–236.

Cohn, W. J., Boylan, J. J., Blanke, R. B., Fariss, M. W., Howell, J. R., and Guzelian, P. S. 1978. Treatment of chlordecone (Kepone) toxicity with cholestyramine. *N. Engl. J. Med.* 298:243–248.

Collins, T. F. X. 1978. Reproduction and teratology guidelines: Review of deliberations by the National Toxicology Advisory Committee's Reproduction Panel. *J. Environ. Pathol. Toxicol.* 2:141–147.

Council on Environmental Quality (CEQ) 1981. *Chemical hazards to human reproduction*. Washington, D. C.: U. S. Government Printing Office.

Davies, A. G. 1980. *Effects of hormones, drugs and chemicals on testicular function*, vol. 1. St. Albans, Vt.: Eden Press.

Dixon, R. L. 1981. The role of pharmacokinetic, adaptive and homeostatic factors in testicular toxicity and risk assessment. In *Proceedings of the Third Life Science Symposium on Risk Analysis*, eds. C. R. Richmond,

P. J. Walsh, and E. D. Copenhaver, p. 196. Philadelphia: Franklin Institute Press.

Dixon, R. L. 1982. Potential of environmental factors to affect development of reproductive system. *Fund. Appl. Toxicol.* 2:5–12.

Dixon, R. L., and Hall, J. L. 1982. Reproductive toxicology. In *Principles and methods of toxicology*, ed. A. W. Hayes, pp. 107–140. New York: Raven Press.

Dixon, R. L., and Lee, I. P. 1981. Pharmacokinetic and adaptive factors as modifiers of testicular toxicity and risk assessment. In *Proceedings of the Third Life Science Symposium on Risk Analysis*, eds., C. R. Richmond, P. J. Walsh, and E. D. Copenhaver, Franklin Institute Press. Philadelphia: pp. 195–212.

Dixon, R. L., and Schrag, S. D. 1984. Industrial chemicals associated with male reproductive dysfunction. *Ann. Rev. Pharmacol. Toxicol.* 25 (in press).

Dougherty, R. C., Whitaker, M. J., Tang, S.-Y., Bottcher, R., Keller, M., and Keuhl, D. W. 1981. Sperm density and toxic substances: A potential key to environmental health hazards. In *Environmental health chemistry: The chemistry of environmental agents as potential human hazards*, ed. J. D. McKinney, pp. 263–278. Ann Arbor, Mich.: Ann Arbor Science Publishers, Inc.

Douglas, W. W. 1980. Histamine and 5-hydroxytryptamine (serotonin) and their antagonists. In *Goodman and Gilman's The pharmacological basis of therapeutics*, 6th Ed., eds. A. G. Gilman, L. G. Goodman, and A. Gilman, pp. 609–646. New York: Macmillan.

Dym, M., and Fawcett, D. W. 1970. The blood–testis barrier in the rat and the physiological compartmentation of the seminiferous epithelium. *Biol. Reprod.* 3:308–326.

Eliasson, R. 1983. Morphological and chemical methods of semen analysis for quantitating damage to male reproductive function in man. In *Methods for assessing the effects of chemicals on reproductive functions*, SCOPE 20, SGOMSEC 1, IPCS Joint Symposia 1, eds. V. B. Vouk and P. J. Sheehan, pp. 263–275. New York: John Wiley & Sons.

Epstein, S. S., Arnold, E., Andrea, J., Bass, W., and Bishop, Y. 1972. Detection of chemical mutagens by the dominant lethal assay in mice. *Toxicol. Appl. Pharmacol.* 23:288–325.

Ettlin, R. A. 1983. Die Untersuchung von Zyto-statika-bedingten Früh- und Folgeveränderungen von maennlichen Ratten, *Schweiz. Med. Wschr.* 113:796–797.

Ettlin, R. A., Bechter, R., and Dixon, R. L. 1982. Assessment of testicular toxicity associated with anticancer agents I. Histopathology. *Proc. West. Pharmacol. Soc.* 25:381–384.

Ettlin, R. A., Bechter R., Lee, I. P., and Hodel, C. 1984. Assessment of testicular toxicity, *Arch. Toxicol.* 7:151–154.

Ewing, L. L. 1983. Cellular and molecular approaches to the study of reproduction: A symposium. *Biol. Reprod.* 28:1–104.

Galbraith, W. M., Voytek, P., and Ryon, M. G. 1982. *Assessment of risks to human reproduction and to development of the human conceptus from exposure to environmental substances.* Springfield, Va.: National Technical Information Service.

Gilman, A. G., Goodman, L. S., and Gilman, A., eds. 1980. *Goodman and Gilman's The pharmacological basis of therapeutics*, 6th Ed. New York: Macmillan.

Gomes, W. R. 1970. Chemical agents affecting testicular function and male fertility. In *The testis*, vol. 3, *Influencing factors*, eds. A. D. Johnson, W. R. Gomes, and N. L. Vandemark, pp. 483–554. New York: Academic Press.

Gomes, W. R. 1977. Pharmacological agents and male fertility. In *The testis*, vol. 4, *Advances in physiology, biochemistry, and function*, eds. A. D. Johnson and W. R. Gomes, pp. 605–628. New York: Academic Press.

Hall, J. L. 1981. Relationship between semen quality and human sperm penetration of zona-free hamster ova. *Fertil. Steril.* 35:457–463.

Hammond, P. B., and Beliles, R. P. 1980. Metals. In *Casarett and Doull's Toxicology: The basic science of poisons*, 2nd Ed., eds. J. Doull, C. D. Klaassen, and M. O. Amdur, pp. 409–467. New York: Macmillan.

Hodel, C., Ettlin, R. A., and Zschauer, A. 1984. Morphologic changes in rat testis by anticancer drugs, *Arch. Toxicol.* 7:147–150.

Hodgen, G. D. 1977. Enzyme markers of testicular function. In *The testis*, vol. 4, eds. A. D. Johnson and W. R. Gomes, pp. 401–423. New York: Academic Press.

Hunt, V. R. 1979. *Work and the health of women.* Boca Raton, Fla.: CRC Press.

Jaffe, J. H. 1980. Drug addiction and drug abuse. In *Goodman and Gilman's The pharmacological basis of therapeutics*, 6th Ed., eds.

A. G. Gilman, L. G. Goodman, and A. Gilman, pp. 535–584. New York: Macmillan.

Jaffe, J. H., and Martin, W. R. 1980. Opioid analgesics and antagonists. In *Goodman and Gilman's The pharmacological basis of therapeutics*, 6th Ed., eds. A. G. Gilman, L. G. Goodman, and A. Gilman, p. 494–534. New York: Macmillan.

James, W. H. 1980. Secular trend in reported sperm counts. *Andrologia* 12:381–388.

James, W. H. 1982. Possible consequences of the hypothesized decline in sperm counts. In *Human fertility factors (with emphasis on the male)*, eds. A. Spira and P. Jouannet, pp. 183–200. Paris: INSERM.

Johnson, L., Petty, C. S., and Neaves, W. B. 1981. A new approach to quantification of spermatogenesis and its application to germinal cell attrition during human spermatogenesis. *Biol. Reprod.* 25:217–226.

Kapp, R. W., Jr., Picciano, D. J., and Jacobson, C. B. 1979. Y-Chromosomal nondisjunction in dibromochloropropane-exposed workmen. *Mutat. Res.* 64:47–51.

Kerr, J. B., and de Kretser, D. M. 1981. The cytology of the human testis. In *The testes,* eds. H. Burger and D. de Kretser, pp. 141–170. New York: Raven Press.

Krasovskii, G. N., Varshavskaya, S. P., and Borisova, A. F. 1976. Toxic and gonadotropic effects of cadmium and boron relative to standards for these substances in drinking water. *Environ. Health Perspect.* 13:69–75.

Lamb IV, J. C., Gulati, D. K., Russell, V. S., Hommel, L., and Sabharwal, P. S. 1984. Reproductive toxicity of ethylene glycol monoethyl ether tested by continuous breeding of CD-1 mice. *Environ. Health Perspect.*, in press.

Lancranjan, I., Popescu, H. I., Gavanescu, I. K., and Serbanescu, M. 1975. Reproductive ability of workmen occupationally exposed to lead. *Arch. Environ. Health* 30:396–401.

Lee, I. P. 1983. Adaptive biochemical repair response toward germ cell DNA damage. *Am. J. Ind. Med.* 4:135–148.

Lee, I. P., and Dixon, R. L. 1972. Effects of procarbazine on spermatogenesis studied by velocity sedimentation cell separation and serial mating. *J. Pharmacol. Exp. Ther.* 181:219–226.

Lee, I. P., and Dixon, R. L. 1973. Effects of cadmium on spermatogenesis studied by velocity sedimentation cell separation technique

and serial mating. *J. Pharmacol. Exp. Ther.* 187:641–652.

Lee, I. P., Suzuki, K., and Nagayama, J. 1981. Metabolism of benzo[a]pyrene in rat prostate glands following 2,3,7,8-tetrachlorodibenzo-p-dioxin exposure. *Carcinogenesis* 2:823–831.

Levine, R. J., Symons, M. J., Balogh, S. A., Arndt, D. M., Kaswandik, N. T., and Gentile, J. W. 1980a. A method for monitoring the fertility of workers 1. Methods and pilot studies. *J. Occup. Med.* 22:781–789.

Levine, R. J., Symons, M. J., Balogh, S. A., Milby, T. H., and Whorton, M. D. 1980b. A method for monitoring the fertility of workers 2. Validation of the method among workers exposed to dibromochloropropane. *J. Occup. Med.* 23:183–188.

Livni, N., and Yaffe, H. 1974. Histochemistry of normal and ethionine-treated rat testis. *Histochemistry*, 40:329–341.

Lu, C. C., and Meistrich, M. L. 1979. Cytotoxic effects of chemotherapeutic drugs on mouse testis cells. *Cancer Res.* 39:3575–3582.

Lucier, G. W., Lee, I. P., and Dixon, R. L. 1977. Effects of environmental agents on male reproduction. In *The testis*, vol. 4, eds. A. D. Johnson and W. R. Gomes, pp. 577–604. New York: Academic Press.

MacKenzie, K. M., and Angevine, D. M. 1981. Infertility in mice exposed in utero to benzo[a]pyrene. *Biol. Reprod.* 24:183–191.

Mann, T., and Lutwak-Mann, C. 1981. *Male reproductive function and semen: Themes and trends in physiology, biochemistry, investigative andrology.* New York: Springer-Verlag.

Marinova, G., Cakarova, O., and Kaneva, Y. 1973. A study on the reproductive function in women working with mercury. *Prob. Akusher. Ginekol.* 1:75. (Abstract)

Marshall, B. E., and Wollman, H. 1980. General anesthetics. In *Goodman and Gilman's The pharmacological basis of therapeutics*, 6th Ed., eds. A. G. Gilman, L. G. Goodman, and A. Gilman, pp. 276–299. New York: Macmillan.

Matter, R. H., Bechter, R., Weber, H., Ettlin, R., and Dixon, R. L. 1983. Differential testicular toxicity associated with anticancer drugs administered during critical periods of postnatal development. *Toxicologist* 3:21. (Abstract)

Mattison, D. R., Nightingale, M. S., and Shiromizu, K. 1983a. Effects of toxic substances on female reproduction. *Environ. Health Perspect.* 48:43–52.

Mattison, D. R., Shiromizu, K., and Nightingale, M. S. 1983b. Oocyte destruction by polycyclic aromatic hydrocarbons. *Am. J. Ind. Med.* 4:191–194.

Mayer, S. E. 1980. Neurohumoral transmission and the autonomic nervous system. In *Goodman and Gilman's The pharmacological basis of therapeutics*, 6th Ed., eds. A. G. Gilman, L. G. Goodman, and A. Gilman, pp. 56–90. New York: Macmillan.

McFarland, R. B., and Reigel, H. 1978. Chronic mercury poisoning from a single brief exposure. *J. Occup. Med.* 20:532–534.

McLachlan, J. A., Newbold, R. R., and Bullock, B. 1975. Reproductive tract lesions in male mice exposed prenatally to diethylstilbestrol. *Science* 190:991–992.

McLachlan, J. A., Newbold, R. R., Korach, K. S., Lamb IV, J. C., and Suzuki, Y. 1981. Transplacental toxicology: Prenatal factors influencing postnatal fertility. In *Developmental toxicology*, eds. C. A. Kimmel and J. Buelke-Sam, pp. 213–232. New York: Raven Press.

McLachlan, J. A., Newbold, R. R., Shah, H. C., Hogan, M., and Dixon, R. L. 1982. Reduced fertility in female mice exposed transplacentally to diethylstilbestrol. *Fertil. Steril.* 38:364–371.

Miller, J. F., Williamson, E., Glue, J. Gordon, Y. B., Grudzinskas, J. G., and Sykes, A. 1980. Fetal loss after implantation: A prospective study. *Lancet* 2:554–556.

Mukhtar, H., Lee, I. P., Foureman, G. L., and Bend, J. R. 1978a. Epoxide-metabolizing enzyme activities in rat testis: Postnatal development and relative activity in interstitial and spermatogenic cell compartments. *Chem. Biol. Interact.* 22:153–165.

Mukhtar, H., Philpot, R. M., Lee, I. P., and Bend, J. R. 1978b. Developmental aspects of epoxide-metabolizing enzyme activities in adrenals, ovaries, and testes of the rat. In *Developmental toxicology of energy-related pollutants*, eds. D. Mahlum, U. Sikov, P. Hackett, and F. Andrew, pp. 89–104. Washington, D. C.: U. S. Department of Energy, Technical Information Center.

Murad, F., and Haynes, R. C. 1980. Androgens and anabolic steroids. In *Goodman and Gilman's The pharmacological basis of therapeutics*, 6th Ed., eds. A. G. Gilman, L. G. Goodman, and A. Gilman, pp. 1448–1465. New York: Macmillan.

Murphy, S. D. 1980. Pesticides. In *Casarett and Doull's Toxicology: The basic science of poisons*, 2nd Ed., eds. J. Doull, C. D. Klaassen, and M. O. Amdur, pp. 357–408. New York: Macmillan.

Nagayama, J., and Lee, I. P. 1982. Comparison of benzo[a]pyrene metabolism by testicular homogenate and the isolated perfused testis of rat following 2,3,7,8-tetrachlorodibenzo-p-dioxin treatment. *Arch. Toxicol.* 51:121–130.

Nelson, W. O., and Patanelli, D. J. 1965. Chemical control of spermatogenesis. In *Agents affecting fertility*, eds. C. R. Austin and J. S. Perry, pp. 78–92. London: Churchill.

Neumann, F., Diallo, F. A., Hasan, S. H., Schenck, B., and Traore, I. 1975. The influence of pharmaceutical compounds on male fertility. *Andrologia* 8:203–235.

Newbold, R. R., and McLachlan, J. A. 1982. Vaginal adenosis and adenocarcinoma in mice transplacentally exposed to diethylstilbestrol. *Cancer Res.* 42:2003–2011.

Nogaki, K. 1958. On action of lead on body of lead refinery workers: Particularly conception, pregnancy, and parturition in case of females and their newborn. *Excerp. Med.*, XVII, 4:515–516. (Abstract #2176)

Okumura, K., Lee, I. P., and Dixon, R. L. 1975. Permeability of selected drugs and chemicals across the blood–testis barrier of the rat. *J. Pharmacol. Exp. Ther.* 194:89–95.

Owen, W. L. 1976. Cancer of the prostate: A literature review. *J. Chron. Dis.* 29:89–114.

Parvinen, L. M., Soderstrom, K. O., and Parvinen, M. 1978. Early effects of vinblastine and vincristine on rat spermatogenesis: Analyses by a new transillumination-phase contrast microscopic method. *Exp. Pathol. (Jena)* 15:85–96.

Parvinen, M. 1982. Regulation of the seminiferous epithelium. *Endocrin. Rev.* 3:404–417.

Parvinen, M., and Vanha-Petulta, T. 1972. Identification and enzyme quantitation of the stages of the seminiferous epithelial wave in the rat. *Anat. Rec.* 174:435–449.

Pedersen, R. A., and Brandriff, B. 1980. Radiation- and drug-induced DNA repair in mammalian oocytes and embryos. In *DNA repair and mutagenesis in eukaryotes*, eds. W. M. Generoso, M. D. Shelby, and F. J. de Serres, pp. 389–410. New York: Plenum Press.

Ritchie, J. M. 1980. The aliphatic alcohols. In *Goodman and Gilman's The pharmacolo-*

gical basis of therapeutics, 6th Ed., eds. A. G. Gilman, L. G. Goodman, and A. Gilman, pp. 376–390. New York: Macmillan.

Robb, G. W., Amann, R. P., and Killian, G. J. 1978. Daily sperm production and epididymal sperm reserves of pubertal and adult rats. J. Reprod. Fertil. 54:103–107.

Russell, L. D. 1983. Normal testicular structure and methods of evaluation under experimental and disruptive conditions, In Reproductive and developmental toxicity of metals, eds. T. W. Clarkson, G. F. Nordberg, and P. R. Sager, pp. 227–252. New York: Plenum Press.

Schrag, S. D., and Dixon, R. L. 1985. Industrial chemicals associated with male reproductive dysfunction. Ann. Rev. Pharmacol Toxicol 25, in press.

Schuler, P., Oyanguren, H., Maturana, V., Valenzuela, A., Cruz, E., Plaza, V., Schmidt, E., and Haddad, R. 1957. Manganese poisoning. Environmental and medical study at a Chilean mine. Indust. Med. Surg. 26:167–173.

Sega, G. A. 1982. DNA repair in spermatocytes and spermatids of the mouse. In Banbury Report, vol. 13, Indicators of genotoxic exposure, eds. B. A. Bridges, B. E. Butterworth, and I. B. Weinstein, pp. 503–513. Cold Spring Harbor, N. Y.: Cold Spring Harbor Laboratory.

Sega, G. A., and Sotomayor, R. E. 1982. Unscheduled DNA synthesis in mammalian germ cells—its potential use in mutagenicity testing. In Chemical mutagens—Principles and methods for their detection, vol. 7, eds. F. J. de Serres and A. Hollaender, pp. 421–445. New York: Plenum Press.

Setchell, B. P., Voglmayr, J. K., and Waites, G. M. H. 1969. A blood–testis barrier restricting passage from blood lymph into rete testis fluid but not into lymph. J. Physiol. 200:73–85.

Shalet, S. M. 1980. Effects of cancer chemotherapy on gonadal function of patients. Cancer Treat. Rev. 7:141–152.

Shen, R. S., and Lee, I. P. 1977. Developmental patterns of enzymes in mouse testis. J. Reprod. Fertil. 48:301–305.

Sieber, S. M., and Adamson, R. H. 1975. Toxicity of antineoplastic agents in man: Chromosomal aberrations, antifertility effects, congenital malformations, and carcinogenic potential. Adv. Cancer Res. 22:57–155.

Skipper, H. E. 1983. Stepwise progress in the treatment of disseminated cancers. In Accomplishments in cancer research, eds. J. G. Fortner and J. E. Rhoads, pp. 48–54. Philadelphia: J. B. Lippincott.

Smith, K. D., and Steinberger, E. 1980. Current status of research on hormonal contraception in the male. In Proceedings of an international workshop on research frontiers in fertility regulation, pp. 169–177, eds. G. I. Zatuchni, M. H. Labbok, and J. J. Sciarra. Hagerstown, Md.: Harper & Row.

Spira, A., and Jouannet, P., eds. 1982. Human fertility factors (with emphasis on the male). Paris: INSERM.

Takeuchi, T. 1970. Biological reactions and pathological changes of human beings and animals under the condition of organic mercury contamination. Presented at the International Conference on Environmental Mercury Contamination, Ann Arbor, Mich.

Tarasenko, N. Y., Kasparov, A. A., and Strongina, O. M. 1972. The effect of boric acid on the generative function of the male organism. Gig. Tr. Prof. Zabol. 16:3. (English Abstract)

Thomas, J. A., and Bell, J. U. 1982. Endocrine toxicology. In Principles and methods of toxicology, ed. A. W. Hayes, pp. 487–507. New York: Raven Press.

Thomas, J. R., Curto, K. A., and Thomas, M. J. 1982. MEHP/DEHP: Gonadal toxicity and effects on rodent accessory sex organs. Environ. Health Perspect. 45:85–88.

Torkelson, T. R., Sądek, S. E., and Rowe, V. K. 1961. Toxicological investigations of 1,2-dibromo-3-chloropropane. Toxicol. Appl. Pharmacol. 3:545–549.

Van Thiel, D. H., Gavaler, J. S., Smith, W. I., and Paul, G. 1979. Hypothalamic–pituitary–gonadal dysfunction in men using cimetidine. N. Engl. J. Med. 300:1012–1015.

Van Thiel, D. H., and Lester, R. 1976. Alcoholism: Its effect on hypothalamo–pituitary–gonadal function. Gastroenterology 71:318–327.

Vernon, R. B., Muller, C. H., Herr, J. C., Feuchter, F. A., and Eddy, E. M. 1982. Epididymal secretion of a mouse sperm surface component recognized by a monoclonal antibody. Biol. Reprod. 26:523–535.

Vitale, R., Fawcett, D. W., and Dym, M. 1973. The normal development of the blood–testis barrier and the effects of clomiphene and estrogen treatment. Anat. Rec. 176:333–344.

Vouk, V. B., and Sheehan, P. J., eds. 1983.

Methods for assessing the effects of chemicals on reproductive functions, SCOPE 20, SGOMSEC 1, IPCS Joint Symposia 1. New York: John Wiley & Sons.

Walsh, D. C., and Egdahl, R. H., eds. 1980. *Women, work and health: Challenges to corporate policy, industry and health care*, Vol. 8. New York: Springer-Verlag.

West, J. D., Frels, W. I., Papaioannou, V. E., Karr, J. P., and Chapman, V. M. 1977. Development of interspecific hybrids of Mus. *J. Embryol. Exp. Morphol.* 41:233–243.

Whorton, D., Krauss, R. M., Marshall, S., and Milby, T. H. 1977. Infertility in male pesticide workers. *Lancet* 2:1259–1261.

Whorton, D., and Milby, T. H. 1980. Recovery of testicular function among DBCP workers. *J. Occup. Med.* 22:177–179.

Wilcox, A. J. 1983. Surveillance of pregnancy loss in human populations. *Am. J. Ind. Med.* 4:285–292.

Willis, J. 1981. Drugs that take the joy out of sex. *FDA Drug Bulletin*, July–Aug., p. 31.

Wong, O., Utidjian, H. M. D., and Karten, V. S. 1979. Retrospective evaluation of reproductive performance of workers exposed to ethylene dibromide. *J. Occup. Med.* 21:98–102.

Woods, J. S. 1984. Drug effects on human sexual behavior. In *Human sexuality in health and illness*, 3rd ed. N. F. Woods, pp. 434–457. St. Louis: C. V. Mosby.

Working, P. K., and Butterworth, B. E. 1984. An assay to detect chemically induced DNA repair in rat spermatocytes. *Environ. Mutagen.* 6:273–286.

Wyrobek, A. J. 1983. Methods for evaluating the effects of environmental chemicals on human sperm production. *Environ. Health Perspect.* 48:53–59.

Wyrobek, A. J., and Bruce, W. R. 1978. The induction of sperm-shape abnormalities in mice and humans. In *Chemical mutagens*, vol. 5, eds. A. Hollacnder and F. J. de Serres, pp. 257–285. New York: Plenum Press.

Zaneveld, J. D. 1982. New developments in spermicidal agents, sperm-immobilizing agents and sperm enzyme agents. In *Research frontiers in fertility regulation*, ed. G. I. Zatuchni. Chicago: Northwestern University.

Zaneveld, J. D. 1982. Sperm enzyme inhibitors for vaginal and other contraception. Res. Front. Fertil. Regul. 2 (3):1–14.

6

Dermatotoxicology

Ronald C. Wester and Howard I. Maibach

The skin is recognized both as a barrier to absorption and as a primary route to the systemic circulation. The skin's barrier properties are often, but not always, impressive. Fluids and electrolytes are reasonably well retained within the body, while at the same time many foreign chemicals are partially restricted from entering the systemic circulation. Despite these barrier properties, the skin is the route by which many chemicals enter the body. In most instances the toxicology of the chemical is slight, and/or the bioavailability (rate and amount of absorption) of the chemical is too low to cause an immediate response. However, some chemicals applied to the skin have the potential to produce toxicity.

Percutaneous absorption is now a primary focal point for dermatotoxicology. It is now recognized that local and systemic toxicity depend on a chemical penetrating the skin. Table 6–1 shows the relationship of percutaneous absorption to toxicologic activity. A local or systemic effect cannot occur unless the chemical has inherent toxicity and the chemical is able to overcome the barrier properties of skin and enter a biologic system (local skin and/or systemic circulation). This chapter explores this concept of percutaneous absorption and inherent toxicity. We briefly review the proper-

Table 6–1. Relationship of Percutaneous Absorption to Toxicologic Activity

Property of chemical		Local or systemic effect
Absorption through skin	Inherent toxicity	
−	−	None
+	−	None
−	+	None
+	+	Reaction

ties of skin and the principles governing percutaneous absorption. Then we explore some chemicals prominent in dermatotoxicology for which percutaneous absorption data are relevant.

Skin Structure

The skin is an organ consisting of two layers derived from different germ layers (Rongone, 1983). These layers are known as epidermis and dermis, and their characteristics are different. The thinner, outer layer (epidermis) is epithelial tissue derived from ectoderm. The thicker, relatively inert inner layer (dermis) consists mainly of connective tissue and has a mesodermal origin. The dermis constitutes approximately 95% of the mass of human skin, whereas the smaller epidermal layer accounts for the major portion of the biochemical transformations occurring in the skin. However, the skin appendages that extend down into the dermal layer, such as sweat glands, hair follicles, and sebaceous glands, are also metabolically important. These appendages are formed during embryonic development from developing epidermal cells that invade the developing dermal layer.

Skin thickness varies with location. The epidermis is approximately 0.1 mm and the dermis 2–4 mm thick. Ths skin on the palms and soles has a much thicker epidermis than that in other areas. This skin at these locations has a thick layer of keratin, whereas the skin at other locations has a relatively thin layer. The dermoepidermal interface is characterized by dermoepidermal ridges and interpapillary pegs. Dermoepidermal ridges provide maximum interface area between the epidermis and dermis. This dermoepidermal relationship is of great importance when one considers that the nutrients for the epidermis must come from the dermis, because there is no blood supply in the epidermis.

The epidermis is a thin layer of cells overlying the dermis. It consists of several types of cells. The innermost type is known as the stratum germinativum (basal cell layer), and is followed by the stratum spinosum (prickle cell layer), stratum granulosum, stratum lucidum, and (the outermost layer) stratum corneum. The combined stratum spinosum and stratum germinativum are often referred to as the Malpighian layer. The basal cell layer consists of one layer of columnar epithelial cells that on division, are pushed up into the prickle cell layer. In humans, the prickle cell layer consists of several layers, believed to be held together by tiny intercellular fibrils known as tonofibrils that pass from one cell to another. As the prickle cells approach the surface, they become larger and form the stratum granulosum, which is two to four cells thick. The keratohyalin granules are formed in this layer. In the stratum granulosum the nuclei are either broken up or dissolved, resulting in the death of the epidermal cell, and the number of cytoplasmic granules increased.

The next layer, stratum lucidum, is ill defined except in areas of thick skin. This layer is said to consist of eleidin, which is presumed to be a transformation product of the keratohyalin present in the stratum granulosum. In the outermost layer, the stratum corneum, the eleidin has been converted into keratin, which represents the ultimate fate of the epidermal cell. Keratin, continuously sloughed off or worn away, must continuously be replaced by the cells beneath it. This sequential transformation and migration of the living basal cells to the dead epithelial cells of the stratum corneum (horny scales) represents a protective action of the skin against foreign objects that penetrate the outer skin barriers. The time required for a basal cell to migrate from the stratum germinativum to the outer part of the stratum corneum has been estimated to be 26–28 days. The extremely metabolically active basal cells lie adjacent to the dermis, which has the only blood supply to the skin and a higher oxygen tension than the other layers of the epidermis.

The dermis is a thick fibrous network of collagen and elastin, which serves as a supporting unit for the epidermis. It is composed of two layers. The outer, thinner one is called the papillary layer because of its prominent papillae, and it merges with the thicker reticular layer. The papillary layer has a finer structure than the reticular layer, because its collagen fibers are not as coarse as those in the reticular layer. The papillae are well nourished by the capillaries that are prominent in them, and the biologically active epidermis is supplied with its essential nutrients by these capillaries. Exchange of nutrients and waste products between the blood and epidermis occurs by diffusion through the dermis, which is thought to serve as a large reservoir of nutrients for the metabolically active epidermis.

The appendages of skin are hair follicles, sebaceous glands, eccrine and apocrine sweat glands, hair, nails, and arrectores pilorum muscle.

Percutaneous Absorption

METHODOLOGY

In vitro techniques involve placing a piece of excised skin in a diffusion chamber, applying radioactive compound to one side of the skin, and then assaying for radioactivity in the collection vessel on the other side (Tregear, 1966). Excised human and animal skin are used, and the skin can be wholly intact or separated into epidermis or dermis. Artificial membranes have been used in place of skin to measure diffusion kinetics. The advantages of the in vitro techniques are that the methodology is easy to use and results obtained quickly. The disadvantage is that the collection bath is saline, which would be compatible with hydrophilic compounds but not with hydrophobic compounds. In vivo, the penetrating compound does not pass completely through the dermis but is removed by capillaries in the dermis.

Franz (1975) evaluated the permeability of 12 organic compounds in vitro using excised human skin and compared the results to those obtained previously in living humans. Care was taken to ensure that his in vitro conditions closely followed those used in vivo, although it was necessary to use human abdominal skin for the in vitro studies. Additionally, the doses employed ranged from 4 to 40 μg/cm^2, with the assumption that the percentage of applied dose absorbed would not be dose dependent. Quantitatively, the in vitro and in vivo data did not agree. The in vitro method was of value to the extent that it tended to distinguish compounds of low permeability from those of high permeability. However, there are notable differences such that the in vitro method alone would not always be a reliable or accurate predictor of percutaneous absorption in living humans. Future work in this area may define the in vitro conditions predictive of in vivo absorption.

Percutaneous absorption in vivo is usually determined by the indirect method of measuring radioactivity in excreta following topical application of the labeled compound. In human studies, plasma levels of compound are extremely low following topical application, often below assay detection level, so it is necessary to use tracer methodology. The labeled compound, usually carbon-14, is applied, and the total amount of radioactivity excreted in urine or urine plus feces is determined. The amount of radioactivity retained in the body or excreted by some route not assayed (CO_2, sweat) is corrected for by determining the amount of radioactivity excreted following parenteral administration. This final amount of radioactivity is then expressed as the percentage of applied dose that was absorbed (Wester and Maibach, 1983b).

The equation used to determine percutaneous absorption is as follows:

$$\text{Percentage percutaneous absorption} = \frac{\text{total radioactivity following topical administration}}{\text{total radioactivity following parenteral administration}} \times 100$$

TEN STEPS TO PERCUTANEOUS ABSORPTION

Multiple factors affecting percutaneous absorption have been summarized by Wester and Maibach (1983a) as 10 Steps (Table 6–2). The reader is referred to this review for details. Some of the steps relevant to this book are summarized below.

The extent of absorption depends on the anatomic site to which the compound is applied. This is true for both humans and animals. Presented in Table 6–3 are data derived from in vivo absorptions of hydrocortisone after application to various human anatomic sites. They are of obvious practical significance in that high total absorption is found for head, neck, and axilla, where both cosmetic and environmental exposure are greater. The female genitalia show greater absorption than forearm skin surfaces (not mucosa), but not so great as scrotal skin. Similar results in anatomic variation have been shown for pesticides. With a variety of chemical moieties examined (steroids, pesticides, and antimicrobi-

Table 6–2. Ten Steps to Percutaneous Absorption[a]

1. Vehicle release
2. Absorption kinetics
   a. Skin site of application
   b. Individual variation
   c. Skin condition
   d. Occlusion
   e. Drug concentration and surface area
   f. Multiple-dose application
3. Excretion kinetics
4. Effective cellular and tissue distribution
5. Substantivity (nonpenetrating surface adsorption)
6. Wash and rub resistance
7. Volatility
8. Binding
9. Anatomic pathways
10. Cutaneous metabolism

[a]This represents our current view. Presumably many steps remain to be discovered.

als), the general pattern of regional variation holds. One important exception is carbaryl, which was extensively absorbed from the forearm, although the other sites were not significantly higher. This finding suggests that carbaryl is extensively absorbed from all body sites.

The percutaneous absorption of hydrocortisone was studied in 18 healthy adult males. The anatomic site was the same, as was the dose (4 μg/cm^2). The mean absorption was 0.9% of the applied dose. However, the absorption for several individuals was one third as much, whereas one subject

Table 6–3. Regional Variation in Percutaneous Absorption of Hydrocortisone in Humans

Skin application site	Percutaneous absorption ratio
Forearm (ventral)	1.0
Forearm (dorsal)	1.1
Foot arch (plantar)	0.14
Ankle (lateral)	0.42
Palm	0.83
Back	1.7
Scalp	3.5
Axilla	3.6
Forehead	6.0
Jaw angle	13.0
Scrotum	42.0

absorbed three times more than the median. The variation was as might be expected in almost any biologic system. Thus, there can be a severalfold difference in absorption even when the site of application, dose, vehicle, and all other factors are the same. However, individual variation is small when compared to variation in studies in which the site, dose, and so on are not controlled.

Percutaneous absorption is increased when the site of application is occluded. Occlusion is a covering of the applied dose, either intentionally, as with bandaging, or unintentionally, as putting on clothing after applying a topical compound. Occlusion changes the hydration and temperature of the skin, and these physical factors affect absorption. Occlusion prevents the accidental wiping or evaporation (volatile compound) of the applied compound, in essence maintaining a higher applied dose. There is more percutaneous absorption with occlusion than even with stripping (Table 6–4). Occlusion is the most practical clinical method to enhance percutaneous absorption.

Behl et al. (1980) showed that hydration of the skin increased penetration of lipid-soluble, nonpolar molecules but had less effect on the penetration of polar molecules. Many drugs belong to this first category, and dermatologists have recognized that hydration increases penetration because occlusion increases penetration and causes endogenous hydration of the stratum corneum.

The reservoir effect (Vickers, 1980) is an example of change in penetration rates as a result of hydration. Initially, a drug applied

Table 6–4. Penetration of Hydrocortisone through Modified Skin

Treatment	Penetration ratio
None	1
Strip	4
Occlude	10
Cantharidine blister	15
Strip + occlude	20

under occlusion enters the stratum corneum. When the occlusive dressing is removed and the stratum corneum dehy-
drates, the movement of drug slows and the
stratum corneum becomes a reservoir. Subsequently, occlusion alone will hydrate the
tissue and increase the rate of movement of
drug, and its pharmacologic action again
becomes apparent.

When a compound comes in contact with
skin, the amount of absorption will depend
on many parameters. Foremost among these
parameters are concentration of applied dose
and surface area. As the concentration of
the applied dose increases, the efficiency of
absorption (percentage) can change. However, a more relevant point is that as the
applied dose is increased, the total amount
absorbed into the body increases. The other
parameter closely associated with dose is
surface area. Increasing the surface area of
the applied dose increases the absorption.
Therefore, the greatest toxicologic potential for percutaneous absorption can occur
when a high concentration of compound is
spread over a large part of the body.

The effect of topical concentration skin
penetration is usually referenced by Fick's
general law of diffusion, commonly written
as

$$J_s = K_p \, \Delta C_s$$

where J_s is the flux across the membrane,
K_p is the permeability constant, and ΔC_s is
the difference in concentration on the two
sides of the membrane. By varying the concentration of the penetrant and observing
the consistency of K_p, one can determine the
extent to which Fick's law is applicable. Data
are usually analyzed from in vitro studies at
steady-state conditions.

Skin Metabolism

Skin is not a passive barrier that only re-
stricts the diffusion of chemical agents into
the body. The skin is a viable membrane
that can metabolize an assortment of topically applied substances before they become systemically available. Because the skin
has many of the same enzymes as the liver,
it is of interest to compare their relative ac-

Table 6–5. Enzyme Activity Ratios in Skin Compared to Liver

Enzyme	Activity ratio (skin:liver) Whole skin	Epidermis[a]
Aromatic hydrocarbon hydroxylase	0.02	0.80
7-Ethoxycoumarin deethylase	0.02	0.80
Aniline hydroxylase	0.06	2.40
NADP-Cytochrome c reductase	0.06	2.40

[a] Assuming epidermis is 2.5% of whole skin.

tivities. This would be important if the activity of the skin were sufficient to allow it
to serve as an alternative metabolic site for
systemically (e.g., iv or orally) administered
drugs. The activities of several cutaneous
enzymes have been measured and compared to hepatic activities. The activities of
these enzymes in skin are low compared to
those in liver, typically 2–6% of the hepatic values. Although these data indicate
that cutaneous metabolism is low, this may
not be representative of the situation in vivo.
If only the metabolically active epidermis is
compared with liver, then the activities are
equal (Table 6–5) (Noonan and Wester,
1983). Any toxic or potentially toxic chemical that penetrates the skin must go through
the metabolically active epidermis before
entering the systemic circulation. Thus, the
chemical can be subject to activation or
deactivation before entering the body.

Where little or no skin metabolism occurs, the chemical that penetrates the skin
barrier is introduced into the systemic circulation. The implication is that some
chemicals may be more toxic after topical
application than when administered orally.
Topically applied hexachlorophene does not
appear to be metabolized. It passes into the
bloodstream unchanged. In contrast, orally
ingested hexachlorophene quickly reaches
the liver through the enterophepatic shunt
system (portal) and is metabolized. Thus,
the only barrier to topical hexachlorophene
toxicity is the barrier to percutaneous absorption. The metabolic detoxification that
occurs after oral absorption is not present
with dermal administration.

Nevertheless, we know that skin metabolism of chemicals does occur. The question is which routes of metabolism occur for a particular chemical and to what extent. This is impossible to assess for every chemical because the information available is insufficient. It is known that the route of metabolism after dermal administration can be different from that after oral administration. After oral administration of [3H]cortisol, the urinary metabolites were mainly corticosteroids, whereas after dermal administration they were mainly oxosteroids. However, cortisol (hydrocortisone) is clinically effective in either case, and this metabolic difference would not be important unless one of the metabolites was an active moiety.

It can probably be assumed that skin metabolism usually deactivates or detoxifies the applied chemical agent. Most skin metabolism studies seem to indicate this. The most notable exception is the case of skin aromatic hydrocarbon hydroxylase (AHH)—activating chemical agents into potent carcinogens.

Cutaneous Metabolic Production of Carcinogens

Much attention has been focused on polycyclic aromatic hydrocarbons because they produce skin carcinomas. Metabolic activation of these compounds is usually the first step toward the induction of skin cancers. The metabolites of benz[a]pyrene (BP) generally fall into three classes: phenols, quinones, and dihydrodiols. It is the dihydrodiols that, when metabolized to epoxide diols, become the more potent carcinogens. The epoxides react with cellular nucleophiles such as DNA, RNA, or proteins. The same is true for other polycyclic aromatic hydrocarbons such as 3-methylcholanthrene and benz[a]anthracene derivatives. These compounds induce skin tumors and this probably is caused by a reactive metabolite (an epoxide).

Knowledge of the binding of BP metabolites to macromolecules has reached a higher level of sophistication. Binding of BP-

dihydrodiol epoxides was found to occur with high stereoselectivity. These investigators isolated the polymer adducts that were formed when [3H]BP was applied to the skin of mice. Figure 6–1 shows that there are two stereochemical configurations for the BP-7,8-dihydrodiols, and they may both be metabolized to the respective 9,10-epoxide. The epoxide may then react with cellular nucleophiles such as DNA, RNA, or proteins. For nucleic acids, the in vivo binding occurred preferentially to guanine at the 2-amino group (in both DNA and RNA). Both stereoisomers bound cellular components, but isomer A formed most of the covalently bound products (Noonan and Wester, 1983).

Thus, any compound such as benzo[a]-pyrene that penetrates the skin must first pass into and through the epidermis and would be subject to an extensive metabolic reaction.

Animal Models and Toxicology

Dermal toxicity is determined in animals to make predictions of human health hazard. It is assumed that the dermal bioavailability (rate and extent of absorption) and skin metabolism between animals and humans are similar. The data in Tables 6–6 and 6–7 show that absorption in the common laboratory animals from which toxicity data are gathered is different from humans (Bronaugh and Maibach, 1983; Wester and Maibach, 1983a). Few (if any) animal toxicity studies include satellite animals, where the dermal bioavailability is determined for

Table 6–6. Percutaneous Absorption of Testosterone in Several Species

Species	Percentage of dose absorbed	Ratio
Human	13.2	1.0
Rhesus monkey	18.4	1.4
Pig	29.4	2.2
Guinea pig	34.9	2.6
Rat	47.4	3.6
Rabbit	69.6	5.3

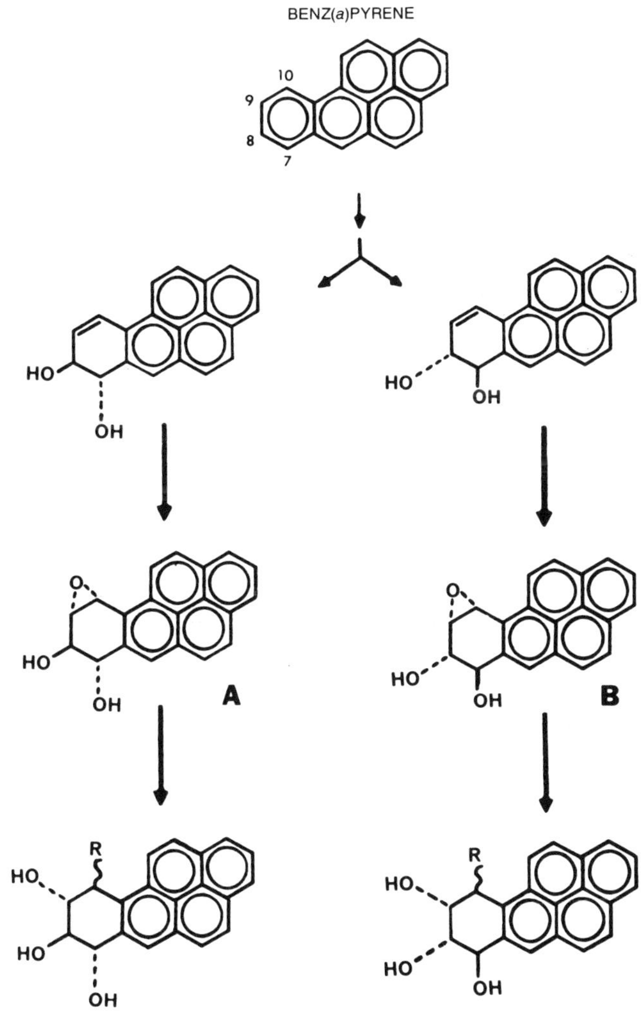

Figure 6–1. Metabolic activation of benz[a]pyrene in mouse skin with stereochemistry indicated; R = OH or cellular nucleophile.

the same dosage forms and conditions. The applied dermal dose that causes laboratory animal toxicity cannot be correlated with the amount of chemical that becomes systemically available, unless corresponding satellite percutaneous absorption studies are also done. Additionally, little information is available on similarities in animal and human skin metabolism.

Neonate and Dermal Toxicity

Little is known about percutaneous absorption in the infant. Yet it is in the infant where the greatest toxicologic response has been seen following topical administration. The main factor governing percutaneous ab-

sorption is the permeability of skin. The critical factor in protection of the infant from the environment is whether the barriers are intact. If the barriers are not intact, any foreign substance coming in contact with the skin may readily be absorbed into the body (Wester and Maibach, 1982).

A 2-week-old infant developed reddish, patchy eczema in the inguinal regions, on the upper part of the thighs, and the axilla. Part of the treatment was to paint the areas with Castellani's solution, an antimicrobial containing phenol and resorcinol. The infant became cyanotic and was in critical condition for days (see Table 6–8).

Infected skin has damaged barrier function, so in the case above there was little

Table 6–7. Permeability of Animal Skin Relative to Human Skin[a]

Compound	Pig	Monkey	Rat	Guinea pig	Hairless mouse	Mouse	Rabbit
N-Acetylcysteine	2.5		1.4				0.8
Benzoic acid		1.4					
Butter yellow	1.9		2.2				4.6
Caffeine	0.7		1.1				1.5
Cortisone	1.2		7.3				9.0
Haloprogin	2.6		3.7				4.4
Hydrocortisone		1.6					
Testosterone	2.2	1.4	3.6				5.3
Ethylene bromide	0.8		2.3	1.5			
Paraoxon	1.4		3.3	3.0			
Thioglycolic acid	3.3		3.0	2.3			
Water	1.4			1.0			3.3
Benzoic acid				0.7			
Hydrocortisone				1.3			
Testosterone				2.6			
Naproxin			2.3				3.5
Butanol					1.8		
Ethanol					1.5		
Octanol					0.6		
Betamethasone					1.3		
5-Fluorouracil					1.1		
Hydrocortisone					1.5		
Acetylsalicylic acid	1.2		1.0		4.9	8.7	
Benzoic acid	0.2		0.6		2.0	2.0	
Urea	1.5		4.8		0.9	5.8	

[a]Values for human skin in all studies were assigned a value of 1.0.

Table 6–8. Infantile Poisoning

Incidence of skin contact	Clinical signs	Possible skin absorption parameter involved
Eczema (inguinal region, thigh, axilla) treated with Castellani's solution	Cyanotic	High absorbancy of damaged skin High absorbancy of application sites Large surface area contact
Phenolic disinfectants in hospital laundry	Death	Large surface area contact Possible occlusive effect of clothing High absorbancy of urorectal area
Bullous lesions treated with hydrocortisone	Cushingoid	Possible borderline preterm High absorbancy of damaged skin Large total chronic dose Enhancement of hydrocortisone absorption via chronic application Possible occlusive effect of clothing
Hexachlorophene in baby powder	Death	Application to large surface area High concentration of hexachlorophene (6.6%) Possible occlusive effect of clothing Chronic application

resistence to absorption. Additionally, the vulva, scrotum, and axilla are sites of enhanced absorption. The situation was further jeopardized in that by painting on the Castellani's solution, the dose was spread over a large surface area; this enhanced the potential for increased systemic availability.

Phenolic disinfectants in the hospital laundry caused death of infants and sickened others. The presence of the toxic compounds in clothing such as diapers allowed these compounds to be spread over a large surface area; thus, two parameters (large surface area and application to the urorectal area) enhanced absorption. Covering the diaper with rubber pants or more clothing would also enhance absorption and enhance the potential for systemic availability.

A male infant born after a 36-week gestation was treated for bullous lesions with 0.25% hydrocortisone. The child developed cushingoid features and edema that cleared only when hydrocortisone treatment was discontinued. It was subsequently learned that at least 120 g of lotion containing a total of 300 mg of hydrocortisone had been applied to the skin over an 8- to 9-day period.

The infant was probably borderline preterm, and its barrier function may not have been intact. This could have resulted in enhanced skin absorption. Percutaneous absorption of hydrocortisone increased with chronic administration. Finally, the addition of clothing over the site of application might have occluded the site and led to further enhanced penetration.

For about 20 years the toxic potential of topically applied hexachlorophene was not recognized. Then, in 1972, there was a hexachlorophene-related baby disaster in France. This involved about 40 deaths from the use of baby powder accidentally contaminated with 6.6% hexachlorophene. The powder normally contains no hexachlorophene. Brain damage occurs in animals when the use of hexachlorophene produces whole-blood levels around 1 μg/ml. Studies showed that newborn babies washed (and rinsed off) for 3–5 days with a 3% hexachlorophene-containing antibacterial sudsing emulsion developed blood levels dangerously close to this (up to 0.8 μg/ml). This provides a small margin of safety, especially if babies are exposed continuously to this procedure by conscientious mothers.

The above clinical cases illustrate that either through error or misjudgment, potentially toxic materials can be applied to infant skin. The parameters that govern skin absorption can have an enhancing effect on skin penetration. The results can be fatal.

Once a compound (and/or metabolites) is absorbed, it is available systemically. In the newborn the ratio of surface area (in square centimeters) to body weight (in kilograms) is three times that of the adult. Therefore, given equal application area of skin per newborn and adult, the systemic absorption seen in the newborn can be much more when based on kilograms of body weight (Table 6–9). Therefore, by topically applying the same-strength compound to both the adult and the newborn, the systemic availability in the newborn is 2.7 times that of the adult. With a different ratio of

Table 6–9. Systemic Availability in Newborn and Adult following Topical Application[a]

Parameter	Adult	Infant
Surface area	17,000 cm^2	2200 cm^2 (13% of adult)
Topical dose	100 mg	13 mg (13% of adult)
Patient weight	70 kg	3.4 kg (neonate)
Systemic dose	$\dfrac{100 \text{ mg} \times 0.2 \text{ abs}}{70 \text{ kg}} = 0.28$ mg/kg	$\dfrac{13 \text{ mg} \times 0.2 \text{ abs}}{3.4 \text{ kg}} = 0.76$ mg/kg

[a]Systemic dose (mg/kg); compound (20% absorbed).

skin surface to body weight, the therapeutic ratio probably is lower in the newborn than in the adult when the compound is applied topically. This increased systemic availability in the newborn would also be interrelated with any differences in systemic metabolism between the newborn and the adult (Wester, Noonan, Cole, and Maibach, 1977).

PCBs and Chloracne

The polychlorinated biphenyls (PCBs), used extensively for industrial purposes for 50 years, are ideal for use in adhesives, paints, varnishes, printing inks, and as general fillers. Because they do not conduct electricity, they found widespread use in electrical equipment such as transformers. This widespread use, coupled with their resistance to degradation in the environment, has resulted in extensive PCB contamination of animal foods and people. During the past 15 years the significance for health has been brought to public attention. Symptoms observed include chloracne.

Chloracne is defined as an acneiform eruption due to poisoning by halogenated aromatic compounds having a specific molecular shape. The degree of halogenation does not necessarily determine toxicity; the position of the halogen atoms on the outside of the molecule (isomerism) is vital (Crow, 1983).

The distribution of chloracne lesions is of considerable diagnostic importance. The most sensitive areas of the human skin are below and to the outer side of the eye (the so-called malar crescent) and behind the ear. They frequently may be affected when the rest of the skin is normal. Furthermore, they are the areas most likely to show residual lesions years after more extensive chloracne has faded. Next in frequency are the cheeks, forehead, and neck, but the nose is almost invariably spared. It should be noted that in the sebaceous gland development of this region, the pathologic basis of chloracne is squamous metaplasia of sebaceous glands into keratin-forming cysts. The male genitalia—both penis and scrotum, but particularly the latter—are sensitive regions. With increasing toxicity the spread of the lesions is to the shoulders, chest, and back, and eventually the buttocks and abdomen. The hands, forearms, feet, legs, and thighs are involved usually only in the worst cases. Previously we discussed the regional variation of percutaneous absorption where the face (forehead, jaw angle) and genitalia (scrotum) were areas of extensive percutaneous absorption. The forearm, foot, ankle, and palm were areas of much lesser absorption. There appears to be some correlation between areas of sensitivity and regional areas of percutaneous absorption.

Experimental data do not indicate whether variation of the route of absorption (oral vs dermal) of a chloracnegen alters the distinctive features of poisoning, but circumstantial evidence suggests that this may be so to a minor degree. A comparison of the Yusho and Taiwan poisonings, where the chloracnegens were ingested without dermal contact or inhalation, shows certain differences from industrial poisonings where contact is known to be by contact and inhalation. Capacitor workers with gross skin contact and inhalation have blood PCB levels as high as the Yusho cases, but no signs of toxicity except chloracne and respiratory changes. In industry, generally, contact appears to make chloracne the most sensitive marker. Pigmentation, ophthalmic signs, and many of the subjective symptoms (often presenting complaints in Japanese and Chinese cases) occur only in severe cases with severe chloracne. It seems possible that these differences and many others may be due not only to different chloracnegens but also to the route of absorption.

The most obvious route of human contamination is considered to be oral consumption of PCBs through the food chain. However, with such extensive use, dermal exposure to PCBs seems obvious. The question then becomes the extent of PCB dermal bioavailability. Table 6–10 gives the dermal absorption and elimination half-lives of PCBs in rhesus monkey and guinea pig (both considered relevant animal models). The PCBs were extensively absorbed, and the elimination from the body was slow, with half-lives in days (Wester et al., 1983). Ta-

Table 6–10. Dermal Absorption of PCBs

Species	PCB[a] (%)	Percentage of dose absorbed[b]	Elimination half-life (days)
Rhesus monkey	42	21.4 ± 8.5	6.9
Guinea pig	42	33.2 ± 6.3	1.9/12.6[c]
Guinea pig	54	55.6 ± 2.6	2.9

[a]Given as percentage chlorine in PCB.
[b]Mean ± SD.
[c]Elimination biphasic; 1.9 is for day 0–10 interval; 12.6 is for day 10–15 interval.

ble 6–11 gives the dermal wash efficiency for PCBs in guinea pig. The wash procedure was twice with water followed by twice with acetone, then repeated. Only 60% of the dermally applied PCB could be removed with immediate washing, and 20% or less was removable 24 hours after application.

Thus, we see that PCBs are extensively absorbed through the skin, are not removed by wash procedures, and are slowly eliminated from the body. There appears to be some correlation between sites of chloracne and regional variation of percutaneous absorption. The PCBs have the inherent toxicity to cause chloracne.

Table 6–11. Dermal Wash Efficiency for PCBs in Guinea Pig

PCB[a]	Wash time	Percentage of dose removed[b]
42	Immediate	58.9 ± 7.5
42	24 Hours postapplication	0.7 ± 0.2
54	24 Hours postapplication	19.7 ± 5.5

[a]Given as percentage chlorine in PCBs.
[b]Mean ± SD for three animals.

Table 6–12. Application Frequency and Percutaneous Absorption of Hydrocortisone

Dose (μg/cm^2)	Application (times/day)	Total dose (μg/cm^2)	Absorption (μg/cm^2)
13.3	1	13.3	0.18
13.3	3	40	0.29
40	1	40	0.84

Dermal Bioavailability and Epidermal Tumors

Wester and co-workers (Wester, Noonan, and Maibach, 1977) determined the effect of frequency of application on percutaneous absorption of hydrocortisone (Table 6–12). When material was applied once or three times per day there was a statistical difference ($p<0.05$) in the percutaneous absorption of hydrocortisone. One application per 24-hour exposure gave a higher percutaneous absorption than if the material was applied at a lower concentration but more frequently, namely, three times per day. This was confirmed with a second chemical, testosterone (Wester et al., 1980).

There is a correlation between frequency of application, percutaneous absorption, and toxicity of applied chemical. Wilson and Holland (1982) determined the effect of application frequency in epidermal carcinogenic assays. Application of a single large dose of a highly complex mixture of petroleum or synthetic fuels to a skin site increased the carcinogenic potential of the chemical compared to smaller or more frequent applications (Table 6–13). This carcinogenic toxicity correlated well with the results of Wester et al. (1980), where a sin-

Table 6–13. Shale Oil–Induced Incidence of Epidermal Tumors

Shale oil	Dose (mg)	Frequency (per week)	Total dose per week (mg)	Number of animals with carcinogenic tumors
OCSO No. 6	10	4×	40	2
	20	2×	40	4
	40	1×	40	13
PCSO II	10	4×	40	11
	30	4×	120	17
	40	1×	160	19

gle applied dose increased the percutaneous absorption of the material compared to smaller or intermittent applications.

Cosmetic Chemicals and Toxicity

The potential toxicity of cosmetics has in the past been dismissed as an event unlikely to occur. The argument was put forth that cosmetics did not contain ingredients that could prove harmful to the body. The argument went further to say that because cosmetics were applied to skin with its "barrier" properties, the likelihood that a chemical would become systemically available was remote. The argument was proven false when carcinogens were shown to be present in cosmetics, and subsequent studies showed that these carcinogenic chemicals could be percutaneously absorbed (Wester, 1982).

N-Nitrosodiethanolamine (NDELA) is an impurity that was found in several cosmetic products. It appears to be formed by a reaction between an amine such as diethanolamine or triethanolamine and a nitrosating agent. In rat feeding tests, NDELA was shown to cause liver cancer. Syrian hamsters injected with NDELA developed liver and skin cancer. Percutaneous absorption studies showed that NDELA readily penetrated swine and monkey skin. When applied in acetone vehicle or commercial lotion, it readily penetrated excised human skin. In a human study with contaminated facial makeup, NDELA was detected in the subjects' urine. The information thus showed the presence of a carcinogen in cosmetics that would become systemically available when the cosmetic was applied to skin. Analytic procedures are available to detect nitrosamines, and every effort should be made in the quality assurance of cosmetics to see that these compounds are not present in the final product.

1,4-Dioxane is an impurity recently detected in some cosmetic raw materials. It can be formed in the synthesis of ethylene glycol polymers and, unless removed by vacuum distillation, will subsequently be detected in commercial products. 1,4-Dioxane is also a carcinogen. Determining its percutaneous absorption has been difficult because the chemical is volatile. With in vitro penetration using diffusion cells and human skin, the absorption was increased 10 times when the application side of the skin was occluded. Dioxane dissolved in a popular lotion and applied to waxed paper disks had evaporated by 90% in 15 minutes, and there was no trace of dioxane present within 24 hours.

The coal tar derivatives used in hair dyes have been implicated as potential carcinogens. Chemicals such as 4-methoxy-m-phenylenediamine, 2,4-toluenediamine, 2-nitro-p-phenylenediamine, and 4-amino-2-nitrophenol have been shown to cause cancer in animals, and some data on skin absorption have been generated for each of these chemicals. To assess the potential risk of these chemicals, it is necessary to have the best estimate of their percutaneous absorption, preferably in humans and under normal-use conditions. This was done using radiolabeled 2,4-diaminoansole (DAA) in Miss Clairol Creme Formula #52, black azure; using radiolabeled p-phenylenediamine (PPD) in Nice 'n Easy #124, blue black; and using radiolabeled HC blue #1 in Loving Care Lotion #795, darkest brown. The study was done in human subjects, and, most importantly, procedural instructions specific for each hair color product were followed. The percutaneous absorption, expressed as percentage of applied dose, was 0.015 for DAA, 0.14 for PPD, and 0.09 for HC blue #1. These are reliable numbers from which the potential risk to humans can be assessed. In addition, the same dyes and procedures were used to dye the hair on rhesus monkey scalps. The percutaneous absorption in the rhesus was 0.02 for DAA, 0.14 for PPD, and 0.12 for HC blue #1. The rhesus monkey is therefore a reliable animal model for percutaneous absorption relevant to humans.

Table 6–14 shows the relationship between percutaneous absorption and erythema for several oils used in cosmetics. The authors attempted to correlate absorbability with erythema. The most absorbed oil,

Table 6–14. Relationship of Percutaneous Absorption and Erythema for Several Oils Used in Cosmetics

Absorbability (greatest to least)	Erythema
Isopropyl myristate	+ +
Glycerol tri(oleate)	−
n-Octadecane	±
Decanoxydecane	+
2-Hexyldecanoxyoctane	−

isopropyl myristate, produced the most erythema. The lowest absorbing oil, 2-hexyldecanoxyoctane, produced the least erythema. Absorbability and erythema for the other oils did not correlate (Suzuki et al., 1978). The lesson to remember with percutaneous toxicity is that a toxic response required both a inherent toxicity in the chemical and the percutaneous absorption of the chemical. The degree of toxicity will depend on the contribution of both criteria.

In the rhesus monkey, the percutaneous absorption of safrole, an hepatocarcinogen, was 6.3% of applied dose. When the site of application was occluded, the percutaneous absorption doubled to 13.3%. Occlusion is a covering of the application site, either intentionally as with bandaging or unintentimnally as by putting on clothing after applying a cosmetic. The percutaneous absorption of cinnamic anthranilate was 26.1% of applied dose, and this increased to 39.0% when the site of application was occluded. The percutaneous absorption of cinnamic alcohol with occlusion was 62.7%, and that of cinnamic acid with occlusion was 83.9% of applied dose. Cinnamic acid and cinnamic aldehyde are agents that elicit contact urticaria (von Krogh and Maibach, 1983), and cinnamic aldehyde is positive for both Draize and maximation methods (Marzulli and Maibach, 1983).

We have thus learned that common cosmetic ingredients can readily penetrate skin and become systemically available. If the cosmetic chemical has inherent toxicity, then that chemical will get into the body of a user and exert a toxic effect.

REFERENCES

Behl, C. R., Flynn, G. L., Kurihara, T., Harper N., Smith, W., Higuchi, W. I., Ho, F. H., and Pierson, C. L. 1980. Hydration and percutaneous absorption: I. Influence of hydration on alkanol permeation through hairless mouse skin. *J. Invest. Dermatol.* 75:346–352.

Bronaugh, R. L., and Maibach, H. I. 1983. In vitro percutaneous absorption. In *Dermatotoxicology*, eds. F. N. Marzulli and H. I. Maibach, pp. 117–129. Washington, D. C.: Hemisphere Publishing.

Crow, K. D. 1983. Chloracne (halogen acne). In *Dermatotoxicology*, eds, F. N. Marzulli and II. I. Maibach, pp. 461–481. Washington, D. C.: Hemisphere Publishing.

Franz, T. J. 1975. Percutaneous absorption. On the relevance of in vitro data. *J. Invest. Dermatol.* 64:190–195.

Marzulli, F. N., and Maibach, H. I. 1983. Contact allergy: Predictive testing in humans. In *Dermatotoxicology*, eds. F. N. Marzulli and H. I. Maibach, pp. 279–299. Washington, D. C.: Hemisphere Publishing.

Noonan, P. K., and Wester, R. C. 1983. Cutaneous biotransformations and some pharmacological and toxicological implications. In *Dermatotoxicology*, eds. F. N. Marzulli and H. I. Maibach, pp. 71–90. Washington, D. C.: Hemisphere Publishing.

Rongone, E. L. 1983. Skin structure, function, and biochemistry. In *Dermatotoxicology*, eds. F. N. Marzulli and H. I. Maibach, pp. 1–70. Washington, D. C.: Hemisphere Publishing.

Suzuki, M., Asaba, K., Komatsu, H., and Mockizuki, M. 1978. Autoradiographic study on percutaneous absorption of several oils useful for cosmetics, *J. Soc. Cosmet. Chem.* 29:265–271.

Tregear, R. T. 1966. *Physical properties of skin.* New York: Academic Press.

Vickers, C. F. H. 1980. Reservoir effect of human skin: Pharmacological speculation. In *Percutaneous absorption of steroids*, eds. P. Mauvais-Jarvis, C. F. H. Vickers, and J. Wepierre, pp. 19–30. New York: Academic Press.

von Krogh, G., and Maibach, H. I. 1983. The contact urticuria syndrome. In *Dermatotoxicology*, eds. F. N. Marzulli and H. I. Maibach, pp. 301–322. Washington, D. C.: Hemisphere Publishing.

Wester, R. C. 1982. Percutaneous absorption and toxicity of cosmetics. *Dermatol. Allergy* 5:8–11.

Wester, R. C., Bucks, D. A. W., Maibach, H. I., and Anderson, J. 1983. Polychlorinated biphenyls (PCBs): Dermal absorption, systemic elimination, and dermal wash efficiency, *J. Toxicol. Environ. Health* 12:511–519.

Wester, R. C., and Maibach, H. 1982. Comparative percutaneous absorption. In *Neonatal skin: Structure and function*, eds. H. I. Maibach and E. K. Boisits, pp. 137–147. New York: Marcel Dekker.

Wester, R. C., and Maibach, H. I. 1983a. Cutaneous pharmacokinetics: 10 steps to percutaneous absorption. *Drug Metab. Rev.* 14:169–205.

Wester, R. C., and Maibach, H. I. 1983b. In vivo percutaneous absorption. In *Dermatotoxicology*, eds. F. N. Marzulli and H. I. Mai-

bach, pp. 131–146. Washington, D. C.: Hemisphere Publishing.

Wester, R. C., Noonan, P. K., Cole, M. P., and Maibach, H. I. 1977. Percutaneous absorption of testosterone in the newborn rhesus monkey: Comparison to the adult. *Pediatr. Res.* 11:737–739.

Wester, R. C., Noonan, P. K., and Maibach, H. I. 1977. Frequency of application on percutaneous absorption of hydrocortisone. *Arch. Dermatol.* 113:620–622.

Wester, R. C., Noonan, P. K., and Maibach, H. I. 1980. Variations in percutaneous absorption of testosterone in the rhesus monkey due to anatomic site of application and frequency of application. *Arch. Dermatol. Res.* 267:229–235.

Wilson, J. S., and Holland, L. M. 1982. The effect of application frequency on epidermal carcinogenesis assays. *Toxicology.* 24:45–54.

7

Respiratory System

Thomas W. Huang

Among the organs of the body, the respiratory system has the most intimate contact with the environment because of its large surface area and the volume of air exchanged with the external environment. The total alveolar surface area of an adult is approximately 70 m^2; the average volume of air exchanged from the environment is approximately 10,000 liters/day, of which 7000 liters reach the alveoli. Clean air contains suspended bacteria, fungi, spores, and a small amount of dust; therefore, the lungs are a major portal of entry for myriad infectious agents. The advent of effective antimicrobial therapy after World War II and improved nutritional and public health standards have effectively controlled infectious diseases such as tuberculosis and pneumonias in the United States. Infectious pulmonary diseases have been replaced by a surge of degenerative and neoplastic diseases caused by environmental chemicals for which there is no effective control and therapy.

During the last two decades, chronic bronchitis, emphysema, and lung cancer have become major public health problems in the United States. Lung cancer alone caused 111,000 deaths in the United States in 1982. Compared to lung cancer, mortality from chronic bronchitis and emphysema

is low. Nevertheless, they can be highly debilitating, and the social and economic costs of medical care and lost productivity are high and increasing. These diseases are all caused by environmental air pollution, due to either industrialization or changing life-styles. The cigarette-smoking habit accounts for more than 85% of lung cancer mortality and the great majority of chronic bronchitis and emphysema morbidity. The shift in importance from infectious to degenerative and neoplastic diseases during the last 40 years is one of the most vivid examples of the impact of environment on human health.

Lung Defenses Against Environmental Agents

Pollutants in the environment are presented to the respiratory system in two physical forms: particulate and gaseous. The former consists of solid particles, such as carbon and mineral dusts, and liquid droplets (mist). The upper respiratory tract (nose, pharynx, and larynx) and airways (trachea and bronchi) have an efficient method of removing particulate inhalants from the inspired air, thus preventing them from reaching the lung parenchyma where they may cause tissue injury. The gaseous toxic materials adsorbed onto particulate inhalants are also removed with the particles. The toxic chemicals remaining in the gaseous phase are removed by an entirely different mechanism, which is generally much less effective.

A prerequisite for the removal of particles from inhaled air is to increase the probability of contact between the particles and the surface of the airway, which is covered with a mucus blanket. Particles, making contact with the mucus blanket, are irreversibly removed from the airstream. Within the airways, interplay of several physical forces on the particles causes them to cross the stream lines of moving air and to be deposited on airway surfaces. Inertial impaction, gravitational sedimentation, and Brownian diffusion are the major forces that exert variable influence on movement of particles, depending on the particle sizes and airway anatomy. Thus, the airways function as an aerodynamic filter (Brain, 1977).

Most particles greater than 10 μm are removed by filtration through vibrissae (hairs) within the nares and by contact with irregular surfaces of turbinates and nasal septa. As the air passage has a sharp-angled turn at the nasopharynx, large particles (10 μm) cannot alter their direction of motion because of inertia, and they impact on the wall of the nasopharynx. The mechanism, referred to as *inertial impaction,* is also effective at each dichotomous branching of airways. Small particles, because they lack sufficient inertia, are not effectively removed by this mechanism. Only 20% of particles of 2 μm are removed by inertial impaction.

Although the diameters of airways become smaller as they branch, the sum of cross-sectional areas of daughter branches is always greater than the stem branch. Since volume flow of air across each level of the airways remains constant, the linear velocity of airstreams and particles decreases as they approach smaller and smaller airways. The gravitational force effectively causes sedimentation of particles toward the bronchial surface as the rate of flow slows down. Sedimentation is an effective mechanism for removal of particles of 5.0 to 0.2 μm in size.

Deposition of particles smaller than 0.1 μm in size is facilitated by Brownian movement as a result of the constant bombardment of the particles by gas molecules. Although the Brownian movement is random in direction, it favors the movement of particles toward the airway surface because of diffusion, and results in deposition of particles on the surface of the mucus blanket. Particles between 0.5 and 0.1 μm in size are least affected by the physical forces discussed above. They are also the particle population that tends to be suspended in the air and inhaled, and are therefore of major concern in environmental health.

The size of particles discussed above refers to the aerodynamic equivalent of spherical water droplets. Thus, very large particles of highly asymmetric shape, such as asbestos fibers up to 300 μm in length, may make their way to alveoli because their equivalent aerodynamic size is only 1 μm of water droplets. The long asbestos fibers can orient themselves parallel to the airstream lines of flow and reach the alveolar spaces.

Contact of particles with the airway surface is followed by transport by a mucociliary escalator from bronchi to trachea, and finally expulsion from the larynx. The mucociliary escalator is composed of a mucus blanket covering the cilia of the airway columnar epithelium. The periciliary space is suffused with a watery (sol) fluid. The faster beating of the cilia toward larger airways moves the gel-like mucus blanket toward the external opening of the respiratory tract. The mucociliary escalator moves at a rate of approximately 3 mm/minute. The particles deposited on the surface of the airways are cleared by this mechanism within 2 hours.

Most of the particulate inhalants that reach the alveoli are phagocytized by alveolar macrophages, primarily derived from circulating monocytes. Adaptation to the local alveolar milieu is necessary for the conversion of circulating monocytes into active alveolar macrophages. The particle-laden macrophages are cleared from the lung mainly by mucociliary transport. The process of migration of dust-laden macrophages from alveoli and alveolar ducts to bronchioles is rather slow, compared with the rate of mucociliary transport. It takes 24 hours to clear 50% of a given dose of particles by this mechanism.

Small fractions of particles eventually gain entrance into the pulmonary tissues. Speculation that some dust-laden macrophages in alveolar spaces may migrate into the alveolar interstitium has never been proven. There are three potential mechanisms for entry of particles into the tissue: (1) Free particles, especially those with needle shape such as asbestos fibers, may conceivably penetrate the delicate alveolar tissue barrier and enter the interstitium. (2) Phagocytosis of particles by type II pneumocytes may also facilitate the entry. (3) The third mechanism is incorporation into the tissue of dusts and dust-laden macrophages over an area of alveolar "ulcer" in alveolar injury. This mechanism will be discussed in detail in the section on pneumoconiosis.

The particles in the interstitium can be again engulfed by macrophages. It is possible that some of the dust-laden macrophages may enter the alveolar spaces, migrate slowly toward a respiratory bronchiole, and ride the mucociliary escalator out of the respiratory tract. The predominant mode of transport, however, is by way of lymphatics to the lymph nodes in the hilus of the lung and in the mediastinum. There are two major interconnecting routes of lymphatic drainage (Nagaishi, 1972). The first is via peribronchial and perivascular lymphatics, which originate around respiratory bronchioles and pulmonary veins. They extend along the bronchovascular tree to the hilus of the lung. The other drainage system originates in the interlobular septa and extends peripherally to the pleura, where it is anastomosed extensively and eventually drains into hilar lymph nodes. Clearance by lymphatics is very slow; the 50% clearance time is 4–5 days. Small numbers of free particles may remain in the lung interstitium along lymphatic drainage systems for 3 to 4 months or even as long as several years. The slow removal of particles from the lung tissue enhances the potential for pulmonary tissue injury from prolonged tissue contact.

In addition to the simple physical removal of particles from lungs to prevent injury, the lungs are also endowed with enzyme systems for metabolic conversion, especially of inorganic chemicals to water-soluble and less toxic compounds. The monooxygenase activity for xenobiosis is normally very low in the lung compared with the liver. The enzyme system, however, is inducible to a much higher level by foreign chemicals present in the inhaled air (Gram, 1973). Clara cells in bronchioles and type I pneumocytes are particularly rich in smooth endoplasmic reticulum, which is known to contain monooxygenase, and may play essential roles in xenobiosis (Huang et al., 1977). Macrophages are also actively involved. If particles are microorganisms, then opsonization, phagocytosis, and killing of microorganisms follow the same mechanisms as with leukocytes in inflammation. Lysozyme, lactoferrin, immunoglobulin A (IgA), and complement are humoral factors present in the airway secretion that exert bacteriostatic and bactericidal activities (Green et al., 1977).

The overall efficiency of the abovementioned defense mechanisms of the lungs is attested to by the fact that the lungs of a normal individual living in an average environment are free of dust and germs.

The respiratory system is poorly equipped to deal with toxic gaseous inhalants in contrast with particulate inhalants. Highly soluble gases, such as ozone, ammonia, and sulfur dioxide, can be effectively removed in the nose, pharynx, and large airways by solubilization in the mucus and serous discharges. The acidity generated is neutralized by the physiologic buffer system in the body fluids and discharges. Another mechanism of minimizing the effect of toxic gases is dilution by airway dead space and functional residual volume of the lung parenchyma, which decreases the concentration of toxic gases reaching small airways and alveoli. The latter mechanism is only effective for short-term exposure.

Toxic chemicals ingested (gasoline, kerosene, 3-methylindole, 4-ipomeanol) may also gain access to the lung by blood circulation. The endothelium, which may also be injured, provides the only effective barrier. Volatility and lipid solubility of these chemicals seem to enhance their exit into the alveolar spaces, and hence injury to the respiratory apparatus.

Toxic Injury to Airways

The structural and physiologic integrity of the airway is indispensable for proper functioning of the aerodynamic filter and mucociliary transport, especially the latter. Any qualitative or quantitative changes in the mucus or disturbances of ciliary movement may interfere with mucociliary transport, thus causing stasis of the mucus. Mucus stasis favors proliferation of microorganisms and predisposes the respiratory tract to infection. Stasis of dust-laden macrophages in alveoli also enhances the injurious effects of dust on the lung parenchyma (Cohen et al., 1979).

Many environmental agents, such as aldehydes, ammonia, ozone, oxides of nitrogen, and sulfur dioxide, are known irritants to the airway epithelium (Green et al., 1977). At lower concentrations they cause transient dysfunction of ciliary motion without structural alterations. Exposure at higher concentrations causes cell degeneration and necrosis. The degeneration of columnar epithelial cells is characterized by cell swelling, dilatation of the endoplasmic reticulum due to redistribution of water and electrolytes among various compartments of the cells, loss of functional organelles such as cilia, and decreased synthetic activities.

With severe injury, necrosis and loss of columnar cells occur. This is followed by proliferation of undifferentiated basal cells of the airway and their eventual differentiation into ciliated or mucin-secreting columnar cells. When the necrosis involves the basal-cell layer as well, the denuded airway surface is covered with a fibrin meshwork containing necrotic cellular debris and neutrophilic infiltrate. Repair is initiated by migration of basal cells from adjacent regions along the denuded basal lamina. Cell pro-

liferation and differentiation follow the same sequence as discussed above. Absence of the ciliary apparatus of columnar cells during the acute phase of injury and early stage of repair severely interferes with the mucociliary transport function, which makes the airway and the entire respiratory system vulnerable to infection.

Acute injury to small airways such as terminal and respiratory bronchioles follows the same sequence of repair as larger airways. During cellular regeneration the nonciliated columnar (Clara) cells appear first, followed by their differentiation into ciliated columnar cells.

With chronic injury to the airways, such as cigarette smoking–related injury, frank cell necrosis is not observed. Non-necrosis-inducing cellular injury presumably shortens the life span of cells, thereby increasing cell proliferation and cell turnover. The proportion of parabasal cells and Kultschitzky cells is increased. Furthermore, squamous metaplasia is frequently observed (Auerbach, Hammond, and Garfinkel, 1979b). There is also hyperplasia and hypertrophy of goblet cells on the surface lining as well as on the bronchial glands in the lamina propria. The consequence is mucociliary transport dysfunction and excessive mucus secretion. This may lead to infection and small-airway obstruction by mucus plugs. Increased cell proliferation may also increase probability of carcinogenesis.

Acute Toxic Lung Injury

There are two major types of alveolar lining cells. Type I pneumocytes are flat, squamous cells covering most of the alveolar surface area. Their cytoplasm is extremely attenuated to facilitate gas diffusion, and their protein synthesis apparatus is poorly developed. They seem to be a population of terminally differentiated cells incapable of replication. The other type of alveolar lining cells, type II pneumocytes, serves as precursor cells to replenish lost type I pneumocytes in the event of physiologic cell turnover or following alveolar injury and large-scale necrosis of type I pneumocytes

(Adamson and Bowden, 1974). Type II pneumocytes are also secretory cells, secreting surfactant and lysozyme. There is persistent interaction between type II pneumocytes and interstitial cells even in adult lungs, suggesting their roles in regulating alveolar tissue turnover and remodeling. A third cell type (type III pneumocyte, brush cells) has been described in alveoli. They are particularly abundant in hamster lungs but are rarely observed in human lungs.

Within the alveolar septa are an anastomosing network of capillaries, lined by endothelium, and interstitial cells. The latter are myofibroblasts, which synthesize the collagen and elastic fibers of the interstitium.

Among the various types of cells in alveolar septa, type I pneumocytes are most susceptible to injury. Endothelium is next most susceptible. The alveolar injury in most cases is characterized by type I pneumocyte injury. The pattern of type I pneumocyte injury, tissue response, and repair follows a similar course irrespective of the nature of the injurious agents (Huang et al., 1977). Degeneration and necrosis of type I pneumocytes caused by pneumotoxin denude the alveolar surface, resulting in increased permeability of the blood–air barrier, because the type I pneumocyte lining of the alveolar space is one of the major permeability barriers. The consequent leakage of plasma fluid and proteins into alveolar space causes pulmonary edema. When the permeability is greatly increased in severe injury, even large protein molecules such as fibrinogen can find their way into the alveolar space. They eventually polymerize into a fibrin meshwork containing necrotic cellular debris, often referred to as the hyaline membrane. The protein-rich edema fluid and hyaline membrane are the hallmark of acute alveolar injury (Figures 7–1 and 7–2).

Hours after injury, DNA synthesis in type II pneumocytes is initiated, and the cells be-

Figure 7–1. Acute toxic lung injury. Alveolar spaces contain edema fluid and hyaline membrane (arrowheads). Small clusters of proliferating type II pneumocytes as a part of reparative process are indicated by arrows.

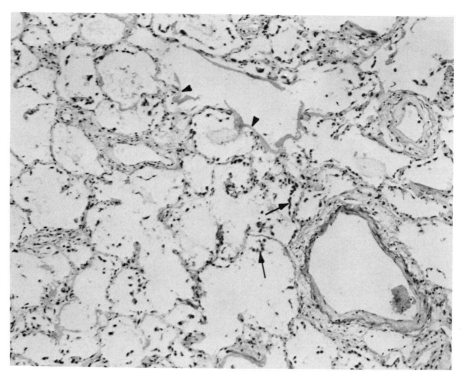

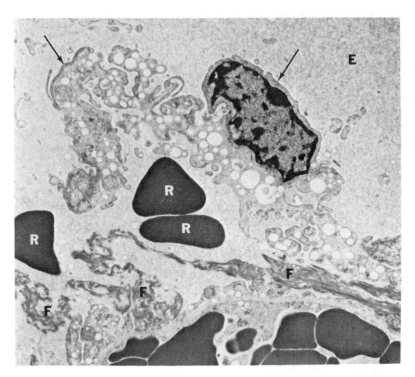

Figure 7–2. Acute toxic lung injury. A degenerating type I pneumocyte (arrow) is sloughed off. The alveolar edema is composed of protein-rich edema fluid (E), red blood cells (R), and fibrin (F). The latter is a component of hyaline membrane.

gin proliferating 24–48 hours after initial injury (Figure 7–3). Five days to one week later, the entire alveolar surface is covered with cuboidal type II pneumocytes.

In the interstitium, edema is seen in the early stage of injury. The interstitial edema often precedes alveolar edema. Later, proliferative activity of interstitial cells is also observed. The increase in interstitial cells is frequently accompanied by an increase in collagen fibers.

In the late, resolving phase of tissue repair, type II pneumocytes seem to transform into flat, squamous type I pneumocytes with concomitant loss of both apical microvilli and cytoplasmic surfactant granules.

In some of the experimental alveolar injuries that we have studied in our laboratories, a nearly complete reconstitution of alveolar structure can be accomplished in 2 to 6 weeks. Physiologic improvement occurs earlier, and function can return to normal within a week after injury.

With injury in which resolution does not follow the pattern presented above, additional changes are observed. Failure of type II pneumocytes to repopulate the alveolar surface within a week or two after injury may lead to emigration of the fibroblasts from the interstitium into the alveolar space. The hyaline membrane thus becomes organized by a poorly vascularized granulation tissue. If this occurs near small bronchioles, bronchiolitis obliterans appears. This is a very characteristic feature of toxic materials injuring respiratory bronchioles and the proximal portion of the alveolar tissues, such as occurs with nitrogen dioxide lung toxicity in silo filler's disease. The results seem to be an irreversible obliteration of lung parenchyma by fibrous tissues. Another type of unsuccessful resolution of injury is that of a diffuse interstitial fibrosis resulting in a loss of alveolar compliance and ventilation–perfusion imbalance (Lamy et al., 1976). Both types of lung fibrosis may be accompanied by simplification of alveolar

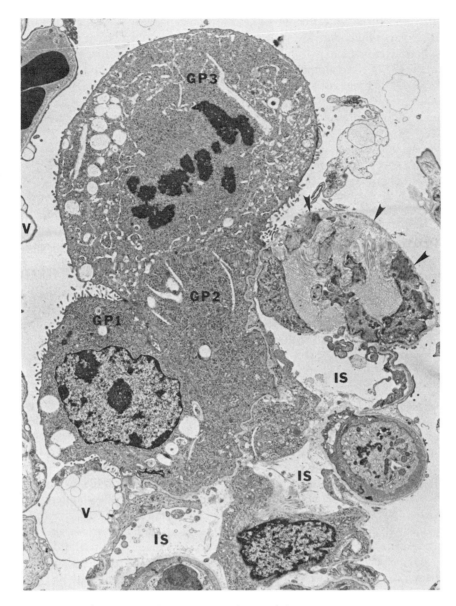

Figure 7–3. Repair of acute toxic lung injury. A cluster of three type II pneumocytes (GP 1, 2, and 3) covers alveolar surface, one of which (GP 3) is in mitosis. Denuded basal lamina (arrowheads) is the consequence of type I pneumocyte necrosis. Interstitial edema (IS) and vesicular degeneration (V) of type I pneumocytes are evident. (From Huang et al., 1977.)

structure and formation of large cystic spaces: honeycomb lungs. The latter represent an irreversible burned-out stage of alveolar injury.

Factors that may cause irreversible lung injury, destruction, and fibrosis are poorly understood. It may be related to the concentration and frequency of exposure to toxic materials. The chemical nature of injurious agents may also play a role.

The endothelium of alveolar capillaries is susceptible to oxidant injury, such as inhalation of high concentrations of oxygen over a prolonged period of time. The resultant tissue change is pulmonary edema and hyaline membrane. The increase in the rate of endothelial cell turnover can only be assessed by tritiated thymidine incorporation by the endothelium. Increases in tritiated thymidine index of the endothelium is also observed with other types of alveolar injury predominantly involving type I pneumocytes. Since endothelial proliferation can be a response of the mesenchyme to a wide variety of tissue injury as a part of the inflammatory process, its significance in a broad spectrum of lung injury is unclear.

When acute alveolar injury causes massive pulmonary edema, the clinical presentation is acute respiratory distress due to intrinsic drowning. However, when the pulmonary edema is minor, the clinical manifestations are usually cough, substernal discomfort, malaise, and fever. In patients whose resolving phase is characterized by pulmonary fibrosis, the clinical presentation may simulate a rapidly progressive fibrosing alveolitis (Hamman-Rich syndrome).

AGENTS CAUSING ACUTE TOXIC LUNG INJURY

The list of agents that may cause acute lung injury is lengthening continuously. This is primarily a result of the introduction of large numbers of new chemical compounds in industries and consumer products. Intensive research during the last decade, resulting from increased awareness of environmental hazards, has helped discover or better define the toxic nature of these compounds when absorbed into the lungs. Therefore, part of the increase is more apparent than real.

Phosgene and Chlorine

The first documented lung toxins are phosgene and chlorine, war gases used during World War I. Soldiers exposed to these gases succumb to acute pulmonary edema due to massive acute injury to type I pneumocytes. The columnar epithelium of small airways is also severely damaged (Pawlowski and Frosolono, 1977). Chlorine gas causes intense airway irritation, which may in itself be incapacitating. Actual injury to airway epithelium and alveolar type I pneumocytes occurs. In modern life, chlorine may be the cause of accidental lung injury due to malfunction of swimming pool chlorination devices, and phosgene by accidental or suicidal exposure in manufacturing industries or laboratories.

Oxides of Nitrogen

Nitrogen dioxide is an oxidant known to cause pulmonary injury in the respiratory bronchioles and proximal portion of alveolar tissue in lung lobules. Nitrogen dioxide and other oxides of nitrogen are liberated by anaerobic bacterial fermentation of nitrate in stored forage, and are the major toxic agent in silo filler's lung disease. Maximum concentration of nitrogen dioxide is usually reached 1–2 weeks after the silo is filled. Farm workers or their families may be exposed to a sufficient concentration of nitrogen dioxide to contract an acute bronchopulmonary illness. Lung lesions are typical of alveolar injury, with pulmonary edema and hyaline membrane in the early stages. In a later stage, intra-alveolar organization in the proximal acinar region gives a classical picture of bronchiolitis obliterans. This may lead to extensive obliteration of lung parenchyma and fibrosis.

Oxides of nitrogen are also extensively used in various industrial processes such as copper and silver dipping, and production of nitrocellulose, and may be the source of lung injury. Mainstream cigarette smoke also contains 250 ppm of nitrogen dioxide or dinitrogen tetroxide, a level far exceeding the general safety limit of 5 ppm. In young cigarette smokers, 80% develop bronchiolitis and proximal acinar lesions that bear striking resemblance to experimental exposure of animals to nitrogen dioxide fumes (Niewoehner et al., 1974). Nitrogen dioxide can also be a product of combustion, especially in burning of nitrocellulose. Electric arc welding produces nitrogen dioxide as a result of oxidation of atmospheric nitrogen at high temperature. Other toxic metal fumes may also be generated in the process. Arc welders working in poorly ventilated rooms may suffer from exposure to nitrogen dioxide and metal fumes.

Sulfur Dioxide and Sulfuric Acid

Sulfur dioxide and sulfuric acid aerosols cause acute bronchitis, bronchiolitis, and proximal acinar alveolar injury similar to nitrogen dioxide (Cockrell et al., 1978). Sulfur dioxide as a general atmospheric pollutant is a product of combustion of sulfer-containing coal or gasoline. Unless the air is heavily polluted, it may not cause symptomatic respiratory system injury. However, as an irritant, it may aggravate symptoms in patients suffering from chronic bronchitis or may trigger extrinsic asthma attacks.

Cadmium and Metal Fume Fever

Aerosols of cadmium chloride solution induce acute toxic pulmonary injury in experimental animals (Strauss et al., 1976). Exposure of workers to cadmium fumes or dust by heating or smelting cadmium produces acute airway irritation and, hours later, cough, fever, general malaise, and dyspnea due to injury to small airways, alveoli, and pulmonary edema. The main toxic compound is the readily volatilized cadmium oxide, which condenses to small particles of 0.02 to 0.25 μm. Emphysema is thought to develop as a sequela of a single acute exposure or repeated chronic exposures. This is not, however, supported by well-documented studies. Repeated cadmium fume inhalation may cause chronic cough and emphysema. Other metal fumes of nickel, manganese, zinc, and selenium can also cause episodes of acute lung injury, collectively called metal fume fever.

Paraquat

Paraquat is an herbicide that may cause severe bronchiolar and alveolar injury (Sykes et al., 1977) as a result of accidental ingestion, attempted suicide, or smoking of marijuana sprayed with the herbicide. Absorp-

tion through skin is also possible. Paraquat ingested or absorbed through the skin becomes highly concentrated in lungs and causes lung injury; injury to the liver and renal tubular epithelium may also occur (Haley, 1979).

Ozone

Ozone is the principal oxidant gas of photochemical smogs. Experimental exposure of animals to ozone causes injury to the small airways and alveoli in the central portions of lobules (Cross et al., 1976). The lesions are those characteristic of bronchiolar columnar cells and alveolar type I pneumocyte injury. Even at concentrations of ozone as low as 0.2 ppm, pulmonary injury is detectable following exposure for 7 days (Schwartz et al., 1976). Therefore, the ubiquitous presence of ozone in our environment poses a potential health hazard. Although a low-grade acute injury such as those caused by ozone does not create any immediate health problem, the long-term health effects of a persistent low-grade acute injury remain unclear. Its additive or synergistic effect with other lung toxins is also largely unknown. This is an area of environmental pathology that requires more research.

Butylated Hydroxytoluene (BHT)

BHT is an antioxidant widely used as a food additive to keep foods fresh. The chemical causes classical type I pneumocyte injury and type II pneumocyte proliferation (Witschi and Cote, 1976; Adamson et al., 1977). Fibrosis is usually mild and does not severely compromise respiratory functions.

Carbon Tetrachloride

Carbon tetrachloride is a widely used haloalkane solvent that may be accidentally inhaled or swallowed, causing acute alveolar injury and pulmonary edema (Chen et al., 1977).

Teflon

Although this polymer of tetrafluoroethylene resin is a widely used coating material of low toxicity, pyrolysis products of Teflon heated to 450°C are highly pneumotoxic when inhaled (Lee et al., 1976). The toxic materials are minute particles of 0.02 to 0.04 μm. The main injury is to the bronchiolar columnar epithelium and type I pneumocytes of alveoli. Pulmonary edema, hemorrhage, and subsequent repair by type II pneumocyte proliferation follow the same pattern as other acute pulmonary injuries. The injury to the endothelium is minimal.

Fire and Smoke Inhalation

Fire causes physical (heat) as well as chemical injury to the human body. The composition of chemicals generated in a fire is a function of oxygen concentration, temperature of fire, and nature and availability of combustible materials (fuel) in a fire. There is no reliable method of predicting the compositions of toxic gases in a particular fire or the actual exposure of a victim (Terrill et al., 1978). Carbon monoxide, which forms a stable carboxyhemoglobin in the victim's blood, and cyanide are among a few compounds that can be reliably measured in victims. The toxic gases can be classified into two major categories. The first group causes systemic poisoning and death, and includes carbon monoxide (CO) and hydrogen cyanide (HCN). The other group causes toxic injury to airways, alveoli, or both. Within this group are nitrogen dioxide and other oxides of nitrogen, sulfur dioxide, hydrogen chloride, isocyanates, ammonia, and acrolein and other aldehyde compounds. Pathologic effects of most of these compounds have been discussed. Acrolein, acetaldehyde, and other aldehydes preferentially cause airway epithelial cell necrosis. It should be noted that high concentration of these irritants may cause severe bronchospasm, which leads to asphyxiation and death before a toxic level in the lung parenchyma is reached.

Some patients who survive the acute phase of injury with pulmonary edema and hemorrhage may eventually succumb to interstitial fibrosis and chronic respiratory failure months or years after smoke inhalation. Many are left with a mild degree of airway obstruction, loss of lung compliance, and alveolar capillary block.

Formaldehyde

Together with urea, formaldehyde is widely used in the plywood industry and in manufacturing of other building materials. It is also a major constituent in urea formaldehyde foam used in house insulation, a practice now prohibited in many parts of the United States. Low concentration of formaldehyde released from building materials and urea formaldehyde foam insulation causes mild to severe upper airway irritation, depending on the concentration, duration of exposure, and individual susceptibility. Irritation to the conjunctiva of the eyes is also frequent. The symptoms are similar to minor colds, with nasal and tracheobronchial discharges. The situation is further aggravated by caulking, which prevents fresh air from entering the house. Poor house ventilation also causes accumulation of other air pollutants generated by cigarette smoking, gas cooking, and unventilated kerosene heaters in the household (Repace and Lowrey, 1980; Spengler and Sexton, 1983). Long-term effects of these pollutants to human health remain to be investigated (White and Froeb, 1980).

3-Methylindole, 4-Ipomeanol, and 3-Substituted Furans

3-Methylindole, also known as skatole, is a foul-smelling metabolite of tryptophan. Fermentation of tryptophan in the rumen of cattle may produce large quantities of 3-methylindole. Its absorption and high concentration in lungs can cause small airway and alveolar injury with massive pulmonary edema and acute respiratory distress (Huang et al., 1977). This naturally occurring disease has been known as acute bovine pulmonary emphysema for over 100 years. The emphysema is of interstitial variety, presumably the consequence of labored breathing secondary to pulmonary edema. There is no comparable human disease except for patients with cirrhosis of the liver and portocaval shunts. 3-Methylindole, absorbed from the intestinal tract, reaches the lungs, bypassing detoxification by the liver because of portosystemic venous shunts. Since 3-methylindole and other indole derivatives are pyrolysis products of tryptophan in cigarette smoke (Wynder and Hoffmann, 1967), they are considered a class of chemicals responsible for cigarette smoking–related pathology of small airways and lung parenchyma. The cigarette smoke contains 0.4–1.4 mg of indole derivatives per 100 cigarettes smoked.

3-Methylindole is not the only lung toxin implicated in acute bovine pulmonary emphysema. 3-Substituted furans have been shown to be even more toxic to bovine and rodent lungs following ingestion (Boyd, 1980). 4-Ipomeanol, a product of mold-damaged sweet potatoes (Ipomoea batatas) caused by common mold, Fusarium solani, has been proven to cause injury to Clara cells in bronchioles at lower doses, and to cause both bronchiolar and alveolar injury at higher doses. Another related compound, perilla ketone in the purple mint plant Perilla frutescens, is also highly toxic to bovine and rodent lungs on ingestion (Wilson et al., 1977). Use of perilla seed oils and leaf extract as flavoring agents in Japanese foods and Chinese herbal medicine may pose a potential hazard for human lungs. However, there have been no recorded cases in humans. Other 3-substituted furans (egomaketone and isoegomaketone) from perilla plants may be equally toxic to lungs (Boyd, 1980). 3-Methylfuran has been reported as a major atmospheric contaminant in certain smogs. It is not generated by automobile exhaust and could be formed by photooxidation and degradation of volatile hydrocarbons (isoprene and other terpenes) released from vegetation. Experimentally, 3-methylfuran can cause bronchiolar epithelial necrosis similar to 4-ipomeanol. Its presence in smog may cause airway irritation and bronchiolitis.

Pharmaceutical Agents

Discussions of acute toxic injury cannot be considered complete without mentioning the large repertoire of chemotherapeutic agents for cancer therapy (Sostman et al., 1977; Weiss and Muggia, 1980). Since the life span of type I pneumocytes is 7–10 days, they are as susceptible to these agents as rapidly proliferating neoplastic cells. Inhibition of type II pneumocyte proliferation by chemotherapeutic agents presumably prevents replenishment of dead type I pneumocytes in physiologic turnover of cells. These agents may also injure type I pneumocytes. Bleomycin, busulfan, methotrexate, carmustine, semustine, zinostatin, mitomycin, and chlorambucil are some of the names on the growing list.

There is also a long list of other drugs that may cause lung injury (Gillett and Ford, 1978). Hydralazine, methysergide, and levodopa are well known for their pulmonary toxicity. The mechanisms of injury, either toxic or immune mediated, are not clear. Pathologic changes in lungs also range from pulmonary edema of acute alveolar injury to fibrosis of sclerosing alveolitis. The differences may only reflect the mode of onset, acute or insidious, and the stages of disease when lung tissues are examined histologically.

Cigarette Smoking–Related Lung Injury

One of the major problems in environmental pathology is that the long-term effects of repeated, minor acute toxic injury to the lung is poorly understood. Each episode of injury is so minor that the tissue-reparative process is capable of reconstituting injured structures. Moreover, resistance (tolerance) to repeated injury is generated in the lung as part of its defense mechanism, which tends to minimize the injurious effects of subsequent exposures. The mechanisms of tolerance include induction of xenobiotic metabolic enzymes for more efficient detoxication and disposal of hydrocarbons (Wiebel et al., 1973; Abramson and Hutton, 1975), and increase in reducing equivalents such as NADPH in antioxidant tolerance. The long-term cumulative effects of injury and response to injury on health of lungs are largely unknown. There have been no readily available experimental models to assess pathologic effects.

Cigarette smoking is a human model for studying long-term effects of repeated minor injury by toxic chemicals of varying compositions (Wynder and Hoffmann, 1967). An average American smoker smokes 30 cigarettes (one and one-half packs) a day. Excluding 8 hours of sleep, a cigarette smoker is exposed to a short period of smoke inhalation every 30 minutes from smoking a cigarette, and he or she usually continues the pattern of exposure for as long as 40 to 60 years. Cigarettes reach a temperature of 400°C at the burning tips. The smoke, in addition to carbon and other dust particles, contains various chemicals, some of which are so unstable that they escape chemical analysis. Most studies of cigarette smoke are based on the analysis of smoke condensate, "tar." It is known to contain airway irritants and lung-toxic chemicals, such as carbon monoxide, nitrogen dioxide, acetaldehyde, 3-methylindole, and ammonia. Large groups of polycyclic hydrocarbons are also present (Wynder and Hoffmann, 1967). On metabolic activation, epoxides are produced. Epoxides may cause nucleophilic attacks on proteins and nucleic acids. The results are cell injury and potential carcinogenesis (Miller, 1970; Boyd, 1980). The clinical and pathologic manifestations are chronic bronchitis, bronchiolitis, emphysema, and cancer.

CHRONIC BRONCHITIS

Repeated impositions of heavy particle load on the airway mucosa by cigarette smoke causes excessive secretion of airway mucus. Increased mucus secretion may be an integral part of accelerated mucociliary escalator activity in response to increased particle load. However, impaired ciliary motility due to toxic chemicals may cause particle stasis

in airways (Cohen et al., 1979) and provide further stimulus for mucus secretion. The increase in mucus-secreting activity is well reflected in the hyperplasia and hypertrophy of mucus-secreting cells in the airway. In normal airways, approximately 90% of mucus is secreted by mucus glands located in the lamina propria of the trachea and major bronchi. The hyperplasia and hypertrophy of mucin-secreting cells within these glands can be quantitatively assessed by calculating the ratio between the thickness of glands and the thickness of the lamina propria as measured from the basement membrane of the surface epithelium to the perichondrium of bronchial cartilages. This ratio is called the Reid index. The index is 0.3 in normal subjects, and increases to 0.6 or more are considered abnormal (Thurlbeck, 1976). The density of mucin-secreting goblet cells in the surface epithelium of the bronchi is also increased. The cells are frequently engorged with cytoplasmic mucin, suggesting increase in mucin-secreting activities. The distribution of surface goblet cells also extends from the bronchi to the bronchioles, which normally are devoid of goblet cells. Goblet cell metaplasia of bronchioles is a prominent pathologic finding in chronic bronchitis. Other pathologic findings include cellular hyperplasia and squamous metaplasia of the airway epithelium (Auerbach et al., 1979b).

The clinical manifestations of chronic airway irritation and excessive mucus secretion include chronic productive (of mucus) cough. When patients have productive cough 3 months of a year for 2 consecutive years, they are considered to suffer from chronic brochitis. Patients with chronic brochitis appear to be more susceptible to viral and bacterial infections of airways and their complication of superimposed bacterial pneumonias. The clinical course of each episode of infection tends to be more portracted. The most commonly encountered bacteria are *Staphylococcus pneumoniae* and *Haemophilus influenzae*. Therefore, chronic brochitics are absent from work more often because of "colds." The period of each episode of absence is longer, presumably because of complicating bacterial infection.

Cigarette smoking is by far the most important etiologic factor in chronic bronchitis in the United States. However, other factors such as general air pollution and regional climate may play important roles in etiology of chronic bronchitis. For example, the United States has the highest cigarette consumption, yet the incidence of chronic bronchitis is estimated to be only a third of that of England and Wales. The incidence is higher in cold, foggy, wet weather. It has been postulated that a general air pollutant such as sulfur dioxide dissolved in water droplets of fog is catalyzed to sulfuric acid. The latter is substantially more irritating and harmful to airways. Dusty conditions in work places are also known to cause or to aggravate existing chronic bronchitis. In byssinosis, chronic bronchitis is the major clinical manifestation. In addition to dust load, immunologic mechanisms may also mediate the airway injury.

CHRONIC RESPIRATORY BRONCHIOLITIS

Inflammatory reaction in respiratory bronchioles due to cigarette smoke–related injury is a pathologic process as prominent as hyperplasia and hypertrophy of mucin-secreting cells of airways. The inflammatory infiltrate, which is present within the wall of respiratory bronchioles and adjacent interstitial space, is composed of predominatly lymphocytes, dust-laden macrophages, and rare plasma cells. Edema is evident (Niewoehner et al., 1974). There are also collections of dust-laden macrophages in alveolar evagination of respiratory bronchioles, as well as in alveolar space in the central portion of the lobules (Figure 7-4). The pattern of injury is similar to that of experimental lung injury induced by nitro-

Figure 7–4. Bronchiolitis in cigarette smokers. Slightly dilated and tortuous terminal and respiratory bronchioles show focal fibrosis and deposition of anthracotic pigment (arrows). The lesion is presumably a precursor of centrilobular emphysema.

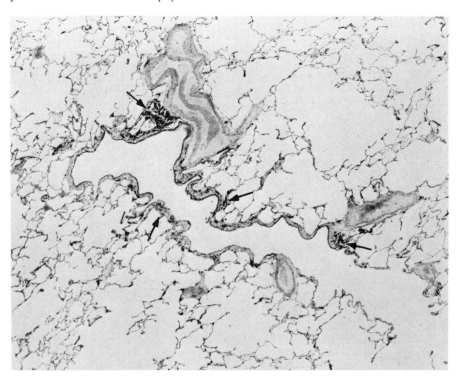

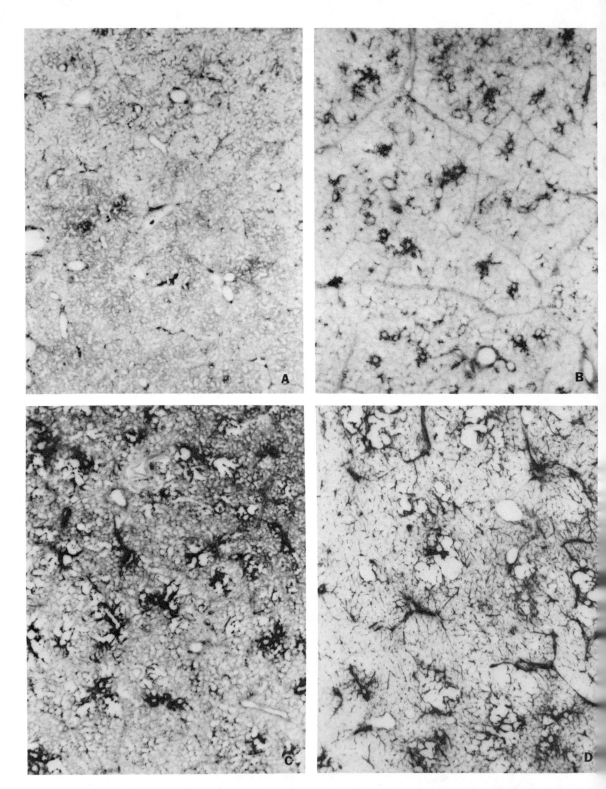

Figure 7–5. Evolution of centrilobular emphysema (Gough preparation). (A) Normal lung. (B) Accumulation of anthracotic pigment in the centrilobular regions around terminal and respiratory bronchioles is noted in cigarette smokers. (C) Dilatation of respiratory bronchioles marks the early stage of centrilobular emphysema. (D) In severe centrilobular emphysema, large irregular emphysematous spaces are the results of dilatation and fusion of respiratory bronchioles.

gen dioxide, sulfur dioxide, ozone, or 3-methylindole.

The inflammatory reaction is particularly evident in cigarette smokers before age 40 (Niewoehner et al., 1974). Thereafter it gradually subsides with attendant gradual loss of smooth muscle cells and increase in fibrous tissues within the wall of respiratory bronchioles. In cigarette smokers after age 60, the inflammatory reaction is rarely found unless there are other intercurrent diseases. The pathologic findings in the respiratory bronchioles at this stage are those of a burnout bronchiolitis, characterized by the loss of smooth muscle bundles, fibrosis, and tortuosity and dilatation of bronchiolar lumens. The latter is mainly due to weakening and destruction of bronchiolar wall constituents and eventual fusion with adjacent bronchiole or alveolar ducts. The result is formation of a large, irregular airspace extending from the midzone to the central region of a secondary lung lobule, corresponding to the proxial portion of an acinus (primary lung lobule). This stage of lung pathology is referred to as centrilobular emphysema (Figure 7-5). Along the adventitia of respiratory bronchioles, there is irregular fibrosis. Some of these exhibit fibrotic nodules containing dust-laden macrophages and free carbon pigments. The pathogenesis of these fibrotic nodules is presumably due to a combination of fibrosis associated with chronic bronchiolitis and incorporation of intra-alveolar dust-laden macrophages into the bronchiolar adventitia. Polarizing microscopic studies of these fibrotic nodules often reveal minute, needle-shaped, birefringent crystal, similar to silica crystals in silicosis. Pulmonary macrophages in cigarette smokers also contain hexagonal platelike inclusions in phagolysosomes, so-called smokers' inclusions. Morphology and electron microprobe analysis suggest that these inclusions are aluminum silicate kaolinite (Brody and Craighead, 1975). These minerals are presumably derived from tobacco leaves and inhaled smoke. They may contribute to lung injury and fibrosis in cigarette smokers, as in other silica-silicate pneumoconiosis.

CENTRILOBULAR EMPHYSEMA

Centrilobular emphysema characteristically involves upper lobes and apical portions of lower lobes. The emphysematous space is surrounded by a mantle of black carbon pigments, an indicator of air pollutants (Figure 7-5). In the early stage of disease, the emphysematous space is more regular and uniformly distributed. In the advanced stage, it is more irregular in shape and variable from lobule to lobule. Concomitant panlobular emphysema is very common.

PANLOBULAR EMPHYSEMA

Although centrilobular emphysema is the predominant type of emphysema associated with cigarette smoking, the incidence of panlobular emphysema is also increased in cigarette smokers. There is a good statistical correlation in North America among cigarette smoking, chronic bronchitis, centrilobular emphysema, and panlobular emphysema, which suggests their common etiology (Auerbach, Hammond, Garfinkel, and Benante, 1972; Thurlbeck, 1976). Panlobular emphysema is due to dilatation of alveolar rather than bronchiolar spaces, associated with destruction of alveolar septa. Alveolar ducts are also proportionately dilated. The distribution of lesions is relatively uniform within a lobule, thus, panlobular (panacinar). During the early stage of disease, the loss of alveolar tissues is manifested by the presence of fenestrae in alveolar septa. These fenestrae are larger in size and more irregular in shape compared with pores of Kohn, which are regarded as physiologic channels for alveolar collateral ventilation. However, the fenestrae and pores may represent a continuum in the evolution of the lesions of panlobular emphysema. As fenestrae enlarge and coalesce, large areas of functioning alveolar tissue are lost, with apparent dilatation of alveolar airspaces.

The basal and anterior zones of lungs are more severely affected. Because of frequent coexistance of panlobular and centrilobular emphysema in cigarette smokers, it is very difficult, if not impossible, to classify severe emphysema with extensive lung destruction.

Unlike centrilobular emphysema, the targets and modes of injury in panlobular emphysema are not clear. Examinations of sputa from cigarette smokers indicate that the flux of macrophages and neutrophils from circulation to alveolar space and broncial lumens is increased, presumably as a result of inflammatory reaction in lungs. Although no significant increase in neutrophils is detectable on histologic examination of lungs, increase in dust-laden macrophages in lungs is evident. The proteolytic theory of tissue injury presumes that the proteolytic enzymes, mostly lysosomal in origin, released by leukocytes may cause tissue digestion if the enzyme activities are unopposed by tissue and serum protease inhibitors. The major components of serum protease inhibitors are α_1-antitrypsin and α_2-macroglobulin. In patients with hereditary α_1 antitrypsin deficiency, ZZ homoygous state of *Pi* locus, panlobular emphysema is one of the major tissue alterations and evolves insidiously over decades. There is experimental evidence that cigarette smoke may inhibit the antitrypsin activities, thus allowing proteolytic injury by lysosomal enzymes to proceed uninhibited. A difficulty with this theory is that the tissues are constantly bathed in antitrypsin, and the inhibition of antiprotease activities in airspace may not have significant impact on the tissue antiprotease activities. An alternative explanation is that cigarette smoke and other environmental pollutants may interfere with the process of maintaining normal alveolar structures. Alveolar structure, which includes septal components and proper alveolar geometry, is probably constantly remodeled in response to injury and in physiologic events of tissue turnover and renewal, a biologic process very similar to constant remodeling of bone in response to changing stress. When the rate of tissue degradation exceeds formation, there is a net loss of tissues, analogous to osteoporosis or osteopenia of bones. Panlobular emphysema is a manifestation of loss of al-

veolar septa. The fundamental biologic process involved in remodeling and maintenance of alveolar structures is largely unknown, although some preliminary observations suggest that cooperative efforts of type II pneumocytes and interstitial cells may play cardinal roles. Elucidation of these basic biologic mechanisms and their vulnerability to modification by environmental agents may hold keys to our understanding of pathogenesis of panlobular emphysema.

Both chronic bronchitis and pulmonary emphysema cause obstruction of small airways during the expiratory phase of pulmonary ventilation, especially during the forced expiration. This is reflected in decrease in FEV_1 (forced expiratory volume in 1 second) of pulmonary function. In chronic bronchitis, the obstruction is presumably caused by inflammatory edema of small-airway mucosa and mucus plugging of small airways. Loss of alveolar tissue and its elasticity, and weakening of mechanical strength of respiratory bronchioles are probably responsible for small-airway obstruction in emphysema.

In the United States, cigarette smoking is the major cause of both chronic bronchitis and emphysema. Although the incidence of emphysema increases with age after age 40, clinically as well as pathologically significant emphysema is rarely observed in nonsmokers. This is particularly true with centrilobular emphysema. Hereditary α_1-antitrypsin deficiency accounts for only a very small fraction of cases of panlobular emphysema. Therefore, smoking accounts for almost all morbidity and mortality related to chronic bronchitis and emphysema. The impact of cigarette smoking is not confined to smokers themselves. Nonsmokers working or living with smokers may also be subjected to substantial risks (White and Froeb, 1980). Children from smoking families are more likely to develop small-airway disease in adult life.

Chronic Toxic Lung Injury

Lungs may suffer chronic injury by repeated exposures to sublethal doses of toxic agents. Agents causing chronic lung injury, however, are characteristically inorganic dusts of low solubility. Slow release of chemicals due to low solubility causes low-grade, nonlethal toxic injury to the lung. The low-grade injury is sustained over a long period of time because of slow clearance of dust particles from alveoli. When dust particles are entrapped in the interstitium, the clearance is further delayed. Therefore, a single exposure to a large dose of inorganic dust may result in persistent lung injury and extensive lung destruction decades after the initial exposure. In experimental silicosis, intratracheal instillation of a large dose of silica causes massive pulmonary edema and acute respiratory distress as seen in acute lung injury, while repeated small-dose exposure results in insidious lung fibrosis and destruction. This supports the concept that the differences between chronic and acute lung injuries are in the dosage and duration of exposures to the toxic materials. As discussed in the acute lung injury, long-term sequelae of certain patients suffering from clinical acute lung injury may have clinical and pathologic features almost identical to chronic lung injury.

In addition to direct chemical toxic injury to the lungs, other pathogenic mechanisms have also been postulated. Mechanical injury due to the shape of dust particles, especially the long needle-shaped particles, may irritate or pierce cells and tissues. The surface of dust particles may also adsorb proteins, causing conformational changes and denaturation of proteins. It is postulated that the denatured proteins may serve as antigens to provoke antibody formation. Subsequent tissue injury is presumably mediated by immune complex or perpetuated by autoimmunity. There is little direct evidence supporting immune-mediated tissue injury.

Although type I pneumocyte injury, necrosis, alveolar edema, hyaline membrane, and type II pneumocyte proliferation as in acute alveolar injury can also be seen in chronic alveolar injury, they are often confined to small foci and inconspicuous. The most prominent features in the early stage

of exposure are collections of dust-laden macrophages in alveolar spaces, forming dust nodules (Figure 7-6). Toxic chemicals released as dust particles are freed into alveolar spaces when macrophages die, as a consequence of normal physiologic turnover or because of the toxic effects of dusts on macrophages. Soluble chemicals released from particles cause a minor episode of acute injury, with attendant pneumocyte injury and necrosis. Release of lysosomal enzymes by macrophages may also mediate the tissue injury. Hyaline membranes are frequently observed in the area of pneumocyte injury, and the alveolar surface may become denuded of pneumocyte covering, forming an alveolar "ulcer." Proliferation of type II pneumocytes may follow. However, healing of these ulcers is presumably incomplete because of the persistent nature of the injury or the chemicals interfering with type II pneumocyte proliferation or migration. As discussed in acute lung injury, the nonhealing alveolar ulcers lead to migration of interstitial cells into the alveolar spaces and organization of intra-alveolar exudate. Dust nodules become laced with randomly oriented, wavy, argyrophilic collagen fibers (reticulin fibers). The proliferating alveolar epithelium eventually grows over the dust nodules and incorporates the nodules into the interstitial compartment (Spencer, 1977). The alveolar space is thus irreversibly obliterated.

Proliferation of interstitial cells and synthesis of collagen and elastic fibers become the most prominent tissue reactions following incorporation of dust nodules into the interstitium. Chemicals released from dust particles become a constant source of irritation to the connective tissue of the lungs and perpetuate the fibrotic reaction. Fibrosis also leads to further effacement of alveolar structure and loss of lung parenchyma. Although lung pathology may vary among various types of penumoconiosis, the common denominators are loss of alveoli, formation of large cystic emphysematous spaces, and fibrosis. Lungs exhibiting a constellation of these features are often called honeycomb lungs.

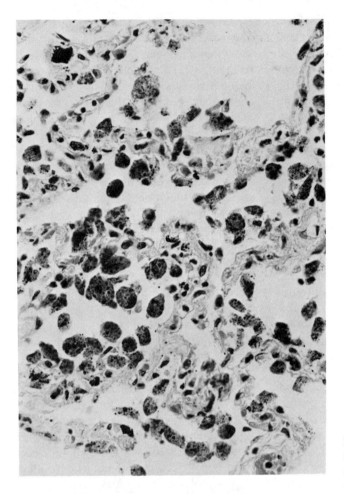

Figure 7–6. Dust-laden alveolar macrophages in pneumoconiosis. (Courtesy of Dr. N. K. Mottet.)

Since fibrosis is one of the most prominent tissue respsonses in chronic alveolar injury, there has been some interest in the types of collagen alteration in lungs. Generally speaking, in the early stages of development of the lesions, argyrophylic collagen fibers (reticulin fibrs) (Huang, 1977) are the most prominent connective tissue elements. There is a relative increase in type III collagen. In late stages, large bundles of collagen fibers develop, some of which appear hyalinized. This is associated with an increase in type I collagen. These are two chemically different classes of collagen. One class may replace the other, but there is no convincing evidence that one class can either mature or transform into the other. The role of type V collagen in fibrotic lung disease is not clear.

AGENTS CAUSING CHRONIC TOXIC LUNG INJURY

Pneumoconiosis is a fibrotic and destructive lung disease due to the inhalation of dust. The dust is characteristically from inorganic chemicals of low solubility.

Asbestos

Asbestos is a group of silicate mineral fibers widely used in industries and modern life because of its physical and chemical inertness. Their resistance to heat, fire, and chemical corrosion prevents them from being replaced by man-made fibers. Chrysotile ($3MgO_2SiO_2H_2O$) has a serpentine form, while the amphiboles are straight, needle-shaped fibers. The amphiboles include amosite, crocidolite, anthophyllite, and tremolite. Because of their widespread use in building materials such as ceiling, tiles, insulation of old houses, and household products, the general population is exposed to asbestos (Sebastien et al., 1982). However, asbestosis as a clinical disease is mainly observed in occupation-related exposure (Becklake, 1976; Kannerstein et al., 1977; Craighead and Mossman, 1982). The list of occupations is very long, including mining, manufacturing of asbestos products, and insulation industries.

Because of the thin fibrous forms, the equivalent hydrodynamic diameters of asbestos fibers are small, which prevents them from being removed by aerodynamic filtration in the airways. Fibers deposited in the small airways and alveoli are not readily removed by macrophages and mucociliary transport, especially the long fibers. Small numbers of asbestos fibers deposited on alveolar sufaces become coated with proteinaceous materials, which are subsequently

mineralized with iron, calcium, and phosphate (Figures 7-7, 7-8, 7-9). The formation of the ferruginous bodies makes fibers visible under the microscope (Figure 7-7). The coating presumably makes fibers less irritating to the tissue and facilitates their encasement by multinculeated giant cells derived from alveolar macrophages. The uncoated fibers, which are many times greater in number, are not detectable under the light microscope. They are very mobile. With the aid of respiratory movement, these long, thin fibers can penetrate into tissues and make their way to the pleural surface. Occasionally they can even penetrate through the diaphragm and enter the peritoneal cavity.

Within alveoli, asbestos fibers cause low-grade but sustained alveolar injury, resulting in fibrosis of alveolar septa and effacement of alveolar architecture. Collections of macrophages containing ferruginous bodies within alveolar spaces are common findings in asbestosis. The ferruginous bodies are frequently engulfed by multinucleated

Figure 7–7. Ferruginous bodies prepared by digestion of lung tissues from patients with history of asbestos exposure.

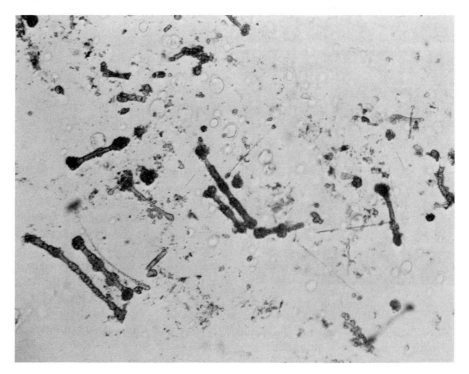

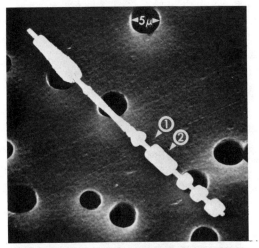

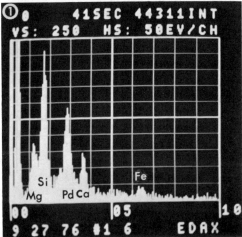

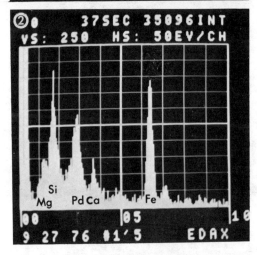

Figure 7–8. Electron microprobe elemental analysis of a ferruginous body. The results indicate the core is composed of asbestos fibers, and beaded coating contains iron. (From Chen and Mottet, 1978. Courtesy of Dr. N. K. Mottet.)

giant cells formed by fusion of alveolar macrophages. In the pleural cavity, they provoke a fibrotic reaction on both the visceral and parietal pleura. Fibrosis on the visceral pleura is relatively mild and diffuse. The fibrotic lesions on the parietal pleura are usually over the ribs of the chest wall or on the diaphragm (Figure 7-9). These lesions are characteristically well-defined geographic areas of dense hyalinized acellular collagenous tissues, with collagen fibers parallel to the pleural surface. They have the appearance of white sugar icing on the cake. Similar lesions are seen in peritoneal cavity, especially on the splenic capsule, which is called hyaline perisplenitis.

Although asbestos may not be carcinogenic, it acts as a potent tumor promoter. The incidence of lung cancer in cigarette smokers is substantially increased by asbestos exposure. Increase in the incidence of mesothelioma, the malignant neoplasm of pleural lining, is well known.

Talc

Talc is a fibrus form of silicate composed of hydrated magnesium silicate, closely related to asbestos. Most of the clinically significant exposures are related to mining and milling of talc. Talc-containing products include cosmetic powders, paints, and roofing materials. In the past, talc used in dusting powders was often heavily contaminated with asbestos fibers. Talc has also been used to cut heroin by drug addicts. As a result, talc can reach lungs by intravenous injections of talc-contaminated heroin.

A characteristic feature of talc pneumoconiosis is the presence of multinucleated giant cells containing birefringent (doubly refractile) crystals in the dust nodules. These crystals can be readily detected by polarizing microscopy. Fibrosis and obliteration of alveolar architecture follows a general pattern seen in pneumoconiosis. Because of frequent contamination by asbestos, ferruginous bodies can also be seen. In certain cases, proper assessement of relative importance of talc or asbestos in causing lung lesions can be very difficult.

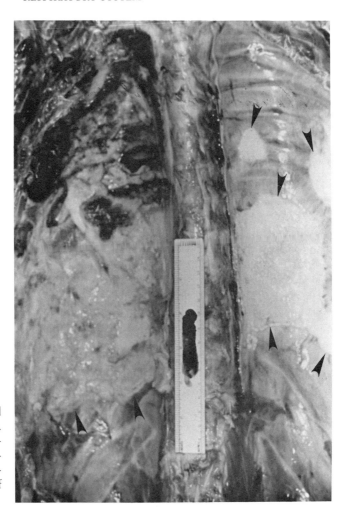

Figure 7–9. Fibrous pleural plaques due to asbestos exposure. The plaques are composed of acellular, dense hyalinized collagenous tissue, which contains uncoated asbestos fiber. (Courtesy of Dr. N. K. Mottet.)

Silica

Silica is silicon dioxide, the most common constituent of the earth's crust. Human endeavors involving cutting, shaping, and polishing of rocks and stones cause risk of exposure to silica, thus silicosis of lungs. The silica content varies with rocks and stones. Sandstones are almost 100% silica; granite is 20% to 70%. Pure limestone and marble are free of silica.

The spectrum of lung injury caused by silica extends from acute alveolar injury with pulmonary edema on one extreme to the chronic fibrotic process developed over decades on the other. Acte silicosis is caused by exposure to a large dose of silica over a very short period of time. The X-ray findings are those of pulmonary edema in acute respiratory distress. Pathologic examination reveals alveolar injury of type I pneumocytes associated with massive alveolar protein-rich edema. The resolution of acute alveolar injury follows the same general pattern of type II pneumocyte proliferation, intra-alveolar organization of hyaline membranes, and diffuse interstitial fibrosis. If patients survive the acute phase of injury, the pathologic pictures are compounded by chronic silicosis due to persistence of silica in lung parenchyma, and consequent chronic alveolar injury.

Chronic silicosis usually develops insidiously over years or decades. The pathologic findings are similar to other chronic alveolar injuries caused by inorganic dusts, that is, intra-alveolar dust nodules composed of collections of silica-laden macrophages, and their incorporation into alveolar septa by emigration of interstitial cells and growth of epithelium over dust nodules. Depending on the forms of silica, small, needle-shaped birefringent crystals are occasionally observed. Because of the small size of the crystals, multinucleated giant cells are rare. One of the characteristics of chronic silicosis is the development of discrete nodules of hyalinized collagenous tissue, which may contain calcium deposits. The acellular collagen fibers tend to be arranged in a concentric manner. The fibrotic nodules may grow from millimeters to centimeters in size, and may also become confluent to occupy an entire lobe (Figure 7-10). Central breakdown and liquefaction of collagen fibers are more commonly seen in concurrent tuberculous infection or in the Caplan syndrome (silicosis and rheumatoid disease). In the latter, the necrotic center of a fibrotic silicotic nodule is heavily infiltrated with polymorphonuclear leukocytes.

Kaolin

Kaolin (porcelain china clay) is a hydrated aluminum silicate widely used in paint, paper, cement, and pharmaceuticals. Occupational exposure occurs during quarrying and packaging of kaolin. Pulmonary lesions are those characteristic of chronic alveolar injury with foci of nodular fibrosis around heavy kaolin deposits.

Other silicates, such as Fuller's earth, cement, and mica, may also cause rare cases of pneumoconiosis. Tissue injury and response are very similar to those of other pneumoconioses.

Coal

Before the late 1960s, little attention had been paid to the hazard of exposure to coal dust. Most textbooks of pathology cited Gardner's assertion that carbon dust was harmless to tissues. However, the argument whether pure carbon is toxic to tissues or not is a moot point, because carbon in na-

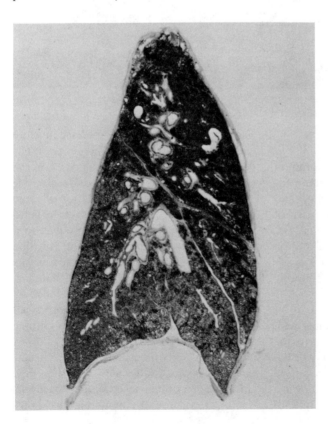

Figure 7–10. Silicosis. Massive fibrosis and obliteration of the lung parenchyma are evident on the upper half of the lung.

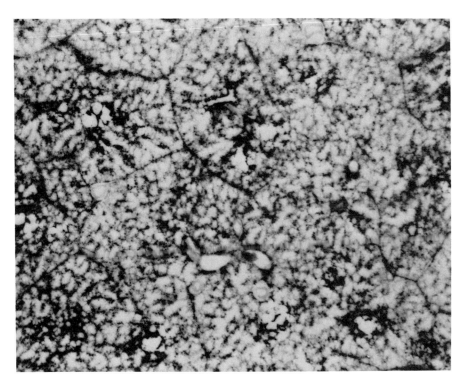

Figure 7–11. Simple coat pneumoconiosis. Heavy deposits of anthracotic pigment in the lung parenchyma, especially in the centrilobular regions, are associated with centrilobular emphysema. The patient is also a cigarette smoker.

ture or as a combustion product is presented to the respiratory system in an impure form. Various chemicals in minute quantity can be adsorbed to the activated carbon and may cause tissue injury as they are slowly released.

Coal miner's lung in its uncomplicated form shows minor tissue changes. The dust-laden macrophages migrate and converge on the peribronchiolar space of the last two generations of respiratory bronchioles, where the lymphatic system of lung parenchyma originates. Although carbon-laden macrophage stasis is seen along the lymphatic drainage system of the lungs, significant pathologic changes are observed mainly in the respiratory bronchioles. The mantle of peribronchiolar carbon-laden macrophages leads to fibrosis, loss of the smooth muscle coat of bronchioles, and eventual weakening and dilatation of bronchioles. Since the respiratory bronchioles are located in the central portion of the secondary lobules of

the lungs, the black anthracotic pigments and associated fibrosis are characteristically centrilobular in distribution (Figure 7-11), similar to those seen in cigarette smokers. The fibrosis in peribronchiolar tissue may extend to adjacent alveolar septa attached to the respiratory bronchiole; it forms nodules of anthracofibrotic lesions called coal macules (Figure 7-12). There is little evidence that injury is inflicted on the alveolar pneumocytes. The anthracofibrotic nodules are rich in argyrophilic collagen fibers. In late-stage lesions, an increase in nonargyrophilic collagen fibers is noted. At this stage of the disease, there is striking similarity between coal pneumoconiosis and cigarette smokers' lungs, especially in heavy smokers. The degree of bronchiolar dilatation (centrilobular emphysema) appears greater in cigarette smokers relative to the centrilobular black pigmentation. Clinically the miners suffer from mild obstructive lung disease, as manifested by decrease in FEV_1

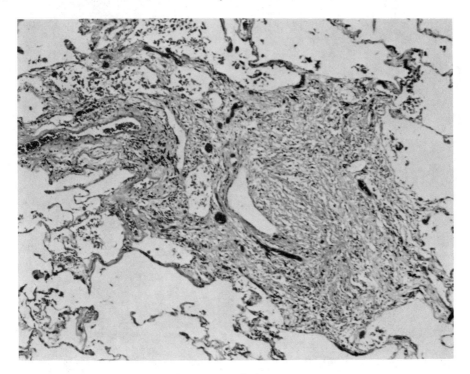

Figure 7–12. A coal "macule" in coal pneumoconiosis.

(forced expiratory volume in 1 second) and productive cough consistent with chronic bronchitis. In this respect, symptoms are very similar to those of cigarette smokers. The decrease in FEV_1 is usually minor, and may vary among different mining regions in the United States. In most regions, no statistically significant difference in FEV_1 is observed. Radiographic findings are those of small coal nodules to larger areas of irregular fibrosis.

Simple, uncomplicated coal miner's pneumoconiosis is a relatively benign process both pathologically and clinically. The process may remain stable after cessation of further exposure to coal dust. However, in a small number of coal miners, rapid progression of lung fibrosis may lead to a severe compromise of pulmonary functions. The process is referred to as complicated coal pneumoconiosis, or progressive massive fibrosis. Pathologically, the lesions consist of fibrotic enlargement of coal nodules, coalescence, massive destruction of lung parenchyma, and formation of cystic spaces filled with muddy coal dust—black honey-

comb. The uninvolved portions of the lungs may show hyperinflation, so-called compensatory emphysema. The posterior aspect of upper lobes and apical segments of lower lobes of the lungs are more severely affected. It may not be possible to draw a sharp line of distinction between simple and complicated forms of coal pneumoconiosis, and the difference may only be quantitative rather than qualitative. Small, coal-filled cysts are occasionally observed in uncomplicated form. Those who believe in a qualitative difference postulate that silica, mycobacterial infection, autoimmunity, or rheumatoid disease may be partly responsible for rapid progression of lung destruction and fibrosis. Support for any of these speculations is lacking. Graphite pneumoconiosis is similar to coal pneumoconiosis in many respects.

Tin

Workers exposed to tin during bagging of concentrated cassiterite (SnO_2) or in smeltering operations may have alveolar deposits of tin in their alveolar macrophages. These deposits tend to be concentrated in certain peribronchiolar alveoli to form dust nodules. However, the evidence of tissue injury is absent, and pulmonary fibrosis, if ever observed, is minimal. Therefore, stannosis represents pulmonary retention of inert foreign materials without significant tissue injury. It is not a form of pneumoconiosis. In this regard, stannosis is very similar to pulmonary deposition of iron oxide and antimony, which are not harmful to the lungs.

Aluminum Powder

Powdered aluminum is used in incendiary bombs and fireworks. Manufacturing and handling of powdered aluminum may pose a potential inhalation hazard. The lung injury is one of acute alveolar injury followed by interstitial fibrosis. Cases are relatively rare.

Workers involved in manufacturing of alumina abrasives may be exposed to aluminum oxide (bauxite). Aluminum oxide deposited in alveoli causes acute alveolar injury with alveolar edema and type II pneumocyte proliferation, which is followed by diffuse interstitial fibrosis. As the chronic phase begins, massive pulmonary fibrosis with obliteration of alveolar structure is the most prominent feature.

Beryllium

Beryllium is a metal highly toxic to the respiratory system. Acute exposure causes irritation and injury to the airway mucosa. In acute injury to the lung parenchyma, pulmonary edema, hyaline membrane, and hemorrhage are the cardinal features, presumably resulting from injury to pneumocytes, endothelium, or both. Beryllium may also be absorbed by skin and transported to lungs by the bloodstream. Fibrois and sarcoid-like granulomas are the hallmark of chronic berylliosis. Fibrosis is often associated with extensive effacement of alveolar structure.

Environmental Lung Diseses Mediated by the Immune Reaction

Organic dusts are normally not very toxic to the lungs by themselves. Unlike inorganic dusts, they are immunogenic and provoke antibody synthesis by the host's immune system. Subsequent re-exposure to antigens results in specific antigen–antibody reactions that may mediate tissue injuries. Four types of immune reaction have been described (McCombs, 1972; Schatz et al., 1979).

Type I is the immediate hypersensitivity reaction mediated by the IgE class of antibodies. IgE is a cytophilic antibody exhibiting a high affinity for cell membranes of mast cells, which are normally present in abundance in the airway mucosa. Exposure to antigens and binding of antigens to antibodies on mast cell membranes initiate exocytosis of mast cell granules. Histamine and release of other active mediators cause vasodilatation, increased vascular permeability, tissue edema, discharge of copious amounts of mucous secretions, and contraction of airway smooth muscles. The latter is responsible for the wheezing characteristic of asthma attacks. Such reactions are immediate and occur within minutes of exposure to antigens. Hay fever of the upper airways and asthma of tracheobrochial trees are classical examples of this type of immune reaction. Antigens usually include pollens, organic dusts, or animal hairs.

Asthma caused by inhaled external antigens as discussed above is called extrinsic asthma and is clearly a disease triggered by exogenous environmental agents. In addition to general environmental conditions, extrinsic asthma is known to occur more often in people in certain occupations, such as millers and bakers, handling grain products. It is not entirely clear if antigens are inherent constituents of grain proteins or contaminants derived from fungi or wheat weevil (*Sitophilus granarius*). Sawmill workers and carpenters may also suffer from asthmatic attack on exposure to sawdusts and other wood products. Cork dust causes bronchial asthma and allergic alveolitis, called suberosis. This is a combination of types I and III immune reaction, similar to asthma with Churg-Strauss granulomatous angiitis of the lungs, occasionally seen in asthma patients. Again, the allergens have not been precisely identified.

Intrinsic asthma attacks are precipitated by factors other than foreign antigens, such as exercise, infection, and emotional stress. Since nonspecific airway irritants discussed in other parts of this chapter can also precipitate asthmatic attacks, intrinsic asthma can also be considered within the scope of environmental disease.

Type II immune reactions are caused by antibodies reacting with cellular or extracellular elements of tissues, an autoimmune reaction. No environmental agents have been implicated in this type of immune reaction in the lungs.

Type III immune reactions are due to formation and tissue deposition of antigen–antibody immune complexes. The consequent tissue injury is called immune complex disease. Immune complexes can be formed in other parts of the body and carried to the lungs by the circulating blood. The lung disease caused by circulating immune complexes, such as rheumatoid disease and systemic lupus erythematosus, are not related to environmental agents and therefore will not be discussed here. Immune complexes formed in situ in the lungs are most relevant to environmental lung diseases.

Inhaled foreign antigens deposited in he lung perenchyma induce inflammation of alveoli mediated by formation of antigen–antibody complexes (Johnson et al., 1979). The immune complex activates complements, some of which are chemotactic to leukocytes, especially products of C5. An influx of neutrophils and phagocytosis of insoluble immune complexes by neutrophils lead to release of lysosomal enzymes and other factors from neutrophils. The released lysosomal enzymes cause injury to lung cells and connective tissue elements (collagen and elastin) when the local and serum α_1-antiproteinase activities are overwhelmed. Activated leukocytes may also release superoxide free radicals, which can cause tissue injury. The alveolar injury increases the permeability of the air–blood barrier, which enhances outpouring of antibody into alveolar space, causing more immune complex formation and tissue injury. The alveolar space is filled with exudate composed of neutrophils, protein-rich edema fluid, and occasionally red blood cells. Abundance of neutrophils in alveolar exudate in early stages of alveolar injury distinguishes immune complex–mediated alveolar injury from that caused by chemical cytotoxic agents in experimental alveolar injury.

Type IV immune reactions are cell-mediated delayed hypersensitivity reactions. Interaction of antigens with immune-competent lymphocytes causes later release of mediators, which immobilize and activate macrophages. The slowly evolving inflammatory infiltrate is composed predominantly of macrophages. This is called granulomatous inflammation. There is a tendency for macrophages to aggregate locally and form tubercles. Activated macrophages, so-called epithelioid histiocytes, secrete lysosomal enzymes and release superoxide free radicals. These can cause tissue injury and extensive tissue necrosis.

In humans exposed to organic dusts, deposition of exogenous antigens in the alveoli causes lung inflammation mediated by immune reaction, the extrinsic allergic alveolitis. Both types III and IV immune reactions are involved. In human case reports of extrinsic allergic alveolitis, the neutrophilic infiltrate has not been a prominent feature. It is possible that this very early event in type III immune reaction may escape pathologic examination. Careful immunopathologic studies searching for immune complexes are required in the future to resolve the problem. The alveolar spaces may be filled with protein-rich edema fluid, hyaline membrane, and occasional macrophages. Lymphocytes and plasma cells infiltrated into the interstitium become the most prominent inflammatory cell infiltrate in the later stage of immune-complex lung injury. The resolution of alveolar injury proceeds by scavenging of cellular debris and proteinaceous exudate by alveolar macrophages, proliferation of type II pneumocytes, and variable organization of alveolar exudate by emigration of interstitial cells, similar to acute toxic lung injury. Granulomas are also frequently observed in extrinsic allergic alveolitis, most likely due to type IV immune reaction, although occasional foreign body–type giant cells containing ingested inorganic dust particles are also observed. In certain cases, the lung lesions are of relatively insidious onset, and lung inflammation is almost exclusively of granulomatous nature, suggesting a predominant role played by type IV immune reaction.

The long-term consequence of extrinsic allergic alveolitis varies, depending on intensity and duration of exposures. Effacement of alveolar structure and fibrosis represents irreversible destruction of lung parenchyma. Clinically, patients have restrictive lung disease, diffusion defect, and airway obstruction. The end-stage lung injury has the gross appearance of a honeycomb lung.

The probability of having clinically significant exposure to antigens that cause extrinsic allergic alveolitis is closely related to the occupational environment. Thus, the clinical diseases are usually named after occupations or special environmental setting, although antigens are similar in many cases. Antigens causing extrinsic allergic alveolitis are either fungi and their derivatives or animal proteins. By far, fungi are the most common source of antigens.

FARMER'S LUNG

Farmer's lung, a prime example of organic-dust lung disease, is caused by massive exposure to fungi, fungal spores, and other fungal derivatives in moldy hay. Spoiled damp hay, with temperatures between 40 and 60°C inside bales, favors prolific growth of fungi, such as *Thermoactinomyces vulgaris*, *Micropolyspora faeni*, and *Coniosporum* spp. When the hay is turned over or raked, a cloud of fungal mycelia and spores

is liberated into the air. Farmers who have been sensitized previously develop fever, chills, dry cough, and shortness of breath 4–8 hours after re-exposure to fungal antigens. X-ray examination of the lungs reveals pulmonary edema similar to alveolar edema seen in acute toxic lung injury. Examinations of lung tissue show alveolar edema, interstitial infiltrate composed of plasma cells and lymphocytes, and bronchiolitis. Occasional non-necrotizing granulomas can also be seen. In late stages of the disease, pathologic features consist of interstitial fibrosis and lymphoplasmocytic infiltrate, mild degree of type II pneumocyte proliferation, intra-alveolar organization of exudate, and simplification (effacement) of alveolar architecture. End-stage honeycomb lungs are seen in farmers who succumb to chronic diseases.

Luxuriant growth of thermophilic *Actinomycetes* also takes place during processing of compost for mushroom (*Agaricus hortensis*) culture. Mushroom workers exposed to mycelia and spores of *Thermoactinomyces vulgaris* and *Micropolyspora faeni* develop lung disease similar to farmer's lung. Peasants who split capsicum pods contaminated by yet unidentified fungal spores during preparation of paprika may suffer from capsicum lung or paprika splitter's lung. The disease is similar to farmer's lung in many respects.

Like farmers, office workers face similar environmental hazards due to growth of fungi in the air-conditioning duct system and humidifers (Fink et al., 1976). Thermophilic *Actinomycetes* and *Aspergillus* spp. are most often implicated. Asthma- and farmer's lung–like symptoms have been described. Similar contamination may occur in heating and air-conditioning systems of an automobile.

MALTWORKER'S LUNG

Aspergillus clavatus is a common fungus contaminating germinating barley in a hot and humid environment. Workers turning malt to release carbon dioxide may inhale mycelia and spore dust and develop allergic alveolitis.

BAGASSOSIS

Bagassosis is similar to farmer's lung. Bagasse, materials left after juice has been expressed from sugar cane, is used in manufacturing paper, cardboard, insulating board, and other building materials. Southern wet and hot climates, such as in Louisiana, favor growth of *Thermoactinomyces vulgaris*, which is the primary cause of extrinsic allergic alveolitis. Histopathology of bagassosis is similar to farmer's lung.

Byssinosis

Byssinosis occurs in workers processing or spinning cotton, flax, hemp, or sisal. Workers typically experience tightness of chest and cough when they return to work on Mondays or following holidays, after they have been working in the industry for several years. This is presumably a period of sensitization. Symptoms usually subside on Tuesday and the rest of the week. As the disease progresses, the cotton workers may develop productive cough and dyspnea that persist throughout the week. The symptoms are those of chronic bronchitis and chronic obstructive lung disease. The pathologic features of byssinosis consist of excessive mucus secretion associated with chronic bronchitis. The lung parenchyma may show small fibrotic nodules containing calcified vegetable fibers surrounded by degenerating macrophages. The immunopathologic basis of byssinosis is unclear and not supported by histopathology. The chronic bronchitic picture may be due exclusively to irritant dust.

SAWMILL WORKER'S LUNG

Fungi grow under tree bark or wood products. Maple-bark stripper's lung is due to exposure to spores of *Cryptostroma corticale*. Sequoiosis is due to exposure to yet unidentified fungi in redwood (*Sequoia sempervirens)* sawdusts. The lung patho-

logical features consist of numerous nonnecrotizing granulomata with foreign body–type giant cells containing fungal spores and wood fiber fragments. Fibrosis also occurs. The overall tissue reactions resemble the delayed hypersensitivity reaction (Figure 7-13).

BIRD FANCIER'S LUNG

Birds are natural protein losers into their intestinal tracts. Incomplete digestion of food proteins also enrich the protein content of bird droppings. Exposures to bird droppings may cause allergic alveolitis similar to farmer's lung. Pigeon, parrot, turkey, and chicken are the most common sources of sensitization (Moore et al., 1974). The diseases are referred to as bird fancier's lung, pigeon breeder's lung, budgerigar fancier's lung, turkey raiser's disease, and chicken raiser's disease.

Bird feathers can also be the origin of antigens and may come from unexpected sources, such as pillows, comforters, or clothing. Other animal proteins, porcine and ox pituitaries, may cause allergic lung disease on inhalation (pituitary snuff taker's lung).

Lung Cancer

Lung cancer is one of a few malignant neoplasms clearly associated with environmental pollution. Urbanization, industrialization, and wide use of combustion engines in transportation are the major causes of general air pollution, which increases the risk of lung cancer. Occupational exposures to radioactive materials in mining industries, chromium, nickel, vanadium, molybdenum, beryllium, and asbestos also contribute to carcinogenesis in selected segments of the population. Workers in occupations likely to be exposed to various chemicals, such as chemical workers, gas workers, carpenters, and painters, also have a higher incidence of lung cancer. However, the most important risk factor is cigarette smoking. It is estimated that the latter accounted for 85% of lung cancer in the United States in

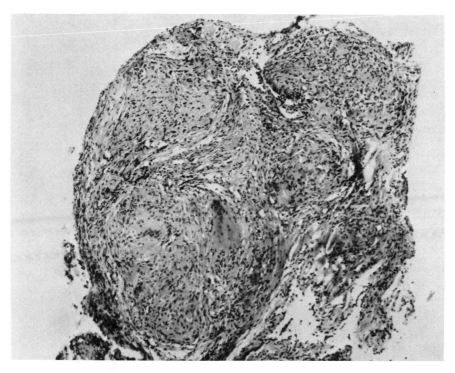

Figure 7–13. Sawmill worker's lung. The granulomatous lesion is composed of epithelioid histiocytes and foreign body–type giant cells. The tissue response is characteristic of type VI immune reaction.

the 1980s. It is also the major cause of cancers of the oral cavity, the larynx, and the esophagus, which are directly or indirectly exposed to cigarette smoke.

The importance of cigarettes as a major public health problem related to changing life-style is clearly demonstrated by the changing incidence of lung cancer in the United States. At the turn of the century, lung cancer was an extremely rare disease. According to the U. S. National Center for Health Statistics and the U. S. Bureau of the Census, the rate of lung cancer in the male population increased from 3 (per 100,000 population) in 1930, to 18 in 1950, and to 47 in 1970. In terms of numbers, lung cancer claimed 18,000 lives in 1950 and 111,000 in 1982. The rate of increase in the incidence of lung cancer in males has slowed down substantially a decade and half after the first surgeon general's report on the potential health hazards of cigarette smoking was released in 1964. However, the rate in females has been increasing steadily over the

last two decades, primarily because of increased cigarette smoking by women. There are no signs that the increase will level off soon. It is projected that lung cancer will claim the lives of 125,000 Americans in 1985. The increase over the 1982 figure will be accounted for mainly by female cigarette smokers.

Cigarette smoke is a complete carcinogen, containing both initiators and promoters (Wynder and Hoffmann, 1967; Hoffmann and Wynder, 1971). The initiator activities of cigarette smoke condensate (tar) reside in the neutral portion, which contains polynuclear aromatic hydrocarbons, N- and O-heteroaromatic compounds, and chlorinated insecticides. Some of the compounds are known carcinogens. The tumor-promoting activities are in the acidic portion of the condensate.

The carcinogens in cigarette smoke require metabolic activation to be biologically active carcinogens (Miller, 1970; Boyd, 1980). The lung tissues are capable of such

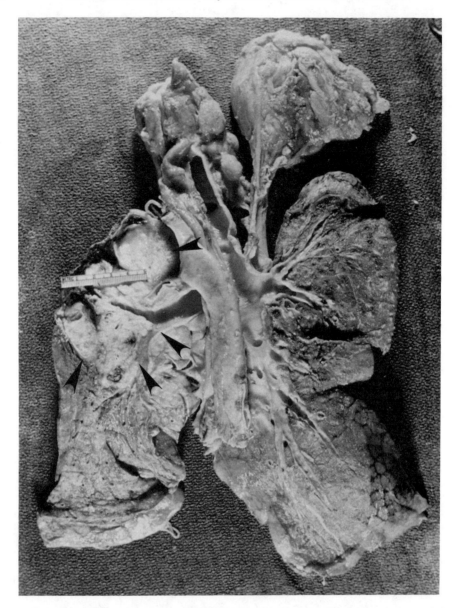

Figure 7–14. Bronchogenic carcinoma. The tumor has destroyed much of the right upper lobe of the lung. (Courtesy of Dr. N. K. Mottet.)

metabolic activation. The enzymes reside mainly in Clara cells of airways and type I pneumocytes of the alveoli (Huang et al., 1977), although other cell types are also active (Gram, 1973).

Carcinomas of the lungs occur more frequently in the large bronchi, and therefore are commonly referred to as bronchogenic carcinomas (Figure 7-14). Peripheral carcinomas account for only 20% of lung can-

cers (Auerbach, Garfinkel, and Parks, 1979a), presumably because of the protective effect of aerodynamic filtration of particulate inhalant via airways and dilution of gaseous pollutants by air in the airway dead space and alveoli. Approximately half of peripheral lung cancers are associated with a scar (Auerbach et al., 1979a). The causal relationship between lung scars and cancers is unclear. One of the explanations is that the convergence of lymphatics due to collapse of lung tissues and scar formation creates a dump site for migrating carcinogen-laden macrophages. Thus, the lung scars are hotspots for carcinogenesis. It is well known that fibrotic lungs predispose to development of peripheral lung cancer. Approximately 70% of peripheral scar carcinomas are adenocarcinomas.

Postmortem studies of tracheobronchial trees in the 1950s reveal that the habit of cigarette smoking, dosage, and duration are correlated with a set of histologic alterations in bronchi: basal cell hyperplasia, loss of cilia with squamous metaplasia, and atypical nuclear changes (Auerbach et al., 1979b). These alterations also correlate with the incidence of invasive lung cancer. Some of the changes are presumably due to cell injury and increased cell turnover. The atypical nuclear changes presumably reflect DNA damage and preneoplastic events. The degree of histologic alterations seems to correlate with the tar and nicotine content of cigarette smoke. Since the surgeon general's report in 1964, there has been a massive switch, first to filtered cigarettes, then to filtered low-tar, low-nicotine cigarettes. When the studies of bronchial histopathology were repeated in the 1970s, it was found that the above-described pathologic changes were less frequent and milder in degree (Auerbach et al., 1979b). This also correlates with a decrease in the incidence of lung cancer.

As the degree of nuclear atypia increases and cellular differentiation decreases, the lesion of carcinoma in situ is produced. Carcinoma in situ may stay in a noninvasive state for a decade before an invasive cancer evolves. Except for well-differentiated squamous cell carcinomas, invasive lung cancer grows rapidly and metastasizes readily. It is one of the most malignant neoplasms known to occur in humans.

According to the WHO classification of lung cancers (Kreyberg et al., 1967; WHO, 1982), squamous cell carcinoma, adenocarcinoma, undifferentiated large-cell carcinoma, and undifferentiated small-cell carcinoma are the four major histologic types.

Other tumors, such as carcinoid tumors and classical bronchoalveolar carcinoma, are uncommon and presumably unrelated to environmental factors.

The neoplastic cells in squamous cell (epidermoid) carcinoma exhibit extensive desmosomal junctions between cells, which prevents cells from separation. Thus, numerous intercellular bridges, representing foci of cytomembranes held together by desmosomes, are observed under the light microscope. In the well-differentiated variety of squamous cell carcinoma, keratinization and keratin-pearl formation are seen. Adenocarcinomas are composed of columnar cells with varying degrees of mucin-secreting activities. Formation of glandular structures is a characteristic feature. Undifferentiated (anaplastic) carcinomas do not have the cellular differentiation of either squamous carcinoma cells or adenocarcinomas. Classification of undifferentiated carcinomas into large-cell and small-cell types depends primarily on cell size and other associated histologic features. Squamous cell carcinoma has the most favorable prognosis within the group; small-cell carcinoma has the least, and adenocarcinoma and large-cell carcinoma, intermediate.

All four major histologic types of lung cancer are related to environmental exposure. There are also associations between various environmental exposures and the relative incidence of different types of lung cancer. This will be discussed with regard to the incidences of small cell carcinoma and adenocarcinoma.

Kultschitzky cells are neuroendocrine cells of the APUD (amine precursors uptake and decarboxylation) system of Pierce. They secrete various peptide hormones, including ACTH, calcitonin, parathyroid-like hormone, and bombesin. In experimental chemical carcinogenesis of the lungs, Kultschitzky cells proliferate. Although they are a minor cell population in large bronchi, they are the major cell type in small-cell carcinoma, which accounts for 20% to 25% of lung cancer (Greco and Oldham, 1979).

In radiation-induced lung cancer in uranium miners, there is a disproportionate increase in small-cell carcinoma. At lower dose levels of radiation exposure, only the incidence of small-cell carcinoma is increased over the control group; at higher dose, both small-cell and squamous cell carcinoma are increased (Archer et al., 1974; Horacek et al., 1977). Carcinoid tumors are low-grade malignant tumors of Kultschitzky cells. It occurs chiefly in a younger age group, and in both sexes, with a female preponderance. Smoking and other environmental factors do not appear to play a role in tumorigenesis of carcinoid tumors.

Adenocarcinomas apparently arise from columnar cells of airways, mucin-secreting cells, or Clara cells. They accounted for 10% to 20% of lung cancer in the past. There is a remarkable difference in incidence of adenocarcinoma between sexes. In the female, adenocarcinoma is the predominant type of lung cancer and may account for 60% of all lung cancer. Because of its preponderance in females and weak association with cigarette smoking, it was thought that induction of lung adenocarcinoma may be due to factors other than smoking or environmental pollution. Recent experience in the United States and elsewhere indicates that the relative incidence of adenocarcinoma proportionate to all lung cancers has been increasing since the late 1960s (Vincent et al., 1977; Valaitis et al., 1981). Since the early 1970s, adenocarcinoma has become the most prevalent type of lung cancer, accounting for 30% to 40% of all lung cancer

(Vincent et al., 1977; Valaitis et al., 1981). The incidence of adenocarcinoma has increased in males over the last two decades. In the female, the increase in the incidence of lung cancer, which correlated with cigarette consumption in the female, is not associated with a decrease in the relative incidence of adenocarcinoma. The fact that female smokers were introduced to filtered, low-tar cigarettes and that there was a mass switch by male smokers from nonfiltered to filtered cigarettes in the mid-1960s suggests that the changing incidence of adenocarcinoma and use of filtered, low-tar cigarettes may be related. Changes in the composition of carcinogens and the pattern of their deposition in the lungs may be responsible for changes in bronchial histopathology (Auerbach et al., 1979b) and the relative incidence of various types of cancers.

Mesotheliomas are rare neoplasms of the pleural lining. Benign mesotheliomas are localized tumors arising from submesothelial mesenchymal cells. There have been no suggestions that these benign neoplasms are related to environmental agents (Scharifker and Kaneko, 1979; Briselli et al., 1981). Malignant mesotheliomas tend to grow rapidly and spread widely along pleural cavities (Figure 7-15). This local aggressive behavior usually claims the lives of patients within a year after the onset of clinical symptoms. The tumors are composed of malignant epithelial (carcinomatous) and mesenchymal (sarcomatous) components.

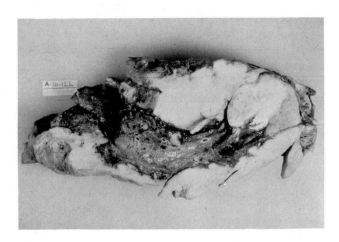

Figure 7–15. Malignant mesothelioma. The massive tumor tissue encases the entire lung along the pleural cavity. (From Chen and Mottet, 1978. Courtesy of Dr. N. K. Mottet.)

Unlike the benign varieties, malignant mesotheliomas are related to environmental exposures, especially in male patients. Approximately half of male and only 5% of female patients give a history of asbestos exposure in insulation and construction industries using asbestos products, asbestos production and manufacturing, shipyards, and mining industries (McDonald and McDonald, 1980). Asbestos also acts as a tumor promoter, thus increasing the incidence of lung cancers in cigarette smokers (Craighead and Mossman, 1982).

REFERENCES

Abramson, R. K., and Hutton J. J. 1975. Effects of cigarette smoking on aryl hydrocarbon hydroxylase activity in lungs and tissues of inbred mice. *Cancer Res.* 35:23–29.

Adamson, I. Y. R., and Bowden, D. H. 1974. The type 2 cell as progenitor of alveolar epithelial regeneration: A cytodynamic study in mice after exposure to oxygen. *Lab. Invest.* 30:35–42.

Adamson, I. Y. R., Bowden, D. H., Cote, M. G., and Witschi, H. 1977. Lung injury induced by butylated hydroxytoluene. Cytodynamic and biochemical studies in mice. *Lab. Invest.* 36:26–32.

Archer, V. E., Saccomano, G., and Jones, J. H. 1974. Frequency of different histologic types of bronchogenic carcinoma as related to radiation exposure. *Cancer* 34:2056–2060.

Auerbach, O., Garfinkel, L., and Parks, V. R. 1979a. Scar cancer of the lung. Increase over a 21 year period. *Cancer* 43:636–642.

Auerbach, O., Hammond, E. C., and Garfinkel, L. 1979b. Changes in bronchial epithelium in relation to cigarette smoking, 1955–1960 vs. 1970–1977. *N. Engl. J. Med.* 300:381–386.

Auerbach, O., Hammond, E. C., Garfinkel, L., and Benante, C. 1972. Relation of smoking and age to emphysema. Whole-lung section study. *N. Engl. J. Med*, 286:853–857.

Becklake, M. R. 1976. Asbestos-related diseases of the lung and other organs: Their epidemiology and implications for clinical practice. *Am. Rev. Resp. Dis.* 114:187–227.

Boyd, M. R. 1980. Biochemical mechanisms in chemical-induced lung injury: Roles of metabolic activation. *CRC Crit. Rev. Toxicol.* August, 7:103–176.

Brain, J. D. 1977. The respiratory tract and the environment. *Environ. Health Perspect.* 20:113–126.

Briselli, M., Mark, E. J., and Dickersin, G. R. 1981. Solitary fibrous tumors of the pleura: Eight new cases and review of 360 cases in the literature. *Cancer* 47:2678–2689.

Brody, A. R., and Craighead, J. E. 1975. Cytoplasmic inclusions in pulmonary macrophages of cigarette smokers. *Lab. Invest.* 32:125–132.

Chen, W. J., Chi, E. Y., and Smuckler, E. A. 1977. Carbon tetrachloride-induced changes in mixed function oxidases and microsomal cytochromes in the rat lung. *Lab. Invest.* 36:388–394

Chen, W. J., and Mottet, N. K. 1978. Malignant mesothelioma with minimal asbestos exposure. *Hum. Pathol.* 9:253–258.

Cockrell, B. Y., Busey, W. M., and Cavender, F. L. 1978. Respiratory tract lesions in guinea pigs exposed to sulfuric acid mist. *J. Toxical. Environ. Health* 4:835–844.

Cohen, D., Arai, S. F., and Brain, J. D. 1979. Smoking impairs long-term dust clearance from the lung. *Science* 204:514–517.

Craighead, J. E., and Mossman, B. T. 1982. The pathogenesis of asbestos-associated diseases. *N. Engl. J. Med.* 306:1446–1455.

Cross, C. E., De Lucia, A. J., Reddy, A. K., Hussain, M. Z., Chow, C. K., Mustafa, M. G., 1976. Ozone interactions with lung tissue. Biochemical approaches. *Am. J. Med.* 60:929–935.

Fink, J. N., Banaszak, E. F., Barboriak, J. J., Hensley, G. T., Kurup, V. P., Scanlon, G. T., Schlueter, D. P., Sosman, A. J., Thiede, W. H., and Unger, G. F. 1976. Interstitial lung disease due to contamination of forced air systems. *Ann. Intern. Med.* 84:406–413.

Gillett, D. G., and Ford, G. T. 1978. Drug-induced lung disease. In *The lung. Structure, function and disease*, eds. W. M. Thurlbeck and M. R. Abell, pp. 21–42. Baltimore: Williams and Wilkins.

Gram, T. E. 1973. Comparative aspects of mixed function oxidation by lung and liver of rabbits. *Drug Metab. Rev.* 2:1–32.

Greco, F. A., and Oldham, R. K. 1979. Small-cell lung cancer. *N. Engl. J. Med.* 301:355–358.

Greene, G. M., Jakab, G. J., Low, R. B., and Davis, G. S. 1977. Defense mechanisms of the respiratory membrane. *Am. Rev. Respir. Dis.* 115:479–514.

Haley, T. J. 1979. Review of the toxicology of Parquat (1,4'-Dimethyl-4,4'-bipyridinium chloride). *Clin. Toxicol.* 14:1–46.

Hoffmann, D., and Wynder, E. L. 1971. A study of tobacco carcinogenesis. XI. Tumor initiators, tumor accelerators, and tumor promoting activity of condensate fractions. *Cancer* 27:848–864.

Horacek, J., Placek, V., and Sevc, J. 1977. Histologic types of bronchogenic cancer in relation to different conditions of radiation exposure. *Cancer* 40:832–835.

Huang, T. W. 1977. Chemical and histochemical studies of human alveolar collagen fibers. *Am. J. Pathol.* 86:81–98.

Huang, T. W., Carlson, J. R., Bray, T. M., and Bradley, B. J. 1977. 3-Methylindole-induced pulmonary injury in goats. *Am. J. Pathol.* 87:647–666.

Johnson, K. J., Chapman, W. E., and Ward, P. A. 1979. Immunopathology of the lung. *Am. J. Pathol.* 95:795–844.

Kannerstein, M., Churg, J., McCaughey, W. T. E., and Selikoff, I. J. 1977. Pathogenic effects of asbestos. *Arch. Path. Lab. Med.* 101:623–628.

Kreyberg, L., Liebow, A. A., and Uehlinger, E. A. 1967. *International classification of tumours.* No. 1. *Histological typing of lung tumours.* Geneva: World Health Organization.

Lamy, M., Fallat, R. J., Koeniger, E., Dietrich, H., Ratliff, J. L., Eberhart, R. C., Tucker, H. J., and Hill, J. D. 1976. Pathologic features and mechanisms of hypoxemia in adult respiratory distress syndrome. *Am. Rev. Respir. Dis.* 114:267–284.

Lee, K. P., Zapp, J. A., and Sarver, J. W. 1976. Ultrastructural alternations of rat lung exposed to pyrolysis products of polytetrafluoroethylene (PTFE, Teflon). *Lab. Invest.* 35:152–160.

McCombs, R. P. 1972. Diseases due to immunologic reactions in the lungs. *N. Engl. J. Med.* 286:1186–1194; 1245–1252.

McDonald, A. D., and McDonald, J. C. 1980. Malignant mesothelioma in North America. *Cancer* 46:1650–1656.

Miller, J. A. 1970. Carcinogenesis by chemicals: An overview. G. H. A. Clowes Memorial Lecture. *Cancer Res.* 30:559–576.

Moore, V. L., Fink, J. N., Barboriak, J. J., Ruff, L. L., and Schlueter, D. P. 1974. Immunologic events in pigeon breeder's disease. *J. Allergy Clin. Immunol.* 53:319–328.

Nagaishi, C. 1972. *Functional anatomy and histology of the lung.* Baltimore; University Park Press.

Niewoehner, D. E., Kleinerman, J., and Rice, D. B. 1974. Pathologic changes in the peripheral airways of young cigarette smoker. *N. Engl. J. Med.* 291:755–758.

Pawlowski, R., and Frosolono, M. F. 1977. Effect of phosgene on rat lungs after single high-level exposure. II. Ultrastructural alterations. *Arch. Environ. Health* 32:278–283.

Repace, J. L., and Lowrey, A. H. 1980. Indoor air pollution, tobacco smoke, and public health. *Science* 208:464–472.

Scharifker, D., and Kaneko, M. 1979. Localized fibrous "mesothelioma" of pleura (submesothelial fibroma). A clinicopathologic study of 18 cases. *Cancer* 43:627–635.

Schatz, M., Patterson, R., and Fink, J. 1979. Immunologic lung disease. *N. Engl. J. Med.* 300:1310–1320.

Schwartz, L. W., Dungworth, D. L., Mustafa, M. G., Tarkington, B. K., and Tyler, W. S. 1976. Pulmonary responses of rats to ambient levels of ozone. Effects of 7-day intermittent or continous exposure. *Lab. Invest.* 34:565–578.

Sebastien, P., Bignon, J., and Martin, M. 1982. Indoor airborne asbestos pollution: From the ceiling and the floor. *Science* 216:1410–1412.

Sostman, H. D., Matthay, R. A., and Putman, C. E. 1977. Cytotoxic drug-induced lung disease. *Am. J. Med.* 62:608–615.

Spencer, H. 1977. *Pathology of the lung.* Phildelphia: W. B. Saunders.

Spengler, J. D., and Sexton, K. 1983. Indoor air pollution: A public health perspective. *Science* 221:9–17.

Strauss, R. H., Palmer, K. C., and Hayes J. A. 1976. Acute lung injury induced by cadmium aerosol. 1. Evolution of alveolar cell damage. *Am. J. Pathol.* 84:561–578.

Sykes, B. I., Purchase, I. F. H., and Smith, L. L. 1977. Pulmonary ultrastructure after oral and intravenous dosage of paraquat to rats. *J. Pathol.* 121:233–241.

Terrill, J. B., Montgomery, R. R., and Reinhardt, C. F. 1978 Toxic gases from fires. *Science* 200:1343–1347.

Thurlbeck, W. M. 1976. *Chronic airflow obstruction in lung disease.* Philadelphia: W. B. Saunders.

Valaitis, J., Warren, S., and Gamble, D. 1981.

Increasing incidence of adenocarcinoma of the lung. *Cancer* 47:1042–1046.

Vincent, R. G., Pickren, J. W., Lane, W. W., Bross, I., Takita, H., Houten, L., Gutierrez, A. C., and Rzepka, T. 1977. The changing histopathology of lung cancer. A review of 1682 cases. *Cancer* 39:1647–1655.

Weiss, R. B., and Muggia, M. F. 1980. Cytotoxic drug-induced pulmonary disease: Update 1980. *Am. J. Med.* 68:259–266.

White, J. R., and Froeb, H. F. 1980. Small-airways dysfunction in nonsmokers chronically exposed to tobacco smoke. *N. Engl. J. Med.* 302:720–723.

Wiebel, F. J., Leutz, J. C., and Gelboin, H. V. 1973. Aryl hydrocarbon (Benzo alpha pyrene) hydroxylase: Inducible in extrahepatic tissues of mouse strains not inducible in liver. *Arch. Biochem. Biophys.* 154:292–294.

Wilson, B. J., Garst, J. E., Linnabary, R. D., and Channell, R. B. 1977. Perilla ketone: A potent lung toxin from the mint plant, Perilla frutescens Britton. *Science* 197:573–574.

Witschi, H., and Cote, M. G. 1976. Biochemical pathology of lung damage produced by chemicals. *Fed. Proc.* 35:89.

WHO, 1982. The World Health Organization histological typing of lung tumors. *Am. J. Clin. Path.* 77:123–136.

Wynder, E. L., and Hoffmann, D. 1967. *Tobacco and tobacco smoke: Studies in experimental carcinogenesis.* New York: Academic Press.

8

Gastrointestinal Tract

Carl J. Pfeiffer

The gastrointestinal tract shares, with the skin and respiratory tract, a relatively direct interaction between the body and external environment. It serves as a partial, protective barrier to prevent internalization of xenobiotics or foreign compounds found in the environment. Mechanisms—often complex, substrate specific, and active metabolic processes—have evolved that facilitate the entry of exogenous compounds that are beneficial to the body, such a digestive products of foodstuffs. Yet exogenous agents can also penetrate the barrier of the gastrointestinal tract, which consists initially of an epithelial cell layer (or multicellular layer found in the stratified squamous epithelium lining the mouth, esophagus, and rectal orifice). Other factors as well tend to make this gastrointestinal barrier more complex than the integumentary or respiratory tract interfaces with the environment, among them the following:

1. The large concentrations of bacteria within certain regions of the gastrointestinal tract, particularly the colon, may modify the character of xenobiotics, making them more or less toxic to the body. Digestive enzymes may also alter ingested foreign compounds.

2. Environmental chemicals, although not transported directly by specific means, may damage the epithelial barrier and thus initiate a series of pathologic events and adverse reactions to other intraluminal chemicals or microbiologic agents.

3. The gut epithelium plays a particularly extensive role, compared to the integumentary and respiratory tracts, in metabolically altering xenobiotics locally in the gut tissue before and during hepatic and renal metabolism.

4. Many environmental agents that can be internalized by any route may later be selectively excreted, usually after minor metabolic transformation, directly into the intestinal lumen as a constituent of bile. These products themselves may exert local toxic effects within the gut, or systemic toxic effects after reabsorption.

5. The storage time, and thus exposure time, of xenobiotics within the gut may be prolonged, and this may enhance their toxic effects.

6. The turnover rate of cellular components comprising the gastrointestinal epithelium is extraordinarily high. Therefore, as also exists for the hematopoietic system, there seems to be greater likelihood for mutagenic alterations to occur in response to selected environmental agents. The high incidence of cancers both in the digestive tract

and hematopoietic systems tends to support this conclusion.

7. Many foreign compounds that are inhaled, as industrial pollutants, following smoking, or after exposure to contaminated air in urban environments, rapidly find their way into the digestive tract by drainage from the sinuses into the distal pharynx and esophagus.

8. Both the active-transport and facilitated-transport mechanisms in the gut, which have evolved with the species, may not be entirely substrate specific, and may enhance entry into the blood or lymphatic circulation of harmful xenobiotics.

Thus, the features enumerated above are important factors with respect to the nature and degree of effect any specific environmental toxin might exert, not only to the gastrointestinal tract but to the body as a whole, when it is presented to the alimentary tract. Coupled with these points are the usual factors relevant to action of environmental agents on any other system, that is, dose of the agent, age, sex, nutritional and health status of the exposed subject, vehicle of administration, dissolution rate of xenobiotic, and so forth.

Further, because the inner surface of the alimentary canal has evolved both morphologically and functionally to transport nutrients, water, and electrolytes, the surface area of the digestive tract has many structural features specialized to increase greatly its surface area. These morphologic features include long length of the digestive tube, grossly visible folds and villi, microscopic-sized surface mucosal convolutions (Pfeiffer, 1971), and long or short microvilli upon the apical surfaces of epithelial cells. Figure 8-1 illustrates the mucosal surface view of the body region of the stomach, showing the typical cobblestone appearance due to epithelial cells, as well as openings to the gastric pits. For a comprehensive collection of electron micrographs of all parts of the digestive tract, in various species, the reader is referred to an extensive atlas on this subject (Pfeiffer, Rowden, and Weibel, 1974).

In considering actions of environmental

Figure 8–1. The surface of the stomach (fundic region) presents a cobblestone appearance and shows the openings to the gastric pits. Surface area of the epithelial cells is greatly increased by presence of microvilli, which can be detected in this scanning electron micrograph (in the center of the field). The small units shown here are individual cells, and the strands are precipitated gastric mucus ($\times 1300$).

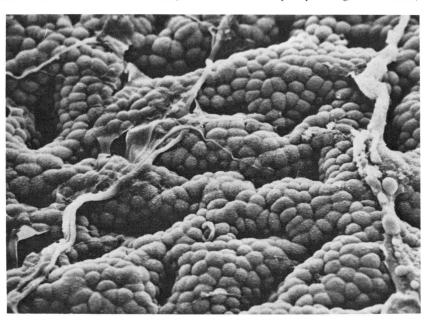

agents on the gastrointestinal tract, one must be aware of possible acute effects (such as the direct irritant actions of plant-derived phorbol esters), possible chronic effects (such as alterations in integrity of the intestinal muscular wall influenced by dietary fiber), or possible long-delayed effects (such as development of gastric carcinoma 15 years after exposure to some ingested chemical carcinogen). Further, the types of environmental agents to be considered must include not only general xenobiotics that enter the gastrointestinal tract even though they possess no special relation to the gut, but also a large group of chemical agents with special reference to foodstuffs. Compounds in the former category include energy-related effluents and hydrocarbons, industrial products and effluents, including organic solvents, phenols, aldehydes, and synthetics (plastics). Compounds in the latter group, which may be either ingested with food or introduced through voluntary exposure, include cosmetics, pesticides, food additives, dyes, sweeteners or preservatives, and alcohol or tobacco. Environmental agents such as aflatoxins or other natural contaminants of microbiologic origin, or trace elements, or radioactive agents must also be considered. In addition, voluntary exposure to chemical agents such as medicinals must be added to the list of environmental agents that the gastrointestinal tract encounters. Earlier reviews by the present author (Pfeiffer, 1977; Pfeiffer and Hänninen, 1977) have summarized many of the adverse gastrointestinal reactions to environmental agents for the period ending with 1973. Finally, it must be borne in mind that all natural chemical, non-nutrient agents found in the environment are not necessarily harmful, and that their absence or deficiency may indeed be associated with pathology of the gastrointestinal tract.

Transport Mechanisms for Xenobiotics in the Gut

A variety of mechanisms exist by which foreign agents could conceivably be trans-ported across the intestinal epithelium; it is known that active transport, facilitated diffusion or solvent drag, passive diffusion, pinocytosis, pore filtration, or persorption mechanisms may exist in the intestines. In fact, however, most nutrients, such as amino acids, sugar, and vitamins, tend to be absorbed primarily by active-transport mechanisms involving some type of biochemical carrier. In contrast, most environmental agents are likely transported by a passive diffusion process, although there may be exceptions, such as the active transport of inorganic lead by the calcium carrier mechanism of transport (Klaassen, 1975). The passive diffusion of environmental agents into the gut epithelial cells is modulated by the usual constraints that would apply to any chemical agent. Thus, greater lipid solubility will enhance absorption, smaller molecules will diffuse more rapidly, and the nonionized form of weak acids or weak bases will be absorbed more readily than ionized forms; moreover, the pH of the lumen of the gut will affect the degree of ionization of such molecules. Once absorbed into the epithelial cell, xenobiotics may undergo chemical transformation, or may be bound by proteins before they exit into the general circulation. Some xenobiotics, such as benzpyrene, 3-methylocholanthrene (3-MC), or DDT, may exit through the lateral-basal aspect of the epithelial cell directly into intestinal lymphatics, and be transported through the lymphatic system before exiting from the thoracic duct into the circulating blood. Accordingly, those agents may exert toxic effects before they are metabolically transformed by hepatic, microsomal drug-metabolizing enzyme systems.

In general, it is considered that most foreign chemicals are absorbed in solution (i.e., in molecular form), although very small particles of nanometer size might be transported into the epithelial cells by pinocytotic mechanisms. Neverhteless, a number of reports have appeared that attest to an additional mechanism of absorption of foreign particles in larger form. This mechanism, termed "persorption," has been studied in detail by Volkheimer and associates (Volkheimer and Schulz, 1968; Volkheimer et al., 1969; Volkheimer, 1974, 1975, 1977), and could play an important role in respect to pathologic reactions resulting from absorption from the gut of polyvinyl chloride particles, metallic iron particles, asbestos, or other hazardous substances that are presented in particulate form. Particulate matter in which the particle diameter reaches 5–150 μm may be internalized by this prosposed persorption mechanism. According to Volkheimer, persorption is accomplished by the passage of undissolved particles in macrocorpuscular form between the epithelial cells. Starch granules, cellulose particles, powdered rabbit hairs, charcoal, pollen, spores, polyvinyl globules, silicate crystals, and other substances were persorbed and transported by both the lymphatic system and portal blood system from the intestinal wall, according to Volkheimer (1974). This phenomenon was reported for several species, including pigs, dogs, chickens, and rats. The persorption ratio (i.e., ratio of persorbed to actually ingested particles) has been estimated at 1:50,000. Although this is only a small percentage, it may have significant implications with respect to toxic reactions, analogous to the marked pathophysiologic reactions to very small quantities of absorbed foreign proteins absorbed, which can produce allergic reactions. Furthermore, asbestos particles have been observed by microscopy to lodge within the intestinal epithelium, perhaps after earlier persorption, and the carcinogenic properties of asbestos are established. Recent studies by LeFevre et al. (1980) attempted to reassess the persorption phenomenon in mice, by utilizing 15.8-and 5.7-μm synthetic spherical particles. These investigators found that the 5.7-μm particles were taken up in Peyer's patches, perhaps by macrophage sequestration, but the larger particles were not, and none of the ingested particles appeared rapidly in blood. Thus, these recent findings do suggest that possible hazards may be associated with enteric exposure to nonsoluble particulate matter (>5 μm), but the true risk and quantitative importance of persorption still remains unclear.

Metabolism of Foreign Compounds by Gastrointestinal Mucosa

Another general concept pertaining to most foreign agents that are presented to the alimentary tract is the fact that considerable metabolism of such agents may occur in the gut mucosa before release of these compounds into the blood and/or lymphatic circulation. Many aspects of this metabolism have been reviewed, with respect to hormones, drugs, and other agents, by Hartiala (1973). An increasing number of reports have appeared in recent years in regard to the gut mucosal metabolism of specific environmental agents. The general classes of metabolic reactions involved in these processes in the mucosa are quite similar to those observed in hepatic and other tissues. For example, gut mucosal microsomal enzymes involve mixed-function monooxygenase systems consisting of cytochrome P-450, which is a terminal oxidase, and NADPH–cytochrome P-450 reductase, which catalyzes reduction of oxidized cytochrome. Hoensch, Woo, Raffin, and Schmid have reported (1976) that benzpyrene hydroxylase, p-nitroanisole O-demethylase, NADPH–cytochrome P-450 reductase, and cytochrome P-450 content were 3–10 times higher in upper villus epithelial cells than in mucosal crypt cells in rat small intestine. Their findings suggested that intestinal drug metabolism was localized primarily to upper villous cells, mainly in the proximal small bowel tissue. Chhabra (1979) also has shown, as depicted in Figure 8-2, decreasing activity of several enzyme systems with increasing aboral distance, such as in the case of benzpyrene hydroxylase, ethylmorphine-N-demethylase, and aniline hydroxylase. Species differences are frequently reported for the activity of various enzymes involved in mucosal metabolism of foreign agents (Aitio et al., 1975). For example, UDP-glucuronyl transferase activity was very low in gastric

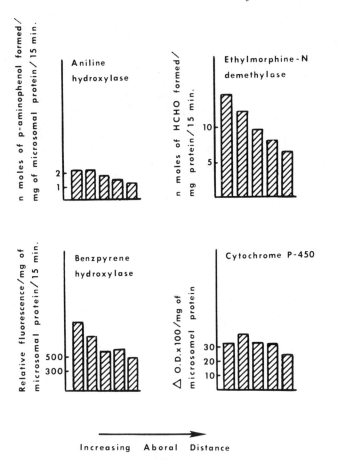

Figure 8–2. Various enzyme systems that metabolize foreign agents in the intestinal mucosa decrease in activity with increasing distance from the gastric pylorus. (Redrawn from data of R. S. Chhabra, 1979.)

and duodenal mucosa of the cat and dog, but was high in both locations in the rat.

Glucuronide synthesis as a component of the mucosal detoxicating capacity has also been documented (Hartiala, 1955; Hänninen, 1968; Hänninen and Aitio, 1968; Hänninen et al., 1968). The glucuronidation of 1-naphthol in the rat intestinal loop has been reported (Bock and Winne, 1975).

Benzpyrene hydroxylase activity in the intestinal mucosa, referred to above, has long been known to exist (Waltenberg et al., 1962), and can be induced by dietary and other means (Wattenberg, 1972; Welch et al., 1972; Zampoglione and Mannering, 1973). Hoensch et al. (1976) also have shown that intestinal mucosal cytochrome P-450 was inducible by administration of 3-methylcholanthrene in the diet (as it is in hepatic tissue), but that cytochrome b_5 was not affected. This is in keeping with the well-established role of the former compound in

oxidative drug metabolism, but a role that has not been established for cytochrome b_5. Several studies have suggested that the behavior of intestinal mucosal drug-metabolizing enzymes is more strictly dependent on diet than the related enzymes in the liver. Polychlorinated biphenyls decrease mucosal enzyme activities, in contrast to stimulation of hepatic enzymes (Hietanen, Laitinen, Lang, and Vainio, 1975). A high-cholesterol diet enhances several mucosal enzyme activities in animals, including aryl hydrocarbon hydroxylase, whereas lipid diets tend to decrease activities of enzyme systems in duodenal mucosa that hydroxylate and glucuronidate foreign compounds (Hietanen, Laitinen, Vaininen, and Hänninen, 1975). Other dietary constituents, such as dried brussels sprouts or cabbage, when added to a complete semisynthetic diet, increased in vitro metabolism of hexobarbital, phenacetin, 7-ethoxycoumarin, and benz[α]pyrene in small-intestinal mucosa (Pantuck et al., 1976). Metals, halogenated hydrocarbons, and cigarette smoking (perhaps because of contained benz[α]pyrene) are also known to induce mucosal cell metabolic activity in animals (Banwell, 1979). Other gut mucosal enzyme activities were also altered by cigarette smoking (Uotila, 1977). The induction, by dietary means, of selective mucosal metabolic pathways is not of course limited to drug-metabolizing systems, but other metabolic routes as well, such as we have shown for the pentose phosphate shunt (Pfeiffer and Debro, 1966).

Microsomes from the intestinal mucosa of human specimens have also been studied (Hoensch, Hutt, and Hartmann, 1979). Monooxygenase activity in the villi of patients with partial villous atrophy was reduced, and in patients with total villous atrophy the monooxygenase activity was absent.

Toxic effects of environmental agents may vary according to the time of day at which exposure occurs, because the intestinal drug-metabolizing enzyme system is influenced by circadian rhythms. Peak activity of mucosal enzyme activity in the rabbit (aryl hydrocarbon hydroxylases, benzphetamine N-demethylase, NADPH–cytochrome C reductase, and cytochrome P-450) occurred around 0600 hours, and minimal activity was observed at around 1200–1500 hours (Tredger and Chhabra, 1977; Chhabra, 1979).

Furthermore, other factors such as age and sex may alter the gut mucosal metabolic response to xenobiotic exposure. In the rabbit, experiments have shown that various hydrolase, reductase, or demethylase activities were very low or absent at birth, and reached adult activity levels by 30–40 days. The enzyme, UDP-glucuronyl transferase was not detectable until birth in the guinea pig intestinal mucosa, but reached adult levels by 3 weeks. In contrast, this enzyme was detected 10 days before birth in the rabbit intestine (Lucier et al., 1977). Also, benzpyrene hydroxylase increased after birth in rabbit intestinal microsomal extracts (Tredger and Chhabra, 1977).

Sex differences in liver but not intestinal mucosal metabolism of xenobiotics have been reported by Chhabra and Fouts (1974). However, insufficient studies have been undertaken to date to allow a conclusion that sex differences do not exist. The observed sex differences in humans to colon and rectal cancers, which may be etiologically related to chemical carcinogenic factors within the intestinal lumen, suggest that further studies on these metabolic factors in relationship to sex may prove worthwhile. Further, in most species studied (including rabbit, guinea pig, rat, mouse, hamster), xenobiotic-metabolizing enzyme systems have tended to show higher activity in liver than in the intestinal mucosa (Chhabra et al., 1974).

The enzyme systems mentioned above may not in all cases detoxify foreign agents presented to the gut; in some instances toxins or chemical carcinogens may be activated or newly formed by gut mucosal enzymic pathways. Free-radical reactions may take place as a consequence of single-electron capture reactions by xenobiotic molecules (e.g., by carbon tetrachloride), with subsequent dissociation into xenobiotic free radicals and anions. Such free radicals may then induce lipid peroxidation reactions of cellular membranes or may induce molecular polymerization. The mixed-function oxidases may convert xenobiotics into epoxides. Epoxides may induce toxicity by covalent binding with tissue macromolecules, although such biologic reactions remain obscure. Oxidation reactions within the cytochrome P-450 system may form toxic compounds that bind to nucleophilic centers in DNA *in vivo* (Reynolds, 1977). Other metabolic reactions with harmful results may also occur, such as intestinal mucosal production of aldehydes, or oxidative dealkylation production of carcinogenic nitrosamines.

Bacterial metabolism within the gut lumen may also alter toxicity of ingested xenobiotics. For example, the glycoside of cycasin found in the cycad plants in Guam is hydrolyzed to methylazoxymethanol, a compound that is both carcinogenic and hepatotoxic. Some bacteria in the colon may convert bile salts into carcinogenic or mutagenic substances, and other bacteria in the stomach and intestines may accelerate the reduction of nitrate to nitrite, and enhance formation of nitrosoamines in the gut. Also, microflora in the gut can hydrolyze sulfamates, such as cyclamate, to produce cyclohexylamine, which may be carcinogenic. Other toxic compounds may be created by the gut microflora as a result of decarboxylation of phenolic carboxylic acids, by reduction of nitro groups, by reduction of azo groups, by reduction of aldehydes and alcohols, and so on. This complex subject has been extensively reviewed by Scheline (1973). Thus, the adverse effects that foreign agents arising from the environment may have on the organism may be directly and indirectly influenced by metabolic events within the gut lumen and mucosal tissue.

Adverse Alimentary Tract Reactions to Pharmacologic Agents

Although foreign compounds of pharmacologic nature are classified by some workers as exogenous agents, their effects on the alimentary canal will not be reviewed in detail in the present chapter. Those pharmacologic agents that are known to induce gastric or intestinal ulcers or bleeding diatheses are summarized in Table 8-1. Another common reaction to drugs is malabsorption, which may result from alteration in physiologic transport mechanisms, from morphologic reduction in intestinal villous size, or from binding with foodstuffs. Drugs that are known to induce intestinal malabsorption are summarized in Table 8-2.

Acute and Delayed Reactions to Nonpharmacologic Chemicals with Irritant Properties

Many chemicals, if ingested, will exert acute corrosive actions on the esophageal, gastric, and intestinal mucosa. Such tissue reactions are nonspecific for the gut epithelium. Included in this category of responses also are mild, direct effects such as astringent activity, or dehydrating effects on sur-

Table 8–1. Drugs and Other Chemical Agents That Can Induce Gastric or Intestinal Ulcers in Human or Animal Systems

Reserpine	Anti-inflammatory agents
Serotonin	Salicylates
Histamine	(e.g., aspirin)
Compound 48/80	Cinchophen
Gastrin-like compounds	Steroids
Catecholamines	Nonsteroidal com-
(e.g., epinephrine)	pounds
Polymyxin B	Phenylbutazone
Caffeine	Indomethacin
KCl (concentrated)	Ibuprofen
Gold thioglucose	Naproxen
Haloperidol	Fenoprofen
Antimetabolic agents	Ketoprofen
Sympatholytic agents	Tolmetin
(e.g., priscoline)	Flurbiprofen
Dimaprit (H-2 agonist)	Sulindac
Promethazine	Oxyphenbutazone
Ethylamine	Flunixin
Cysteamine	
Cystamine	
Propionitrile	
n-Butyronitrile	
Miscellaneous short-	
chain alkanes and	
alkenes	

Table 8–2. Intestinal Malabsorption Induced by Pharmacologic Agents

Drug	Absorption defect[a]
Surface-active agents	
Alcohol	Folic acid
Cholestyramine	Fat, bile acids, vitamins
Antibacterial agents	
Kanamycin	Fat, protein electrolytes
Neomycin	Fat, vitamin B_{12}
Polymycin	Fat, protein
Miscellaneous agents	
Calcium carbonate	Fat
Clorfibrate	Sterols
Cholchicine	Fat, vitamin B_{12}, xylose
Contraceptives (oral)	Xylose, folic acid
Indomethacin	Xylose
Methotrexate	Xylose, vitamin B_{12}, vitamin K
Phenformin	Fat, xylose, folic acid
Phenindandione	Fat, xylose
Phenytoin	Xylose, folic acid
Phenolphthalein	Fat
PAS	Fat, vitamin B_{12}, xylose
Quinacrine	Fat
Sulfasalazine	Folic acid
Triparanol	Fat, protein, carotene

Source: Modified from data of Banwell (1979).
[a]It should be noted that the absorptive defects listed are those established by standard absorption tests and materials; it is likely that numerous other substances are also malabsorbed.

face epithelial cells such as can be anticipated with alcohols. These acute responses may be characterized initially as mucosal bleeding and inflammatory responses, such as gastritis, but may be associated with greatly delayed effects such as increased susceptibility to cancer. Thus, lye-induced strictures of the esophagus are often associated with development of esophageal carcinoma 15–20 years later, and the initial and acute erosive actions on the gastric epithelium of animals treated with the mutagen, N-methyl-N^1-nitro-N-nitrosguanidine (MNNG), may later be followed by intestinal metaplasia of the stomach, and gastric cancer. A summary of many of the documented gastrointestinal manifestations to various common organic and inorganic poisons, many of which are corrosive, is presented in Table 8-3. Similarly, the acute gastrointestinal responses to a number of metallic poisons are delineated in Table 8-4.

Actions of Pesticides in the Alimentary Canal

Organic pesticide residues have long been an environmental contaminant to which humans are exposed. Because of body storage and concentration of some types of these agents, the concentrations of pesticides may be greater in ingested animal food than in plant food. The organophosphate type of pesticide, which is more acutely toxic to human beings than chlorinated hydrocarbons, is more readily degraded in the environment and constitutes a lesser hazard from the standpoint of body storage and food chain concentration. Dichlorodiphenyl-trichloroethane (DDT) and dichlorodiphenyl-dichloroethylene (DDE) residues have been found in body fat of most subjects evaluated in the United States, and were present in 62% of U.S. samples of cow's milk tested (Pfeiffer, 1977). DDT is degraded, under aerobic conditions only, by *Aerobac-*

Table 8–3. Adverse Gastrointestinal Reactions to Toxic Actions of Nonpharmacologic Chemicals

Chemical agent	Gastrointestinal manifestations
Corrosive poisons	
Strong acids (H_2SO_4, HCl)	Charring of gastric mucosa, ulceration, chemical peritonitis, gastric stenosis, similar effects in duodenum
Iodine	Corrosion of gastric mucosa, vomiting, and diarrhea
Sodium fluoride	Corrosion of gastric mucosa
Alkaline corrosives (KOH, NaOH)	Strictures of esophagus and pylorus
Organic corrosives (phenol, lysol)	Visceral congestion, coagulation necrosis of the gastric mucosa
Volatile organic poisons	
Ethyl alcohol	Gastritis, fatty degeneration and cirrhosis of liver, acute pancreatitis
Methyl alcohol	Gastritis, acute pancreatitis
Chloroform	Fatty metamorphosis of liver, cirrhosis, gastric ulcers
Gasoline and kerosene	Gastrointestinal edema and ulceration
Nonvolatile organic poisons	
Dimethylhydrazines	Colon cancer
Nitrosoguanidines	Acute gastritis and erosions
MNNG, ENNG, and	Intestinal metaplasia of the stomach
other nitrosamines	Carcinogenesis in stomach, esophagus, or intestines
Nonmetallic inorganic poisons	
Phosphorus	Acute symptoms: gastric mucosal corrosion, vomiting, nausea Subacute symptoms: fatty metamorphosis of liver
Nitrites	Gastric and intestinal irritation and hemorrhage, diarrhea
Miscellaneous compounds	
Insecticides (chlorinated hydrocarbons)	Gastrointestinal edema and congestion
Poisonous mushrooms (Amanita)	Gastrointestinal submucosal hemorrhage, diarrhea, vomiting, jaundice

Table 8–4. Pathophysiologic Responses in the Gut to Metallic Poisons, after Ingestion or Absorption

Chemical agent	Gastrointestinal manifestations
Arsenic	Gastrointestinal edema and congestion, vomiting, diarrhea, ulceration, liver degeneration, inhibition of intestinal enzyme activity
Bismuth	Necrotizing colitis, gastro-enteritis
Cadmium	Competition with calcium absorption
Copper salts	Gastric mucosal corrosion, intestinal ulcers, fatty liver degeneration
Gold compounds	Ulcerative enteritis and colitis, central necrosis of liver
Iron salts	Gastric or intestinal irritation
Lead	Hemorrhagic gastritis and colitis, vomiting, and diarrhea
Manganese	Corrosive gastroenteritis
Mercury	Mucosal sloughing, acute hemorrhagic colitis, diarrhea, vomiting
Nickel	Ecchymosis in gastrointestinal mucosa, vomiting, diarrhea
Thallium	Acute gastric and intestinal inflammation, vomiting, diarrhea
Vanadium	Gastrointestinal inflammation, diarrhea, and nausea
Zinc salts	Congestion, necrosis, and ulceration of upper alimentary tract

ter aerogenes in the gut, and also coliform bacteria of the rat intestinal flora can degrade DDT to DDD [1,1 dichloro-2,2-bis (*p*-chlorophenyl) ethane]. Chlorinated or polychlorinated hydrocarbons are rapidly absorbed in the gut. Dieldrin is mainly transported out of the gut in the portal vein, and aldrin and endrin, malathion, carbaryl, dimethoate, DDT, and dieldrin readily penetrate all regions of the intestinal tract (Shah and Guthrie, 1973). Several insecticides tested have shown that transport into the intestinal epithelium is by a passive process. They appear to be relatively nontoxic to the alimentary tract. Although it is of little rel-

evance to human toxicity, the glycogen content in the midgut epithelium of the American cockroach is increased by oral treatment with pyrethrum, and degeneration of the epithelium lining in the fish intestine has been observed after DDT exposure. Also, intestinal water and electrolyte transport are altered in DDT-treated fish (Pfeiffer, 1977). The increased toxicity of organophosphate pesticide to young mammals has been attributed partly to the increased rate of intestinal absorption in young animals (mice). The phosphate and carbamate insecticides, but not chlorinated hydrocarbons, showed greater penetration into the colon of mice (Shah and Guthrie, 1973).

Polychlorinated Biphenyls and Triphenyls and the Gut

For many years human foodstuffs such as cereals, milk, poultry, eggs, and salmon meat have been found to be contaminated by polychlorinated biphenyls (PCBs), which are industrial agents used as sealants, adhesives, heat-transfer agents, and dielectric fluids in transformers and capacitors. Many toxic reactions in human beings have been observed following PCB exposure, including diarrhea, vomiting, weakness, nail pigmentation, and skin eruptions. In monkeys, oral PCB administration induced gastric hyperplasia and dysplasia, and gastric submucosal mucous cysts (Allen and Norback, 1973). In rats the physiologic assimilation and excretion of biphenyls depends on the compound in question, as biliary excretion of 2,5,2',5'-tetrachlorobiphenyl (TCB) may exceed 42% in 24 hours, in contrast to 1% for PCB (Peterson et al., 1976). Detailed information about the effects of PCBs on the intestinal mucosa are not yet available.

Adverse Effects of Polyvinyl Chloride on the Gut

In recent years the use of various organic plasticizers and stabilizers such as polyvinyl chloride (PVC) has increased, and consequently industrial exposure and environmental contamination with PVC have occurred. Rawls has recently conducted epidemiologic studies on 10,173 workers in 37 plants producing polyvinyl chloride, and found that cancers of the digestive tract were more common in PVC-exposed workers than in a control population (Rawls, 1980). PVC is also known to be mutagenic to bacteria, and to be a mutipotent carcinogen in rodents. Orally administered plasticizers and polyvinyl chloride stabilizers have been shown to induce congestion of the small intestines and mucosal sloughing in the stomach and intestines (Nikonorow et al., 1973). Volkheimer (1975) has reported that PVC particles can be persorbed by intestinal enterocytes. More experimental studies on the carcinogenic or cancer-promoting effects of PVC in the mammalian gastrointestinal tract are required to evaluate this problem.

Asbestos Exposure and Alimentary Tract Disease

During the past 25 years considerable attention has been paid to the possible association of occupational exposure in asbestos and cancer. Asbestos fibers are also known to be present in some sources of drinking water, beer, wine, and other beverages. A positive epidemiologic correlation has been found between exposure to asbestos and respiratory tract cancers, and pleural and peritoneal mesotheliomas. More recently, epidemiologic studies have suggested that gastrointestinal tract cancers are also increased in populations exposed to asbestos. Small-intestinal cancers were more common in males residing in asbestos-mining counties in Quebec. Also, colon cancer, rectal cancer, and gastric cancer were increased in incidence among asbestos insulation workers in New York and New Jersey, and this adverse trend became accentuated in recent years (Graham et al., 1977). Further, the notion that the high incidence of gastric cancer in Japan was associated with talc-treated rice (talc, like some forms of asbestos, is a hydrous silicate of magnesium) has been raised, but has not been supported by all investigators. Because of these epidemiologic findings, experimental animal in-

vestigations have been undertaken to elucidate this possible mode of carcinogenesis.

Oral administration of asbestos fibers (containing 53% chrysotile asbestos) to rats induced a significant number of tumors in 14–18 months, but little organ specificity was observed. Other studies in rats fed 6% chrysotile for 3 months revealed that chrysotile particles were found in colonic goblet cell mucus, within the cytoplasm of the epithelial cells, and down within the smooth muscle layers. Evans and co-workers (1973) reported, after inhalation exposure of rats to crocidolite fibers, that most of this contaminant was later excreted via the feces. The penetration of the gastrointestinal tract mucosa of the rat by chrysotile asbestos was not found to occur in experiments of Gross et al. (1974), but Pontefract and Cunningham (1973) clearly observed, after oral administration of chrysotile asbestos to rats, the appearance of asbestos in blood (mostly cleared after 4 days), the omentum, and other organs. A number of pathophysiologic changes and morphologic alterations in gastrointestinal mucosal tissue have been reported in animals subjected to prolonged exposure to chrysotile asbestos. This material was cytotoxic to small-intestinal epithelial cells, and reduced the active transport of radiolabeled glucose into the intestine (Jacobs and Richards, 1980). Gastric physiologic changes, such as mucin, acid, or pepsin secretion, were not altered in the guinea pig fed asbestos fibers. DNA synthesis in the rat gastrointestinal tract was altered by chrysotile in a complex manner dependent on dose and time after exposure. Workers in several laboratories reported that tritium incorporation into DNA was increased, after asbestos, in the gastric, small and large intestinal mucosa, and rectum, but was decreased in the liver. In the monkey pancreas, chrysotile asbestos stimulated DNA synthesis, but this was not observed in rat pancreas. Chrysotile asbestos induced signs of morphologic cytotoxicity in the small intestine such as vacuolation of epithelial cells and derangement of surface microvilli in the ileum (Figures 8-3 and 8-4), and separation of epithelial cells. Be-

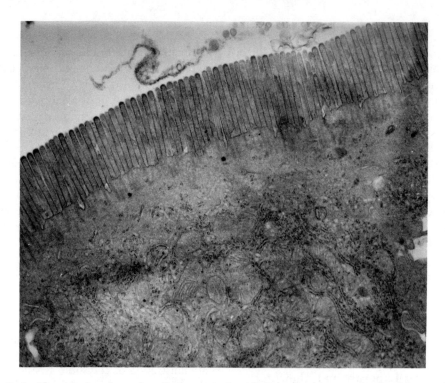

Figure 8–3. The apical surface of an ileal, mucosal epithelial cell of a control-treated (normal diet) rat has densely packed, long microvilli, which are the structures upon which digestion and absorption occur ($\times$ 7000). (Courtesy of Dr. R. Jacobs, University College, Cardiff, Wales.)

Figure 8–4. In contrast to Figure 8–3, the surface epithelial cells in the ileal mucosa of the chrysotile-treated rat (14 months treatment at 50 mg/day) demonstrate several pathologic alterations, including cellular vacuolization and irregular-shaped and reduced numbers of microvilli ($\times$ 10,500). (Courtesy of Dr. R. Jacobs, University College, Cardiff, Wales.)

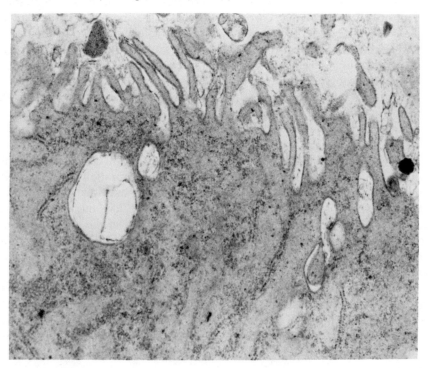

cause of the widespread human exposure to asbestos, continued investigation of its gastrointestinal toxicity is warranted.

Drinking Water Contaminants and Gastrointestinal Pathology

The most common contaminants of drinking water that contribute to gastrointestinal pathology are various bacterial and viral organisms that cause enteritis, diarrhea, vomiting, and water and electrolyte imbalance. This type of natural contaminant is beyond the scope of the present review and will not be considered here. The presence of multiple trace elements in drinking water may be of great importance, and will be reviewed under the following section. However, there are other organic contaminants that may be present in drinking water and that may be of pathophysiologic significance. Recently attention, mostly made up of speculations, has been brought to reaction products of chlorine that potentially could be carcinogenic, following the addition of chlorine to water for disinfection of microbial organisms. Chlorine readily reacts with humic substances to form various trihalomethane (THM) species that are considered to be carcinogenic. Epidemiologic studies until 1980, in which human alimentary tract cancer incidence rates have been correlated with THM levels in drinking water in selected regions of the United States, have shown that a significant positive correlation existed for male pancreatic cancer but not cancers of other sites. These preliminary data, which did not show significance for females, did not strongly support the above hypothesis, but additional investigations on this problem are worthwhile. Chlorine has been used as an additive to drinking water for many years, although only in recent years has pancreatic cancer been increasing in incidence in North America and several other countries.

Tannic acid is a polymer of hydroxybenzoic acids and in some locations is a common component of drinking water, particularly in rural regions where surface water draining coniferous forests is ingested. Although relatively nontoxic to human beings, its known toxic effects include liver necrosis, acute gastroenteritis, induction of necrosis of mucosal glands, and congestion of the lamina propria and submucosa of the digestive tract. It can be ulcerogenic in animals, and it reduces gut absorption of glucose and methionine. The tannin content of drinking water tends to be higher in several, but not all, countries (e.g., Romania and Newfoundland) that have exceptionally high incidence rates of gastric or esophageal carcinoma, and some experimental evidence has suggested that tannin may promote carcinogenesis in different sites. Its true role as an environmental factor that contributes to the pathology of the human digestive tract remains an intriguing question that has not been satisfactorily evaluated at this time.

Environmental Trace Elements and Gastrointestinal Pathology

Living tissues are composed principally of 11 elements, but small amounts of numerous other elements are required as essential trace elements in a variety of biochemical reactions, mainly as catalysts or as components of enzymes. Foodstuffs, drinking water, and other beverages supply all of these elements, but in certain geographic settings the supply of specific elements may be either deficient or excessive. Furthermore, industrial exposure of workers (e.g., to cadmium, nickel, or copper), exposure of populations to bioconcentrated environmental contamination of heavy metals in food or water (e.g., methylmercury), may result in toxic effects of selected trace elements. Although many of the acute toxic effects have been well characterized in humans and animals, the more subtle effects of chronic excess or deficiency of several trace elements remain partially obscure. There are many unproven hypotheses about these latter reactions, and in spite of definite evidence, there is increasing general belief that many chronic diseases such as cardiovascular diseases and cancers of various sites may be modulated by dietary trace elements.

The absolute amounts of ingested trace elements may be greater in foodstuffs than in drinking water, but because of food factors that may delay absorption of elements (e.g., precipitation of calcium or iron in the gut lumen by phytates), elements in water may be more readily absorbed in the absence of food. The heavy metals are particularly toxic, because at very low concentrations they inhibit enzyme systems; they may interact with imidazole, carboxyl, or sulfhydryl groups on proteins, with amino acid residues, or they may chelate with phosphoryl groups of nucleic acids.

LEAD

Lead has been found to be present in animal and plant tissues to a greater extent than mercury, cadmium, aluminum, or other trace metals, and it is readily absorbed and accumulated. Most high concentrations in the gut tissue have been observed in humans in the cecum and duodenum. Peptic ulcer can be caused by lead intoxication, and gastric hypoacidity has been seen in patients with plumbism. Animal experiments have demonstrated that gastric evacuation and gut motility are depressed by lead intoxication. The gastrointestinal absorption of lead has been reviewed elsewhere (Pfeiffer, 1977). An inverse relationship has been found between particle size and lead absorption; absorption of lead chromate and lead octoate from dried paint films is enhanced when the particle size is reduced from 1000 to 50μm. Studies with radioactive ^{203}Pb in the rat have in most but not all cases shown that oral or parenteral administration of chelating agents, such as calcium disodium ethylenediaminetetraacetate or 2,3-dimercaptopropanol significantly increase intestinal lead absorption (Jugo et al., 1975). The absorption of lead salts in solution is relatively low, ranging from 8% to 12% in human beings, and with increasing age, the gastrointestinal absorption of lead decreases. In the body, organic forms of lead such as diethyl, triethyl, or tetraethyl lead may be partially converted into inorganic lead. The comparative rates of gastrointestinal absorption of these various compounds are not yet established, but time lengths of survival after oral administration of these lead alkyls in rats are similar except after triethyl lead chloride, which is more toxic.

MERCURY

Mercury-containing compounds create a significant public health hazard, expecially in recent years as water pollution and use of mercury-containing seed disinfectants have increased, and in view of the numerous mercury compounds used in industrial processes. Methyl mercury is greatly concentrated (up to 8000-fold in liver) in biologic systems, and this compound remains unchanged in transport from one animal to another. It is highly lethal because of its low excretory rate.

The toxicity of mercurial compounds depends on the degree of intestinal absorption, and the following compounds show an increasing order of toxicity: methyl and ethyl mercury dicyandiamides, methyl and ethyl mercury chloride, phenylmercury benzoate, and $HgCl_2$. Chronic mercury poisoning in human beings is associated with diarrhea and recurrent attacks of abdominal pain, though symptoms in humans and animals differ, depending on whether the cause is organic or inorganic mercurial compounds. Phenylmercuric acetate and ethylmercuric chloride are absorbed from the intestines in an unchanged form, and the absorption rate of the former compound exceeds that of mercuric acetate.

ZINC AND CADMIUM

Because of chemical similarities of zinc and cadmium (tetrahedral configuration and isoelectronic valence shells), these two elements compete physiologically. Cadmium is a cumulative poison, and food can become contaminated with cadmium from galvanized water pipes. With respect to the gastrointestinal tract, cadmium may inhibit absorption of phosphorus and impair the digestion of protein and fat, and may inhibit enzyme systems such as carboxypeptidase. Acute cadmium toxicity in humans is accompanied by severe gastroenteritis. Increasing dietary levels of calcium inhibit the absorption of cadmium. Also, cadmium absorption is reduced in the presence of dietary zinc as a result of competition for absorption sites. Several studies have demonstrated that the intestinal mucosa is a good barrier for cadmium.

Large doses of zinc may cause enteritis, but parenteral administration of zinc sulfate (up to 88 mg/kg) to animals significantly inhibits experimental gastric ulcers induced by reserpine, restraint, cold-water immersion, or other stimuli (Pfeiffer, Cho, Cheema, and Saltman, 1980). Preliminary studies of patients with peptic ulcer suggest that orally administered zinc may accelerate ulcer healing, but published results are somewhat equivocal. Zinc acts at the level of cellular membranes, increasing the stability and reducing permeability of membranes (Pfeiffer and Cho, 1980). As well, it reduces gastric acid secretion, and mucosal mast cell histamine release. Zinc deficiency states have been associated with several pathologic findings, including esophageal lesions, an increased incidence of esophageal cancer in human beings, and increased susceptibility to experimental esophageal cancer in rats induced by methylbenzylnitrosamine (MBN). Thus, environmental exposure either to excessive zinc, such as occupational exposures, or to chronic zinc deficiency may be associated with adverse alimentary tract reactions.

COPPER AND MOLYBDENUM

In the intestinal tract, copper competes with cadmium and zinc for absorptive sites. Gastroesophageal erosions have been observed in swine that were poisoned by copper compounds, and acute gastrointestinal erosions have been reported in humans after acute copper intoxication. Both of the above reactions may, however, be nonspecific to copper. The physiologic handling of copper by the digestive tract has been reviewed elsewhere by the author (Pfeiffer, 1977).

Molybdenum is of toxicologic interest because it is an industrial contaminant and is found in high enough concentrations in certain wild plants ingested by cattle and sheep to cause toxicity in such foraging species. Molybdenum, which is rapidly absorbed in the gut in low quantities, can cause diarrhea and other toxic symptoms in cattle, sheep, and rats.

OTHER TRACE ELEMENTS

The gastrointestinal physiologic effects, including absorption, secretion, and actions on motor activity, of many other trace elements have been frequently reported. Some of these gut responses are reviewed elsewhere (Pfeiffer, 1977), but their specific pathologic effects on the alimentary tract are not well studied. It is likely that excesses or deficiencies of some of these trace elements, either individually or in combination with other elements, modify disease responses within the gut. One of the lines of evidence that supports this hypothesis but does not prove it is the epidemiologic correlation of disease, such as gastric cancer, with the natural geochemical environment. Minerals in the natural chemical background of particular populations can be expected to become evident in plants and animal food grown in the same environment, as well as in the air and drinking water. Marked correlations of this type have already been reported for cancer of the stomach (Pfeiffer, Fodor, and Canning, 1973; Malnasi et al., 1976). A comparative study by the author (Pfeiffer and Fodor, 1979) on multiple trace elements in drinking water, as correlated with gastric cancer mortality in high- and low-risk zones in Iceland, Japan, and Newfoundland revealed that of 23 trace elements studied, only lead and nitrate were significantly correlated with gastric cancer mortality. This type of investigation, in which diverse populations were investigated, also emphasized the importance of ruling out spurious associations.

N-Nitroso Compounds

Nitrosamines were first reported to be toxic to humans in 1937, and since the 1960s interest in the carcinogenic properties of nitrosamines has greatly increased. Many different natural and synthetic nitrosamines have subsequently been shown to be carcinogenic to the alimentary tract and other sites in experimental animals, and it is believed that humans would respond similarly. Interestingly, different N-nitroso compounds elicit site specificity with respect to particular regions of the alimentary tract. Nitrosamines may be presented to the human digestive tract in two ways. They may enter as contaminants present on ingested foodstuffs, particularly on preserved meats or fish, or in beer, but they may be present also in a wide variety of foods. Second, nitrosamines may be formed in vivo through reactions of ingested amines (present in meat, some drugs, food additives, contaminants of food by agricultural chemicals, etc.) with nitrite. The nitrite may be derived by reduction of dietary nitrate, a reaction facilitated by some bacterial enzyme systems (in oral microflora), or nitrite may be ingested directly as a food preservative or other compound. This reaction readily takes place in gastric juice at low pH, but may also occur elsewhere in the more distal digestive tract. By 1980 more than 13 commonly ingested amines, including aminopyrine, morpholine, disulfiram, methylbenzylamine, and heptamethyleneimine, had been identified that were tumorigenic in rats if given when nitrite was present (Lijinsky, 1980). It has been proven experimentally that carcinogenic nitrosamines, such as dimethylnitrosamine (DMNA), can be formed on formaldehyde and sodium benzoate-preserved fish (Koppang, 1974). Thus, nitrite preservatives are not the only preservatives that have been incriminated in association with carcinogen formation on foodstuffs.

Other Environmental Factors and Digestive Tract Pathology

Normal constituents of food, including level of dietary fiber, content of fat, protein, or starch, have long been considered in relationship to cancer, diverticulosis, and other diseases of the alimentary tract, but nutritional factors are beyond the scope of the present review. Recent studies have shown by comparison of different regions within one country (e.g., Japan, Greece) that the incidence of diverticulosis varies in relation to factors other than dietary fiber intake, and it has been suggested that urban-related environmental factors are responsible for elevated incidence (Manousos et al., 1973). Nevertheless, such environmental agents have not yet been identified. Similarly, colon cancer is elevated in urban and northeastern regions of the United States, although the specific and supposed environmental factors remain unidentified (Haenszel and Dawson, 1965).

Inhalation of the multiple carcinogens and possible cancer-promoting agents in air contaminated by tobacco smoke, by smokers and nonsmokers alike, is another risk factor for alimentary tract cancers, and for peptic ulcer disease. Indeed, cigarette smoking is one of the most well-established risk factors for cancers of most sites, including all alimentary tract sites. The role of smoking has been documented extensively in numerous treatises elsewhere. Intestinal brush border enzymes such as lactase, sucrase, maltase, or alkaline phosphatase are reduced by tobacco leaf extracts (Mitra et al., 1980). The same enzymes are altered after prenatal exposure of rats to hydrazine or 1,2-dimethylhydrazine, of which the latter compound is a colon-specific carcinogen. Depending on the enzyme, however, enhanced or decreased activity was observed. Other environmental agents, such as arsenic or the herbicide contaminant, 2,3,7,8-tetrachlorodibenzo-p-dioxin, also affect these intestinal brush border enzymes (Schiller, 1979). It should be borne in mind, as has been demonstrated by quantitative analysis (Jayant et al., 1977), that the influence of tobacco smoke or other environmental factors on the pathologic responses of the gastrointestinal tissues may interact in a synergistic manner with a complex of other exogenous or nutritional factors (Jayant et al., 1977).

REFERENCES

Aitio, A., Hietanen, E., and Hänninen, O. 1975. Mucosal drug metabolism and drug-induced ulcer. In *Experimental ulcer*, ed. T. Gheorghui, pp. 17–21. Baden-Baden, W. Germany: G. Witzstrock.

Allen, J. R., and Norback, D. H. 1973. Polychlorinated biphenyl and triphenyl-induced gastric mucosal hyperplasia in primates *Science* 179:498–499.

Banwell, J. G. 1979. Environmental contaminants and intestinal function. *Environ. Health Perspect.* 33:107–114.

Bock, K. W., and Winne, D. 1975. Glucuronidation of 1-naphthol in the rat intestinal loop. *Biochem. Pharmacol* 24:859–862.

Chhabra, R. S. 1979. Intestinal absorption and metabolism of xenobiotics. *Environ. Health Perspect.* 33:61–69.

Chhabra, R. S., and Fouts, J. R. 1974. Sex differences in the metabolism of xenobiotics by extrahepatic tissue in rats. *Drug Metab. Dispos.* 2:375–379.

Chhabra, R. S., Pohl, R. J., and Fouts, J. R. 1974. A comparative study of xenobiotic-metabolizing enzymes in liver and intestine of various animal species. *Drug Metab. Dispos.* 2:443–447.

Evans, J. C., Evans, R. J., Holmes, A., Hounam, R. F., Jones, D. M., Morgan, A., and Walsh, M. 1973. Studies on the deposition of inhaled fibrous material in the respiratory tract of the rat and its subsequent clearance using radioactive tracer techniques. *Environ. Res.* 6:180–201.

Graham, S., Blanchet, M., and Rohrer, T. 1977. Cancer in asbestos-mining and other areas of Quebec. *J. Natl. Cancer Inst.* 59:1139–1145.

Gross, P., Harley, R. A., Swinburne, L. M., Davis, J. M. G., and Greene, W. B. 1974. Ingested mineral fibers. Do they penetrate tissue or cause cancer? *Arch. Environ. Health* 29:341–347.

Haenszel, W., and Dawson, E. A. 1965. A note on mortality from cancer of the colon and rectum in the United States. *Cancer* 18:265–272.

Hänninen, O. 1968. On the metabolic regulation in the glucuronic acid pathway in the rat tissues. *Ann. Acad. Sci. Fenn. A.* 2(142):1–96.

Hänninen, O., and Aitio, A. 1968. Enhanced glucuronide formation in different tissues following drug administration. *Biochem. Pharmacol.* 17:2307–2311.

Hänninen, O., Aitio, A., and Hartiala, K. 1968. Gastrointestinal distribution of glucuronide synthesis and the relevant enzymes in the rat. *Scand. J. Gastroenterol.* 3:461–464.

Hartiala, K. 1973. Metabolism of hormones, drugs, and other substances by the gut. *Physiol. Rev.* 53:496–534.

Hartiala, K. J. W. 1955. Studies on detoxication mechanisms. III. Glucuronide synthesis of various organs with special reference to the detoxicating capacity of the mucous membrane of the alimentary canal. *Ann. Med. Exp. Fenn.* 33:240–245.

Hietanen, E., Laitinen, M., Lang, M., and Vainio, H. 1975. Inducibility of mucosal drug-metabolizing enzymes of rats fed on a cholesterol-rich diet by polychlorinated biphenyl, 3-methylcholanthrene and phenobarbitone. *Pharmacology* 13:287–296.

Hietanen, E., Laitinen, M., Vainio, H., and Hänninen, O. 1975. Dietary fats and properties of endoplasmic reticulum: II. Dietary lipid induced changes in activities of drug metabolizing enzymes in liver and duodenum of rat. *Lipids* 10:467–472.

Hoensch, H. P., Hutt, R., and Hartmann, F. 1979. Biotransformation of xenobiotics in human intestinal mucosa. *Environ. Health Perspect.* 33:71–78.

Hoensch, H., Woo, C. H., Raffin, S. B., and Schmid, R. 1976. Oxidative metabolism of foreign compounds in rat small intestine: Cellular localization and dependence on dietary iron. *Gastroenterology* 70:1063–1070.

Jacobs, R., and Richards, R. J. 1980. Distribution of 6-6 (n)-[^{3}H] sucrose and its radiolabeled degradation products from isolated perfused rat small intestine loops following prolonged ingestion of chrysotile asbestos. *Environ. Res.* 21:423–431.

Jayant, K., Balakrishnan, V., Sanghvi, L. D., and Jussawalla, D. J. 1977. Quantification of the role of smoking and chewing tobacco in oral, pharyngeal, and oesophageal cancers. *Br. J. Cancer* 35:232–235.

Jugo, S., Maljkovic, T., and Kostial, K. 1975. Influence of chelating agents on the gastrointestinal absorption of lead. *Toxicol. Appl. Pharmacol.* 34:259–263.

Klaassen, C. D. 1975. Absorption, distribution and excretion of toxicants. In *Toxicology:*

The basic science of poisons, eds. L. J. Casarett and J. Doull, p. 32. New York: Macmillan.

Koppang, N. 1974. Dimethylnitrosamine-formation in fish meal and toxic effects in pigs. *Am. J. Pathol.* 74:95–106.

LeFevre, M. E., Hancock, D. C., and Joel, D. D. 1980. Intestinal barrier to large particulates in mice. *J. Toxicol. Environ. Health* 6:691–704.

Lijinsky, W. 1980. Significance of *in vivo* formation of N-nitroso compounds. *Oncology* 37:223–226.

Lucier, G. W., Sonawane, B. R., and McDaniel, O. S. 1977. Glucuronidation and deglucuronidation reactions in hepatic and extrahepatic tissues during perinatal development. *Drug. Metab. Dispos.* 5:279–287.

Malnasi, G., Jakab, S., Incze, A., Apostol, A., Csapo, J. M., Szabo, E., Csapo, J. J., and Jakab, K. 1976. An assay for selecting high risk population for gastric cancer by studying environmental factors. *Neoplasma* 23:333–341.

Manousos, O. N., Vrachliotis, G., Papaevangelou, G., Detorakis, E., Doritis, P., Stergiou, L., and Merikas, G. 1973. Relation of diverticulosis of the colon to environmental factors in Greece. *Dig. Dis.* 18:174–176.

Mitra, G., Poddar, M. K., and Ghosh, J. J. 1980. Effect of tobacco-leaf extract administration on liver, lung, intestine, and serum enzymes. *Toxicol. Appl. Pharmacol.* 52:262–266.

Nikonorow, M., Mazur, H., and Piekacz, H. 1973. Effect of orally administered plasticizers and polyvinyl chloride stabilizers in the rat. *Toxicol. Appl. Pharmacol.* 26:253–259.

Pantuck, E. J., Hsiao, K. -C., and Loub, W. B. 1976. Stimulatory effect of vegetables on intestinal drug metabolism in the rat. *J. Pharmacol. Exp. Ther.* 198:278–283.

Peterson, R. E., Seymour, J. L., and Allen, J. R. 1976. Distribution and biliary excretion of polychlorinated biphenyls in rats. *J. Toxicol. Appl. Pharmacol.* 38:609–619.

Pfeiffer, C. J. 1971. Mucosal surface convolutions: cellular aggregates observed on the enteric surface of various species. *Biol. Gastroenterol. (Paris)* 3:225–229.

Pfeiffer, C. J. 1977. Gastroenterologic response to environmental agents—absorption and interactions. In *Handbook of physiology—reactions to environmental agents,* eds.

D. H. K. Lee, H. L. Falk, S. D. Murphy, and S. R. Geiger, pp. 349–374. Bethesda, Md.: American Physiological Society.

Pfeiffer, C. J., and Cho, C. H. 1980. Modulating effect by zinc on hepatic lysosomal fragility induced by surface-active agents. *Res. Commun. Chem. Pathol. Pharmacol.* 27:587–598.

Pfeiffer, C. J., Cho, C. H., Cheema, A., and Saltman, D. 1980. Reserpine-induced gastric ulcers: Protection by lysosomal stabilization due to zinc. *Eur. J. Pharmacol.* 61:347–353.

Pfeiffer, C. J., and Debro, J. R. 1966. Stress and dietary influence on the direct oxidative pathway of carbohydrate metabolism in the intestine. *Arch. Int. Biochem. Physiol.* 84:97–105.

Pfeiffer, C. J., and Fodor, J. G. 1979. Gastric cancer mortality and water trace elements: International study of Iceland, Newfoundland and Japan. In *Gastric cancer—etiology and pathogenesis,* ed. C. J. Pfeiffer, pp. 45–59. New York: G. Witzstrock.

Pfeiffer, C. J., Fodor, J. G., and Canning, E. 1973. An epidemiologic analysis of mortality and gastric cancer in Newfoundland. *Can. Med. Assoc. J.* 108:1374–1380.

Pfeiffer, C. J., and Hänninen, O. 1977. The alimentary excretion of environmental agents and unnatural compounds. In *Handbook of physiology—reactions to environmental agents,* eds. D. H. K. Lee, H. L. Falk, S. D. Murphy, and S. R. Geiger, pp. 513–535. Bethesda, Md.: American Physiological Society.

Pfeiffer, C. J., Rowden, G., and Weibel, J. 1974. *Gastrointestinal ultrastructure: An atlas of scanning and transmission electron microscopy.* New York: Academic Press.

Pontefract, R. D., and Cunningham, H. M. 1973. Penetration of asbestos through the digestive tract of rats. *Nature* 243:352–353.

Rawls, R. 1980. Studies update on vinyl chloride hazards. *Chem. Eng. News* 58:27–28.

Reynolds, E. S. 1977. Environmental aspects of injury and disease: liver and bile ducts. *Environ. Health Perspect.* 20:1–13.

Scheline, R. R. 1973. Metabolism of foreign compounds by gastrointestinal microorganisms. *Pharmacol. Rev.* 25:451–523.

Schiller, C. M. 1979. Chemical exposure and intestinal function. *Environ. Health Perspect.* 33:91–100.

Shah, P. V., and Guthrie, F. E. 1973. Penetration

of insecticides through isolated sections of the mouse digestive system: Effects of age and region of the intestine. *Toxicol. Appl. Pharmacol.* 25:621–624.

Tredger, J. M., and Chhabra, R. S. 1977. Circadian variations in microsomal drug-metabolizing enzyme activities in rat and rabbit tissues. *Xenobiotica* 7:481–489.

Uotila, P. 1977. Effects of single and repeated cigarette smoke-exposure on the activities of aryl hydrocarbon hydroxylase, epoxide hydratase and UDP-glucuronosyltransferase in rat lung, kidney, and small intestinal mucosa. *Res. Commun. Chem. Pathol. Pharmacol.* 17:101–114.

Volkheimer, G. 1974. Passage of particles through the wall of the gastrointestinal tract. *Environ. Health Perspect.* 9:215–225.

Volkheimer, G. 1975. Hematogenous dissemination of ingested polyvinyl chloride particles. *Ann. N.Y. Acad. Sci.* 246:164–170.

Volkheimer, G. 1977. Persorption of particles: physiology and pharmacology. *Adv. Pharmacol. Chemother.* 14:163–187.

Volkheimer, G., and Schulz, F. H. 1968. The phenomenon of persorption. *Digestion* 1:213–218.

Volkheimer, G., Schulz, F. H., Lindenau, A., and Beitz, U. 1969. Persorption of metallic iron particles. *Gut* 10:32–33.

Wattenberg, L. W. 1972. Dietary modification of intestinal and pulmonary aryl hydrocarbon hydroxylase activity. *Toxicol. Appl. Pharmacol.* 23:741–748.

Wattenberg, L. W., Leong, J. L., and Strand, P. J. 1962. Benzpyrene hydroxylase activity in the gastrointestinal tract. *Cancer Res.* 22:1120–1125.

Welch, R. M., Cavallito, J., and Loh, A. 1972. Effect of exposure to cigarette smoke on the metabolism of benzo [a] pyrene and acetophenetidin by lung and intestine of rats. *Toxicol. Appl. Pharmacol.* 23:749–758.

Zampoglione, N. G., and Mannering, G. J. 1973. Properties of benzpyrene hydroxylase in the liver, intestinal mucosa and adrenal of untreated and 3-methylcholanthrene-treated rats. *J. Pharmacol. Exp. Ther.* 185:676–685, 1973.

9

Liver and Biliary Tree

Edward S. Reynolds and Mary Treinen Moslen

Criteria to Establish the Hepatotoxicity of Environmental Chemicals

The scientific literature contains numerous reports of liver and biliary tract injury in humans exposed to environmental chemicals in the diet, home, occupation, and through voluntary consumption of analgesics, laxatives, vitamins, alcohol, and contraceptive hormones. Some of these reports provided the first evidence that liver injury could result from exposure to specific chemicals or classes of chemicals, for example, acute necrosis in aircraft factory workers exposed to 1,1,2,2-tetrachloroethane (Willcox et al., 1915), cirrhosis in research laboratory workers exposed to dimethylnitrosamine (Barnes and Magee, 1954), porphyria in Turkish men, women, and children who had eaten wheat contaminated with hexachlorobenzene (Ockner and Schmid, 1961), jaundice in women with inherited or acquired defects in bile excretion after use of C-17 alkylated oral contraceptives (Mowat and Arias, 1969), liver cell adenoma in young women with a history of oral contraceptive use (Baum et al., 1973), and angiosarcoma in polymerization plant workers exposed to vinyl chloride (Creech and Johnson, 1974).

When liver injury develops in identifiable groups of exposed persons or the type of liver injury is relatively rare, as in the above reports, the hepatotoxicity of a specific chemical in humans can be readily established. But the type of injury often is not distinctive, and although the incidence is higher in people exposed to specific suspect compounds, individual cases may also be attributed to viruses or other known toxins. A problem that has become evident in recent years is that sequential or concurrent exposure to different chemicals can markedly exacerbate the hepatotoxicity of relatively weak toxins. A good example of this synergism is the enhancement of acetaminophen liver injury by chronic alcohol consumption (McClain et al., 1980).

Five criteria for the identification of environmentally associated liver injury in humans are outlined in Table 9-1. There must be either biochemical or histologic evidence of liver injury. There must not be evidence that a viral agent, trauma, hypoxia, or another nonchemical agent caused the liver injury. There must be a well-documented history of exposure to one or more suspect environmental chemicals before the onset of injury. One should look for a "cause-and-effect" temporal relationship. Sometimes, but not always, the type of acute or chronic liver injury or tumor is distinctive for the

Table 9–1. Criteria to Establish the Hepatotoxicity of an Environmental Chemical

1. Evidence of liver injury
2. Absence of evidence for viral or other nonchemical cause
3. History of exposure to chemical
4. Identification of toxic chemical or its metabolites in breath, blood, urine, intestinal contents, or tissues
5. Hepatotoxicity of chemical in experimental animals

agent. Ideally, toxic levels of the agent, or its metabolites, should be demonstrated in the blood, urine, stool, or tissues of patients at the time of discovery of injury. Finally, by analogy to Koch's postulates, the agent suspected of causing the patient's disease should produce a similar type of injury in experimental animals. Compliance with this final criterion may be rather difficult, because some chemicals produce liver injury in experimental animals only under specific conditions or after the animals have been pretreated with specific enzyme inducers.

Mechanisms of Liver Injury by Environmental Chemicals

The liver and biliary tract are responsible for (1) the uptake, synthesis, storage, and release of glucose to blood, (2) the uptake, storage, utilization, and transport of fat, (3) the synthesis of proteins that control the distribution of extracellular water (albumin), transport and regulate amounts of essential metals (e.g., transferrins and metallothionein), clot blood (e.g., fibrinogen), and participate in host defense (e.g., components of complement), and (4) the uptake, synthesis or metabolism, and excretion of bile constituents, including bile acids and heme degradation products (e.g., bilirubin). The liver has a central role in regulating the homeostasis of the internal milieu of the body through deactivation of hormones, conversion of ammonia to urea, and detoxification of bacterial products absorbed from the intestine, which if released to the sys-

temic circulation would have a deleterious effect on the function of other organs. The liver is a flexible organ that has an enormous functional reserve and the capacity to respond to dietary and hormone changes as well as to the presence of xenobiotics (chemicals foreign to the body). A rich supply of nonspecific enzymes give the liver the ability to metabolize a broad spectrum of organic materials. This ability to metabolize almost any organic material renders the liver particularly prone to injury by chemicals.

Figure 9-1 schematizes mechanisms by which environmental chemicals can detrimentally affect the functional integrity of the liver. Trophic effects can be indirectly injurious. A chemical or its metabolites may bind competitively or noncompetitively at receptor sites on the cell surface or within the cytoplasmic matrix. Binding at such sites can stimulate, exaggerate, or abolish the cellular response controlled by that locus and result in acute or chronic injury. Interference by a chemical or its metabolite with a specific cellular pathway can deplete energy sources or detrimentally alter a synthetic or degradative process. Direct interactions between a chemical or its metabolite and components of an organelle can impair the functions of the organelle and result in acute or chronic injury. Interactions between a chemical or its metabolites and either chromosomes or cell constituents that maintain chromosome integrity can initiate or promote the process of carcinogenesis.

Functional Organization of the Liver

Grossly, the liver is a big, bulky, rather amorphous organ whose size is carefully maintained in adults at 2.0% to 2.2% of body weight. Structurally and biochemically, the parenchyma of the liver is a fantastically organized reception, metabolism, distribution, and excretion system. The specialized functions of the liver are responsive to alterations in hormones, diet, and chemicals absorbed from the environment but foreign to the body.

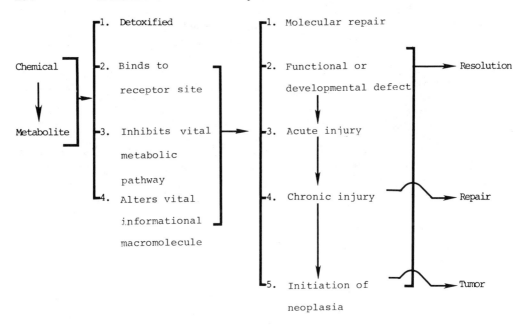

Figure 9–1. Schematic of mechanisms by which environmental chemicals may injure liver and biliary tract.

ANATOMY

The liver receives directly, via the portal venous circulation, all water-soluble materials—glucose, amino acids, bile salts, minerals, bacterial products, and water-soluble xenobiotics—that are present in food or other materials ingested and absorbed from the intestine. Eventually, via an indirect pathway, the lymphatic and systemic circulation, the liver also receives the bulk of the non-water-soluble materials—fatty acids, cholesterol, bilirubin, steroids, and lipid-soluble vitamins and xenobiotics. Many of these materials are processed by parenchymal cells. Some processed materials, including bile salts and conjugates of bilirubin and xenobiotics, are excreted in the bile.

Under normal circumstances, the liver receives blood from both the portal vein (~60%) and the hepatic artery (~40%) (Figure 9-2). After the blood is directed and redirected into ever smaller vessels, it traverses the sinusoids of the liver lobule, the major functional subunits of the liver. As it percolates through the vascular sinusoids of the lobule, the blood exchanges nutrients and delivers body wastes and absorbed xeno-

biotics. Revitalized blood exits the lobule via the central vein; it eventually emerges from the liver by the hepatic vein and re-enters the systemic circulation.

Human liver contains approximately 50,000 lobules (Figure 9-3), which are irregular polygonal prisms 2–3 mm in diameter. At the center of each lobule is a central efferent vein, while around the periphery are four to six portal triads (or tracts). Each portal triad contains a bile duct and terminal branches of the portal vein and hepatic artery within a connective tissue sheath. This is the "classic" lobule that pathologists conventionally use, because the pattern is readily recognized grossly and microscopically. Alternatively, Rappaport (1975) proposed that the functioning liver lobule or acinus is centered about a portal tract and is bounded at its periphery by multiple central veins.

In the classic lobule, plates of polyhedral parenchymal cells, or hepatocytes, radiate from the central vein out to the periphery of the lobule. These plates are one cell thick, are irregular, and freely interconnect (Figure 9-4). On one or more aspects, the hepatocyte plates abut vascular sinusoids,

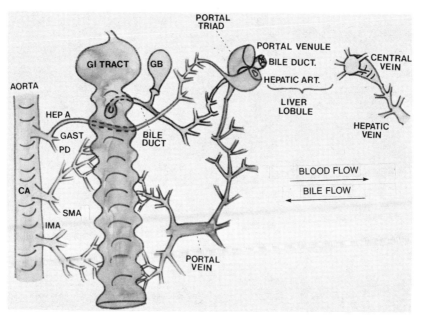

Figure 9–2. Schematic of the orientation of the liver and its functional unit, the lobule, to arterial hepatic (HEP A) and portal venous blood inputs, and to bile duct and hepatic venous outputs. PD, pancreatoduodenal artery; CA, celiac artery. Portal blood, from the superior and inferior mesenteric arteries (SMA, IMA), enters the liver via the portal vein after traversing the capillary nets of the intestinal mucosa. Thus, nutrients and other substances taken up by the intestinal epithelium are directly conveyed to the liver. A portion of the aortic blood enters the liver via the hepatic artery. Blood enters the lobule at its periphery from portal triads each of which contains a bile duct and terminal branches of the portal vein and hepatic artery. The lobule is drained by the central vein. After exiting from the liver, blood flows from the hepatic vein into the inferior vena cava, and then after transit through the lung re-emerges in the aorta. Bile is secreted by parenchymal cells of the liver lobule, collected and stored in the gallbladder (GB), and secreted into the duodenum on demand. Many of the chemical components of the bile are readily reabsorbed by the intestinal epithelium, transferred to the portal blood, and redelivered to the liver where they are taken up by parenchymal cells and re-excreted in the bile. This cycle is called the enterohepatic circulation.

which are lined by flat, fenestrated endothelial cells, by star-shaped phagocytic Kupffer cells, and by an occasional fat-storing cell.

Bile canaliculi (Figures 9-4 and 9-5) are capillary networks of interfacial canals that form between parenchymal cells and that are isolated from sinusoidal blood by "tight" but not impermeable junctions. The walls of the bile canaliculi are composed of specialized regions of the plasma membranes of adjacent parenchymal cells. The canalicular network eventually connects with the terminal branches of bile ducts in the portal triads at the periphery of the lobules. Although the lumens of bile canaliculi are continuous with those of the bile ducts in the portal triads, the junctions are so attenuated that they are not readily demonstrable by either light or electron microscopy. Called ductules, or cholangioles, these connections dilate on obstruction of bile ducts and may rupture. Lumens of smaller branches of bile ducts in portral triads are lined by a cuboidal epithelium. As the ducts become larger, their lining cells become columnar.

Approximately 500–1000 ml of bile are actively secreted daily by liver parenchymal cells across the bile canalicular membranes into the interfacial canals. The secreted bile enters the bile duct system in the portal triads and exits from the liver through the hepatic ducts (Figure 9-2). When there is no food

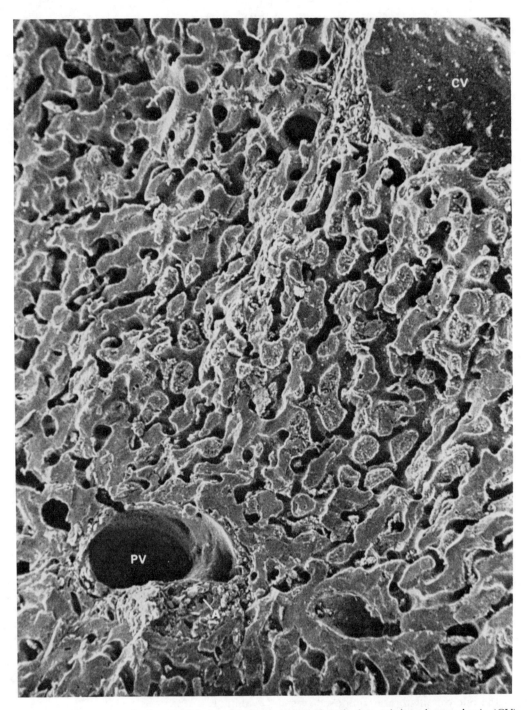

Figure 9–3. A sector of a hepatic lobule with the portal triad at the lower left and central vein (CV) at upper right. Parenchymal cells form irregular branching, reanastomosing plates of cells separated by a labyrinthine network of sinusoidal capillaries through which blood percolates on its way from the portal triad to the central vein. Branches of the portal vein (PV) and an interlobular artery (A) are seen clearly in the portal triad at lower left. (Scanning electron micrograph, × 400). (Courtesy of Dr. M. Moto, Department of Anatomy, Nigata University Medical School, Nigata, Japan.)

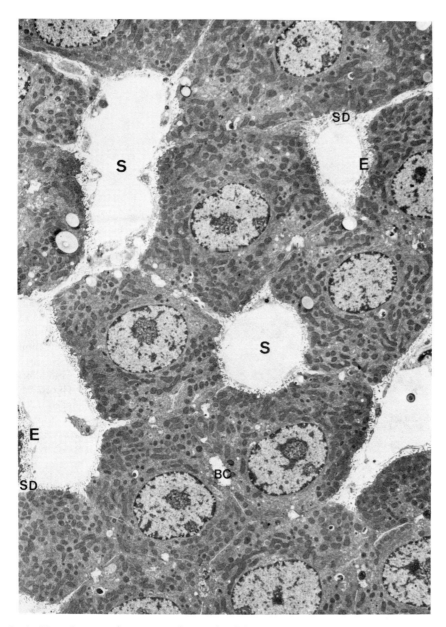

Figure 9–4. Hepatic parenchyma is made up of polyhedral parenchymal cells arranged in irregular plates or "cords"—one cell thick—that border endothelium (E)-lined blood sinusoids (S). The space between the microvilli-lined surfaces of parenchymal cells and the overlying endothelium is known as the space of Disse (SD). The walls of bile canaliculi (BC) are formed from the plasma membrane of adjacent parenchymal cells (rat liver, perfusion fixed, × 4000).

in the upper gastrointestinal tract, most of the bile is stored and concentrated in the gallbladder. The stored bile is secreted on demand into the duodenum.

The normal anatomic configuration of the liver develops early in life, and beyond a certain point of maturation, lobules cease to increase in number and thereafter merely hypertrophy. The regenerative capacity of the liver's parenchymal cells and endothelium is phenomenal. When two thirds of the liver is removed surgically or destroyed

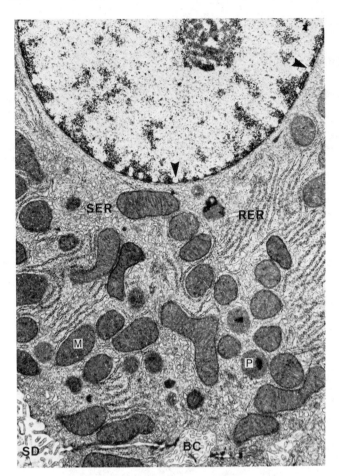

Figure 9–5. Portion of liver parenchymal cell. Nucleus at top. Space of Disse (SD) at lower left, bile canaliculus (BC) at bottom. The cytoplasm of parenchymal cells is rich in organelles with stacks of parallel arrays of rough endoplasmic reticulum (RER), tubular tangles of smooth endoplasmic reticulum (SER), mitochondria (M), and peroxisomes (P) arrayed in an orderly and presumably interactive manner. The nucleus, which contains a nucleolus, communicates with the cytoplasm via nuclear pores (arrows) that traverse the nuclear envelope (rat, ×22,000).

through chemical or hypoxic injury, the remnant will grow and restore the liver's original size within 2 weeks.

PARENCHYMAL CELLS

The workhorses of the liver are its polyhedral parenchymal cells, which comprise the vast bulk (90–95%) of its mass. These parenchymal cells (Figures 9-4 and 9-5) are more specialized than the endothelial and phagocytic cells that line the sinusoids, and thus warrant a detailed description.

Parenchymal cells contain one or more round nuclei, each with at least one prominent nucleolus. Nuclei are usually in the interphase configuration, as the cells are relatively long-lived. Nuclei contain DNA and the enzymatic apparatus required for its replication and repair, and for the synthesis

of RNA transcripts and their processing into functional messenger (mRNA), ribosomal (rRNA), and transfer (tRNA) RNA species. The nuclei are bound on their periphery by a well-formed nuclear envelope, a specialized cisterna of the endoplasmic reticulum that surrounds the nucleoplasm, isolating it from the cytoplasm. The inner surface of the nuclear envelope is coated by heterochromatin, while the cytoplasmic surface is studded by polysomes. The nuclear envelope is perforated by pores—structured portals through which the nucleus communicates with the cytoplasm and through which substances controlling DNA transcription such as steroid and thyroid hormones bound to their cytoplasmic receptors pass inward. These pores may also be the intracellular "highways" through which electrophilic metabolites of xenobiotics gain access to DNA.

Plasma membranes of the parenchymal cells with their many surface specializations form the morphologic and functional interface between the cell, its immediate extracellular environment, and neighboring cells. Surfaces of the plasma membrane border on the space subjacent to sinusoidal lining cells (the space of Disse) and that line bile canaliculi are irregularly microvillous, while the surfaces that abut one another are relatively smooth. Protein constituents of the parenchymal plasma membrane sufaces differ, apparently in accord with their specific functions.

The external plasma membrane surface is coated with glycoproteins and glycolipids involved in attachment recognition and in cell–cell interactions. Also on the surface are receptor sites for specific substances in the cell's environment that regulate its function. Receptor sites on the plasma membranes of liver parenchymal cells include those for insulin and glucagon. Adjacent parenchymal cells are connected to one another by zones of attachment that run along the borders of the bile canaliculi. These zones are sealed at their inner edges by tight junctions or "zonulae occludens" (where the outer layers of plasma membranes of adjoining cells fuse), and are reinforced at their lateral edge by a zonulae adherens, a parallel strip, where intermediate "prekeratin" filaments (tonofibrils) present in the adjacent cytoplasm insert on the inner surface of the plasma membranes. At this location, an additional dense band(s) forms in the intracellular space. Actin, clathrins, ankrin, intermediate filaments, and other proteins line the cytoplasmic surface of plasma membranes, either stabilizing or deforming it with the formation of specialized surface structures such as microvilli, coated pits, phagosomes, and secretory vacuoles.

Mitochondria account for one-fourth of the parenchymal cell volume. They are bound by a double membrane, the inner one of which encloses the mitochondrial matrix. The inner membrane has an electron transport system localized to its hydrophobic core, which is tightly coupled via ion translocation to high-energy phosphate (ATP) synthesis. The outer mitochondrial membrane is the intracellular site of monoamine oxidase activity.

Endoplasmic reticulum accounts for one-third to one-half of the parenchymal cell volume. This organelle consists of a continuous network of smooth-surfaced tubules and flattened envelopes coated on their cytoplasmic surface by polyribosomes. The latter, the rough endoplasmic reticulum, is usually arrayed in many layered stacks called ergastoplasm, while the loose branching tubular tangles of smooth endoplasmic reticulum permeate the cytoplasmic matrix. Lamellae of rough and smooth endoplasmic reticulum often appear to envelop mitochondria. The cisternae of the endoplasmic reticulum connect with the cisternae of the perinuclear envelope and with the Golgi. Endoplasmic reticulum is the site of the assembly of very-low-density lipoprotein complexes (VLDL) excreted in the blood, the synthesis of triglycerides, phospholipids, cholesterol, and the elongation and desaturation of fatty acids. The polyribosome aggregates on the outer surface of the rough endoplasmic reticulum are the sites of protein synthesis. Specialized liver functions localized to the endoplasmic reticulum of hepatocytes include the terminal dephosphorylation of glycogen via glucose 6-phosphatase for liberation of glucose from the cell, conjugation of bilirubin via glucuronyl transferase, and the oxidation of many lipid-soluble xenobiotics via the cytochrome P-450 system (see next section).

Golgi apparatus, situated about bile canaliculi in hepatocytes, consist of stacks of smooth-surfaced, membrane-bound envelopes functionally interposed between the endoplasmic reticulum, secretory granules, plasma membrane, peroxisomes, and lysosomes. Golgi carry out the post-transcriptional modification of proteins synthesized by the endoplasmic reticulum and package them into secretory vacuoles, primary lysosomes, or peroxisomes. Enzyme activities localized to Golgi include the terminal N- and O-glycosylation of oligosaccharide groups of proteins, and the glycosylation and sulfation of glycolipids destined for incorporation in the external face of the plasma membrane.

Lysosomes are also oriented near the bile canaliculi of hepatocytes. These single membrane-bound structures function within the cell as "digestors." Their enzymes include acid hydrolases, which digest proteins, nucleic acids, lipids, carbohydrates, and glucosaminoglycans to their basic molecular constituents. Lysosomal enzymes, synthesized by the endoplasmic reticulum, are packaged into primary lysosomes by the Golgi. Primary lysosomes then fuse with phagosomes containing the material to be digested, forming the digestive vacuole or secondary lysosome. Phagosomes may contain materials taken up from outside the cell or from within the cell by autophagocytosis—a walling off and removal through digestion of cytoplasm and/or organelles that are no longer needed. This latter process of autophagocytosis is a striking functional adaptation and can be stimulated in hepatocytes by glucagon and partial hepatectomy.

Another single membrane-bound structure found in hepatocytes is the peroxisome or microbody. This organelle contains catalase, one or more flavin oxidases, and urate oxidase enzymes. Peroxisomal oxidases reduce molecular oxygen to hydrogen peroxide, which in turn is consumed in peroxidation reactions or dismutated to water and oxygen by catalase. This organelle also carries out amino acid hydroxylation and α oxidation of fatty acid acyl coenzymes A (CoA).

The cytoplasmic matrix, the ground substance of the hepatocyte within which all organelles reside, is normally rich in glycogen particles and relatively free of triglyceride droplets. The cytoplasmic matrix contains specialized enzymes and webworks of structural proteins that maintain the internal organization of the cells. Enzymatic constituents include those that carry out the synthesis, intermediary metabolism, and degradation of amino acids, fatty acids, and glycogen. The cytoplasmic matrix is also the site of function of constitutive proteins of the cell, including superoxide dismutase, glutathione S-transferases, calmodulin, metallothionein, and the enzymes involved in anaerobic glycolysis, urea synthesis, and alcohol oxidation.

Structural elements in the hepatocyte cytoplasmic matrix include microtubules, intermediate filaments, and actin microfilaments. Microtubules, long cylindrical rods formed by the polymerization of tubulins a and b, are considered to maintain internal configurations appropriate to optimal function. They may also function as guides along which organelles may be pulled or pushed. Intermediate filaments in liver parenchymal cells are prekeratin bundles or "tonofibrils," which form in association with the zonula adherens, which stabilizes cells in regions of intercellular contact. Disordered aggregates of intermediate filaments are now recognized to be a prominent component of "alcoholic hyaline," a filamentous aggregate that appears in parenchymal cells in several pathologic conditions, including the exposure of animals to the antifungal agent griseofulvin. Microfilaments, bundles of polymerized actin, are prominent in the cytoplasmic matrix beneath the microvillous surfaces of the cell that border the space of Disse and the bile canaliculus.

Not all parenchymal cells are equivalent. Those closer to the portal triad (periportal) have a greater number of mitochondria and higher respiratory enzyme activities, whereas those closer to the central vein (centrolobular) are richer in NADPH-dependent enzymes. Periportal hepatocytes take up, conjugate, and excrete the majority of the bile acids processed by the liver. Centrolobular hepatocytes have the major responsibility for the metabolism of drugs and xenobiotics, and have a richer supply of many of the enzymes involved in these processes including cytochrome P-450 isozymes (Baron et al., 1978). In addition, the extracellular environments of the hepatocytes across the lobule are not equivalent. Periportal hepatocytes, closer to the site of blood entry, receive a greater supply of nutrients and apparently function at higher O_2 tension than the centrolobular hepatocytes.

Acute liver injury rarely disturbs the

overall lobular architecture of the liver, whereas chronic disorders usually either partly or entirely destroy it. However, acute liver injury can markedly alter specific subcellular components of hepatocytes. For example, the first definitive electron-microscopic observation of the effects of a liver toxin revealed that carbon tetrachloride rapidly causes dispersion, vacuolization, and degranulation of the rough endoplasmic reticulum (Oberling and Rouiller, 1956). Phalloidin, a mushroom-derived toxin, has a marked effect on the structure and functional integrity of the bile canaliculi (Elias et al., 1980).

Biotransformation of Environmental Chemicals

Very few environmental chemicals initiate the process of liver cell injury without metabolic activation. The liver contains a rich supply of nonspecific enzymes that metabolize xenobiotics, often via a multiphase sequence of steps, to more water-soluble and more readily excretable forms. Occasionally the metabolic process converts a xenobiotic to a reactive electrophile that is capable of injurious interactions with liver cell constituents (Reynolds, 1977).

MECHANISMS OF XENOBIOTIC BIOTRANSFORMATION

Williams (1959) divided the process of xenobiotic metabolism into phase I and phase II–type reactions (Figure 9-6). Phase I reactions are oxidations, reductions, or hydrolyses, while phase II reactions are conjugations with glutathione, glucuronides, or other water-soluble groups. Many xenobiotic compounds sequentially undergo phase I and phase II reactions, whereas others undergo only phase I or phase II reactions.

The NADPH–cytochrome P-450 system, commonly known as the mixed-function oxygenase system, is the most important enzyme system involved in phase I reactions. This system, localized in the endoplasmic reticulum, consists of a flavoprotein NADPH–cytochrome P-450 reductase and a heme-containing enzyme cytochrome P-450 (Figure 9-7). Cytochrome P-450 is not a single enzyme but is a family of an as yet unknown number of isozymes that have different but overlapping substrate specificities. Cytochrome P-450 isozymes are versatile proteins that catalyze numerous types of reactions including aliphatic and aromatic hydroxylations and epoxidations, N-oxidations, sulfoxidations, N-, S-, and O-dealkylations, deaminations, dealkylations, desulfurations, and dehalogenations, and reductive reactions involving direct electron transfer, such as the reduction of azo, nitro, N-oxide, and epoxide groups (see review of Wislock et al., 1980).

Other hepatic enzymes that catalyze phase I reactions are the amine oxidases, esterases, amidases, and azo reductases. In addition, aliphatic alcohols and aldehydes are metabolized by the cytosolic alcohol and aldehyde dehydrogenases and oxidases.

Figure 9–6. Two-phase process of xenobiotic metabolism according to Williams (1959). Phase I reactions convert the xenobiotic to an active "primary," often potentially toxic metabolite, which is then detoxified by phase II conjugation reactions. By this mechanism the liver converts lipophilic xenobiotics to more water-soluble and excretable metabolites. Although considered a detoxication pathway, some primary and secondary metabolites are reactive electrophilic species capable of injurious interactions with cell constituents.

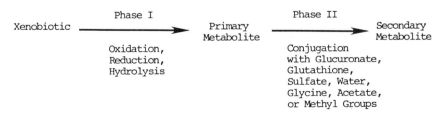

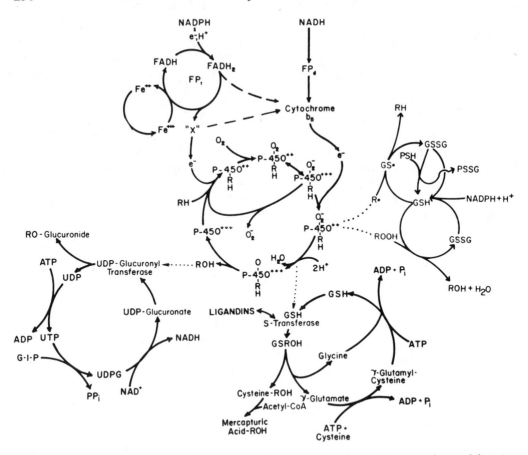

Figure 9–7. A schematization of the reactions of the cytochrome *P*-450-centered mixed-function oxygenase system of the liver endoplasmic reticulum and related conjugation systems. In the primary phase I reaction with cytochrome *P*-450 (center wheel), substrate (RH) binds to oxidized cytochrome *P*-450, is reduced by an electron transferred via a flavoprotein (FP) from reduced nicotinamide adenine dinucleotide phosphate (NADPH), and then complexes with molecular oxygen. The complex is then reduced by a second electron derived from reduced nicotinamide adenine dinucleotide (NADH) (or NADPH). The triplex of substrate, cytochrome *P*-450, and O_2 decomposes, with one atom of oxygen reduced to water and the other atom incorporated into the substrate. Oxidized substrates—that is, primary metabolites (alcohols, aldehydes, phenols, epoxides)—may then undergo phase II conjugation reactions via a glutathione *S*-transferase (lower center) or a UDP-glucuronyl transferase (lower left). Alternatively, the substrate may be released as a free radical (R·) or peroxide or hydroperoxide (ROOH). Peroxides would react with cellular glutathione (GSH) via glutathione peroxidase (right), leading, respectively, to RH and ROH. In addition (not shown), epoxides may be hydrolyzed to diols by epoxide hydrase. Adequate intracellular contents of the cofactors NADPH, NADH, O_2, ATP, glucose 1-phosphate (G1P), cysteine, glutathione (GSH), or phosphoadenosine phosphosulfate (PAPS) are required for one or more reactions. Also essential for efficient, safe biotransformation of compounds with reactive primary metabolites is an adequate activity of the appropriate enzyme for the phase II conjugation reaction. (From Reynolds and Moslen, 1980.)

Table 9-2 summarizes the major phase II reactions with regard to the types of conjugations, the enzymes that catalyze the conjugations, and the donor substrates and acceptors for the conjugations. Also listed are representative compounds that undergo the different types of conjugations. Several of the enzymes that catalyze these conjugations, notably the glutathione *S*-transferases, UDP-glucuronyl transferases, and sul-

Table 9–2. Phase II Reactions

Type of conjugation	Enzymes	Donor substrate	Acceptors	Examples
Hydration	Epoxide hydrase	Water	Aliphatic and aromatic epoxides	Bromobenzene epoxide Benz[α]pyrene epoxide
Glycosidation	Glucuronyl transferases	UDP-glucuronate	Aliphatic and aromatic alcohols, phenols, carboxyls, and amines	Trichloroethanol Acetaminophen
Glutathione (GSH)	GSH S-transferases	GSH	Strong electrophiles including epoxides, esters of strong acids, acyl chlorides	Vinyl chloride 1,2-Dibromoethane Acetaminophen
Sulfation	Sulfotransferases	Phosphoadenosine phosphosulfate (PAPS)	Aromatic amines, phenols	Acetaminophen 2-Acetylaminofluorene
Acylation	Acetylases	Acetyl-CoA	Aliphatic and aromatic amines	Aminofluorine Isoniazid
Methylation	Methylases	S-Adenosyl-methionine	Polyhydric phenols, thiols, amines, nitrogen heterocyclics	Hydrogen sulfide
Amino acid	Amino acid transferase	Glycine, glutamine, taurine	Carboxylic acids (CoA derivatives)	Phenoxyacetic acids (2,4-D, 2,4,5-T)

fotransferases, are families of isozymes with different but overlapping substrate specificities. Hepatic epoxide hydrase and UDP-glucuronyl transferase are endoplasmic reticulum membrane enzymes, whereas most of the other hepatic phase II enzymes are predominantly located in the cytoplasmic matrix.

The process of xenobiotic metabolism by liver constituents can be quite complex as illustrated by the schematization of cytochrome P-450 and related conjugation systems in Figure 9-7, and the pathways of trichloroethylene (Figure 9-8) and acetaminophen (Figure 9-9) metabolism. The metabolic processes can involve two or more enzymes that are located in different parts of the cell, require multiple cofactors, proceed via several different intermediates, and lead to the formation of a variety of end products.

Although the hepatic enzymes that catalyze phase I and II reactions are primarily thought of as enzymes that detoxify xenobiotics, these enzymes also function in the metabolism or detoxication of endogenous substrates. For example, the UDP-glucuronyl transferases convert bilirubin to a water-soluble and excretable glucuronyl conjugate. The neurotransmitter serotonin

is a substrate for the acetylases. The hormone testosterone is deactivated by cytochrome P-450. The S-methylases detoxify hydrogen sulfide formed by anaerobic bacteria in the intestinal tract. Therefore, chemicals or conditions that modulate the activity of the phase I and phase II enzymes can affect the metabolism of normal physiologic substances.

CONSEQUENCES OF XENOBIOTIC BIOTRANSFORMATION

Ideally the biotransformation of lipophilic xenobiotics by phase I and II reactions would first introduce a polar group (e.g., a hydroxyl) that could then be efficiently conjugated with another polar entity to produce a stable, water-soluble, and readily excretable compound. Some xenobiotic compounds excreted into the bile as conjugated metabolites are too polar to be reabsorbed from the intestine and do not re-enter the circulatory system. A few xenobiotics excreted into bile, such as the heavy metal hepatotoxins, arsenic and copper, undergo extensive enterohepatic circulation (Klaassen, 1977). Numerous hepatotoxins are converted to unstable reactive metabolites by phase I or phase II reactions.

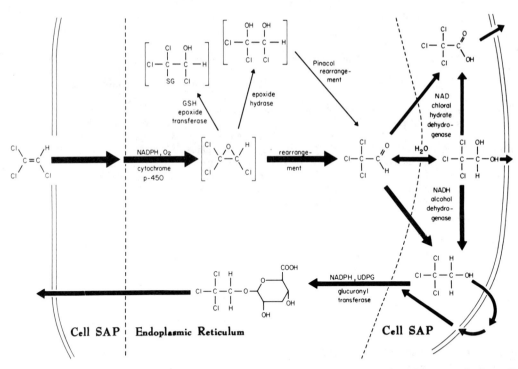

Figure 9–8. Biotransformation of trichloroethylene is assumed to occur by phase I and phase II reactions chiefly along the metabolic route indicated by the largest arrows. NADPH-dependent oxidation by cytochrome *P*-450 produces an epoxide as the primary metabolite, which rearranges with chloride migration to form trichloroacetaldehyde as the major secondary metabolite. Trichloroacetaldehyde is converted to a tertiary generation of metabolites through hydration, enzymatic oxidation, and enzymatic reduction to an alcohol. Trichloroethanol subsequently is conjugated to a glucuronide—the major urinary metabolite. Smaller arrows indicate possible involvement of epoxide hydrase in the rearrangement of the primary epoxide intermediate.

Table 9-3 lists examples of hepatic biotransformation mechanisms by which xenobiotics are converted to reactive electrophilic species. If these reactive species are not detoxified by subsequent metabolic processes or by interaction with cell defense systems, then the reactive electrophiles may interact with a nucleophilic site in a vital cell constituent in an injurious manner (see Figure 9-1). If the alteration is not repaired, acute injury, chronic injury, or neoplasia could result.

What evidence is there that such activations and subsequent molecular alterations actually occur? All of the compounds listed in Table 9-3 (except paraquat) have been demonstrated to bind irreversibly (covalently) to various macromolecular constituents of liver cells. For several of these

compounds the sites of macromolecular binding are consistent, although not necessarily directly linked, with the characteristics of the ensuing hepatic lesion. For example, carbon tetrachloride, which rapidly causes structural, functional, and compositional alterations to the endoplasmic reticulum of hepatocytes, covalently binds to lipid components of the liver endoplasmic reticulum (Reynolds and Moslen, 1980). Diethylnitrosamine, which is a potent animal carcinogen, ethylates the phosphate backbone of liver DNA in a very slowly repaired, persistent manner (Floot et al., 1979).

Evidence for the critical role of the metabolic activation of environmental hepatotoxins to reactive electrophilic intermediates has accumulated from animal studies employing inducers or inhibitors of the

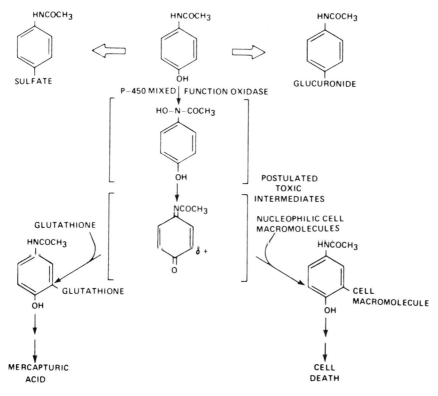

Figure 9–9. Biotransformation of acetaminophen occurs by three alternative pathways. Therapeutic doses of the compound are usually metabolized to glucuronide and sulfate conjugates. With higher doses of acetaminophen, these conjugation reactions become saturated, and increasing amounts of acetaminophen penetrate to the mixed-function oxygenase of the endoplasmic reticulum and the n-H bond of the amido nitrogen is oxidized to a hydroxyl group. This potentially toxic metabolite can be detoxified through a GSH S-transferase-mediated GSH conjugation. However, when large quantities of the toxic metabolite form and then deplete GSH supplies, the reactive metabolite reacts with its macromolecular environment, injuring the cell. Thus, acetaminophen's ability to produce injury depends on the rates of its conjugation by two different saturable pathways, the rate of metabolism by cytochrome *P*-450 and the rate of detoxication of a reactive metabolite by conjugation with GSH. (From Mitchell et al., 1974.)

presumptive activation reaction (Figure 9-10). For example, the sulfuric acid ester metabolite of 2-acetylaminofluorene (Table 9-3, part E) was determined to be the ultimate carcinogenic form for 2-acetyl-aminofluorene (Miller and Miller, 1981) by a series of studies on the liver neoplastic effects of 2-acetylaminofluorene using conditions associated with varying activities of hepatic sulfotransferases. The enlightening studies of Jollow and colleagues (Jollow et al., 1974; Mitchell et al., 1974) with the model hepatotoxin bromobenzene and with acetaminophen (see Figure 9-9) demon-

strated how uses of inducers and inhibitors of the suspect activation and detoxification processes could clarify the mechanisms by which these agents caused liver injury. These studies provided a scientific rationale for the administration of glutathione precursors as an antidote for acetaminophen overdose.

Liver cells are not solely reliant on the detoxification enzymes for protection against reactive electrophilic forms of xenobiotic and endogenous compounds. An antioxidant "line of defense" also provides protection. The major constituents of the antioxidant defense are vitamine E, glutathione, molec-

Table 9–3. Examples of Xenobiotic Biotransformation to Reactive Electrophilic Intermediates

A. Catalyzed by NADPH-cytochrome *P-450* system reactions:
   1. Reductive dechlorination of carbon tetrachloride to a free radical

$$CCl_4 + e^- \rightarrow \bullet CCl_3 + Cl^-$$

   2. Hydroxylation of chloroform to phosgene

$$CHCl_3 + O_2 \rightarrow [HOCCl_3] \rightarrow O{=}CCl_2$$

   3. Monooxidation of vinyl chloride to epoxide

   4. Monooxidation of bromobenzene to an epoxide

   5. Monooxidation of aflatoxin to epoxide

   6. Monooxidative dealkylation of diethylnitrosamine to an ethonium ion

   7. Monooxidative desulfuration of carbon disulfide to reactive-singlet sulfur

B. Catalyzed by cytochrome *P-450* reductase reaction:
   Paraquat-mediated activation of molecular oxygen to superoxide and hydroxyl radicals

$$O_2^{-\bullet} \xrightarrow{SOD} H_2O_2 + O_2$$

$$O_2^{-\bullet} + H_2O_2 \rightarrow H_2O + O_2 + HO\bullet$$

C. Catalyzed by NAD-alcohol dehydrogenase system reactions:
  1. Oxidation of ethanol to acetaldehyde

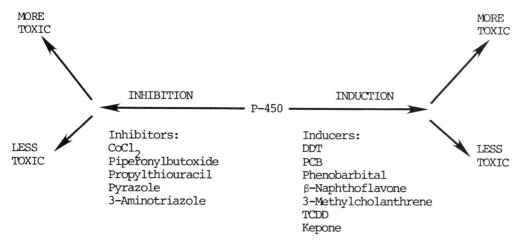

  2. Oxidation of allyl alcohol to acrolein

D. Catalyzed by glutathione S-transferase reaction:
  Glutathione conjugation of 1,2-dibromoethane to a halonium ion

E. Catalyzed by sequential cytochrome P-450 and sulfotransferase reactions:
  Sulfate conjugation of the 2-acetylaminofluorene N-OH metabolite to a
  reactive sulfate ester

Figure 9–10. Schematic of usual effects of cytochrome *P*-450 inducers and inhibitors on the toxicity of xenobiotics. (1) When inhibitors increase toxicity, it is likely that *P*-450 is the site of detoxification, and/or the parent compound or a metabolite formed by an alternate pathway is the toxin. (2) When inhibitors decrease toxicity, then *P*-450 is the likely site of toxification, and the parent compound is less toxic than the metabolite. (3) When *P*-450 inducers increase toxicity, then the metabolite is likely to be more toxic than the parent compound. (4) When inducers decrease toxicity, then the metabolite is less toxic than the parent compound, or a detoxifying metabolic pathway has been induced that forms less toxic metabolites, or the toxic metabolite is more readily detoxified than the parent compound.

MORE
TOXIC

MORE
TOXIC

INHIBITION   INDUCTION

P-450

LESS
TOXIC

LESS
TOXIC

Inhibitors: Inducers:
CoCl$_2$ DDT
Piperonylbutoxide   PCB
Propylthiouracil   Phenobarbital
Pyrazole   β-Naphthoflavone
3-Aminotriazole   3-Methylcholanthrene
                                TCDD
                                Kepone

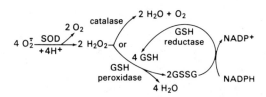

Figure 9–11. Schematic of the interrelationships between four important enzymatic components of the cellular antioxidant defense system. Superoxide dismutase (SOD) catalyzes the dismutation of superoxide (O_2^-) to peroxide. Catalase reduces peroxide to H_2O. GSH peroxidase also detoxifies peroxide by reducing it to H_2O. GSH reductase re-reduces the oxidized glutathione (GSSG) to GSH. The NADPH required for the reduction of GSSG to GSH is primarily supplied by the oxidation of glucose via the pentose phosphate pathway.

ular oxygen, and the series of enzymes that detoxify reactive species of oxygen generated (Figure 9-11).

Vitamin E (α-tocopherol), a lipophilic compound present in liver cells at a 0.05 mM concentration, acts to protect the lipid membranes from electrophilic species by undergoing reversible redox reactions. The principal role of vitamin E apparently is to protect the lipid constituents of membranes against free radical-initiated peroxidation reactions. Evidence for this role of vitamin E in the defense of liver cells against xenobiotic hepatotoxins comes from animal studies with the free-radical toxin carbon tetrachloride. Livers of animals fed diets deficient in vitamin E are more vulnerable to lipid peroxidation following poisoning with CCl_4 (see Reynolds and Moslen, 1980).

Glutathione (GSH), the most abundant water-soluble member of the intracellular antioxidant defense, is present in liver cells at a concentration of 4–7 mM. GSH has a nucleophilic sulfhydryl group that can react with and thus detoxify reactive electrophilic species (Van Bladeren et al., 1980). Glutathione can also donate its sulfhydryl hydrogen to a reactive free radical. The glutathione radical formed is sufficiently stable to undergo annihilation reactions with other glutathione radicals to form stable oxidized GSSG. Reduced glutathione is regenerated

from GSSG by an NADPH-dependent reaction catalyzed by a glutathione reductase (Figure 9-11).

Under normal physiologic conditions, significant concentrations of the active oxygen species—superoxide hydroxyl radical and peroxide—do not accumulate intracellularly. Thus, molecular oxygen may be viewed as a member of the antioxidant defense (Fee, 1981). However, when stable xenobiotic radicals are produced, and superoxide or hydrogen peroxide are formed in excess of the cell's capacity to detoxify them, then radical oxygen-mediated processes of cell injury will ensue.

The occasional observation of liver injury in humans exposed to the broad-spectrum herbicide paraquat (Bullivant, 1966) could potentially be related to deficiencies of constituents of the liver antioxidant "defense." As outlined in Table 9-3 (part B), the metabolism of paraquat can lead to the formation of superoxide. Animal studies have demonstrated that a given dose of paraquat that does not cause liver injury in control mice, will cause liver injury in mice pretreated with a diet deficient in selenium (an essential constituent of GSH peroxidase) or with diethylmaleate (a GSH depletor) (Cagen and Gibson, 1977). Both GSH peroxidase and GSH are involved in the detoxication of superoxide (see Figure 9-11).

Control of Specialized Liver Functions

A variety of physiologic, hormonal, dietary, and xenobiotic compounds exert control over the rate, and specificity of specialized function of the liver. This flexibility to modulate its functions allows the liver to adapt to changes in the external environment (Conney et al., 1977).

GLUCOSE

The liver is the primary reservoir, salvager, and synthesizer of glucose for the body. Blood glucose content is regulated chiefly by the antagonistic actions of insulin and glucagon. Insulin and glucagon bind to specific receptors on the hepatocyte plasma membrane and trigger a series of metabolic processes. Insulin binding leads to increased hepatocyte retention and storage of glucose as glycogen. Insulin activates glucokinase, which phosphorylates glucose (forming glucose 6-phosphate, which cannot diffuse out of the cell) and also activates glycogen synthetase and inhibits glycogen phosphorylase. In contrast, glucagon binding leads to increased hepatocyte release of glucose by stimulating the breakdown of glycogen (glycogenolysis) to free glucose, which passes into the blood through the cell's plasma membrane.

Gluconeogenesis that is, the conversion of amino acids, lactate, and glycerol to glucose—is stimulated by glucagon and inhibited by insulin. This adaptation, in the case of food deprivation, occurs more slowly than those associated with glycogen synthesis and lysis. Rates of gluconeogenesis reach a peak after about 4 days of fasting and decline thereafter as fatty acids become the primary source of energy. In periods of starvation, glucagon converts the liver to a producer of ketones, which are an alternative energy source for the brain.

At any one time the ratio of insulin and glucagon released into the portal blood from the islets of Langerhans controls glucose uptake, storage, synthesis, utilization, and release by the liver. This is essentially a first-pass effect, in that proteolytic enzymes in blood, liver, lung, and other organs readily deactivate these hormones. In chronic liver disease, the delicate antagonistic balance of insulin and glucagon can become disordered. For example, in cirrhotics a significant part of the portal blood may be diverted away from the liver, and serum glucagon levels become abnormally elevated.

Normally the insulin–glucagon control maintains a sufficient liver glycogen supply to regulate blood glucose and to provide for hepatic glucose-dependent function. However, other hormones, notably catecholamines released in response to stress, can stimulate liver glycogen breakdown and rapidly deplete the liver of glycogen.

Environmental chemicals can affect, and be affected, by body glucose homeostasis in several different ways. "Hypoglycin," a chemical present in the seeds of unripe ackee fruit, inhibits gluconeogenesis and produces hypoglycemia in "Jamaican vomiting sickness," a syndrome that does not occur in well-nourished people with adequate liver stores of glycogen (Zimmerman, 1978). Poisoning with carbon tetrachloride rapidly deactivates hepatic glucose 6-phosphatase by damaging the enzymes' membrane environment. Trichloroethylene and several other compounds that are metabolized by the liver to glucuronyl conjugates are more hepatotoxic to fasted animals than fed animals. Low hepatic glycogen contents may also contribute to the greater vulnerability of fasted animals to xenobiotics such as acetaminophen, whose metabolism is associated with depletion of the GSH component of the hepatic antioxidant defense system. Reduction of oxidized GSSG to GSH (see Figure 9-11) requires NADPH; the major source of reducing equivalents for NADPH, which is oxidation of glucose via the pentose pathway, can be compromised by limited availability of hepatic glucose stores.

LIPIDS

Metabolism of lipids by the liver is under strict hormonal regulation. Fatty acids, normally a major source of energy, virtually become the sole source under conditions of physical stress, injury, undernutrition, and starvation. The liver has the major role in fatty acid metabolism through (1) oxidization of fatty acids to ketone bodies, which can be utilized by the brain as a substitute for glucose, (2) converting excess sugars and amino acids into fatty acids and transporting them as "lipoprotein" complexes to adipose tissue for storage, and (3) trapping fatty acids released by adipose tissue and either utilizing or returning them.

Fatty acids are released from adipose tissue through the action of hormones that stimulate activation of lipases. Norepinephrine and epinephrine are the most important physiologic activators of lipases. This activity can also be stimulated by glucagon, ACTH, and other pituitary hormones through common pathways involving increased cyclic adenosine monophosphate (cAMP). In contrast, insulin inhibits hormone-sensitive lipase activity within adipose tissue and suppresses fatty acid oxidation within the liver.

Transport of triglycerides from liver to adipose tissue and other organs is accomplished by its assemblage into very-low-density lipoproteins (VLDL), which consist of a hydrophobic core of triglycerides and cholesterol esters surrounded by an amphophilic layer of phospholiped, cholesterol, and protein. VLDL are assembled within the cisternae of the endoplasmic reticulum, stored in the Golgi, and excreted by "reverse" endocytosis. Normally the rates of fatty acid uptake and synthesis by liver cells do not exceed their capacity to excrete triglyceride as VLDL.

Therefore, although the liver has a crucial role in the economy of fatty acids and triglycerides within the body, a little triglyceride is usually present as recognizable droplets of fat within liver cell cytoplasm. However, as will be discussed in the section on steatosis, accumulation of fat in parenchymal cells is a relatively common response of the liver to almost any form of injury.

CONTROL OF BILE SECRETION

Bile is a yellow fluid, iso-osmolar with plasma, that is formed by the liver. The major constituents of bile are mineral salts (largely Na^+ and Cl^-), bile salts, bile pigments (chiefly bilirubin conjugates), lecithin, and cholesterol. The bile salts, bile pigments, and lipids are packaged as macromolecular aggregates called micelles. The gallbladder concentrates bile about 10-fold by absorption of water and salts. If the gallbladder epithelium is damaged or irritated, the ability to concentrate bile is compromised.

Bile secretion can be altered or controlled by a variety of physiologic and nonphysiologic stimuli. Presence of food in the upper gastrointestinal tract stimulates contraction of the gallbladder and secretion of bile into the duodenum. Approximately 95% of the bile salts secreted into the duodenum are rapidly returned to the liver by the enterohepatic circulation, extracted by hepatocytes, and resecreted into bile. Because bile salts are a major constituent of bile, the concentration of bile salts in portal blood influences the amount of bile acids and bile secreted. Synthetic bile salts, which do not form micelles as efficiently as endogenous bile salts, enhance bile secretion. Some xenobiotic agents that inhibit active sodium transport inhibit bile secretion.

Bile formation is mediated neither solely by a diffusion process (as is urine formation), as was once thought, nor solely by an osmotic gradient generated by an ion pump between the canaliculus and the liver cell (Klaassen, 1977; Boyer, 1980). Liver parenchymal cells actively secrete bile at a higher pressure than sinusoidal blood flow by a sodium-dependent process that is not completely understood.

Boyer (1980) has proposed a new model of bile formation based on the concept that the "hepatocyte is a polar cell in which transport processes are directed to the uptake of solutes across the basolateral or sinusoidal membranes and the secretion of solutes across the small apical surface that lines the lumen of the bile canaliculus." Critical to Boyer's model is the localization of the Mg^{2+}-ATPase responsible for sodium–potassium exchange to the lateral and sinusoidal plasma membranes and the determination that the canalicular plasma membranes had a different type of Mg^{2+}-ATPase, possibly a myosin ATPase activated by the action of the pericanalicular microfilaments (Oda and Phillips, 1975; Blitzer and Boyer, 1978).

Bile salts are proposed to be actively taken up by a sodium-coupled carrier, bound to intracellular transport proteins, packaged into micelles, and then actively secreted into the canaliculi lumen. This type of transcellular pathway with active transport, carrier proteins, and/or secretion of membrane-bound vacuoles is apparently involved in the secretion of a number of bile solutes including bilirubin conjugates.

Time-lapse cinephotomicrography of cultured primary hepatocytes by Oshio and Phillips (1981) demonstrated that bile canaliculi forcefully contract and expel their contents. The contractions were associated with pericanalicular vacuolar movements. One of the few proteins present in bile at high concentrations relative to its plasma concentration is immunoglobin A (IgA), which is secreted into the bile in an endocytic vesicle.

Osmotic forces produced by bile acids and other solutes transported into the bile by the transhepatocyte pathway "pull" water and other solutes into the canaliculi lumen through the semipermeable junctional complexes between hepatocytes that form the barrier between the canaliculi lumen and the sinusoidal space. This paracellular pathway accounts for the bulk of the water and ions present in bile.

Control of Xenobiotic Biotransformation

The capacity of the liver to metabolize environmental chemicals can vary depending on genetic differences, circadian rhythm, diet, hormones, and exposure to xenobiotics.

Clinical studies with twins or families indicate that interindividual differences in the metabolism of a variety of xenobiotics, chiefly drugs, are largely under genetic control, and in some instances are controlled by multiple genetic loci (Atlas and Nebert, 1976). Marked differences in hepatic metabolism have been associated with altered responses or toxicities. For example, an "atypical" genetic variant of hepatic alcohol dehydrogenase with high activity has been found in a high percentage of Japanese persons and may account for the marked immediate sensitivity of many Asiatics to alcohol (Stamatoyannopoulos et al., 1975). Liver injury following treatment with the tuberculostatic agent isoniazid has been linked to the polymorphic phenotype

of "rapid acetylators" of hydrazine-type compounds (Atlas and Nebert, 1976). Rapid acetylators, which are either homozygous or heterozygous for a dominant gene, more rapidly convert isoniazid to a reactive acetylhydrazine metabolite.

Circadian variabilities occur in the rate of xenobiotic metabolism by humans (Vesell, 1977). For example, subjects metabolize ethanol more slowly at night than during the day. Rodents have marked circadian rhythms; activities of hepatic enzymes and contents of cofactors involved in xenobiotic metabolism are higher during the night. For the night-feeding rodent, the timing of this higher capacity for metabolism and presumably detoxification of xenobiotics potentially encountered in food should be beneficial. Indeed, rodents have been found to be more resistant to the hepatotoxic effects of several halogenated hydrocarbons during the night than during the day.

Given the central role of the liver in the processing of dietary nutrients, it should not be surprising that variations in diet can alter the activities of many liver constituents, including those involved in phase I and phase II reactions. A study in which each subject also served as control demonstrated that shifts from "usual home diet" to a low-carbohydrate, high-protein diet increased the hepatic metabolism of representative xenobiotic drugs (Conney et al., 1977). Animal studies indicate that dietary deficiencies in protein or fat markedly diminish liver cytochrome P-450.

Hormones can influence xenobiotic metabolism. Hyperthyroid patients, for example, metabolize aminoantipyrine faster than normal controls, while hypothyroid patients metabolize the drug more slowly (Vessell, 1977). Natural and synthetic steroids with an alkylated C-17 position and a phenolic A ring cause a predictable decrease in hepatic biliary excretory function in all tested subjects (Mowat and Arias, 1969). Sex differences in the vulnerability of rodents to hepatotoxins may be related to hormonal regulation of metabolic pathways in the liver.

Repeated or prolonged exposure to many

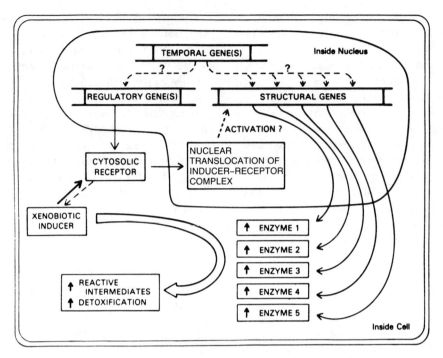

Figure 9–12. Schematic of genetic mechanism of enzyme induction proposed to occur in response to a xenobiotic inducer. Diagram depicts the Ah complex (aryl hydrocarbon hydroxylate) (from Nebert et al., 1981). Major product of the regulatory gene is the cytosolic receptor, which binds the xenobiotic. Various induced enzymes expressed represent products of different structural genes of the complex. Induced enzymes detoxify xenobiotics. Temporal genes control expression of the genetic locus during development, sexual maturation, and aging. Note that the interaction of the inducer–receptor complex with genetic material results in the synthesis of multiple enzymes. (From Nebert et al., 1981.)

xenobiotics metabolized by the liver enhances the rates of biotransformation of the same agent on subsequent exposure. This capacity of environmental chemicals to induce enzymes responsible for their own clearance should, in general, be beneficial. However, the extension of this enhanced metabolic capacity to other compounds can enhance the toxicity of other environmental chemicals.

Induction is not a simple phenomenon. Chemical inducers are known to enhance the synthesis of one or more forms (isozymes) of hepatic enzymes involved in the phase I and II reactions, including cytochrome *P*-450, glutathione *S*-transferase, alcohol dehydrogenase, monoamine oxidase, and UDP-glucuronyl transferase. The various isozymes have different molecular weights, substrate specificities, subunits,

and/or cellular locations. Different inducers "induce" different patterns of phase I and II enzyme activities; some are broad based and others relatively specific.

Figure 9-12 schematizes events thought to occur in response to xenobiotic inducers (Nebert et al., 1981). After the inducer passively diffuses across the cell membranes, it binds with a cytosolic receptor that is the product of a regulatory gene. The receptor–inducer complex translocates across the nuclear envelope, interacts at a promoter site on a chromosome, and activates sequences of structural genes responsible for the synthesis of multiple gene products. Interaction of the receptor–inducer complex at several different promoter sites would lead to the synthesis of multiple groups of gene products.

It is difficult to believe that receptors specific for the recently developed products of modern chemistry have existed since the beginning of biologic time. Rather, xeno-biotics must effectively compete with endogenous substates for binding on specific receptors and then stimulate a serendipitous, factitious, or otherwise inappropriate response. Some critical unanswered questions include these: What are the endogenous substrates for the receptors that bind to xenobiotics? What are consequences that result from the inhibition of binding of the natural endogenous substrates to their receptors?

Pathologic Responses to Environmental Chemicals

A number of different systems have been proposed to classify the types of injury that occur in the liver and biliary tract following exposure to environmental agents. For example, Popper and Schaffner (1959) grouped pathologic responses into five morphologically distinguishable groups: (1) zonal hepatocellular reactions (necrosis and/or steatosis) without inflammatory reactions, (2) intrahepatic cholestasis (primarily stasis of bile in bile canaliculi), (3) hepatic necrosis with inflammatory reactions ("viral hepatitis-like"), (4) hepatic cancer, and (5) unclassified (i.e., morphologic patterns that do not fit into the first four types).

Zimmerman (1978) devised a system of classification based on the postulated mechanism of action of the toxic chemical, the morphologic features of injury, and the circumstances of exposure. A modification of this system is presented in Table 9-4. Zimmerman proposed that all hepatotoxins could be classified as either predictable "intrinsic hepatotoxins" or nonpredictable "host idiosyncratic hepatotoxins." Predictable hepatotoxins reliably produce injury in appropriately exposed persons, have toxic manifestations that exhibit a dose dependency, and readily produce similar lesions in experimental animals. In contrast, the toxic responses of nonpredictable hepatotoxins are highly dependent on the condition of the host, occur at a very low fre-

quency, lack apparent dose dependency, and are not readily replicated in experimental animals. On the basis of their mechanisms of action, predictable hepatotoxins can be further subdivided into agents that chiefly cause cytotoxicity or cholestatis, while nonpredictable toxins can be subdivided into agents that do or do not elicit an allergic response. Both predictable and nonpredictable toxins may produce types of injuries that are similar morphologically (Reynolds and Moslen, 1980).

For a few predictable cytotoxic hepatotoxins, the specific biochemical mechanism by which an agent causes cell injury is quite well understood. For example, ethionine, the ethyl analog of methionine, rapidly depletes cellular ATP by trapping the methyl donor S-adenosylmethionine as S-adenosylethionine. However, for most hepatotoxins, the specific cause-and-effect chain of molecular events critical to the process of initiation of liver injury remains to be unraveled—despite the characterization of numerous biochemical, functional, and/or structural aberrations that occur early in the course of injury. The extensively studied model hepatotoxin carbon tetrachloride has been demonstrated to produce specific early aberrations in the lipid composition, enzyme function, and configuration of the endoplasmic reticulum (Reynolds and Moslen, 1980), yet the linkages between these aberrations and the resulting cell death are not clear. Because the present level of knowledge rarely allows classification of hepatotoxins on the basis of primary critical interference with the function of a specific pathway or organelle, we feel more secure with broad classifications based on predictability of pathogenetic response (Table 9-4) or based on type of morphologic response (Table 9-5).

A classification of diseases in the liver and biliary tract promulgated by the International Association for the Study of Liver and the World Health Organization (U.S., DHEW, 1977) attempts a combined morphologic and pathogenetic classification.

The morphologic classification given in Table 9-5 lists representative xenobiotics that

Table 9–4. Pathogenetic Classification of Liver Responses to Hepatotoxins

Hepatotoxin category	Postulated mechanism	Pathologic lesion	Incidence of injury after exposure	Dose dependency	Latent period	Time course	Replication of lesion in animal
Predictable							
Cytotoxic	Compound or its metabolite damages or interferes with cell compo-nent(s) or pro-cess(es), leading to structural or functional ah-normality.	Often distinctive	High	Apparent	Usually brief	Predictable	Relatively easy
Cholestatic	Compound or its metabolites interfere with bile-excretory mechanisms or pathways.	Distinctive	High	Apparent	Usually brief	Predictable	Relatively easy
Nonpredictable							
Metabolic idiosyncrasy	Rate of generation or detoxica-tion of toxic metabolite is highly depen-dent on variable host factors.	Usually not distinctive	Low	Not apparent	Variable	Predictable when under-stood	Difficult
Hyper-sensitivity	Allergic reactions to chemical or its covalently bound adducts occur.	Usually not distinctive	Very low	Not apparent	Variable	Not predictable	Difficult

Source: Modified from Zimmerman (1978).

have been associated with each type of change in humans and/or experimental animals. This classification system differs from the three previously mentioned systems in several ways. Adaptive responses and metabolic derangements are listed as separate categories. Acute zonal and nonzonal hepatocellular necroses, although morphologically distinct, are included together under the category of toxic hepatitis.

A note of caution must be sounded before these morphologic entities are discussed. Similar alterations can occur as a consequence of multiple conditions. For example, the accumulation of large and small droplets of triglycerides in liver parenchy-mal cells with or without occasional foci of necrosis or fibrosis or association with conspicuous pleomorphism of hepatocytic nuclei may be observed in a person exposed to fumes of various hepatotoxic solvents as well as in persons with early alcoholic hepatitis. Centrolobular necrosis observed at autopsy in the absence of other specific lesions may well be the result of diminished blood flow or congestive heart failure or both, and is not necessarily attributable to a primary hepatotoxic event per se. Confusing, often conflicting nomenclature, as well as inadequate characterization of the lesions produced, including preneoplastic changes, interfere with the diagnosis of hepatic injury

Table 9–5. Morphologic Classification of Liver Responses to Hepatotoxins

Response	Representative toxin
Adaptation	
Steatosis	Alcohol, hydrazine
Proliferation of smooth endoplasmic reticulum	DDT, polychlorinated biphenyls
Microbody increase	Clofibrate
Metallothionein increase	Cadmium
Metabolic derangement	
Porphyria	Hexachlorobenzene, TCDD
Other metabolic derangements	Ethionine, ethanol
Acute toxic hepatitis	
Zonal necrosis	Allyl alcohol, nitrosamines, carbon tetrachloride, elemental phosphorus, copper, poisonous mushrooms (genus *Amanita*)
Diffuse "viral hepatitis-like" focal necrosis	Isoniazid
Intrahepatic cholestasis	
Pure cholestasis without inflammation	C-17 Alkylated anabolic steroids
Cholestasis with inflammation	Chlorpromazine
Vascular diseases	
Veno-occlusive disease	Pyrrolidizine alkaloids from senecio plants
Budd-Chiari syndrome	Oral contraceptives, radiation
Chronic liver injury	
Active viral "diffuse hepatitis"	Oxyphenistatin
Fibrosis	Vitamin A, vinyl chloride
Cirrhosis	Aflatoxin, alcohol
Neoplasia	
Liver cell adenoma	Oral contraceptives
Malignant hemangioendothelioma	Arsenic, Thorotrast, vinyl chloride
Cholangiosarcoma	Thorotrast
Hepatocellular carcinoma	Cycasin, aflatoxin

from environmental factors. This problem will diminish as improvements are made in the characterization of the biochemical and morphologic consequences of environmental chemical exposure as well as through increased clinical vigilance.

ADAPTATION

Adaptations are responses of the liver to physiologic and xenobiotic stimuli wherein the cells themselves are not destroyed and the biochemical, functional, and/or morphologic changes are (potentially) reversible. Cells are considered to be responding to humoral and other pathophysiologic events in their environment in an effort to maintain homeostasis.

Steatosis

Fatty liver, or steatosis, is characterized biochemically by a triglyceride (lipid) content greater than 5% by weight and histologically by the appearance of an excessive amount of stainable fat droplets. Usually, the accumulation of an amount of fat sufficient to displace a significant amount of the functioning parenchyma is regarded as a pathologic change. However, fat accumulation can also stem from dietary or hormonal perturbations in the liver's central role in the metabolism and distribution of fatty acids and triglycerides. Thus, fat can be stored in the liver as an energy source analogous to glycogen.

Fatty liver can result from single or multiple defects in the normal process of fat metabolism, including the following:

1. Stimulation of excessive entry of free fatty acids into the liver may occur as a consequence of starvation, stress (catecholamine release), and endogenous or therapeutic excess of corticosteroids.

2. Interference with the synthesis of phospholipids from triglycerides through nutritional lack of precursors, such as the methyl group donors methionine and choline, is a defect seen in animals given ethionine (which traps the methyl donor S-adenosylmethionine) or choline-deficient diets.

3. Increased fatty acid synthesis may occur when there is an increase in β-glycerophosphate, the carbohydrate backbone of triglycerides.

4. Decrease in fatty acid oxidation is a defect that can occur when other sources provide reducing equivalents normally formed by fat oxidation.

5. Decreased synthesis of apoproteins necessary for the excretion of triglycerides as lipoproteins may occur.

6. Coupling of triglycerides or cholesterol with apoproteins in the assembly of secreted VLDL may be impaired.

7. Secretion of assembled VLDL from the liver may be impaired.

Thus, accumulation of fat in liver parenchymal cells can be the consequence of multiple causes ranging from a response to physiologic signals to outright destruction of the VLDL-excretion pathway.

Under some circumstances, extreme steatosis may be injurious per se. However, usually when the nutritional or metabolic defect is corrected, the process leading to fat accumulation is readily reversed and the accumulated fat cleared from the liver. Steatosis is such a common adaptive response to dietary/metabolic abnormalities, as well as such a common consequence of many toxic agents (even those that do not primarily involve the liver) that fat accumulation cannot be considered as a specific response to any environmental agent.

Proliferation of Smooth Endoplasmic Reticulum

Exposure to many xenobiotics leads to an increase in liver cytoplasmic contents of endoplasmic reticulum. This increase chiefly involves smooth components of this organelle and occurs predominantly in centrolobular hepatocytes, which become strikingly enlarged. Most of the xenobiotics that cause this proliferation are metabolized by the endoplasmic reticulum NADPH–cytochrome P-450 system and induce increases in one or more activities catalyzed by this system.

Chemicals that induce proliferation of the endoplasmic reticulum constituents include synthetic steroids, ethanol, the widely used solvent 1,1,1-trichloroethane, and the environmentally persistent polyhalogenated aromatics, including DDT, polychlorinated or brominated biphenyls (PCB,PBBs) and tetrachlorodibenzo-dioxin (TCDD). This change is considered primarily as an adaptive response, because the capacity of a xenobiotic to induce the enzymes that metabolize the xenobiotic should result in its accelerated clearance from the body.

Noninvasive tests are available to determine if humans have increased liver NADPH–cytochrome P-450 activities. Two useful tests are the measurement of the exhalation of ^{13}C- or ^{14}C-labeled CO_2 derived from the hepatic oxidative demethylation of [^{13}C] or [^{14}C] aminopyrine and the measurement of blood clearance of sulfobromophthalein, which is oxidatively debrominated and glucuronidated in the liver, and before secretion in bile. Clinical studies have documented elevated liver NADPH–cytochrome P-450 activities by such noninvasive tests in multiple occupational groups compared to control groups, for example, New York state workers exposed to PCBs at a capacitator-manufacturing plant (Alvares et al., 1977), Swedish sprayers of lindane and DDT (Kolmodin-Hedman, 1974), and Australian petrol pump attendants (Harman et al., 1981).

The adaptive phenomenon of induction of endoplasmic reticulum components is not without pathologic implications. Factitious increases in enzyme systems that accelerate the deactivation of endogenous compounds may alter the internal milieu of the body. For example, estrogens and testosterone may be cleared more rapidly. Environmental chemicals may be more rapidly activated or more slowly detoxified. Animal studies have demonstrated that pretreatments with potent inducers of the NADPH–cytochrome P-450 system (e.g., PCBs, phenobarbital) enhance both the metabolism and the hepatotoxicity of carbon tetrachloride, bromobenzene, halothane, trichloroethylene, and acetaminophen (see Jollow et al., 1974; Mitchell et al., 1974; Reynolds and Moslen, 1980).

In the next section on acute toxic hepatitis, case histories (see legends of Figures 9-13 and 9-17) will be presented of two individuals who were long-standing users of chemicals that modulate the hepatic constituents involved in xenobiotic metabolism before their exposure to the presumptive xenobiotic hepatotoxins.

Microbody Increase

Microbodies, or peroxisomes, increase in number in liver cells as a respone to clofibrate and other hypolipidemic drugs (Reddy, 1973). The mechanism of increased number is unknown. Microbodies, which contain peroxidase and catalase, provide part of the intracellular defense against active oxygen species such as superoxide and peroxide. Thus, this adaptive response may be of potential benefit to the liver.

Metallothionein Increase

Metallothionein, a cytosol matrix protein with a high cysteine content, has a high affinity for certain metals, notably Cd, Zn, Hg, Ag, and Sn. Exposure of animas to low levels of Cd and Zn induces marked increases in the metallothionein content of liver cells. This adaptive response can have protective consequences, because induced animals with high hepatic metallothionein contents are protected against the toxic effects of subsequent administration of large doses of Cd (Leber and Miya, 1976). The usual environmental sources of cadmium are inhaled tobacco smoke and Cd-rich shellfish, liver, and kidney.

Metabolic Derangement

Derangements of specific metabolic pathways in the liver can affect the functional integrity of the organ and the health of the person. Environmental chemicals can cause metabolic derangements that deplete energy sources or detrimentally alter synthetic or degradative processes. Some common dietary constituents can damage the livers of people with inherited metabolic defects; others when consumed in excess can perturb multiple hepatic functions.

Porphyria

The porphyrias are a group of disorders in which inborn or chemically induced derangements of enzymes involved in protoheme biosynthesis result in an increased formation of the porphyrins or their precursors. Where derangements of porphyria synthesis result in accumulation of excess porphyrin, the condition is called hepatic porphyria.

Hexachlorobenzene residues in seed grain used for food gave rise to an epidemic of porphyria in Turkey from 1955 to 1959 (Ockner and Schmid, 1961; Courtney, 1979). Most of the injured Turks were children aged 5 to 16. Photosensitivity with subsequent skin lesions and red urine were the most common symptoms. About one-third of the patients had hepatomegaly. Excess porphyria formation by hexachlorobenzene has been linked to a progressive decrease in uroporphyrinogen decarboxylase, the enzyme that decarboxylates uroporphyrinogen III, an intermediate porphyrin species. Uroporphyrinogen III accumulates, and the synthesis pathway does not proceed to form the final product protoheme, which exerts feedback repression over the key regulatory enzyme ALA synthetase. The consequence is an activation of the whole synthetic process, and a massive excess of uroporphyrinogen III. Exposures to other persistent polyhalogenated aromatics including TCDD and endrin have also been associated with cases of porphyria.

Other Metabolic Derangements

Galactosemia is an example of an inherited defect wherein reversible liver injury can result from a common dietary consituent. People with galactosemia have a deficiency in galactose 1-phosphate uridyl transferase, the enzyme that converts galactose to glucose. Galactose and galactose 1-phosphate accumulate in tissues. When newborns with this deficiency are given galactose-containing cow's milk, marked steatosis, bile stasis, bile duct proliferation, and large liver lobes develop within the first month of life. Removal of galactose from the diet relieves the symptoms and results in remission, whereas continued galactose consumption can lead to cirrhosis.

Ethanol is an example of a voluntarily consumed drug that can cause myriad metabolic alterations in the liver (see review of Lieber, 1980). When alcohol is present it becomes the preferred fuel for the liver and displaces up to 90% of all other substrates. Oxidation of alcohol by the NAD–alcohol dehydrogenase system results in the formation of more NADH than the liver can reasonably utilize and a relative deficiency of the oxidized cofactor NAD. The enhanced NADH:NAD ratio contributes to an increased lactate:pyruvate ratio. Hyperlactacidemia can result from a decreased utilization of lactate. Hypoglycemia may result from impaired gluconeogenesis. Mitochrondria use reducing equivalents from ethanol and oxidize fewer fatty acids, which normally are the chief energy source of the liver. Fat accumulates, and protein synthesis is impeded.

An additional possible consequence of the biotransformation of large amounts of chemicals such as ethanol, by processes that require large amounts of molecular oxygen or perturb normal balances of energy equivalents, is that cells may become metabolically stressed. Severe metabolic stress where the cellular supply of energy equivalents or oxygen drops below that required to maintain functions essential to cell survival such as membrane (Na, K) pumps, may account for the centrolobular foci of necrotic cells observed subsequent to alcohol binges and in alcoholic hepatitis.

ACUTE TOXIC HEPATITIS

Liver cell injury characterized by rapid onset of parenchymal degeneration or overt necrosis is called acute toxic hepatitis. The cellular changes are accompanied by an inflammatory reaction—increased blood flow, edema and cellular infiltrations, and regeneration of lost parenchymal mass. The clinical signs and symptoms of acute toxic hepatitis—that is, malaise and anorexia in mild cases and jaundice, hemorrhage, and coma in severe cases—are consequences of the inability of the injured liver cells to carry out their normal functions. Injury can be so slight that it is apparent functionally but not morphologically. Environmental chemicals can cause localized, zonal injury to cells in parts of the lobule or produce a nonlocalized, focal injury to scattered cells.

Zonal Necrosis

The acute and subacute liver necrosis caused by environmental chemicals is predominantly zonal, involving centrolobular, midzonal, or periportal parenchyma—depending on the specific toxin. Centrolobular necrosis is by far the most frequent form. Acetaminophen (Figure 9-13), cadmium, the industrial solvent trichloroethylene (Figure 9-14), and the anesthetic Fluroxene (Figure 9-15) are centrolobular parenchymal cell toxins, whereas the industrial copolymer 1,1-

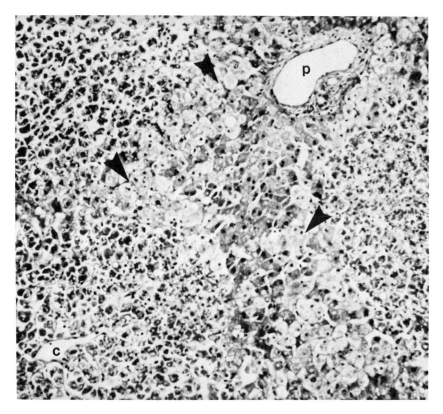

Figure 9–13. Acute toxic hepatitis with centrolobular necrosis following acetaminophen use in a middle-aged man with a long history of alcohol abuse. He took approximately 50 g of acetaminophen over a 3-day period for severe abdominal pain. On admission he was febrile and jaundiced, and he proceeded to develop hypotension. SGOT rapidly rose to 7720 IU. X-Ray examination revealed free air in the abdomen. At laparotomy, a ruptured bladder was repaired and the liver biopsied. Recovery was gradual, and the patient was eventually discharged. This representative portion of the biopsy specimen reveals acute centrolobular necrosis. Portal area (p) at upper right; central veins (c) at lower left. Vacuolated cells (arrows) are present at the interface between necrotic centrolobular hepatocytes and viable periportal areas. [Case: courtesy of Dr. Craig J. McClain (McClain et al., 1980).]

dichloroethylene, the diuretic agent furosemide, and the diagnostic agent radioactive colloidal gold are midzonal toxins. Periportal parenchymal cell necrosis follows ingestion of the poisonous mushroom *Amanita phalloides* (Figure 9-16) and white phosphorus (Figure 9-17). Steatosis of parenchyma in any zone can accompany the necrosis (Figure 9-18).

Reasons for the zonal hepatotoxicity of environmental toxins include transzonal gradients of one or more of the following:

Entry rate of the xenobiotic into the liver cell.

Persistence of the xenobiotic within the cell,

Specificities of enzymes or isozymes involved in the activation or detoxification of the xenobiotic,

Availability of cofactors for activation or detoxification processes,

Availability of molecular oxygen.

The zonal hepatotoxicity of some environmental chemicals is consistent with zonal differences in the activities of enzymes that activate the chemical. For example, most chemicals that are primarily activated by the preponderantly centrolobular NADPH–cy-

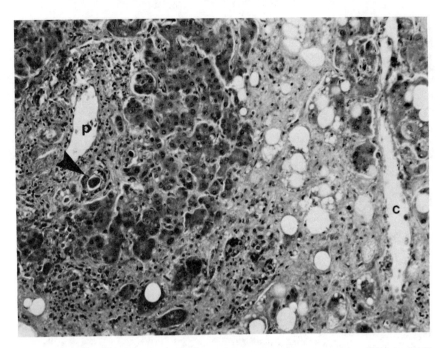

Figure 9–14. Subacute toxic hepatitis with centrolobular necrosis, stromal collapse, and fibrosis in a middle-aged tool manufacturer exposed to "trichloroethylene" fumes. The man was in good health until he exposed himself to the vapors over a heated vat purported to contain trichloroethylene. Three days later he noted a sore throat, malaise, then anorexia and vomiting. By the seventh day after exposure he was jaundiced, had an ecchymotic rash, hepatomegaly, and ascites. Renal failure ensued. He lapsed into coma and died on day 22 after exposure. This history is unusual for trichloroethylene toxicity, in that people exposed to high concentrations of this chlorocarbon usually are narcotized long before sufficient trichloroethylene is absorbed to produce liver injury. The actual contents of the vat were not determined.

The liver obtained at autopsy reveals overall preservation of hepatic architecture with portal area (p) on left and central vein (c) on right. Parenchymal cells are absent from the centrolobular area, and its stroma is collapsed, trapping within it some large fat vacuolated hepatocytes. Bile ducts are increased in portal areas, and some ducts contain bile plugs (arrows). Loss of parenchymal cells and stromal collapse focally connect, that is, "bridge" portal areas and central veins. This case imperfectly fulfills criteria 1, 3, and 5 of Table 9–1.

tochrome *P*-450 system cause centrolobular necrosis (e.g., carbon tetrachloride, bromobenzene, and the nitrosamines), whereas allyl alcohol, which is activated to allyl aldehyde (acrolein) by the predominantly periportal alcohol dehydrogenase, causes periportal injury. More extensive uptake of phalloidin by the periportal cells (possibly via the same active uptake process responsible for the efficient liver extraction of bile acids from portal blood) may account for the periportal injury caused by the phalloidin.

Diffuse Focal Necrosis

A few toxins cause acute or subacute focal hepatic necrosis wherein dead cells with acidophilic cytoplasm and pyknotic nuclear remnants are scattered randomly in the parenchymal cell plates in all lobular zones. Macrophages and other inflammatory cells including leukocytes often, but not always, surround these cells. Centrolobular cholestasis may be a prominent feature. Because this form of acute or subacute hepatocellular injury resembles viral hepatitis both

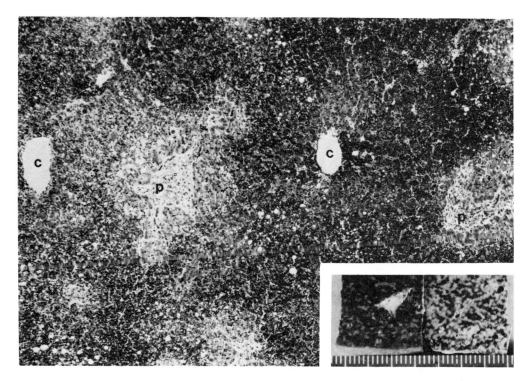

Figure 9–15. Acute toxic hepatitis with massive hepatocellular necrosis following Fluroxene administration in an older woman with a long history of diphenylhydantoin, phenobarbital, and phenylbutazone treatment, and a 4-year history of gastric ulcer. She developed massive hematemesis responsive to transfusions. Seizures recurred, which responded to high doses of diphenylhydantoin (2400 mg/day). Twenty days later she underwent subtotal gastrectomy. Immediately before surgery, liver function tests were normal. The anesthetic was 6% Fluroxene. The operation lasted 6 hours, and hypertension and hypoxia were *not* complications. Postoperatively, the patient was alert. Fourteen hours later she was in shock, and SGOT was 3000 IU. At the time of death, 36 hours after operation, SGOT had risen to 8640 IU, and prothrombin time was prolonged to 60 seconds. Grossly hemorrhagic necrosis (dark areas in gross photograph in inset) involved the centrolobular half in the block on the right and almost all the parenchyma on the left. Massive predominantly centrolobular necrosis was confirmed microscopically. P, portal area; C, central vein.

clinically and morphologically, the latter must be ruled out as a possible cause. Diffuse "hepatitis-like" necrosis has been associated with the widely prescribed tuberculostatic compound isoniazid, and several other drugs including iproniazid, chlorpromazine, and other phenothiazines.

INTRAHEPATIC CHOLESTASIS

Cholestasis is a decrease or absence of bile secretion from the liver coupled with an accumulation of biliary constituents in bile canaliculi. The disease frequently presents with steatorrhea which is characterized by frequent fatty stools, pruritis or skin itchiness, and jaundice. These symptoms are consequences, respectively, of inadequate biliary secretion of bile acids needed for dietary fat absorption, elevated blood contents of bile acid, and systemic increases in bilirubin glucuronide. The bilirubin that accumulates in the blood of persons with uncomplicated xenobiotic-induced intrahepatic cholestasis is chiefly bilirubin diglucuronide; this is bile pigment that may have leaked back into the blood from the distended obstructed bile canaliculi. Intrahe-

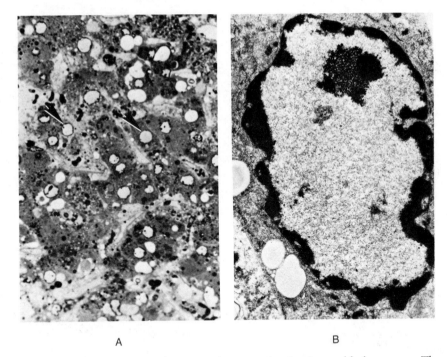

A   B

Figure 9–16. Acute toxic hepatitis due to mushroom poisoning in an elderly woman. The woman picked mushrooms near her home, and cooked and ate them. Persistent vomiting and watery diarrhea ensued within 10 hours, and by 48 hours she was in shock. She died 2 days later. The symptoms and clinical course are characteristic of the phallotoxin, α-amantine, produced by the *Amanita* genus of mushroom. α-Amantine, which inhibits DNA-dependent RNA polymerase II, affects nuclei of hepatocytes. (A) By light microscopy, nuclei appear centrally vacuolated like "Orphan Annie eyes" (arrows). (B) By electron microscopy, nuclear components segregate and fragment. Chromatin is dispersed and deposits as dense clumps against the inner layer of the nuclear envelope. [Case: Courtesy of Dr. Robert Kisilevsky (Kisilevsky, 1974).]

patic cholestasis must always be distinguished from extrahepatic cholestasis caused by impacted gallstones, tumors involving the extrahepatic biliary tract, bacterial infection of the biliary tract, or other causes of bile duct obstruction.

Pure Cholestasis without Inflammation

Cholestasis is morphologically manifest by the appearance of yellow-orange-brown branching bile plugs in canaliculi and sometimes in small bile ducts, and by the absence of overt cell necrosis or inflammatory cell infiltrates. Bile canaliculi are dilated, are surrounded by a dense material, and have shortened or absent microvilli. This condition is most commonly observed in women taking oral contraceptives. Mowat

and Arias (1969) demonstrated that administration of C-17 alkylated steroids with a phenolic A ring caused a predictable, reversible reduction in hepatic excretory function. When excretory function was decreased by more than 90%, jaundice occurred. Women with the Dubin-Johnson syndrome, an inherited defect in hepatic excretory function associated with a mild hyperbilirubinemia, rapidly develop jaundice during the first or second cycle of oral contraceptives.

Several natural constituents, including a South African plant constituent icterogenin, the fungal toxins sporidemin and cytochalasin B, and the mushroom toxin phalloidin, cause cholestasis in domestic and experimental animals. Icterogenin is a C-17 alkylated steroid-like compound that may

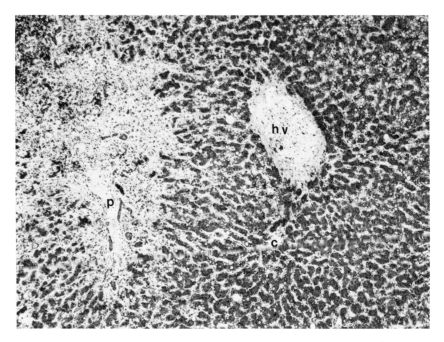

Figure 9–17. Toxic hepatitis with periportal necrosis following exposure to white phosphorus in a seaman. One day out of port the seaman developed a flulike syndrome that progressed to delirium over the next 4 days. On evacuation from his ship he was found to be febrile, disoriented, and jaundiced. SGOT was 1600 IU and blood ammonia 168 mmol/liter. His condition continued to deteriorate; he went into shock and died on the seventh day of his illness. Autopsy revealed a periportal pattern of acute hepatocellular necrosis. Portal area (p) to the left, central lobular vein (c) and sublobular hepatic vein (h.v.) to the right. Gas chromatography–mass spectrometry analysis of liver extracts revealed a peak at 124 MW, characteristic of tetrameric phosphorus (P_4).

act by a mechanism similar to that of the C-17 alkylated oral contraceptives. Phalloidin, which binds to F actin and prevents its depolymerization, causes a thickening of the actin microfilament matrix around bile canaliculi and increased paracellular permeability of the bile canaliculi (Elias et al., 1980).

Cholestasis with Inflammation

Cholestasis with overt cell necrosis and inflammatory cell infiltration frequently occurs as a consequence of acute parenchymal cell injury (see Figure 9-18). Occasionally, the syndrome may occur as a result of primary injury to the bile canaliculi or bile ducts. Cholestasis has been associated with occupational exposure to 4′,4-diamino-diphenylmethane and in numerous people taking the widely used phenothiazine tran-

quilizer chlorpromazine. Histologic findings have included bile "thrombi" in canaliculi, bile staining in parenchymal and Kupffer cells, scattered foci of cell necrosis, and portal inflammatory exudate.

VASCULAR DISEASES

Veno-Occlusive Disease

Veno-occlusive disease is characterized by acute and/or chronic occlusion of the centrolobular and sublobular hepatic veins by loose fibrous tissue. The larger veins are not affected. The major environmental factor associated with this disease is ingestion of pyrrolizidine alkaloids, which are components of several hundred species of plants (Zimmerman, 1978). Cases in Jamaica have been associated with drinking "bush tea," a folk remedy for acute illness that is made

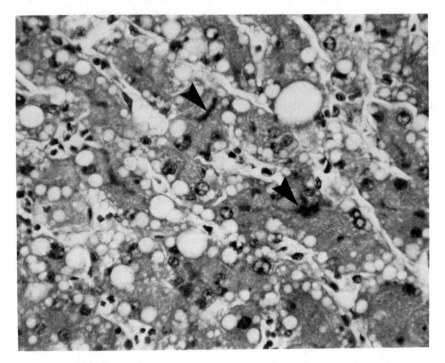

Figure 9–18. Intrahepatic cholestasis and fatty metamorphosis in white phosphorus poisoning. Arrows point to bile plugs in distended bile canaliculi. The large numbers of clear cytoplasmic vacuoles contain triglycerides.

from the *Senecio jacoboea* plant, in South Africa with eating senecio-contaminated bread, in central Asia with eating cereal grains contaminated by seeds of *Heliotropium lasiocarpium,* and in central India with eating cereals contaminated by *Crotalaria* seeds. The pyrrolizidine alkaloid phytotoxins produce scarring and obliteration of hepatic veins with blockage of the hepatic venus outflow tract.

The clinical features of veno-occlusive disease depend on the amount and duration of pyrrolizidine alkaloid exposure. The disease can be acute, subacute, or chronic. Acute veno-occlusive disease begins with the abrupt onset of hepatomegaly and ascites. Centrolobular necrosis may be a concomitant of injury. Recovery may occur in a matter of weeks, or the disease may progress to a fatal outcome. As the chemical course becomes more protracted and centrolobular scarring about the central vein becomes a more prominent feature, the pathologic picture progresses to a "conges-

tive" cirrhosis. "Megalocytosis," enlargement of hepatocytes by as much as 30 times their normal size, is a feature of chronic disease due to these agents. his nuclear aberration is considered to result from the antimitotic activity of pyrrolizidine alkaloids.

When the disease has occurred in a given area, the incidence has been greater in poor people. However, it is not known whether the poor are more likely to ingest contaminated foods or have a greater propensity (possibly due to protein deprivation) to activate the pyrrolizidine alkaloids to reactive intermediates.

Budd-Chiari Syndrome

Budd-Chiari syndrome is a rare disorder characterized by partial or complete obstruction of the inferior vena cava or hepatic veins and their tributaries. The acute type of this syndrome usually presents with abdominal pain, nausea, an enlarged tender liver, and severe ascites. Esophageal varices may quickly develop. Usually there is no jaundice. In the chronic type of this syndrome, the same symptoms develop more slowly. Usually the hepatic veins are both sclerosed and thrombosed. There is a proliferation of fibrous tissues in the veins plus extreme congestion of the lobule. Prognosis is usually grave. The liver scintiscan is a valuable noninvasive test that can aid in establishing the diagnosis of this syndrome.

Oral contraceptives have been linked to the Budd-Chiari syndrome. A cause–effect relationship has not yet been established; however, the incidence of venous thrombosis is 3 to 10 times higher in women using oral contraceptives. A review of Budd-Chiari syndrome by Lockhat et al. (1981) noted that before the commercial introduction of oral contraceptives, the syndrome occurred with equal frequency in males and females, whereas after that time the syndrome has been reported in twice as many women as men. Radiation has also been associated with the syndrome.

CHRONIC LIVER INJURY

Repeated or continued exposure to environmental chemicals can cause slowly evolving or delayed liver necrosis and scarring.

Diffuse Hepatitis

A number of people who were prolonged users of the laxative preparations containing oxyphenisatin have been reported to develop acute or chronic hapatitis, which sometimes progressed to cirrhosis and occasionally resulted in death from hepatic failure (Klatskin, 1975). A large number of nonprescription laxatives used to contain oxyphenisatin before the hepatotoxicity of this chemical was recognized. In most cases of chronic oxyphenisatin poisoning, hepatitis occurred after a latent period of more than 1 year. Clinical, laboratory, and morphologic features frequently resembled those of viral hepatitis. Withdrawal from the laxative preparations usually led to a slow but complete recovery. Invariably, re-exposure

caused a recurrence within days to weeks. Based on the prompt recurrence on challenge and the frequent finding of serologic markers of an immunologic reation in people taking this laxative, the mechanism of oxyphenisatin-induced hepatitis is considered to be an allergic sensitization reaction (Klatskin, 1975).

Fibrosis

Fibrosis is characterized by the deposition of excessive amounts of collagen such that the features of the hepatic lobules are accented, but neither the architecture of the liver nor the portocentral flow of blood are disrupted. Evidence for regeneration of hepatic parenchyma in nodular growth patterns (i.e., regenerative nodules) is minimal. Presinusoidal portal hypertension is sometimes present. The extrahepatic portion of the portal vein is often dilated and tortuous, while the intrahepatic radicals are narrow and tapering. Collagen accumulation can result from the collapse of preexisting lobular connective tissue stroma or be from the formation of new fibers. The biosynthesis of collagen fibers is often accelerated by sustained liver cell injury. Pericellular fibrosis hampers liver function by impeding the exchange of materials between blood and hepatocytes.

Hepatic fibrosis associated with exposure to environmental chemicals usually is a consequence of recurrent injury following repetitive exposure or continuous injury following prolonged low-level exposure. Significant numbers of cases of fibrosis were encountered during World Wars I and II in defense industry workers repeatedly exposed to tetrachloroethane, dinitrobenzene, and chlorinated naphthalenes (Zimmerman, 1978). Portal fibrosis with portal hypertension has also been found in humans repeatedly exposed to arsenic compounds or vinyl chloride (Popper et al., 1978). Excessive dietary or supplemental intake of vitamin A has been linked to hepatic fibrosis with striking perisinusoidal fibrosis and obliteration of the space of Disse by swollen fat-storing Ito cells. The swollen

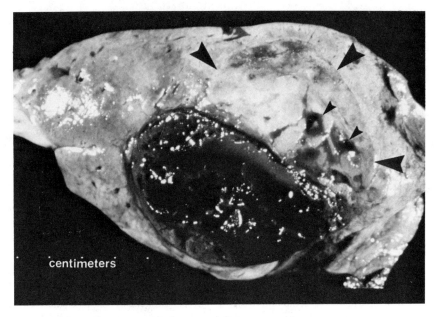

A

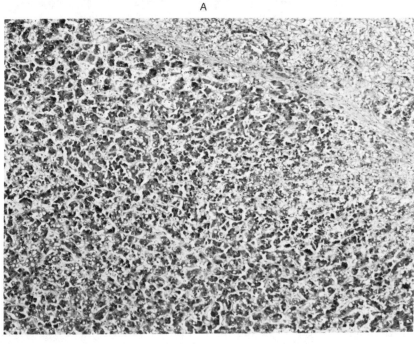

B

Figure 9–19. Liver cell adenoma in a young woman who had taken oral contraceptive pills containing estrogens ethylated at the C-17 position for 8 years. This person had a sudden onset of acute right upper quadrant abdominal pain that radiated to the right shoulder. On admission there was a leukocytosis and she was explored. A large subcapsular hematoma of the liver was found and evacuated. Symptoms were not alleviated, the patient was re-explored 10 days later, and a liver adenoma was found on biopsy. Because of an aggressive peritonitis, sepsis, and progressive respiratory insufficiency, the patient died on the twenty-ninth hospital day. At autopsy, the liver was markedly enlarged, fatty, and contained eight liver cell adenomas. Adjacent to the largest one in the right lobe was a large organizing hematoma that extended through the capsule of the liver. (A) The gross picture is a cross section through the level of the largest adenoma (delineated by large arrows) and its adjacent hema-

Ito cells in one case (Jacques et al., 1979) contained green fluorescence that faded to blue, which is characteristic of vitamin A fluorescence. Thus, this case meets hepatotoxicity criterion 4 in Table 9-1.

Cirrhosis

Cirrhosis, the end stage of all acute, subacute, and chronic liver diseases, shows partial or total obliteration of lobular architecture and regenerative nodules, in addition to prominent fibrosis. When the regenerative nodules are small (< 1 cm in diameter) and few normal vascular markings are retained, the process is termed micronodular cirrhosis. When the regenerative nodules are large (> 1 cm) and retain some normal lobular vascular markings (i.e., portal triads and central veins within the nodules), the process is called macronodular cirrhosis. Neither of these two types of cirrhosis is a specific sequela of any type of environmental chemical. The most common chemical cause of micronodular cirrhosis is prolonged alcohol abuse.

Neoplasia

Liver neoplasia can involve a series of processes in which one or more chemicals act as initiator, promoter, and/or cocarcinogen (see review of Farber, 1982). *Initiators* interact with chromosomes or the cell constituents that maintain chromosome integrity in ways that alter the composition, structure, and/or fidelity of DNA replication or repair. A mutation may be introduced, or an oncogene may be activated. A critical consequence of the genomic alterations produced by initiators is that such altered cells can subsequently act as sites of origin for the development of neoplasia. *Promoters* stimulate replication of cells.

Several chemical promoters of liver neoplasia have been reported to stimulate preferentially replication of liver cells with altered genomes (Schulte-Hermann et al., 1981). *Cocarcinogens* may act in several ways, including enhancing the rate of activation of the responsible chemical to its ultimate carcinogenic form, diminishing the rate of detoxification of the active species generated from the proximate carcinogenic form, or diminishing the rate and/or efficiency of DNA repair. A key distinction between promoters and cocarcinogens is that exposure to promoters must occur after exposure to the initiator, whereas exposure to the cocarcinogen can occur before or at the same time as exposure to the initiator. Exposure to an initiator or cocarcinogen can be solitary or brief, whereas repeated or prolonged exposure to a promoter is necessary.

Four types of liver tumors whose induction is considered to be significantly influenced by environmental chemicals are liver cell adenomas, angiosarcomas, cholangiosarcomas, and hepatocellular carcinomas.

Liver Cell Adenoma

Liver cell adenomas are rare benign tumors composed of mature, often vacuolated hepatocytes, arranged in cords, but without recognizable lobular architecture or portal areas. Fibrous capsules may (but not always) separate the adenoma from normal parenchyma. These tumors tend to be large, are often multiple, are highly vascular, usually occur in otherwise normal (i.e., noncirrhotic) liver, and contain multiple areas of recent or old hemorrhage. A significant proportion become manifest as an abdominal catastrophe due to hemorrhage into the tumor, which may have ruptured into the peritoneum (Figure 9-19).

toma (lower center). The hematoma approaches the liver capsule at the lower right. Small areas of hemorrhage can also be seen within the adenoma (small arrows). (B) Microscopically, liver cell adenoma consists of cells resembling hepatocytes in parenchymal cell cords. Portal triads and central veins are virtually absent. The adenoma is partially surrounded by a fibrous capsule, a portion of which is at upper right.

Most liver cell adenomas reported recently have been found in premenopausal women with a history of oral contraceptive steroids use. Two epidemiologic findings support a cause–effect relationship between oral contraceptives and liver cell adenoma: the marked increase in the incidence of this tumor after the oral contraceptives were introduced commercially in the 1960s and the increased risk of this tumor with increasing duration of oral contraceptive use. Rooks et al. (1979) estimate that 88% of the 320 cases of liver cell adenoma diagnosed each year in the United States are attributable to oral contraceptives. The mechanisms by which oral contraceptive use leads to liver cell adenoma are not known. Results of animal studies, however, indicate oral contraceptive steroids may promote liver neoplasia (Taper, 1978; Yager and Yager, 1980).

Malignant Hemangioendothelioma

Malignant hemangioendotheliomas, commonly referred to as angiosarcomas, are malignant liver tumors composed of spindle cells lining and/or projecting into the lumina of blood vessels. Tumor nodules are usually multiple and highly vascularized with a spongy or multicystic appearance (Figure 9-20). Portal fibrosis (accompanied by extensive bile duct proliferation), focal hyperplasia, and dysplasia of sinusoidal epithelium are often precedents and concomitants of angiosarcoma development. Clinical signs and symptoms of the tumors are those of portal hypertension (i.e., splenomegaly, ascites, edema, and esophageal varices).

A relatively rare tumor, angiosarcoma occurs in significantly increased frequency in people occupationally exposed to vinyl chloride or to inorganic arsenicals (Popper et al., 1978). Indeed the high frequency of this rare tumor in certain populations of industrial workers accounted for the rapid etiologic association between vinyl chloride and angiosarcoma (Creech and Johnson, 1974). This relationship was documented concurrently in experimental animals. Angiosarcomas have also been observed

in a number of people who had been exposed 20 or more years previously to Thorotrast during diagnostic radiology. Thorotrast, first used clinically in 1928 for visualization of liver, spleen, and cerebral arteries, is a colloidal solution of thorium dioxide that contains the natural radioactive isotope ^{232}Th. ^{232}Thorium releases α and β particles and γ rays during its decay to the stable element lead (^{208}Pb). Estimated biologic half-life of ^{232}Th is 400 years; approximately 70% of the Thorotrast dose given is taken up and permanently retained by liver reticuloendothelial (Kupffer) cells. Thorotrast was first recognized as a neoplastic agent in 1947, 19 years after its first clinical trials.

Cholangiosarcoma

Cholangiosarcomas (bile duct carcinomas) are malignant tumors that arise from the epithelium of small and large bile ducts. Tumor cells resemble biliary epithelium, grow in tubular or papillary arrays, and may be accompanied by an abundant fibrous stroma. Most tumors secrete mucus but not bile. Grossly, these tumors are usually firm, white nodules. Cirrhosis is commonly absent. The incidence of this tumor is highest in areas of the Far East where people are endemically parasitized by the bile fluke *Clonorchis sinesis*. Cholangiosarcomas have also developed in people following treatment with Thorotrast.

It is curious that more associations have not been found between exposure to chemical agents in the environment and cholangiocarcinoma or other types of injury to the biliary tract. Bile excreted by animals given several environmental chemicals metabolized by the liver has been found mutagenic in bacterial test systems (Connor et al., 1979). In the case of the widely used gasoline additive and fumigant 1,2-dibromoethane (see Table 9-3, part D), the mutagenic metabolite excreted in the bile has been presumptively identified as a bromoethane–glutathione conjugate, which rearranges to a reactive halonium ion (Rannug and Beije, 1979; Van Bladeren et al., 1980).

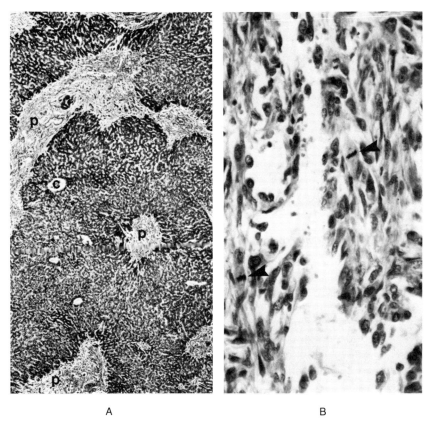

A   B

Figure 9–20. Angiosaroma arising in a vinyl chloride polymerization plant operator. This person developed increasingly frequent and progressively severe bouts of upper GI pain accompanied by hematemesis and production of black tarry stools during the year preceding death. Hepatospleno-megaly and ascites developed. Death was caused by rupture of esophageal varices. At autopsy there were multicentric foci of angiosarcoma in the liver arising against a background of portal fibrosis, bile duct proliferation, and focal sinusoidal dilation and dysplasia of sinusoidal lining cells. p, Portal area; c, central vein. (A) Severe portal fibrosis and bile duct proliferation are visible; (B) the angio-sarcoma with plump dysplastic "endothelium" containing mitotic figures (arrows) lining vascular spaces. (Case courtesy of Dr. Joe Suyemoto, Dept. of Pathology, Leominster Hospital, Leominster, Ma.)

Only a few chemicals, such as the antineo-plastic nitrogen mustard derivative CCNU [1-(2-chloroethyl)-3-cyclohexyl-1-nitro-sourea] are known that produce acute ne-crosis of the bile duct epithelium. There-fore, the bile duct epithelium must have a remarkable protective system that guards against the potentially injurious milieu passing through its lumen!

Hepatocellular Carcinoma

Hepatocellular carcinomas are malignant tumors composed of cells resembling hepa-tocytes, usually arranged in broad cords that typically are two to eight cells thick. The tumor cells may be highly pleomorphic with bizarre giant nuclei, may be associated with broad trabeculae of fibrous tissue, and/or may form pseudo-acini. Some hepatomas consist mainly of hepatocyte-like cells with a clear, often vacuolated cytoplasm. Pro-duction of bile by tumor cells and invasion of branches of portal and hepatic veins are characteristic features. Unlike the three pre-viously discussed forms of liver neoplasia, cirrhosis is usually but not invariably a con-comitant of hepatocellular carcinoma.

Despite its relative rarity in the United States and Europe, primary hepatocellular carcinoma is the most common malignant tumor in males in the world. The incidence in women is significantly less. Environmental factors are thought to be responsible for at least part of the striking geographic variations in the incidence of hepatocellular carcinoma. Infection with hepatitis B virus is considered a major cause of hepatocellular carcinoma (London, 1981). However, data from animal and epidemiologic studies support the hypothesis that natural chemical carcinogens may be responsible for at least some of the human cases of hepatocellular carcinoma. A number of myco- and phytotoxins, which are carcinogenic for experimental animals, are present in significant quantities in foodstuffs eaten by humans and other animals when those foodstuffs are stored under less than optimal conditions. Aflatoxins, cycasin, and pyrrolizidine alkaloids are the most likely candidates. The high incidence of hepatocellular carcinoma in equatorial Africa and in parts of southeast Asia has, for instance, been associated with improper storage of grains and contamination of foods with the fungal product aflatoxin. Peers et al. (1976) found a significant correlation between the calculated daily intake of aflatoxin and the incidence of primary liver cancer in adult males in different parts of Swaziland.

Also regarded as potential human liver carcinogens are the dialkylnitrosamines, which are potent liver carcinogens in animals, and can be present in or synthesized from nitrite precursors in the environment. Human liver DNA from a suspected victim of dimethylnitrosamine poisoning was found to be methylated at the 7- and O-6 positions of guanine (Herron and Shank, 1980). This finding indicates that humans, like rodents, metabolically activate dialkylnitrosamines to strong alkylating agents (see Table 9-3, part A, 6).

High incidences of liver tumors have been found in several studies of alcoholics (see Lieber et al., 1979). Consequently, because of the liver enzymatic and metabolic alterations and the cytotoxicity associated with alcoholism, alcohol could act as a cocarcinogen or a promoter in liver neoplasia. Animal studies indicate ethanol is a cocarcinogen in vinyl chloride-induced liver neoplasia (Radike et al., 1981). It is possible that chemicals and viruses act synergistically in the development of hepatocellular neoplasia. Repeated exposure to a cytotoxic, cirrhotic chemical could enhance the neoplasia process initiated by a carcinogen, or infection with a cytotoxic virus could enhance the carcinogenic process initiated by a chemical.

Conclusions

Alert clinicians, often in collaboration with other scientists, have identified large numbers of chemicals that are hepatotoxic. This identification is easier for agents that reliably cause acute injury or cause an unusual or distinctive form of chronic injury or neoplasia than for agents that cause less predictable, more common, or less distinctive forms of injury. In fact, known acute hepatotoxic agents are now used so sparingly in industry, and then under such controlled conditions, that occupationally acquired acute hepatic injury has become a relatively rare event. Acute hepatic injury due to chemicals in the environment now occurs chiefly through exposure in the home, in the diet, and as a consequence of life-style or medical treatment.

Recognition and prevention of the more elusive chemical causes of nonpredictable or nondistinctive hepatotoxicity will require more careful inquiry by clinicians into possible exposures to suspect toxins, and more precise characterization of the biochemical and morphologic consequences of such chemicals. A problem of great current concern is the identification of environmental chemicals and conditions that are nontoxic or only minimally toxic, but that can enhance the potential of other chemical or nonchemical agents to cause acute, chronic, or neoplastic liver or biliary tract injury. At the present time only a limited number of persons at risk for liver or biliary tract injury from environmental chemicals can be identified. Hopefully, this situation will gradually be rectified as those concerned with health in the environment acquire a better scientific understanding of the processes that initiate and modulate injury to the liver and biliary tract.

Acknowledgments

This work was supported in part by NIH Grants ES 02102 and AM 27135. We thank Diane Pugh for her diligent and constructive preparation of the manuscript.

REFERENCES

Alvares, A. P., Fischbein, A., Anderson, K. E., and Kappas, A. 1977. Alterations in drug metabolism in workers exposed to polychlorinated biphenyls. *Clin. Pharmacol. Ther.* 22:140–146.

Atlas, S. A., and Nebert, D. W. 1976. Pharmacogenetics and human disease. In *Drug metabolism—from microbe to man*, pp. 393–430. London: Taylor and Francis, Ltd.

Barnes, J. M. and Magee, P. M. 1954. Some toxic properties of dimethylnitrosamine, *Br. J. Ind. Med.* 11:167–174.

Baron, J., Redick, J. A. and Guengerich, F. P. 1978. Immunohistochemical localization of cytochromes P-450 in rat liver. *Life Sci.* 23:2627–2632.

Baum, J. K., Bookstein, J. J., Holtz, F., and Klein, E. W. 1973. Possible associations between benign hepatomas and oral contraceptives. *Lancet* 2:926–929.

Blitzer, B. L., and Boyer, J. L. 1978. Cytochemical localization of (Na$^+$, K$^+$)-ATPase in the rat hepatocyte. *J. Clin. Invest.* 62:1104–1108.

Boyer, J. L. 1980. New concepts of mechanisms of hepatocyte bile formation. *Physiol. Rev.* 60:303–326.

Bullivant, C. M. 1966. Accidental poisoning by paraquat: Report of two cases in man. *Br. Med. J.* 1:1272–1273.

Cagen, S. Z., and Gibson, J. E. 1977. Liver damage following paraquat in selenium-deficient and diethylmaleate-pretreated rats. *Toxicol. Appl. Pharmacol.* 40:193–200.

Conney, A. H., Pantuck, E. J., Kuntzman, R., Kappas, A., Anderson, K. E., and Alvares, A. P. 1977. Nutrition and chemical biotransformation in man. *Clin. Pharmacol. Ther.* 22:707–719.

Connor, T. H., Forti, G. C., Sitra, P., and Legator, M. S. 1979. Bile as a source of mutagenic metabolites produced *in vivo* and detected by Salmonella typhimurium. *Environ. Mutagen.* 1:269–276.

Courtney, K. D. 1979. Hexachlorobenzene (HCB): A review. *Environ. Res.* 20:225–266.

Creech, J. L, Jr., and Johnson, M. N. 1974. Angiosarcoma of liver in the manufacture of polyvinyl chloride. *J. Occup. Med.* 16:150–151.

Elias, E., Hruban, Z., Wade, J. B., and Boyer, J. L. 1980. Phalloidin-induced cholestasis: A microfilament-mediated change in junctional complex permeability. *Proc. Natl. Acad. Sci.* 77:2229–2233.

Farber, E. 1982. Sequential events in chemical carcinogenesis. In *Cancer*, vol. 1, 2nd Ed. ed. F. F. Becker, pp. 485–506. New York: Plenum Press.

Fee, J. A. 1981. Is superoxide toxic and are superoxide dismutases essential for aerobic life? in *Oxygen and oxyradicals in chemistry and biology*, eds. M. A. J. Rodgers and E. L. Powers, pp. 205–239. New York: Academic Press.

Floot, B. G. J., Phillippus, E. J., Hart, A. A. M., and Den Engelse, L. 1979. Persistence and accumulation of potential single strand breaks in liver DNA of rats treated with diethylnitrosamine or dimethylnitrosamine. *Chem. Biol. Interact.* 25:229–242.

Harman, A. W., Frewin, D. B., and Priestly, P. G. 1981. Induction of microsomal drug metabolism in man and in the rat by exposure to petroleum. *Br. J. Ind. Med.* 38:91–97.

Herron, D. C., and Shank, R. C. 1980. Methylated purines in human liver after probable dimethylnitrosamine poisoning. *Cancer Res.* 40:3116–3117.

Jacques, E. A., Buschmann, R. J., and Layden, T. J. 1979. The histopathologic progression of Vitamin A-induced hepatic injury. *Gastroenterology* 76:599–602.

Jollow, D. J., Mitchell, J. R., Zampaglione, N., and Gillette, J. R. 1974. Bromobenzene-induced liver necrosis. Protective role of glutathione and evidence for 2,3-bromobenzene oxide as the hepatotoxic metabolite. *Pharmacology* 11:151–169.

Kisilevsky, R. 1974. Hepatic nuclear and nucleolar changes in amanita poisoning. *Arch. Pathol.* 97:253–258.

Klaassen, C. D. 1977. Biliary excretion. In

Handbook of physiology. Section 9, *Reactions to environmental agents*, ed. D. H. K. Lee, pp. 537–553. Bethesda, Md.: American Physiological Society.

Klatskin, G. 1975. *Toxic and drug-induced hepatitis.* in *Diseases of the liver*, 4th Ed., ed. L. Schiff, pp. 604–710. Philadelphia: J. B. Lippincott.

Kolmodin-Hedman, G. 1974. Decreased plasma half-lives of antipyrine and phenylbutazone in workers occupationally exposed to lindane and DDT. In *Drug interactions*, eds. D. L. Morselli, S. Garattini, and S. N. Cohen, pp. 249–257. New York: Raven Press.

Leber, A. P., and Miya, T. S. 1976. A mechanism for cadmium- and zinc-induced tolerance to cadmium toxicity: Involvement of metallothionein. *Toxicol. Appl. Pharmacol.* 37:403–414.

Lieber, C. S. 1980. Alcohol, protein metabolism and liver injury. *Gastroenterology* 79:373–390.

Lieber, C. S., Seitz, H. K. Garro, A. J., and Worner, T. M. 1979. Alcohol-related diseases and carcinogenesis. *Cancer Res.* 39:2863–2886.

Lockhat, D., Katz, S. S., Lisbona, R., and Mishkin, S. 1981. Oral contraceptives and liver disease. *Can. Med. Assoc. J.* 124:993–999.

London, W. T. 1981. Primary hepatocellular carcinoma—etiology, pathogenesis and prevention. *Hum. Pathol.* 12:1085–1097.

McClain, C. J., Kromhout, J. P., Peterson, F. J., and Holtzman, J. L. 1980. Potentiation of acetaminophen hepatotoxicity by alcohol. *J.A.M.A.* 244:251–253.

Miller, E. C., and Miller, J. A. 1981. Searches for ultimate chemical carcinogens and their reactions with cellular macromolecules. *Cancer* 47:2327–2345.

Mitchell, J. R., Thorgeirsson, S. S., Potter, W. Z., Jollow, D. J., and Keiser, H. 1974. Acetaminophen-induced hepatic injury: Protective role of glutathione in man and rationale for therapy. *Clin. Pharmacol. Ther.* 16:676–684.

Mowat, A. P., and Arias, I. M. 1969. Liver function and oral contraceptives. *J. Reprod. Med.* 3:45–55.

Nebert, D. W., Eisen, H. J., Negishi, M., Lang, M.A., Hjelmeland, L. M., and O'Key, A. B. 1981. Genetic mechanisms controlling the induction of polysubstrate monooxygenase (P-450) activities. *Ann. Rev. Pharmacol. Toxicol.* 21:431–462.

Oberling, C., and Rouiller, C. 1956. Les effets de l'intoxication aigue au tetrachlorure de carbone sur le foie du rat; etude au microscope electronique. *Ann. Anat. Pathol. (Paris)* 1:401–427.

Ockner, R. K., and Schmid, R. 1961. Acquired porphyria in man and rat due to hexachlorobenzene intoxication. *Nature (Lond.)* 189:499.

Oda, M., and Phillips, M. J. 1975. Electron microscope cytochemical characterization of bile canaliculi and bile ducts *in vitro. Virchos Archiv. (Cell Pathol.)* 18:109–118.

Oshio, C., and Phillips, M. J. 1981. Contractivity of bile canaliculi: Implications for liver function. *Science* 212:1041–1042.

Peers, F. G., Gilman, G. A., and Linsell, C. A. 1976. Dietary aflatoxins and human liver cancer. A study in Swaziland. *Int. J. Cancer* 17:167–176.

Popper, H., and Schaffner, F. S. 1959. Drug induced hepatic injury. *Ann. Intern. Med.* 51:1230–1252.

Popper, H., Thomas, L. B., Telles, N. C., Falk, H., and Selikoff, I. J. 1978. Development of hepatoangiosarcoma in man induced by vinyl chloride, Thorotrast and arsenic. *Am. J. Pathol.* 92:349–376.

Radike, M. J., Stemmer, K. L., and Bingham, E. 1981. Effect of ethanol on vinyl chloride carcinogenesis. *Environ. Health Perspect.* 41:59–62.

Rannug, U., and Beije, B. 1979. The mutagenic effect of 1,2-dichloroethane on Salmonella typhimurium. II. Activation by the isolated perfused liver. *Chem. biol. Interact.* 24:265–285.

Rappaport, A. M. 1969. Anatomical considerations. In *Diseases of the liver*, 4th ed. L. Schiff, pp. 1–50. Philadelphia: J. B. Lippincott.

Reddy, J. K. 1973. Possible properties of microbodies (peroxisomes). Microbody proliferation and hypolipidemic drugs, *J. Histochem. Cytochem.* 21:967–971.

Reynolds, E. S. 1977. Environmental aspects of injury and disease: Liver and bile ducts. *Environ. Health Perspect.* 20:1–13.

Reynolds, E. S., Brown, B. R., Jr., and Vandam, L. D. 1972. Massive hepatic necrosis after fluroxene anesthesia—a case of drug interaction? *N. Engl. J. Med.* 286:530–533.

Reynolds, E. S., and Moslen, M. T. 1980. Environmental liver injury: Halogenated hydrocarbons. In *Toxic injury of the liver*, eds.

E. Farber and M. F. Fisher, pp. 541–596. New York: Marcel Dekker.

Rooks, J. B., Ory, H. W., Ishak, K. G., Strauss, L. T., Greenspan, J. R., Hill, A. P., and Tyler, C. W., Jr. 1979. Epidemiology of hepatocellular adenoma: The role of oral contraceptive use. *J.A.M.A.* 242:644–648.

Schulte-Hermann, R., Ohde, G., Schappler, J., and Timmermann-Trosiener, I. 1981. Enhanced proliferation of putative preneoplastic cells in rat liver following treatment with tumor promoters, phenobarbital, hexachlorocyclohexane, steroid compounds and nafenopin. *Cancer Res.* 41:2556–2562.

Stamatoyannopoulos, G., Chen, S. -H., and Fuki, M. 1975. Liver alcohol dehydrogenase in Japanese: High population frequency of an atypical form and its possible role in alcohol sensitivity. *Am. J. Hum. Genet.* 27:789–796.

Taper, H. S. 1978. The effects of estradiol-17-phenylpropionate and estradiol benzoate on N-nitrosomorpholine-induced liver carcinogenesis in ovariectomized female rats. *Cancer* 42:462–467.

U.S., Dept. of Health, Education and Welfare, PHS, NIH. 1977. *Disease of the liver and biliary tract.* Washington, D.C.: U.S. Government Printing Office.

Van Bladeren, P. J., Briemer, D. D., Rotteveel-Smijs, G. M. T., de Jong, R. A. W., Buijs, W., Van der Gen, A., and Mohn, G. R. 1980. The role of glutathione conjugation in the mutagencity of 1,2-dibromoethane. *Biochem. Pharmacol.* 29:2975–2982.

Vesell, E. S. 1977. Genetic and environmental factors affecting drug disposition in man. *Clin. Pharmacol. Ther.* 22:659–679.

Willcox, W. H., Spilsbury, B. H., and Legge, T. M. 1915. An outbreak of toxic jaundice of a new type amongst aeroplane workers—its clinical and toxicological aspect. *Trans. Med. Soc. Lond.* 38:129–156.

Williams, R. T. 1959. *Detoxication mechanism,* 2nd Ed. London: Chapman and Hall, Ltd.

Wislocki, P. G., Miwa, G. T., and Yu, A. Y. H. 1980. Reactions catalyzed by the cytochrome P-450 system. In *Enzymatic basis of detoxication,* vol. 1, ed. W. B. Jakoby, pp. 135–182. New York: Academic Press.

Yager, J. D., Jr., and Yager, R. 1980. Oral contraceptive steroids as promoters of hepatocarcinogenesis in female Sprague-Dawley rats. *Cancer Res.* 40:3680–3685.

Zimmerman, H. J. 1978. *Hepatotoxicity.* New York: Appleton-Century-Crofts.

10

Urinary System

Robert A. Goyer

Chronic renal failure is an important cause of morbidity, mortality, and economic loss. In the United States, it is the fifth most common disease-related cause of death after cardiovascular disease, cancer, diabetes mellitus, and cirrhosis of the liver. The crude U.S. death rate is about 5 per 100,000 per year without selection for age or race; it approaches 10 per 100,000 for nonwhite males. A report of the geographic distribution of diseases according to state economic areas shows patches of high mortality rates from nephritis and nephrosis extending through the mid-South and into the Northeast (Mason et al., 1981). Patterns of this nature suggest a role for environmental factors, but definitive data are not available. Age-standardized mortality rates compiled in England for males and females aged 60 years and over indicate that from 1971 onward there has been a trend of increasing mortality from renal diseases (Sorahan et al., 1982). Factors contributing to this trend may be increasing recognition of renal failure as a cause of death, or a change in natural history of renal disease following the introduction of kidney transplants. The rising trend might also reflect an increase in drug- or chemical-related disease.

As greater numbers of persons seek therapy for end-stage renal disease, costs rapidly increase. From data derived from Medicare payments for treatment of patients with end-stage renal disease in the United States, the Social Security Administration reports that in 1974, 3099 renal transplants were performed and 15,749 patients underwent dialysis at a cost of $286 million. Cost for maintenance dialysis treatment and kidney transplantation in 1981 was about $1.5 billion. For 1984 it is estimated that 5231 transplants will be performed, and 55,360 patients will undergo dialysis at a cost of $3.057 billion (Salvatierra et al., 1979). On a nationwide basis the direct medical cost of kidney disease is estimated at $5.5 billion annually.

Although the proportion of renal disease that is attributable to environmental or occupational factors cannot be determined precisely, there is increasing understanding of the renal metabolism and pathology related to specific toxic substances. Knowledge of the causes of renal disease provides opportunity for prevention. This chapter summarizes the pathophysiology of the kidney that might occur from exposure to environmental factors. Selected drugs and chemicals that may produce such effects are also considered, with particular emphasis on mechanisms of injury.

Renal Excretion of Toxins

The kidney is the principal organ for excretion of toxins, both endogenous and exogenous. Twenty-five percent of cardiac output is delivered to the kidney. Afferent blood is filtered by the glomerulus, and components of the filtrate undergo net absorption or excretion. The large number of nephrons provides a very extensive surface of endothelial cells for toxins to contact. Optimal mechanisms for excretion must not only be selective to conserve essential metabolites but must also transport toxins in a manner that reduces the potential for cell injury. Mechanisms such as degradative metabolism and intracellular sequestration or protein binding help prevent toxicity (Shreiner and Maher, 1965; Maher, 1976).

CELLULAR TRANSPORT

Drugs and other chemicals including metals may be transported across proximal tubular cells, that is, from renal capillaries across tubular cells to be excreted in tubular lumen or vice versa (absorption). Many cationic substances are excreted against concentration gradients at rates that exceed glomerular filtration. This implies an active carrier-mediated transport process. Such a process requires energy obtained from oxidative metabolism located in mitochondria. An active process for transporting solutes in renal tubular cells has certain implications regarding susceptibility of tubular cells to effects of toxins. If cationic drugs or chemicals are actively transported, there is the immediate problem of competition with transport of essential cations. Active transport with the capability of concentrating absorbed material may concentrate potential nephrotoxins as well as essential solutes in the renal cortex. The same toxins that impair energy metabolism will impede the cellular transport of essential solutes (Rennick, 1978). Other toxic substances may be concentrated in the medulla or the papillae probably as a consequence of the physiologic mechanism that concentrates urine.

METABOLIC DEGRADATION

Metabolic degradation or transformation most often occurs in the liver, but many of the same enzyme systems are present in the kidney as well. The metabolism of drugs and chemicals within the kidney may result in substances that are either more or less toxic. Those drugs and chemicals that are metabolized by the mixed-function oxidase system have received the most attention. For example, several low-molecular-weight chlorinated alkyl hydrocarbons such as carbon tetrachloride and trichloromethane may be transformed into reactive, toxic products that bind covalently to renal tissue, producing membrane injury. In addition, low-level exposure to other substances such as polychlorinated biphenyls (PCBs) that activate the enzyme systems may enhance the production of toxic products (Kluwe et al., 1979). Similarly, pretreatment with phenobarbital enhances the activity of mixed-function oxidase enzymes and, hence, the toxicity of compounds like methoxyflurane whose metabolic products are fluoride and oxalate, two substances potentially toxic to the kidney. Fluoride ion is toxic to cell membranes, whereas oxalate may precipitate within the lumen of nephrons (Mazze, 1976).

INTRACELLULAR PROTEIN BINDING

Intracellular concentration of toxins may be influenced by protein binding. The soluble cytoplasmic protein, metallothionein, and insoluble acidic protein complexes forming nuclear inclusion bodies are examples of a phenomenon that concentrates two different groups of metals.

Metallothionein is a low-molecular-weight protein capable of intracellular binding to a number of metals (Cherian and Goyer, 1978). Synthesis in renal tubular cells may be induced by cadmium, zinc, mercury, copper, gold, and silver. Properties of metallothionein are summarized in Table 10-1. It contains 6–11% metal and 30% cysteine, and does not contain any aromatic amino acids. The metal ion is bound to the

Table 10–1. Properties of Metallothionein

1. Synthesis induced by certain metals
2. Low molecular weight (6000–10,000)
3. High content of cysteine (30%) and affinity for metals
4. Absence of disulfide bonds and aromatic amino acids
5. Absorption maximum at 250 nm; Cd-cysteine bond, minimum absorption at 280 nm
6. Heat stability

protein by mercaptide linkages. The unusual absorption properties in the ultraviolet range provide a method for in vitro detection. The principal biologic role of metallothionein is not known for certain, but a number of functions have been suggested. Because this protein can bind with various essential and nonessential metals, it may have an important function in regulating their metabolism and toxicity. Metallothionein is an intracellular protein that can act as a storage site. Thus, the specific binding of cadmium to this intracellular protein could explain the long biologic half-life of cadmium in humans. Although the half-life of the protein moiety of metallothionein is only 4–5 days, similar to other tissue proteins, cadmium transfers to newly formed protein in the cell.

Lead and bismuth accumulate in renal tubular cells bound to a complex of acidic proteins that form morphologically discernible inclusion bodies (Goyer and Cherian, 1977). As with metallothionein, the sequestering of toxic metals by the protein complex is thought to reduce the intracellular toxicity of these metals.

MEMBRANE REACTIONS AND PINOCYTOSIS

Macromolecular substances are transported by pinocytosis and inclusion in intracellular vacuoles. Proteins that are normally included in glomerular filtrate are taken up by the cell membrane by pinocytosis (Figure 10-1). Such pinocytotic vesicles are identified as phagosomes and fuse with primary lysosomes, which contain lysosomal enzymes. Secondary lysosomes are

formed, and the macromolecular material is degraded or broken down. The low-molecular-weight products then leave the lysosome in order to prevent increase in osmolarity and lysosome swelling (Jacques, 1975).

Potential nephrotoxins that may be taken into renal tubular cells in this manner include chelating agents like nitrilotriacetic acid, EDTA, and the metal-binding protein metallothionein. Membrane binding of EDTA administered as the calcium–EDTA chelate persists with dislocation of the calcium to other cellular components but not the EDTA. This suggests the manner in which EDTA may sequester cellular lead or other metals for exretion (Schwartz et al., 1970).

Pathogenic Mechanisms of Renal Disease

Nephrotoxic drugs and chemicals have been used experimentally to produce most of the recognized pathologic processes occurring in the kidney. The major pathogenic mechanisms involve either an immunologically induced process or direct toxicity to some component of the kidney, the glomerulus, tubules, and/or interstitium (Roxe, 1980; Curtis, 1979; Davis et al., 1981).

IMMUNOLOGIC RENAL DISEASE

Immunologically Induced Glomerular Lesions

The etiology of membranous glomerulonephritis is obscure in most cases, but specific antigens associated with nephrotoxins have been identified as part of immune-complex deposits. A proposed mechanism is that circulating immune complexes passively become trapped in different areas of the nephron (glomeruli, tubulointerstitial areas, or blood vessel walls), giving rise to an immune-complex glomerulonephritis or membranous glomerulonephropathy. Also, circulating autoantibodies may actively react with specific components of the glomerular and/or tubular basement membrane.

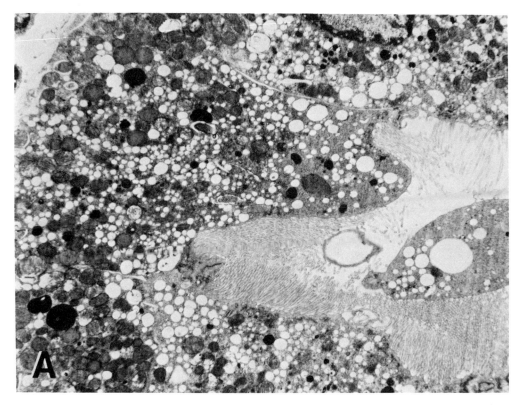

Figure 10–1. Proximal renal tubular lining cell of rat 4 hours after ip injection of metallothionein. The cytoplasm contains multiple pinocytotic vesicles characteristic of absorption of anionic macromolecules (EM, ×5200). (From Cherian et al., 1976.)

Acute Interstitial Nephritis

Acute interstitial nephritis (AIN) occurs as a cell-mediated immune response to a variety of drugs, particularly penicillin and related antibiotics, but is also reported after therapy with thiazides, furosemide, salts of gold, and occupational exposure to mercury (Table 10-2) (Kleinknecht et al., 1978). Clinical symptoms reflect a systemic hypersensitivity reaction including fever, skin rash, and eosinophilia. Renal involvement is manifested by mild proteinuria and hematuria. AIN tends to be more severe, with a high incidence of renal failure in adult patients, and is usually milder in patients under 15 years of age. It has also been pointed out that absence of prior allergic reaction to a drug (penicillin) does not alter risk to AIN. Kidneys are usually swollen as visualized radiographically because of edema

Table 10–2. Drugs Associated with Acute Interstitial Nephritis

Drug class	Examples
Antibiotics and other chemotherapeutic agents	Penicillins, methicillin, ampicillin, oxacillin, nafcillin, cephalosporins, gentamicin, kanamycin, colistin, polymyxin B, chloramphenicol, glafenin, carbenicillin, sulfonamides
Antitubercular drugs	Rifampin
Diuretics	Furosemide, thiazides, chlorthalidone
Other drugs	Phenylbutazone, phenindione, allopurinol, phenytoin, azathioprine, antipyrine, phenobarbital, carbimazol

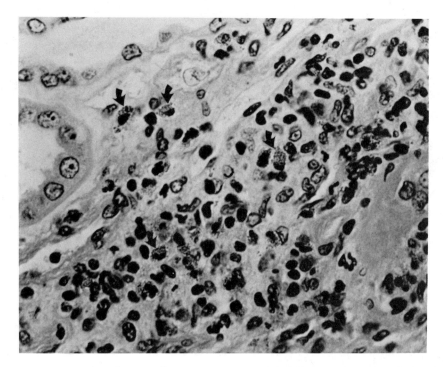

Figure 10–2. Interstitial nephritis with numerous eosinophils (arrows) admixed with lymphocytes, occasional histiocytes, and a few plasma cells (H&E, ×600). (Courtesy of Dr. Charles Jennette, University of North Carolina, Chapel Hill.)

fluid and cellular infiltration, composed most commonly of lymphocytes and plasma cells as well as eosinophilic and polymorphonuclear neutrophils (Figure 10-2). In some instances the histologic appearances may suggest chronic inflammation, and macrophages and giant cells may be present (Figure 10-3). Renal tubular cell damage is always present, but there is no fibrosis in the acute stages. Glomerular and vascular lesions are uncommon, and the lesions are usually reversible. However, persistent loss of renal function indicates progression to fibrosis and chronic interstitial disease in an undetermined number of cases. Deposits of IgG and C3 may be detectable along tubules in biopsies during the acute phase. IgE may be elevated in the serum to confirm the allergic or hypersensitivity process. The reaction can be further suggested by tests of cell-mediated hypersensitivity (lymphocyte transformation test) or antibody-mediated hypersensitivity (circulating antibodies reacting with the drug).

DIRECT TOXICITY TO COMPONENTS OF THE KIDNEY

Direct Glomerular Toxicity

Glomerular lesions may be caused by the direct toxicity of drug or chemical. Direct toxicity to components of the glomerular apparatus are relatively uncommon but have been described following therapeutic use of some drugs such as puromycin or by materials that may be deposited in basement membrane (Caulfield et al., 1976). Particulate substances such as gold and silica and immune complexes may become deposited in mesangial cells (Burkholder, 1982). Whether material within mesangial cells is actually phagocytosed is unclear, but the reaction to such deposits may be proliferation of glomerular cells and inflammatory cells response. Injury to the mesangium may alter glomerular permeability. Solutes and water move across glomerular capillary walls through an extracellular pathway that con-

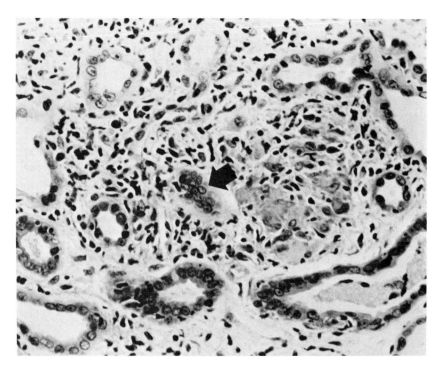

Figure 10–3. Interstitial nephritis with granulomatous inflammation including multinucleated giant cell (arrow) (H&E, ×360). (Courtesy of Dr. Charles Jennette, University of North Carolina, Chapel Hill.)

sits sequentially of endothelial fenestrae, glomerular basement membrane, the pores of slit diaphragms, and the filtration slits. Water permeability is determined by total area of epithelial slit pores. Contraction of the glomerular mesangium shortens and narrows glomerular capillaries, in turn narrowing epithelial slit pores and reducing glomerular filtration. Some particulate materials such as asbestos fibers have been observed in transit through glomerular pores without being deposited in glomerular cells or evoking any apparent cellular reaction (Auerbach et al., 1980).

Acute Tubular Toxicity

Acute tubular effects of toxins may vary from necrosis of tubular cells leading to acute renal failure to subtle subcellular lesions and functional effects. Injury to proximal tubular lining cells is manifest by increased excretion of substances normally resorbed by these cells such as glucose, amino acids, phosphate, and sodium. Extension of the lesion to distal portions of the tubule is accompanied by loss of ability to acidify the urine and to maintain water and electrolyte balance. Tubular toxicity may be accompanied by glomerular effects, and if the process is persistent may lead to a chronic interstitial nephropathy, as in lead and cadmium toxicity.

Chronoic Interstitial Nephritis

Chronic interstitial nephritis generally has fewer distinguishing morphologic features than most forms of acute renal disease. Morphologically it is characterized by infiltration with mononuclear cells, prominent interstitial fibrosis, and tubular atrophy. Chronic interstitial disease may occur as a sequela to severe acute tubular disease, or acute interstitial nephritis, or as an expression of chronic low-dose exposure to specific nephrotoxins. The term "tubulointerstitial disease" may be preferable, because it better identifies the primary sites of the pathologic process. Progressive fibrosis of the interstitial tissue results in a decreasing number of functional nephrons with eventual reduction in glomerular filtration rate and azotemia. There may be few symptoms preceding the onset of renal failure.

The contribution of chronic interstitial nephritis to the overall morbidity and mortality due to renal disease may be substantial, although it is difficult to express quantitatively at the present time (Cotran, 1979). Reasons for this are lack of agreement on systems of classification (etiology versus descriptive morphology) and the nonspecific clinical findings. On the basis of morphology, there is the uncertainty as to how much of kidney disease diagnosed as chronic pyelonephritis is the result of bacterial infection and how much is due to a toxin or some associated disease. The identification of chronic pyelonephritis is made more precise by following established criteria. This includes the presence of gross irregular scarring, inflammation, fibrosis, and deformity of calyces underlying parenchymal scars, predominant tubulointerstitial histologic damage, and relative sparing of glomeruli. In a review of kidney histology obtained by bilateral nephrectomy before renal transplantation, Schwartz and Cotran (1976) found evidence of bacterial residues (by immune fluorescence) in only a few of the large number of kidneys diagnosed as having chronic pyelonephritis. This suggests that most cases identified at least in the past as chronic pyelonephritis are not caused by bacterial infection, particularly in the absence of pelvocalyceal lesions. It is possible that local humoral and cell-mediated reactions directed against bacteria and bacterial antigens are responsible for the persistent mononuclear cell infiltrate, but there is no evidence that the morphology identified as chronic pyelonephritis is the result of autoimmune and antibody-mediated immunologic injury. It is likely, therefore, that some percentage of chronic interstitial nephritis labeled as chronic pyelonephritis is due to something other than bacterial infection.

In those studies that have classified chronic interstitial nephritis on the basis of etiologic agents, analgesic abuse, heavy metals (lead, cadmium, and mercury), and chronic exposure to certain industrial solvents appear to lead to renal disease. Chronic interstitial nephritis may also be seen in certain miners (silica) and heroin addicts, possibly as the sequela to acute interstitial nephritis and immune-induced disease or glomerulonephritis. The contribution of direct toxicity from therapeutic drugs to chronic interstitial nephritis is not clear.

Although the discussions that follow in this chapter are largely organized on the basis of exposure to specific substances, it must be recognized that interactions or synergisms between various toxic agents and associated diseases are likely, and the retrospective identification of precise etiologic factors may not be possible.

Drug and Chemical Causes of Renal Disease

METALS
Lead

The renal effects of lead are primarily tubular or tubulointerstitial and they may be both acute and chronic (Table 10-3). However, the acute effects of lead differ from

Table 10–3. Characteristics of Lead Nephropathy

Early effects (reversible, epithelial cell)	Late effects (irreversible, interstitial)
Morphologic, proximal tubular cell	Tubular cell atrophy/hyperplasia
Nuclear inclusion bodies, cytomegaly, swollen organelles, distorted mitochondria	Progressive fibrosis, glomerular sclerosis, loss of nephrons
	Azotemia
Functional	Neoplasia, rodents (humans?)
Decreased absorption of amino acids, glucose, phosphate, sodium	
Increased renin production	

effects of most other metals in that cell injury is for the most part reversible and necrosis is uncommon. Cells of the proximal tubule are most severely affected, and this effect is characterized by reduction in resorptive function manifested by a generalized aminoaciduria, glycosuria, and hyperphosphaturia. These components of the Fanconi syndrome have been observed in children with acute lead toxicity, usually in children who also have overt symptoms of central nervous system toxicity and in rats with exposure to lead. Proximal tubular dysfunction has been more difficult to demonstrate in workers with chronic lead nephropathy (Goyer and Rhyne, 1973).

The effects of lead on renal tubular cells and sodium reabsorption are less clear. Increase in plasma renin and aldosterone while consuming a low-sodium diet has been observed in a group of men with a history of "moonshine" ingestion and occult lead toxicity (Sandstead et al., 1970). In contrast, recent studies on the effect of minimally toxic levels of lead exposure in rats showed a reduction in plasma renin activity in spite of a significant increase in blood

pressure (Victery et al., 1982). These differences may reflect a difference in time–dose relationship.

The renal effects of lead may also be influenced by interactions with calcium. Decreasing dietary calcium increases lead retention, possibly because of a decrease in lead excretion. Increased blood lead in children is associated with decreased 1,25-dihydroxyvitamin D (synthesized in the kidney) and may reflect impaired synthesis (Mahaffey, 1980).

The proximal renal tubular cells of persons with lead poisoning and experimental animals are characterized morphologically by the presence of intranuclear inclusion bodies. In conventional paraffin-embedded hematoxylin and eosin-stained sections of renal tissue, the inclusions appear as dense, homogeneous, and eosinophilic bodies (Figure 10-4), and by electon microscopy have a characteristic fibrillary margin around a dense central core (Figure 10-5). Morphologically they are always separate and distinct from nucleoli and may be multiple in the same nucleus. The inclusion bodies are a protein–lead complex, and they may

Figure 10–4. Lead-induced inclusion body (arrow) in nucleus of renal tubular cell of lead-toxic rat (H&E, ×800).

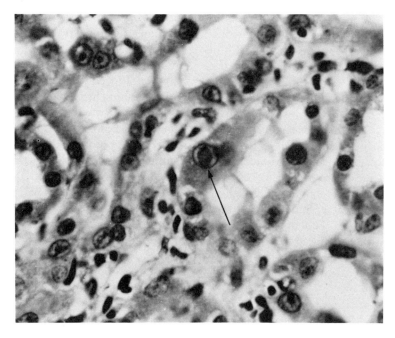

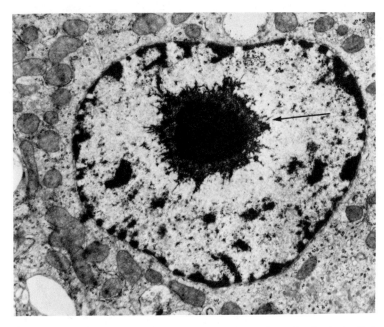

Figure 10–5. Lead-induced inclusion body (arrow) in nucleus of proximal tubular lining cell of lead-toxic rat. Ultrastructure consists of dense core and outer, irregular fibrillary zone ($\times$ 12,000).

be isolated by differential centrifugation. The protein is a nonhistone protein rich in glutamic and aspartic acids and glycine, and may be a mixture of acidic proteins with similar physicochemical properties (Moore et al., 1973). The origin and nature of the protein has not yet been determined, but recent studies of formation of inclusion bodies in renal cell cultures suggest that they form initially in cytoplasm and migrate into the nucleus (McLachlan et al., 1980). The major fraction of lead in the kidney during the acute phase of lead toxicity is bound in the inclusion bodies. For this reason, the inclusion bodies have been interpreted as serving as an intracellular depot for lead. Nevertheless, proximal renal tubular cells during the acute phase of lead toxicity are usually swollen, and mitochondria show dilution of matrical granules and altered cristae (Figure 10-6). Functional studies of mitochondria show reduced respiration and oxidative phosphorylation. Lysosomes do not seem to have a role in sequestering intracellular lead.

Chelation therapy of lead toxicity produces a marked increase in lead excretion. This is accompanied by reversal of acute morphologic effects of lead on proximal renal tubular cells with loss of inclusion bodies from nuclei and restoration of normal renal cell morphology and function (Goyer and Wilson, 1975).

Both experimental animals and people with chronic exposure to lead may develop a progressive interstitial nephropathy. In laboratory animals, progression from acute tubular to chronic tubulointerstitial disease may be followed as a continuum. There is an increase in chronic interstitial renal disease in workers with long histories of occupational exposure, but the nonspecific nature of the morphologic changes makes it difficult to identify lead as the etiologic agent except by association. There is a progressive increase in fibrosis, beginning in peritubular areas extending into the interstitium (Cramer et al., 1974). Inflammatory cells are uncommon and are probably not a primary component of the process. There is eventual atrophy of tubules and hyperplasia of surviving tubules. There is little evidence that the glomerulus is directly affected by excessive exposure to lead except

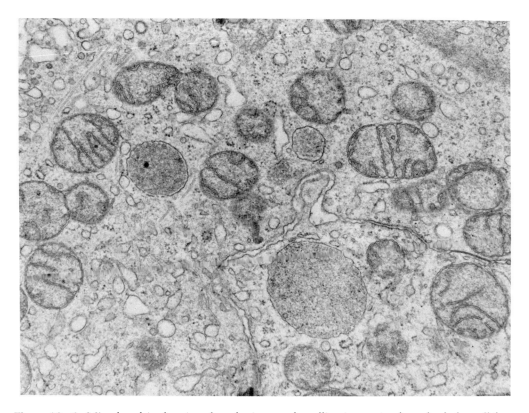

Figure 10–6. Mitochondria showing altered cristae and swelling in proximal renal tubular cell from renal biopsy of man with 6-week history of excessive occupational exposure to lead. In some mitochondria the inner membrane divides the inner compartment, resulting in cleavage ($\times 26,000$). (From Cramer et al., 1974.)

for some nonspecific swelling of mesangial and epithelial cells. In the terminal or end stage, glomeruli become sclerotic. An immunologic basis for the progression of lead-induced nephropathy as suggested following gold and mercury exposures might be suspected, but at the present time there is no published documentation of antirenal antibodies or immune-complex formation in the pathogenesis of lead nephropathy. One recent study suggests that lowered glomerular filtration rate occurs in occupational exposure to lead that does not produce clinical toxicity (Wedeen et al., 1979). The pathophysiologic basis for this observation is not yet determined but may be a consequence of direct toxicity to epithelial cells of the glomerular apparatus.

Intranuclear inclusion bodies are uncommon in the late stages of lead nephropathy, although they may be seen in renal biopsy or autopsy as a manifestation of a superimposed severe acute exposure. A recent study has shown that inclusion bodies may be found in urine of workers with occupational exposure to lead, but their presence or absence in urine has not been related to severity of lead nephropathy (Schumann et al., 1980).

Cadmium

Cadmium accumulates in the kidney with age, and if exposure is excessive cadmium will induce a progressive form of chronic renal tubular disease (Friberg et al., 1974). Unlike many nephrotoxins, including other heavy metals such as lead and mercury, there are virtually no acute effects of inorganic cadmium salts on the kidney, except perhaps for some nonspecific effects that have been seen in animals given near-lethal doses.

Table 10–4. Characteristics of Cadmium Nephropathy

Early effects	Late effects
Increase in cadmium in renal cortex (critical concentration)	Renal tubular acidosis
	Hypercalciuria
	Glomerular proteinuria
Increase in urinary cadmium excretion	Nephrocalcinosis, renal stones
Decreased absorption of amino acids, glucose, phosphate, low-molecular-weight proteins (e.g., β_2-microglubulin, retinol-binding protein)	Interstitial fibrosis

Cadmium nephropathy has only been recognized in the past 30–40 years, but it has been intensely studied, particularly in persons with heavy occupational exposures, and is dependent on increasing cadmium content of the renal cortex.

Some of the characteristics of cadmium nephropathy are listed in Table 10-4. Normally, less than 1 or 2 μg of cadmium is excreted in urine per day. The effects of cadmium on proximal renal tubular function are manifest by increased cadmium in the urine, low-molecular-weight proteinuria, aminoaciduria, glucosuria, and decreased renal tubular reabsorption of phosphate. With chronic exposure to toxic levels, renal tubular acidosis, hypercalciuria, and calculi formation occur. There are few reports of morphologic effects in humans, but the changes appear to be nonspecific and consist of tubular cell degeneration in the initial stages (reversible), progressing to tubular atrophy and interstitial fibrosis (irreversible). Nephrocalcinosis may also occur in severe cases of chronic exposure (Kazantzis, 1979).

The proteinuria is principally tubular, consisting of low-molecular-weight proteins whose tubular absorption has been impaired by cadmium injury to proximal tubular lining cells. The predominant protein is a β_2-microglobulin. This protein is normally absorbed by proximal renal tubular lining cells. Although increased urinary excretion might be expected to reflect

a nonspecific index of proximal renal tubular cell injury, its presence in urine has been most closely related in a quantitative way with cadmium nephropathy (Kjellstrom and Nordberg, 1978); and, with current availability of radioimmune assay procedures, it is probably, next to cadmium determination per se, the single most useful index of cadmium-induced renal disease. It is widely used to monitor excessive cadmium exposure in populations at risk. A number of other low-molecular-weight proteins have been identified in the urine of workers with excessive cadmium exposure, such as retinol-binding protein, lysozyme, ribonuclease, and immunoglobulin light chains (Buchet et al., 1981).

Aminoaciduria in cadmium toxicity is generalized, reflecting increased excretion of amino acids normally reabsorbed by proximal tubular lining cells. It increases in severity in cadmium workers with increasing exposure to cadmium. Glucosuria and decreased tubular reabsorption of phosphate parallel the occurrence of low-molecular-weight proteinuria and aminoaciduria, reflecting the proximal tubular cell injury.

Although most information available to date related to cadmium exposure and cadmium nephropathy has been obtained from workers with occupational exposure, there is some evidence now that persons in the general population with nonoccupational exposure to cadmium may also have cadmium-related renal tubular dysfunction. Among inhabitants of cadmium-polluted areas of Japan where dietary content of cadmium is increased, the prevalence of proteinuria and glucosuria is higher than in control areas, and there is some association between increased excretion of low-molecular-weight proteins in urine and level of cadmium pollution (Nogawa et al., 1979). Also, a study in Belgium found that a group of women living near a nonferrous metal smelter had a higher body burden as reflected by an increased excretions of cadmium in urine and a higher prevalence of signs of renal dysfunction than women from a control area (Lauwerys et al., 1980).

With the awareness that cadmium-induced nephropathy may even occur in persons in the general population, it becomes of major public health importance to know what is the maximum level of cadmium exposure that a person can be exposed to without risk of renal tubular dysfunction and cadmium nephropathy. The concept of a critical concentration of cadmium has very important implications with regard to establishing maximum levels of cadmium that human populations may be exposed to with some margin of safety. A World Health Organization (WHO, 1977) task force established the critical concentration of cadmium in the renal cortex of humans to be about 200 $\mu g/g$ or renal tubular dysfunction. This level is based on a limited number of cadmium measurements from autopsy and biopsy material and may be a minimal level, because in recent vivo measurements in persons with renal cadmium concentration in the 300- to 400-$\mu g/g$ range have been observed in the absence of discernible renal disease (Nomiyama, 1980).

One of the most challenging questions regarding the metabolism of cadmium has been the role of metallothionein in cellular metabolism and potential toxicity. Nordberg and co-workers (1975) made the very interesting observation that the intravenous injection of cadmium bound to metallothionein protects mice from the texticular necrosis that occurs following injection of a similar dose of inorganic cadmium. This supports the notion that the binding of cadmium to metallothionein protects from cadmium toxicity. This mechanism, however, has a limited capacity, because continued exposure to cadmium does produce renal tubular cell injury.

Mercury

Mercury may produce different effects on the kidney depending on the biochemical form of the metal and nature of exposure (Table 10-5). Inorganic mercury compounds are classic examples of agents that cause acute tubular necrosis. Bichloride of mercury was used as a suicidal agent during the nineteenth and early part of the twen-

Table 10–5. Renal Effects of Mercury

Acute, high-dose effects (mercuric chloride)
  Tubular cell necrosis
  Acute renal failure

Chronic, low-dose effects (inorganic salts of mercury, elemental mercury, mercury vapor)
  Immunologically induced membranous glomerulopathy
  Proteinuria
  Nephrotic syndrome

Alkyl mercury (methyl mercury)
  Mild proximal tubular cell injury
  Exocytosis of membranous bodies into urine

tieth centuries but was unpopular for this purpose because of the painful accompanying corrosive injuries it produced. Regardless of the route of administration, however, mercuric chloride produces acute tubular necrosis within hours of administration, resulting in anuria and death. If the patient can be maintained by dialysis, regeneration of tubular lining cells is possible. These may be followed by ultrastructural changes consistent with irreversible cell injury, including actual disruption of mitochondria, release of lysosomal enzymes, and rupture of cell membranes.

The necrosis of the epithelium of the pars recta kidney following injection of mercuric chloride has been described in detail in the rat. Cellular changes include fragmentation and disruption of the plasma membrane and its appendages, vesiculation and disruption of the endoplasmic reticulum and other cytoplasmic membranes, dissociation of polysomes and loss of ribosomes, mitochondrial swelling with appearance of amorphous intramatrical deposits, and condensation of nuclear chromatin. These changes are common to renal cell necrosis due to various causes (Gritzka and Trump, 1968).

Although exposure to high dose of mercuric chloride is directly toxic to renal tubular lining cells, chronic low-dose exposure to mercuric salts or even elemental mercury vapor levels may induce an immunologic glomerular disease. This form of mercury injury to the kidney is clinically the most common form of mercury-induced

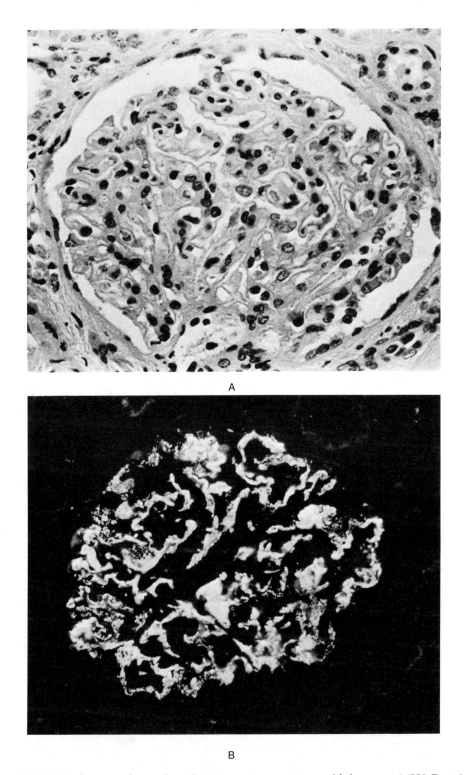

A

B

Figure 10–7. Membranous glomerulonephritis in patient receiving gold therapy. (a) (H&E, ×400); (b) immunofluorescence microscopy, anti-IgG (×400). (From Dr. Charles Jennette, University of North Carolina, Chapel Hill.)

nephropathy. Exposed persons may develop a proteinuria that is reversible after workers are removed from exposure. It has been stated that mercury-induced nephropathy seldom occurs without sufficient exposure to produce detectable mercury neuropathy as well.

Experimental studies have shown that the pathogenesis of mercury nephropathy has two phases: an early phase characterized by an anti-basement membrane glomerulonephritis followed by a superimposed immune-complex glomerulonephritis (Roman-Franco et al., 1978). The pathogenesis of the nephropathy in humans appears similar, although antigens have not been characterized. Also, the early glomerular nephritis may progress in humans to an interstitial immune-complex nephritis (Tubbs et al., 1982).

Gold

Use of gold in the form of organic salts to treat rheumatoid arthritis may be complicated by development of proteinuria and the nephrotic syndrome. Morphologically, the kidney shows an immune-complex glomerulonephritis with granular deposits along the glomerular basement membrane and in the mesangium (Figures 10-7 and 10-8). The pathogenesis of the immune-complex disease is not known for certain, but gold may behave as a hapten and generate the production of antibodies with subsequent disposition of gold protein–antibody complexes in the glomerular subepithelium. Another hypothesis is that antibodies are formed against damaged tubular structures, particularly mitochondria, providing immune complexes for the glomerular deposits (Viol et al., 1977).

The pathogenesis of the tubular cell lesions induced by gold therapy is probably initiated by the direct toxicity of gold with tubular cell components. From experimental studies it appears that gold salts have an affinity for mitochondria of proximal tubular lining cells, which is followed by autophagocytosis and accumulation of gold in

Figure 10–8. Membranous glomerulonephritis in patient receiving gold therapy showing typical wedge-shaped subepithelial deposits ($\times 3000$). (From Dr. Charles Jennette, University of North Carolina, Chapel Hill.)

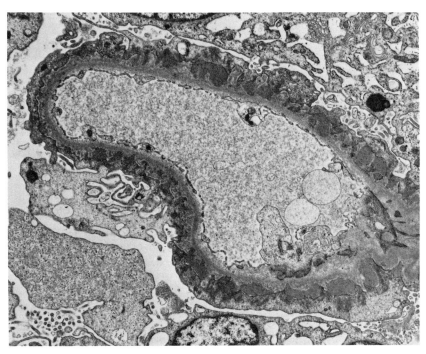

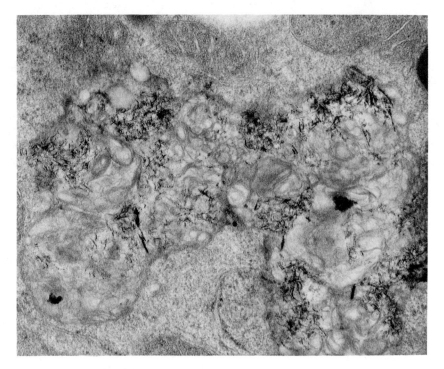

Figure 10–9. Gold spicules in tubular epithelial cell mitochondria ($\times 30,000$). (From Dr. Charles Jennette, University of North Carolina, Chapel Hill.)

amorphous phagolysosomes (Stuve and Galle, 1970), and gold particles can be identified in degenerating mitochondria (Figure 10-9), in tubular lining cells, and in glomerular epithelial cells by X-ray microanalysis (Ainsworth et al., 1981).

Bismuth

The effects of bismuth on the kidney are similar to those of lead, but it is not nearly as important as lead as a cause of renal disease because it is not present in such large amounts in the ambient environment, nor is it as important industrially. However, bismuth has been used therapeutically to treat a variety of ailments, most importantly for syphilis. Bismuth administration results in the formation of characteristic nuclear inclusion bodies in proximal renal tubular lining cells that are similar to the lead-induced bodies and are composed of a bismuth–protein complex (Figure 10-10). The protein is an acidic protein with amino acid composition similar to that forming the lead inclusion bodies. However, there is a slight difference in morphology between the lead- and bismuth-induced inclusion bodies. Also, bismuth–protein complexes are observed in mitochondria of proximal tubular lining cells (Fowler and Goyer, 1975). The bismuth content of the inclusion bodies has been confirmed by X-ray microanalysis of tissue sections. Whether bismuth produces a chronic interstitial nephropathy like lead is not documented. However, bismuth inclusions have been found at autopsy more than 30 years after a course of bismuth therapy.

Uranium

Exposure to compounds of uranium in humans and experimental animals results in injury and necrosis of proximal renal tubules. The most sensitive site is the pars recta (like mercury), but injury and necrosis may extend to other parts of the proximal tubule depending on dose. Acute injury is followed by regeneration of tubular epithelial

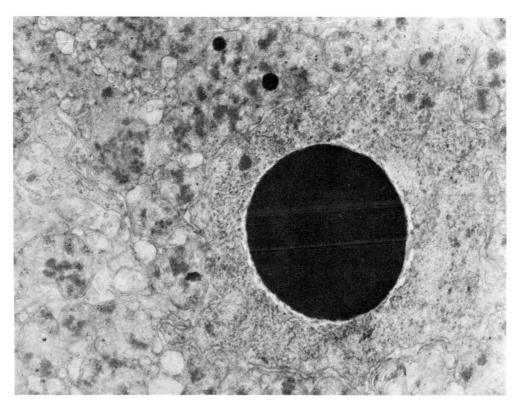

Figure 10–10. Bismuth-induced inclusion body in nucleus of proximal tubular lining cell of rat following administration of bismuth subnitrate. Smaller inclusions are present in adjacent mitochondria (×26,000). (From Goyer and Rhyne, 1973.)

cells. Chronic effects have not been reported.

THERAPEUTIC AGENTS

Nonsteroidal Anti-Inflammatory Drugs

Interstitial nephritis has been associated with the use of several nonsteroidal anti-inflammatory drugs, particularly analgesic mixtures (Table 10-6). Salicylates and phenacetin used in combination have been most strongly suggested as etiologic agents, but a number of other nonsteroidal anti-inflammatory agents have been implicated, including phenylbutazone, indomethacin, fenoprofen, tolmetin, naproxen, and ibuprofen (Shelly, 1978; Warren and Mosley, 1983).

The prevalence of analgesic-associated nephropathy varies worldwide, probably related to patterns of analgesic use, and has been found most often in women aged 45–55 years. The entity has been reported more frequently in Australia and Switzerland, less frequently in the United States, Canada, and Germany. It is estimated that more than 37

Table 10–6. "Analgesic-Associated" Nephropathy[a]

Functional effects	Morphologic effects
Distal tubular changes	Microangiopathy
Loss of sodium-concentrating ability	Degeneration of distal tubular cells, collecting tubules
Acidosis	Papillary necrosis (infarction)
	Interstitial fibrosis, sclerosing glomerulopathy, and azotemia

[a]Chronic ingestion of mixtures containing phenacetin, less commonly other nonsteroid anti-inflammatory agents.

million people in the United States have ar- thritis and use these drugs. This is indeed a very large population at risk. Analgesic ef- fects are said to be a factor in as much as 20% to 30% of cases of interstitial nephri- tis in the southeastern United States (Mur- ray and Goldberg, 1975). Whether the re- moval of phenacetin as an ingredient of these drugs actually will result in a decline in in- terstitial nephritis, as expected, is not clear to date.

The pathologic changes observed in analgesic-associated nephropathy involve tubular epithelial cells and interstitial tissue with absence of primary glomerular dis- ease. Papillary necrosis may also occur. A sketchy history of use of headache powders over a period of many years is said to be typical in some patients, but uncertainties regarding pathogenesis and confounding factors have given preference to the de- scriptive term analgesic-associated neph- ropathy. Functional changes include loss of concentrating ability, urinary sodium de- pletion, and decreased ability to acidify ur- ine. Frank tubular acidosis, however, only occurs in severe cases where glomerular fil- tration is reduced.

The primary pathology of analgesic- associated nephropathy is degeneration and necrosis of tubular cells of the medulla, vasa rectae, loops of Henle, and collecting tu- bules, and it is most severe in the tips of the papillae with resultant papillary necrosis (Prescott, 1970). Renal tubular celluria is common and reflects exfoliation of epithe- lial cells. The celluria may provide a nidus for calculus formation. There is a reduction of cells in the interstitial tissue, with pro- gressive fibrosis extending into the cortex, eventually resulting in periglomerular fi- brosis and glomerular sclerosis.

The tubular cell necrosis and fibrosis is thought to result from toxic injury to tu- bular interstitial cells and ischemia, and has the appearance of infarction with coagula- tive necrosis resulting from a slow ischemic process or microangiopathy. The necrotic papillae may have sharp edges of demarca- tion and may contain a brownish black ap- pearance grossly thought to be related to

deposits of breakdown products of phena- cetin.

Nonsteroidal anti-inflammatory agents have been found experimentally to reduce medullary perfusion. Aspirin interferes with a number of aspects of cellular metabolism including oxidative phosphorylation, mu- copolysaccharide synthesis, and depletion of cellular glutathione. Phenacetin is thought to be converted to a cytotoxic metabolite that binds covalently to tissue proteins, leading to irreversible cell injury. Aspirin, phenacetin, and other nonsteroidal anti- inflammatory agents are thought to be syn- ergistic, hence the greater frequency of an- algesic nephropathy among persons using combination analgesics.

Diagnosis is most often made by cou- pling the history of analgesic abuse with morphologic evidence of chronic interstitial nephritis. Necrotic papillae may be voided in urine, and the resultant lesions can be recognized by X-ray examination. About 12% of cases progress to terminal renal failure (Nanra, 1980).

Other nonsteroidal anti-inflammatory agents may produce hypersensitivity reac- tions (Figure 10-11), lipoid nephrosis, and interstitial nephritis (Finkelstein et al., 1982).

Antibiotics

Nephrotoxicity related to antibiotics is most often due to drugs not primarily prescribed for problems of the kidney (Curtis, 1979). Nevertheless, the kidney becomes the ma- jor site of toxicity because of transport, concentration, and excretory functions. All parts of the nephron or kidney may be af- fected, but usually there is some specificity in site of action. Particular toxins affect specific portions of the nephron; some nephrons are affected whereas others re- main unaffected.

Mechanisms of injury span a broad spec- trum of potential lesions. The most com- mon effect is direct toxicity to renal tubular cells manifested by cell injury and necrosis. Direct toxicity to glomeruli is not as con- spicuous but does occur. Immunologically

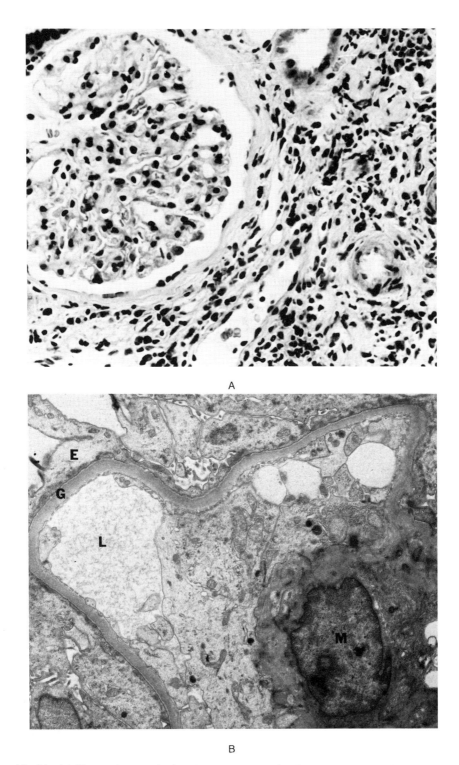

A

B

Figure 10–11. (a) Photomicrograph showing an interstitial inflammatory cell infiltrate rich in lymphocytes but with scattered eosinophils, and a light-microscopically normal glomerulus in a patient with fenoprofen nephropathy (H&E, ×300). (b) Electron micrograph of a glomerulus from the same patient showing extensive visceral epithelial foot process fusion. E, Visceral epithelial cell; G, glomerular basement membrane; L, capillary lumen; M, mesangial cell (×3200). (From Dr. Charles Jennette, University of North Carolina, Chapel Hill.)

induced lesions in glomeruli and interstitial tissue may also occur.

AMINONUCLEOSIDES. Aminonucleosides, particularly gentamicin, and tobramycin, most commonly produce acute toxicity to proximal tubular lining cells, sometimes without oliguria. There is a relationship between dose accumulation in proximal tubular lining cells and cellular necrosis. Concentration in tubular cells results in cortical ratios of 5 to 20 times concentration in the medulla. The antibiotic becomes selectively localized in lysosomes, accounting for the concentration in renal cortex and resulting in lysosomal overload and inhibition of lysosomal hydrolases. The pattern of enzyme inhibition differs for gentamicin and streptomycin. Alteration of lysosomal function and membranes may contribute to the cellular toxicity of these antibiotics. Proximal tubular necrosis may be detected by lysosymuria, β-microglobulinuria, and decreased concentrating ability. A tubular syndrome may occur characterized by loss of potassium, magnesium, calcium, and sometimes glucosuria. Pathologically the tubular changes vary from cloudy swelling to frank necrosis with tubular casts and desquamated cells. Interstitial edema with some cellular infiltrate occurs, but blood vessels appear normal (Fabre et al., 1978).

Direct toxicity of the aminoganglioside, puromycin, to glomerular components may also occur and may be a factor in renal failure. Experimental studies of the effects of puromycin have provided considerable basic information regarding the pathogenesis of direct chemical injury to glomerular structures. The effects are nonspecific. Epithelial cells become swollen with increase in lysosomes and pinocytotic activity, fusion and loss of foot processes, and reduction in number of filtration slits. As the lesion progresses, epithelial cells become detached, leaving "naked" basement membrane in direct contact with Bowman's capsule, which may account for the severe proteinuria (Caulfield et al., 1976). It is suggested that as the lesion progresses there is increase in basement membrane synthesis, mesangial cell proliferation and fusion, and crescent formation leading to the light-microscopic appearance of focal glomerular sclerosis (Gärtner, 1980).

The glomerular lesions produced by puromycin do not appear to invoke an immunologic response, so that the resulting alterations are entirely related to the direct toxicity of the drug.

CEPHALOSPORINS. The nephrotoxicity of cephalosporins was first noted when this drug was used in combination with aminonucleosides, but it is now recognized that cephalosporins, particularly cephalothin and cephaloridine, may produce degeneration and necrosis of proximal tubular lining cells and acute renal failure. It has been suggested that the cellular toxicity is the result of metabolic activation of the five-member thiophene ring present in cephalothin and cephaloridine, the only two cephalosporins that seem capable of producing direct nephrotoxicity (Mitchell et al., 1977). Toxicity is dose dependent. Necrosis occurs when concentration exceeds 1000 μg/g wet tissue. The correlation between dose and response as well as the localization of the lesion in the proximal portion of the nephron may be explained by a striking corticomedullary gradient in tissue concentration. The mechanism of toxicity is complex and not well defined. Direct mitochondrial toxicity as well as inhibition of cytochrome P-450 oxidase has been observed. The cellular uptake of cephaloridine and nephrotoxicity has been modified or eliminated in experimental animals by pretreatment with either probenecid or p-aminohippuric acid. In a few patients treated with cephalosporins, an allergic interstitial nephritis occurs manifested by hematuria and eosinophilia similar to that observed in penicillin nephropathy.

AMPHOTERICIN B. The increasing use of immunosuppressive therapy and attendant systemic mycotic infections has resulted in an increased administration of amphotericin B. This drug is almost always associated with some degree of toxicity to the distal renal tubule with accompanying acidosis, hypokalemia, and polyuria (Butler, 1966; Douglas and Healy, 1969). Reduced renal blood flow and glomerular filtration rate may also occur. Pretreatment of experimental animals with furosemide or sodium protects against amphotericin B nephrotoxicity, suggesting that incorporation of amphotericin B into the luminal membranes of distal tubular cells increases chloride permeability, activating tubuloglomerular feedback (via chloride flux in the macula densa), resulting in renal ischemia and reduction in the glomerular filtration rate.

Hypokalemia is manifested morphologically by empty vacuoles in the basilar cytoplasm of cells of proximal and distal tubules. Hypokalemic vacuolation consists of invaginations of the basilar membrane and is reversible.

TETRACYCLINES. Nephrotoxicity of tetracycline incited considerable interest in the early 1960s, shortly after its introduction. Persons, particularly children, developed a reversible proximal tubular dysfunction after receiving outdated drugs. The nephrotoxicity was found to be due to a degradation product, anhydro-4-epitetracycline. The problem has disappeared with the substitution of citric acid for lactose as a vehicle (Curtis, 1979).

Other rare effects of tetracycline that have been reported are impairment of renal-concentrating ability by demethylchlorotetracycline and rare occurrence of acute interstitial nephritis after minocycline. More important to current usage is the awareness that the serum half-life of the two most commonly used drugs, tetracycline and oxytetracycline, is greatly prolonged in renal failure, and the antianabolic effect of the tetracyclines, which inhibit the incorporation of amino acids into protein, may further contribute to negative nitrogen balance and uremia by raising blood urea nitrogen.

Penicillamine

Penicillamine (β-β-dimethylcystein) was first used clinically as a copper-chelating agent to treat Wilson's disease. Because of the drug's potential for decreasing collagen formation, its use has been extended to a number of clinical disorders in which fibrosis is a major component such as rheumatoid arthritis, pulmonary fibrosis, and liver disorders.

It has been hypothesized that the drug acts by reducing disulfide linkage, which inhibits polymerization of macromolecules with subsequent impairment of collagen formation. Use of the drug has been tempered by the occurrence of side effects in as many as 30% of patients. The most important side effect (20% of cases) is proteinuria. The morphologic appearance of the glomerular lesions is typically that of perimembranous glomerulonephritis with segmental subepithelial immune-complex deposits. These changes are best demonstrated as granular immunofluorescent deposits of IgG and C3. Withdrawal of penicillamine therapy has resulted in disappearance of the proteinuria and repair of the basement membrane changes in 60% of cases (Gärtner, 1980).

Immune-complex glomerulonephritis with granular deposits along basement membrane and in the mesangium can be produced experimentally, confirming the role of an immunologic mechanism in the pathogenesis of the nephropathy.

Cis-Platinum

Cis-Platinum (cis-dichlorodiamminiplatinum II), one of the platinum compounds with antitumor activity, produces proximal and distal tubular cell injury mainly in the corticomedullary region where the concentration of platinum is highest (Madias and Harrington, 1978). Although 90% of administered cis-platinum becomes tightly bound to plasma proteins, only unbound platinum seems to exert tumor cytotoxicity. However, unbound platinum is rapidly filtered by the glomerulus and has a half-life of only 48 minutes. Within tissues, platinum is protein bound with largest concentrations in kidney, liver, and spleen, and has a half-life of 2 or 3 days. Tubular cell toxicity seems to be directly related to dose, and prolonged weekly injection in rats causes atrophy of cortical portions of nephrons and cystic dilatation of inner cortical or medullary tubules, as well as chronic renal failure due to tubulointerstitial nephritis (Choie et al., 1981).

VOLATILE HYDROCARBONS

Volatile hydrocarbons, particularly chlorinated compounds such as carbon tetrachloride and trichloroethylene, may produce glomerular lesions leading to nephrotic syndrome and renal failure.

The relationship of volatile hydrocarbon exposure to the development of glomerulonephritis in populations is not clear. It has been determined that among patients with glomerulonephritis there are more persons with history of exposure to hydrocarbon solvents than would be expected. Attempts to produce the glomerular lesions observed in patients have only been partially successful (Zimmerman and Norbach, 1980). Solvent-exposed rats had increased proteinuria and glomerular sclerosis, but proliferative lesions and significant immune deposits were not observed. Of 15 patients studied in Sweden with poststreptococcal glomerulonephritis, 6 had history of brief exposure to organic solvents before development of their disease, suggesting to these investigators that solvent exposure may influence the outcome of an infection with streptococci. Prior exposure to hydrocarbon-containing solvents has been identified in a number of patients with Goodpasture's syndrome (Gärtner, 1980). Apart from the pulmonary manifestation of cough, shortness of breath, and hemoptysis, there may be hematuria and proteinuria. Renal morphology consists of a proliferative glomerulonephritis with IgG and C3 in glomerular basement membrane.

An autoimmune mechanism following chronic exposure is probably responsible for the glomerular lesions. In patients who have the Goodpasture's syndrome, the primary site of damage may be the alveolar basement membrane of lung, which is damaged by inhalation of the solvents, and antibodies to altered alveolar basement membrane may cross-react with glomerular basement membrane. Alternatively, autoimmunity may follow direct toxic injury to renal tubular or glomerular structures. Acute exposure to these solvents does produce acute tubular necrosis, and it is likely that prolonged exposures to low levels that do not result in cell necrosis may produce cell injury sufficient to damage renal cell membranes and provide the antigen for the immune reaction (Gärtner, 1980).

Experimental studies have shown that trichloroethylene and carbon tetrachloride-induced tubular cell injury is potentiated by polyhalogenated biphenyl exposure—for example, polychlorinated biphenyls (Kluwe et al., 1979).

SILICON

An association between occupational exposure to free silica (SiO_2) and a chronic nephropathy has been suspected for several years, but the number of reported cases is few. Clinically, lung fibrosis is the primary problem, but in an early study from Italy chronic renal failure was found in 40% and proteinuria in 20% of 20 patients with chronic silicosis. To date, measurement of silicon (Si) content of kidney tissue of patients with proteinuria and chronic silicon exposure has shown that renal silicon content is greatly elevated over levels in control cases, and there appears to be a direct relationship between level of exposure and probability of renal disease. Animal studies have demonstrated that silicon is excreted with glomerular filtrate, and morphologic study of experimental animals and human biopsy material has demonstrated silicon deposits in subepithelial and subendothelial areas of basement membrane and in epithelial cells. Human biopsy materials show a mild focal or segmental proliferative glomerulonephritis and absence of significant immune-complex deposits. These findings suggest a direct toxic effect on the glomerulus. These cases also have varying degrees of tubular cell degeneration. Animal studies demonstrate a dose-related nephropathy that

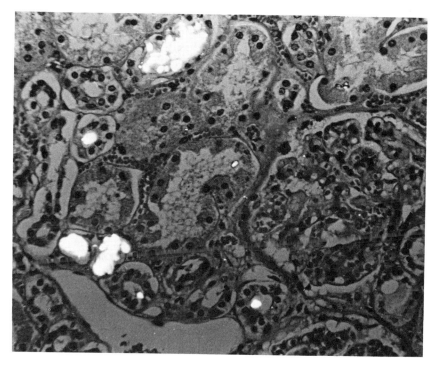

Figure 10–12. Oxalate crystals in tubules of patient with ethylene glycol toxicity (polarized light microscopy, H&E, ×200). (From Dr. Charles Jennette, University of North Carolina, Chapel Hill.)

is primarily tubular, with an interstitial inflammatory reaction and fibrosis. The proliferative glomerular lesions observed in humans are not seen in animals, but this difference in response may be related to dose or species (Hauglustaine et al., 1980).

ETHYLENE GLYCOL

Ethylene glycol, a constituent of antifreeze, is occasionally ingested and causes severe acute toxicity to brain and kidney. Acute tubular necrosis is followed by renal failure. Exposure often leads to permenent renal damage. A morphologic feature of mild ethylene glycol toxicity is cytoplasmic vacuolation, which may suggest hypokalemic nephropathy or osmotic nephrosis due to mannitol. Most ethylene glycol is excreted unmetabolized, but about 2% is metabolized to oxalic acid accompanied by deposition of calcium oxalate crystals in the kidney, which may contribute to a persistent inflammatory reaction and interstitial fi-

brosis (Figure 10-12). Excessive urinary excretion of oxalate and crystal formation may also be seen following administration of halogen-containing anesthetic agents, particularly methoxyflurane and halothane (Roxe, 1980). Treatment of acute ethylene glycol toxicity is with ethanol, which competes as a substrate for alcohol dehydrogenase (Peterson et al., 1981).

HEROIN

Heroin deserves brief mention, because it is estimated that about 1% of heroin addicts develop hematuria, proteinuria, or even the nephrotic syndrome (Cunningham et al., 1980). Morphologically, the renal lesion has been described as focal sclerosing glomerulonephritis. In the absence of proliferative lesion or immune deposits, a direct toxic effect of heroin or even a contaminant or solvent employed in the administration of heroin has been suggested as the major pathogenetic mechanism. However, heroin-related increases in IgM titers have been regarded as evidence that an immunologic mechanism may actually play some role in this disorder.

BALKAN NEPHROPATHY

A high frequency or endemic of a chronic interstitial nephritis has been recognized since 1957 in localized areas of Bulgaria, Rumania, and Yugoslavia. The disease may have been present as long ago as the 1920s. Families with affected persons are confined to villages located in valleys between hilly areas near the Danube River as it passes through portions of the three countries.

Balkan nephropathy is an interesting case study of an environmentally related chronic renal disease. At this time the etiology is unknown, but a number of factors have been implicated. Mycotoxins, particularly ochratoxin-A, have been implicated because of similarities with disease in animals and identification of the mycotoxin in food where nephrotoxicity is most frequent. Silicates have been suggested because of the proximity of villages with affected families to streams and rivers. Drinking water containing silicate and also nickel and chromium produces chronic nephropathy and renal tumors in experimental animals.

There also seems to be an association between incidence of nephropathy and urinary tract tumors. Inhabitants of the 15 villages in the Vratza region of northern Bulgaria have a 30–40% mortality rate from chronic nephropathy; urinary tract tumors comprise 25–30% of all neoplasms in males and females in these geographic areas (Markovic, 1972).

Cancer of the Urinary Tract

Tumors of the renal parenchyma, pelvis, and ureters are uncommon, accounting for less than 2% of all human cancers. Nevertheless, these are usually lethal tumors, and the survival rate for renal cancer remains essentially unchanged over the past 20 years. A compilation of trends in cancer rates in the United States indicates that the incidence of

Table 10–7. Trends in Kidney and Urinary Bladder Cancer Rates, Incidence per 100,000 (Whites)/Year

		1969	1976	Average annual percentage change
Kidney	M	9.0	9.6	1.2
	F	4.3	4.8	1.3
Bladder	M	23.8	26.4	2.3
	F	6.3	7.3	2.5

Source: Data from Pollack and Horm (1980).

both kidney and bladder cancer is increasing (Table 10-7) (Pollack and Horm, 1980). In contrast to renal cancer, however, mortality from bladder cancer is decreasing, probably reflecting earlier diagnosis and improvements in therapy. The role of environmental factors is unclear, but cancer of these sites is most common in certain industrialized nations (Sweden) and in persons in higher socioeconomic groups. It is nearly twice as common in males as in females, and there is perhaps a slowly increasing incidence in females, probably reflecting the increase in smoking among women.

The ratio between tumors of renal parenchyma and pelvis is fairly constant, about five to one, and the parallel trends in increasing incidence argues for some commonality in the etiology of tumors at both sites, although some factors may be site specific.

RENAL ADENOCARCINOMA

Renal cortical adenomas and adenocarcinomas tend to be circumscribed, ranging in size from microscopic lesions to large neoplasms (Hamilton, 1975). These tumors are believed to arise from proximal renal tubular epithelium, and the spectrum from small benign lesions to clearly malignant lesions suggests a continuous pathologic process, so that it is often difficult to label smaller tumors as benign or malignant. In the absence of invasion of surrounding tissue, features such as frequent mitotic figures, cellular pleomorphism, and hemorrhage and necrosis generally indicate a malignant potential regardless of size (Fig-

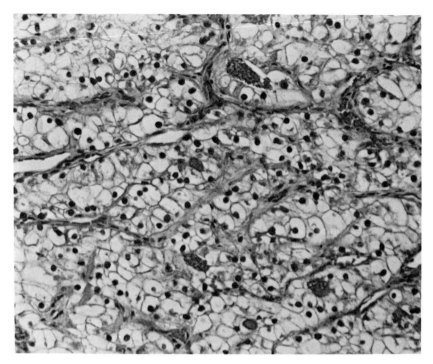

Figure 10–13. Photomicrograph of renal cell carcinoma showing neoplastic cells with clear cytoplasm and a scantily fibrovascular stroma (H&E, ×200). (From Dr. Charles Jennette, University of North Carolina, Chapel Hill.)

ure 10-13). Calcification may be detected by X-ray examination in about 15% of cases. Although 2–3% may be cystic, the commonest form is a solid tumor that is usually composed of clear cells rich in lipid, glycogen, or both, but may contain granular cells or even tightly packed eosinophilic cells referred to as oncocytes. Cell pattern may be trabecular, solid, or mixed, but it is doubtful that cell type or structural pattern has any clinical significance. Grading is difficult and has not been shown to be clinically useful. These tumors usually grow slowly, and overall survival is 20–25% after nephrectomy. The presence of multiple tumors, renal vein invasion, or regional lymph node metastases indicates a poorer prognosis.

Tumors of the renal pelvis form a spectrum from benign papillomas to frank papillary carcinomas and, like bladder tumors, are generally low-grade cancers, but they tend to recur regardless of their morphology.

The role of specific environmental factors in the etiology of urinary tract tumors has been difficult to define. Apart from increases in renal tumors in asbestos workers and the identification of some occupationally related bladder tumors, there does not appear to be a clearly defined association with specific chemicals or environmental factors, but rather a combination of exposure to substances in the environment, and life-style practices such as tobacco use. This suggests that there may be interactions between substances or that the urinary tract, like the lung, must cope with a number of substances with promoter activity. Cigarette smokers have a twofold increase in risk to urinary tract tumors, and an increase associated with alcohol and coffee usage is suggested. Also, chronic interstitial nephritis may predispose to urinary tract tumors. People with endemic (Balkan) nephropathy have an increase in renal tumors and a possible relationship between chronic interstitial nephritis and renal neoplasia, as has been demonstrated experimentally for lead and nitrilotriacetic acid. Yet human populations with excessive exposure to these and other known carcinogens (cycasin in Guam, aflatoxins in Africa and Asia) have not yet been shown to have an increase in kidney cancer (Sufrin and Beckley, 1980).

A number of case reports and epidemiologic studies have linked heavy use of analgesic mixtures and transitional cell carcinoma of the renal pelvis and, less commonly, tumors of the ureter. Phenacetin is an aromatic amide with N-hydroxylated amines. One of these metabolites, N-hydroxyphenacetin, has been shown to be a potent liver carcinogen and is suspected of being the carcinogen responsible for the renal tumors due to chronic analgesic abuse (Gonwa et al., 1980). Renal tumors may be induced in laboratory animals by various natural products and biologic and chemical agents, but in most instances linkage of exposure of these substances to renal cancer in humans is lacking or, at best, only suspected. Tumors of the kidney have been produced experimentally in rodents by several investigators over the past 30 years by the ingestion of various inorganic compounds of lead (Van Esch and Kroes, 1969). Renal tumors have even been observed in wild rats presumably exposed to lead fumes from burning refuse. The tumors arise from tubular epithelial cells in kidneys and are similar to renal cortical tumors found in humans. Production of tumors requires continuous exposure to relatively large concentrations of lead in diet or drinking water for 1 to 2 years. The tumors occur in a background of severe interstitial nephritis characterized by tubular atrophy as well as focal areas of hyperplasia. They are usually multifocal and vary from microscopic adenomas to large renal adenocarcinomas that may invade contiguous structures or metastasize to lungs. Intranuclear inclusions, usually present in proximal tubular epithelial cells, are absent in neoplastic cells, and, as expected, the tumors contain much less lead than adjacent renal parenchyma (Mao and Molnar, 1967). Tumor cells are pleomorphic, and ultrastructural studies have shown marked morphologic alterations in mitochondria.

As association between renal cancer and excess exposure to lead in people has not been clearly established, but a study of lead smelter and battery workers found a significant excess of malignancies at all sites combined, mostly lung tumors, but not specifically kidney (Cooper and Gaffey, 1975). However, case reports of renal tumors in workers with lead nephropathy have recently appeared (Baker et al., 1980; Lilis, 1981).

Renal cancer occurs after injection of crystalline nickel subsulfide (Ni_3S_2) into the kidney of rats, but renal cancer does not occur following treatment with amorphous nickel sulfide (NiS). Also, no experimental evidence indicates that nickel compounds are carcinogenic in experimental animals when administered by oral or subcutaneous routes (Sunderman, 1981).

Nitrilotriacetic acid, a polyamino polycarboxylic acid with chelating properties similar to EDTA (used to treat lead poisoning), produces chronic interstitial nephropathy in rodents. A spectrum of tubular cell histology occurs from hyperplasia to small adenomas to adenocarcinomas (Goyer et al., 1981).

URETERAL TUMORS

Primary tumors of the ureter are very rare and are usually well-differentiated papillomas covered with transitional epithelium (Hamilton, 1975). Associations with specific chemicals or environmental factors have not been reported.

TUMORS OF THE URINARY BLADDER

Tumors of the urinary bladder usually develop at multiple sites, suggesting that each site is the result of a separate event, each site being derived from an individual cell that has been transformed by urine-borne carcinogens. Hicks (1980) suggests that

the induction of human bladder cancer may occur as the result of prolonged or repeated expo-

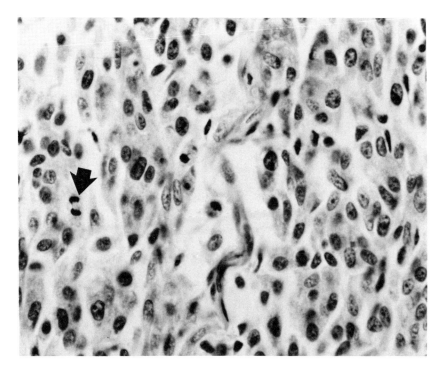

Figure 10–14. Photomicrograph of a high-grade transitional cell carcinoma showing disorganized elongated cells with plemorphic nuclei having coarse chromatin (arrow, mitotic figure) (H&E, ×470). (From Dr. Charles Jennette, University of North Carolina, Chapel Hill.)

sure to large doses of a single carcinogen such as β-naphthylamine but far more bladder tumors probably result either from exposure to low doses of two or more carcinogens that have a synergistic effect, or from initiation of the neoplastic process by a low dose of carcinogen followed by promotion with cofactors that may not be complete carcinogens per se.

Tumors of the urinary bladder are nearly always transitional cell papillomas (Figure 10-14) extending from well-differentiated, benign-appearing lesions to frank malignant carcinomas. However, because of the tendency of all urinary bladder papillomas to recur, regardless of histologic appearance, all tumors of the urinary bladder epithelium are considered malignant or potentially malignant.

Aniline Dye Tumors

The occurrence of excessive urinary bladder cancers among workers in the aniline dye industry at the end of the last century is one of the classic accounts of chemical carcinogenesis in a human population.

Benzidine and β-naphthylamine are potent mutagens, and benzidine is now linked to the occurrence of malignant lymphomas as well as bladder cancer. Carcinogenesis related to β-naphthylamine has been found to be due to a specific metabolite, an *ortho*-hydroxylamine, 2-amino-R-naphthol, which is water soluble. The ortho-hydroxylated metabolites are excreted in urine as sulfated glucuronate complexes and are split in urine by glucuronidases. Both benzidine and β-naphthylamine produce toxic effects in proximal renal tubular lining cells at levels of exposure in which tumors occur, and it has been suggested that they may in fact be promoters rather than primary carcinogens (IARC, 1982).

Saccharin and Bladder Cancer

Saccharin is a prime example of the problem of proving an effect of a weakly carcinogenic substance in humans. Saccharin is a non-nutritive sweetener that was discovered in 1879, and shortly after the turn of the century it was introduced as a substitute for sugar in canned products. Usage through the 1950s and 1960s was fairly well limited to dietetic foods mixed with cyclamates. Following the ban on cyclamate use in 1969, per capita consumption of saccharin has increased steadily, principally as a sweetener in diet soft drinks. In 1976 the U.S. Food and Drug Administration reported that approximately 2.7–3.5 million kg of saccharin were used in the United States. Earlier long-term animal feeding studies indicated formation of bladder tumors, but there was uncertainty as whether this effect was due to saccharin itself or to an impurity, *ortho*-toluene sulfonamide (OTA). A subsequent study in Canada in which two generations of rats were fed saccharin or OTA, beginning with the weaning of the first generation, demonstrated an increased incidence of bladder tumors in second-generation rats fed saccharin but not OTA.

Continued studies of the carcinogenic properties of saccharin have not shown conclusively that it is mutagenic (Batzinger et al., 1977). Epidemiologic studies have likewise been negative in spite of the large populations that have been at risk and available for study (Morrison and Buring, 1980). One possible explanation for the lack of positive epidemiologic studies is that the large usage of saccharin only began about 10 years ago, so that the usual latency period of 20 or more years that elapses between exposure and tumor formation has not yet occurred.

Experimental induction of bladder tumors occurs in a diet containing saccharin in which the urinary bladder had been previously exposed to a nontumorigenic dose of the carcinogenic nitrosamide, *N*-methyl-*N*-nitrosourea. These experiments suggest the carcinogenic action of saccharin is by way of promotion of previously initiated cells (Hicks et al., 1978).

REFERENCES

Ainsworth, S. K., Swain, R. P., Watabe, N., Brackett, N.C., Pilia, P., and Hennigar, G. R. 1981. Gold nephropathy, ultrastructural fluorescent and energy-dispersive x-ray microanalysis study. *Arch. Pathol. Lab. Med.* 105:373–378.

Auerbach, O., Constan, A. S., Garfinkel, L., Parks, V. R., Kaslow, H. D., and Hammond, E. C. 1980. Presence of asbestos bodies in organs other than the lung. *Chest* 77: 133–137.

Baker, E. L., Goyer, R. A., Fowler, B. A., Khettery, U., Bernard, D. B., Adler, S., White, R. deV., Babayan, R., and Feldman, R. G. 1980. Occupational lead exposure, nephropathy, and renal cancer. *Am J. Ind. Med.* 1:139–148.

Batzinger, R. P., Ou, S. L., and Bueding, E. 1977. Saccharin and other sweeteners: Mutagenic properties. *Science* 198:944–946.

Buchet, J-P., Roels, H., Bernard, A., and Lauwerys, R. 1981. Assessment of renal function of workers simultaneously exposed to inorganic lead and cadmium. *J. Occup. Med.* 23:348–352.

Burkholder, P. M. 1982. Functions and pathophysiology of the glomerular mesangium (editorial). *Lab. Invest.* 46:239–241.

Butler, W. T. 1966. Pharmacology, toxicity, and therapeutic usefulness of amphotericin B. *J.A.M.A.* 195:371–375.

Caulfield, J. P., Reid, J. J., and Farqubar, M. G. 1976. Alterations of the glomerular epithelium in aminonucleoside nephrosis. *Lab. Invest.* 34:43–59.

Cherian, M. G., and Goyer, R. A. 1978. Metallothioneins and their role in the metabolism and toxicity of metals. *Life Sci.* 23:1–10.

Cherian, M. G., Goyer, R. A., and Richardson, L. D. 1976. Cadmium-induced nephropathy. *Toxicol. Appl. Pharmacol.* 38:399–406.

Choie, D. D., Longenecker, D. S., and Del Campo, A. A. 1981. Acute and chronic cisplatin nephropathy in rats. *Lab. Invest.* 44:397–402.

Cooper, W. C., and Gaffey, W. R. 1975. Mortality of lead workers. *J. Occup. Med.* 17:100–107.

Cotran, R. S. 1979. *Interstitial nephritis in kidney disease—present status.* Baltimore: Waverly Press, pp. 254–280.

Cramer, K., Goyer, R. A., Jagenburg, R., and Wilson, M. 1974. Renal ultrastructure, renal function and parameters of lead toxicity in workers with different periods of lead exposure. *Br. J. Ind. Med.* 31:113–127.

Cunningham, E. E., Brentjens, J. R., Zielezrey, M. A., Andres, G. A., and Veruto, R. C. 1980. Heroin nephropathy: A clinic-pathologic and epidemiologic study. *Am. J. Med.* 68:47–53.

Curtis, J. R. 1979. Drug-induced renal disease. *Drugs* 18:377–391.

Davis, B. B., Mattammal, M. B., and Zenser, T. V. 1981. Renal metabolism of drugs and xenobiotics. *Nephron* 7:187–196.

Douglas, J. B., and Healy, J. K. 1969. Nephrotoxic effects of amphotericin B, including renal tubular acidosis. *Am. J. Med.* 46:154–162.

Fabre, J., Tillastre, J-P., Morin, J-P., and Rudhardt, M. 1978. Nephrotoxicity of gantamicin. Action on subcellular organelles and pharmacokinetics in the kidney. In *Contributions to nephrology*. vol. 10, *Toxic nephropathies*, pp. 53–62, eds. G. M. Berlyne, S. Giorannetti, and S. Thomas. Basel: S. Karger.

Finkelstein, A., Fraley, D. S., Stachura, I., Feldman, H. A., Gandy, D. R., and Bourke, E. 1982. Fenoprofen nephropathy: Lipoid nephrosis and interstitial nephritis. *Am. J. Med.* 72:81–86.

Fowler, B. A., and Goyer, R. A. 1975. Bismuth localization within nuclear inclusions by x-ray microanalysis: Effects of accelerating voltage. *Histochem. Cytochem.* 23:722–726.

Friberg, L., Piscator, M., Nordberg, G. F., and Kjellstrom, T. 1974. *Cadmium in the environment*, 2nd Ed. Cleveland: Chemical Rubber Co. Press.

Gärtner, H. V. 1980. Drug-associated nephropathy. In *Drug-induced Pathology*. Vol. 69, *Current topics in pathology*, eds. C. L. Berry, E. Grundmann, and W. H. Kirsten, pp. 144–174. New York: Springer-Verlag.

Gonwa, T. A., Corbett, W. T., Schey, H. M., and Buckalew, V. M. 1980. Analgesic-associated nephropathy and transitional cell carcinomas of the urinary tract. *Ann. Intern. Med.* 93:249–252.

Goyer, R. A., and Cherian, M. G. 1977. Tissue and cellular toxicology of metals. In *Clinical chemistry and chemical toxicology of metals*, ed. S. S. Brown, pp. 89–103. Amsterdam: Elsevier-North Holland.

Goyer, R. A., Falk, H. L., Hogan, M., Feldman,

D. D., and Richter, W. 1981. Renal tumors in rats given trisodium nitrilotriacetic acid in drinking water for 2 years. *J.N.C.I.* 66:869–880.

Goyer, R. A., and Rhyne, B. C. 1973. Pathological effects of lead. *Int. Rev. Exp. Pathol.* 12:1–77.

Goyer, R. A., and Wilson, M. H. 1975. Lead-induced inclusion bodies: Results of EDTA treatment. *Lab. Invest.* 32:149–156.

Gritzka, T. L., and Trump, B. F. 1968. Renal tubular lesions caused by mercuric chloride. *Am. J. Pathol.* 52:1225–1277.

Hamilton, J. M. 1975. Renal carcinogenesis. *Adv. Cancer Res.* 22:1–56.

Hauglustaine, D., Van Damme, B., Daenens, P., and Michielsen, P. 1980. Silicon nephropathy: A possible occupational hazard. *Nephron* 26:219–224.

Hicks, R. M. 1980. Multistage carcinogenesis in the urinary bladder. *Br. Med. Bull.* 36:39–46.

Hicks, R. M., Chowaniec, J., and Wakefield, J. St. J. 1978. Experimental induction of bladder tumors by a two-stage system in carcinogenesis. In *Mechanisms of tumor promotion and cocarcinogenesis*, vol. 2, eds. T. J. Slaga, A. Sivak, and R. K. Boutwell, pp. 475–489. New York: Raven Press.

International Agency for Research on Cancer. 1982. *Some aromatic amines, anthraquinones, and nitro compounds and inorganic fluorides used in drinking water and dental preparations.* IARC Monographs on the Evaluation of Carcinogenic Risk of Chemicals to Humans, vol. 27, pp. 39–61. Lyons, France: World Health Organization.

Jacques, P. J. 1975. The endocytic uptake of macromolecules. In *Pathology of cell membranes*, vol. 1, eds. B. F. Trump and U. A. Arstilla, pp. 225–276. New York: Academic Press.

Kazantzis, G. 1979. Renal tubular dysfunction and abnormalities of calcium metabolism in cadmium workers. *Environ. Health Perspect.* 28:155–159.

Kjellstrom, T., and Nordberg, G. T. 1978. The kinetic model of cadmium metabolism in the human body. *Environ. Res.* 16:248–269.

Kleinknecht, D., Kanfer, A., Morel-Maroger, L., and Mery, J. P. 1978. Immunologically mediated drug-induced acute renal failure. *Contrib. Nephrol.* 10:42–52.

Kluwe, W. M., Herrmann, C. L., and Hook, J. B. 1979. Effects of dietary polychlorinated biphenyls and polybrominated biphenyls on the renal and hepatic toxicities of several chlorinated hydrocarbon solvents in mice. *J. Toxicol. Environ. Health* 5:605–615.

Lauwerys, R., Roels, H., Bernard, A., and Buchet, J-P. 1980. Renal response to cadmium in a population living in a non-ferrous smelter area in Belgium. *Int. Arch. Occup. Environ. Health* 45:271–274.

Lilis, R. 1981. Long-term occupational lead exposure, chronic nephropathy and renal cancer: A case report. *Am. J. Ind. Med.* 2:293–298.

Madias, N. E., and Harrington, J. T. 1978. Platinum nephrotoxicity (review). *Am. J. Med.* 65:307–314.

Mahaffey, K. R. 1980. Nutrient-lead interactions. In *Lead toxicity,* eds. R. L. Singhal and J. A. Thomas, pp. 425–460. Baltimore: Urban and Schwarzenberg.

Maher, J. F. 1976. Toxic nephropathy. In *The kidney,* eds. B. M. Brenner and F. C. Rector, Jr., pp. 1355–1384. Philadelphia: W. B. Saunders.

Mao, P., and Molnar, J. J. 1967. The fine structure and histochemistry of lead induced renal tumors in rats. *Am. J. Pathol.* 50:571–603.

Markovic, B. 1972. Endemic nephritis and urinary tract cancer in Yugoslavia, Bulgaria and Rumania. *J. Urol.* 107:212–219.

Mason, T. J., Fraumeni, J. F., Hoover, R., and Blot, W. J. 1981. *An atlas of mortality from selected diseases,* NIH Publication No. 81-2397. Washington, D.C.: U.S. Dept. of Health and Human Services.

Mazze, R. I. 1976. Methoxyflurane nephropathy. *Environ. Health Perspect.* 15:111–119.

McLachlin, J. R., Goyer, R. A., and Cherian, M. G. 1980. Formation of lead-induced inclusion bodies in primary rat kidney epithelial cell cultures. *Toxicol. Appl. Pharmacol.* 56:418–431.

Mitchell, J. R., McMurtry, R. J., Statham, C. N., and Nelson, S. D. 1977. Molecular basis for several drug-induced nephropathies. *Am. J. Med.* 62:518–526.

Moore, J. R., Goyer, R. A., and Wilson, M. H. 1973. Lead-induced inclusion bodies: Solubility, amino acid content, and relationship to residual acidic proteins. *Lab. Invest.* 29:488–494.

Morrison, A. B., and Buring, J. E. 1980. Artificial sweeteners and cancer of the lower urinary tract. *N. Engl. J. Med.* 302:537–541.

Murray, T., and Goldberg, M. 1975. Chronic interstitial nephritis: Etiologic factors. *Ann. Intern. Med.* 82:453–459.

Nanra, R. S. 1980. Clinical and pathological aspects of analgesic nephropathy. *Br. J. Clin. Pharmacol.* 10:3595–3685.

Nogawa, K., Kobayashi, E., and Honda, R. 1979. A study of the relationship between cadmium concentrations in urine and renal effects of cadmium. *Environ. Health Perspect.* 28:161–168.

Nomiyama, K. 1980. Recent progress and perspectives in cadmium health effects studies. *Sci. Total Environ.* 14:199–232.

Nordberg, G. F., Goyer, R. A., and Nordberg, M. 1975. Comparative toxicity of cadmium-metallothionein and cadmium chloride on mouse kidney. *Arch. Pathol.* 99:192–197.

Peterson, C. D., Collins, A. J., Hines, J. M., Bullock M. L., and Keane, W. F. 1981. Ethylene glycol poisoning: Pharmacokinetics during therapy with ethanol and hemodialysis. *N. Engl. J. Med.* 304:21–23.

Pollack, E. S., and Horm, J. W. 1980. Trends in cancer incidence and mortality in the United States, 1969–76. *J.N.C.I.* 64:1091–1103.

Prescott, L. F. 1970. Phenacetin nephropathy. *Br. Med. J.* 4:493.

Rennick, G. 1978. Renal excretion of cationic drugs: Tubule transport and metabolism. In *Nephrotoxicity interaction of drugs with membrane systems, mitochondria-lysosomes,* ed. J. P. Fillastre, pp. 1–41. New York: Masson Publishing.

Roman-Franco, A. A., Twirello, M., Albini, B., Ossi, E., Milgrom, F., and Andres, G. A. 1978. Anti-basement membrane antibodies and antigen-antibody complexes in rabbits injected with mercuric chloride. *Clin. Immunol. Immunopathol.* 9:404–481.

Roxe, D. M. 1980. Toxic nephropathy from diagnostic and therapeutic agents. *Am. J. Med.* 69:759–766.

Salvatierra, O., Feduska, N. J., Vincenti, F., Duca, R., Potter, D., Nolan, J., Cochrum, K. C., and Amend, W. J. C. 1979. Analysis of costs and outcomes of renal transplantation at one center. *J.A.M.A.* 241:1409–1473.

Sandstead, H. H., Michelakis, A. M., and Temple, T. E. 1970. Lead intoxication. Its effect on the renin-aldosterone response to sodium deprivation. *Arch. Environ. Health* 20:356–363.

Schumann, G. B., Lerner, S. I., Weiss, M. A.,

Gawronski, L., and Lohiya, G. K. 1980. Inclusion-bearing cells in industrial workers exposed to lead. *Am. J. Clin. Med.* 74:192–196.

Schwartz, M. M., and Cotran, R. S. 1976. Primary renal disease in transplant recipients. *Hum. Pathol.* 7:455–459.

Schwartz, S. L., Johnson, C. B., and Doolan, P. D. 1970. Study of the mechanism of renal vasculogenesis induced in the rat by EDTA. Comparison of the cellular activities of calcium and chromium. *Mol. Pharmacol.* 6:54–59.

Shelly, J. H. 1978. Pharmacological mechanisms of analgesic nephropathy. *Kidney Int.* 13:15–26.

Shreiner, G. E., and Maher, J F. 1965. Toxic nephropathy. *Am. J. Med.* 38:409–449.

Sorahan, T., Kokoszynska, R., and Adams, R. G. 1982. Trends in mortality from nephritis and nephrosis. *Lancet* 1:567.

Stuve, J., and Galle, P. 1970. Role of mitchondria in the handling of gold by the kidney. *J. Cell Biol.* 44:667–676.

Sufrin, G., and Beckley, S. A. 1980. *Renal adenocarcinoma*, technical report, vol. 49, International Union Against Cancer, pp. 133–144.

Sunderman, F. W., Jr. 1981. Present research on nickel carcinogenesis. *Environ. Health Perspect.* 40:131–142.

Tubbs, R. R., Gephardt, G. N., McMahon, J. T., Pohl, M. C., Vidt, D. G., Barenberg, S. A., and Valenzuela, R. 1982. Membranous glomerulonephritis associated with industrial mercury exposure. *Am. J. Clin. Pathol.* 77:409–413.

Van Esch, G. J., and Kroes, R. 1969. The induction of renal tumors by feeding basic lead acetate to mice. *Br. J. Cancer* 23:765–771.

Victery, W., Vander, A. J., Shulak, J. M., Schoeps, P., and Julius, S. 1982. Lead, hypertension and the renin-angiotension system in rats. *J. Lab. Clin. Med.* 99:354–362.

Viol, G. W., Minielly, J. A., and Bistricki, T. 1977. Gold nephropathy: Tissue analysis by x-ray fluorescent spectroocopy. *Arch. Pathol. Lab. Med.* 101:635–640.

Warren, S. E., and Mosley, C. 1983. Renal failure and tubular dysfunction due to zomepirac therapy. *J.A.M.A.* 249:396–397.

Wedeen, R. P., Mallik, D. K., and Batuman, V. 1979. Detection and treatment of occupational lead nephropathy. *Arch. Intern. Med.* 139:53–57.

World Health Organization. 1977. WHO environmental health criteria for cadmium. *Ambio* 6:287–290.

Zimmerman, S. W., and Norbach, D. H. 1980. Nephrotoxic effects of long-term carbon tetrachloride administration in rats. *Arch. Pathol. Lab. Med.* 104:94–99.

11

Immune System

Robert Burrell

The most obvious environmental effect on the immune response is that which initiates the response, that is, the antigen. Although survival of an individual depends on mounting effective immune responses against toxic or infectious agents, the same responses may be directed against innocuous materials as well. If the immune response to such materials is accompanied by certain types of inflammatory sequelae, immune injury or immunopathology can result. A second way in which environmental agents affect the immune response is by inhibiting normal responses or producing abnormal ones. This chapter will review the mechanisms of both the immune injury-generating and the immune-interference effects induced by environmental agents.

Mechanisms of Immune and Immune-like Injury

The body receives antigens primarily through three portals of entry: inhalation, direct skin contact, and ingestion. The route of such contact in part determines the type of immune response produced. For instance, inhalation of antigen primarily favors IgA and IgE responses, whereas direct skin contact favors cell-mediated immune responses. Often, such contact results in a demonstra-

ble immune response, but with no accompanying injury. For reasons not sufficiently understood, contact with antigen in certain individuals results in enough inflammation to be noticed. A number of mechanisms of immune injury are currently recognized.

IMMEDIATE ALLERGY

Immediate-type allergy or hypersensitivity is IgE dependent (Ishizaka, 1971) and is thus called because the signs and symptoms of reactivity occur within seconds or minutes after antigen contact. IgE may be found free in both plasma and secretions, but it is in the form bound to basophils and mast cells that is most significant clinically. IgE antibodies have a molecular weight of about 190,000, have a relatively fast gamma, electrophoretic mobility, and are present in normal serum in concentrations of only about 250 ng/ml. These concentrations may rise to nearly 700 ng/ml in severely allergic individuals, but it must be remembered that these circulating levels of IgE represent levels over and above those molecules bound to mast cells and basophils. The IgE is bound to the cell membranes by means of the Fc portion of the antibody's heavy chains, and from 5000 to 27,000 molecules may be bound per cell in the nonallergic individual and from 15,000 to 40,000 in the highly allergic. It is this property of IgE that has led to the synonyms, skin-sensitizing or cytotropic antibody.

IgE-producing plasma cells may be found widely dispersed in the secretory surfaces, especially in the bronchial and gastrointestinal mucosa, but very rarely in systemic lymphoid organs. When two or more IgE molecules per cell react with antigen, a stress is transmitted to the cell membrane, and certain stored pharmacologic mediators and enzymes are metabolically released from granules of the mast cell (Austen, 1978). Histamine, leukotrienes (LTD), heparin, serotonin, and various plasma kinins are among those substances known to be released by such IgE–antigen reactions. In addition, certain factors are released (e.g., platelet-activating factor and an eosinophil chemotactic factor) that in turn cause these target cells to release other mediators or controlling substances. The function of moderate, controlled amounts of these mediators is to facilitate tissue growth and repair as well as to induce modest amounts of inflammation to act in a positive, defensive way. When present in higher amounts, however, these mediators bring about the clinical signs and symptoms of allergy. The chief target tissues are smooth muscle and capillary endothelium, but the effect on these tissues may differ with the type of mediator primarily released. Smooth muscle contraction, capillary dilatation, and increase in capillary permeability are the classic signs of allergic reactions.

However, these mediators are not the only molecules important in the allergic reaction. Certain inhibitory mediators are released by eosinophils, which in turn have been attracted to the reaction via mast cell mediator release. Eosinophils release enzymes capable of degrading histamine and LTD's, and phagocytize immune complexes. Moreover, the mechanism is in part controlled by agonists of the sympathetic and parasympathetic nervous systems. The equilibrium of these two systems maintains homeostatic tone and function of organs.

These systems regulate mediator release in allergic reactions and, consequently, degree of responsiveness of the principal organ affected ("shock organ") (Frick, 1984). If this balance is upset, the organ loses tone, and dysfunction results. Knowledge of these actions permits artificial pharmacologic intervention to restore tone.

An important aspect of the allergic reaction that is often overlooked is the allergy-prone or atopic individual. In spite of uniform opportunity for sensitization in everyone to certain ubiquitous allergens (e.g., ragweed pollen), comparatively few become clinically hypersensitive. Atopy is partly due to inheritance, that is, the allergic tendency is inheritable and may be HL-A linked in part; however, atopy is also a function of the relative balance of IgE helper and suppressor cells in an individual. If, for reasons not entirely known—although partly genetic and partly environmental—the number of IgE helper cells increases, the result will be an increase in IgE production and binding to mast cells. Such an "allergic breakthrough" from the normal suppressor cell damping mechanism will result in the clinical manifestations of immediate allergy (H. D. Katz et al., 1979).

An extensive treatment of allergy is beyond the scope of this chapter, but well-recognized IgE-generating allergens can be categorized into large general classes such as pollens, animal danders, feathers, dusts, molds, organic dusts, industrial chemicals, and foods (Table 11-1). Except for foods, all of these materials are capable of generating IgE reactions in susceptible individuals when inhaled. Dermal manifestations of IgE-dependent reactions may arise following inhalation or ingestion, and may appear as urticaria or atopic dermatitis, although the latter involves other pharmacologic and physiologic abnormalities as well (Baer and Gigli, 1979). Gastrointestinal allergy is often blamed for many food-induced disturbances of the GI tract, but it is a very difficult diagnosis to detect (T. P. King and Norman, 1978). Egg and fish protein sensitivity, and milk allergy in infants in the absence of malabsorption causes, do seem

Table 11–1. Representative Antigens That
May Cause Respiratory Allergy

Antigen category	Examples
Pollens	Timothy, orchard, June, and Burmuda grasses Maple, birch, oak, and elm trees Ragweed, plantain, pigweed, lambs quarters, sheep sorrel
Organic dusts	Coffee dusts, sawdust, seed meals, flour
Foods	Fish M, egg white, milk proteins
Molds	*Alternaria, Aspergillus, Helminthosporium, Hormodendrum, Mucor, Rhizopus*
Epidermoids	Horse, cat, rabbit, and other animal danders Avian dander and feathers Wool Insect and mite exoskeleta, egg cases, etc.
Industrial chemicals	Platinum, and nickel salts Penicillin Pyrethrum Plasticizers

to be notable exceptions (T. P. King and
Norman, 1978).

CYTOTOXIC ANTIBODIES

If humoral antibodies of the classes other
than IgE react with cell surface antigens, the
result could lead to cytotoxicity, lysis, or
phagocytic engulfment of the target cell.
Complement may be involved in some of
these reactions, although not necessarily.
There are three general ways in which cell
surface substances become antigenic. In one,
there is a coincidental specificity between an
environmental agent and a host substance
as in the well-studied example of the similarity between streptococcal cell membrane
antigen and myofibrillar antigen of heart
muscle in rheumatic fever (Espinosa et al.,
1969). An immune response to the extrinsic
antigen from the environment induces an
antibody that cross-reacts with intrinsic tissue antigens.

Another way that cytotoxic antibodies
arise is when an extrinsic substance, usually
a hapten of low molecular weight, couples
to host cell surfaces and induces an antibody response. Although the antibody is reacting with an extrinsic substance, there is
a resultant toxicity to the cell to which it is
attached. Drugs such as quinidine, sulfonamides, digitoxin, aspirin, novobiocin, ri-
fampin, and stibophen are just a few of the
many drugs known to combine to platelets
(McMillan and Gardner, 1977). The resulting destruction of platelets when antibody
reacts with the platelet-bound drug leads to
an immune thrombocytopenia (Cimo et al.,
1977). A similar mechanism is thought to
be responsible for certain forms of acquired
hemolytic anemia where certain antibiotics
(e.g., penicillin) have been shown to bind to
red cells and to induce cytotoxic antibodies. Such erythrocytes are Coombs' positive, but care must be taken in the interpretation of positive Coombs' tests. Certain
extrinsic agents such as cephalosporin and
vital dyes affect erythrocyte stroma nonspecifically, so that nonimmunologic proteins
bind to the cell surfaces (Frank et al., 1977).
A similar result is known to follow cardiac
surgery, where blood has been circulated
through artificial devices for lengthy periods of time.

The third way cytotoxic antibodies may
arise is when environmental agents affect cell
membranes in such a way as to expose hidden determinants. Such hidden antigens that
develop protected from immune response-
forming capability during embryogenesis are
thought to be regarded as "foreign" when
encountered later in life. Although largely a
theoretical mechanism, some evidence exists that cold agglutinins and panagglutin-
ins against erythrocytes arise in this manner.

Antibodies directed against glomerular,
skin, or alveolar basement membranes are
generally considered cytotoxic, although no

cells are involved; the antigen is an acellular membrane. Although abundant information exists that antibodies exist against these membranes, that they do deposit on them in vivo, fix complement, attract neutrophils and macrophages, and that the resulting inflammation damages these membranes, it is not clear how environmental or infectious agents are responsible for the production of membrane antibodies (Unanue and Dixon, 1967). A final, albeit hypothetical cytotoxic mechanism of injury involving humoral antibodies is through the possible mediation of antibody-dependent cell-mediated cytotoxicity (ADCC) (Roitt et al., 1976). In this instance an environmental agent could adsorb to a host cell or membrane and induce an antibody response. Subsequent deposition of antibodies on these cell-bound antigens could bind to Fc receptors on killer or K lymphocytes and result in cellular destruction. Research on ADCC to date has largely focused on innate cellular antigens or antigens from infectious agents.

IMMUNE-COMPLEX DISEASE

Immune-complex disease results from the deposition of antigen–antibody complexes in or on certain vulnerable sites, reacting with complement and subsequently causing damage through macrophage and neutrophil mediation (Randadive and Movat, 1979). The ratio of antigen to antibody in the complex seems to be important in causing the inflammation; that is to say, if formed at equivalence, the complexes would become particulate and be phagocytized, but soluble complexes formed in antigen excess resist phagocytosis and seem to generate more inflammation (Dixon et al., 1961). The renal glomerular basement membrane is the most well-known site of immune-complex deposition. Here, immune complexes localize within and on the epithelial side of the basement membrane (Dixon et al., 1961). The penetration of the complexes into the membrane is thought to be due to the proteolytic action of enzymes liberated from inflammatory cells drawn to the area as a result of complement activation by the complexes. Immune complexes also bind to platelet membranes, causing the release of stored basoactive amines. Immune-complex glomerulonephritis is most well known as a secondary phenomenon to certain bacterial, viral, and parasitic infections (e.g., poststreptococcal glomerulonephritis), or associated with autoantibody–antigen complexes in systemic lupus erythematosus. However, the possibility that immune-complex renal disease might be due to environmental agents complexing with host proteins to become antigens certainly cannot be excluded.

The idea of immune-complex disease resulting from contact with environmental agents has been most commonly discussed with regard to the inhalation disease, hypersensitivity pneumonitis (HP), a disease that is caused by the inhalation of respirable organic dusts of vegetable or animal origin (Emanuel et al., 1964). The prototype, farmer's lung, is produced in susceptible individuals following inhalation of dense aerosols of spoiled hay containing various species of thermophilic actinomyces. It has been postulated (Pepys, 1969) that antigens from these materials stimulate precipitating antibodies such that on subsequent inhalation, the intrapulmonary antigen–antibody reactions result in an Arthus reaction or allergic vasculitis in the lung. Unfortunately, there is very little evidence available to support this hypothesis (Burrell and Rylander, 1981). The only evidence that was used to establish this idea consisted of observations that many affected individuals possessed precipitating antibody to antigens in the offensive dust, the appearance of pulmonary function changes following bronchoprovocation testing occurred at a time coincident with the appearance of what has been called an Arthus skin reaction in humans, and an early report of a severe atypical case of farmer's lung characterized by pulmonary vasculitis (Barrowcliff and Arblaster, 1968). Against this view are observations that precipitins occur in many exposed individuals with no history or evidence of clinical disease, precipitins do not always occur in affected patients, repeated experimental studies have failed to produce evidence of an immune-complex etiology, and the pathology is not characteristic of a vasculitis reaction (Emanuel et al., 1964). The Arthus reaction was originally described in rabbits and is due to intravascular deposition of immune complexes involving the formation of thrombi, fibrin, and neutrophils, which leads to necrosis. The histologic characteristic of acute lesions in human HP is primarily a mononuclear infiltrate of the alveolar spaces with granulomata developing in the walls of the alveoli and bronchiole, whereas chronic disease is characterized by more local destruction of alveoli, large focal areas of fibrosis, and some dilatation of the bronchioles (Emanuel et al., 1964; Seal, 1975).

Intravascular formation of immune complexes may adsorb to formed elements in the blood and result in acquired hemolytic anemia or immune neutropenia and thus resemble the cytotoxic mechanism (Petz and Fudenberg, 1975; Frank et al., 1977). In the former, there seems to be an association of drugs like quinine and phenacetin with direct causality.

CELL-MEDIATED IMMUNE INJURY

The distinguishing feature of this form of immune injury is the participation of lymphocytes in bringing about inflammation (Hay, 1979). Specific antigen receptors are bound to lymphocyte cell membranes, and when they react with antigen, macromolecular mediators called lymphokines are released. Lymphokines have a variety of defensive functions, among which are chemotactic, mitogenic, and cytotoxic properties (David, 1976). This type of immunity is very effective against infectious agents that are either cell bound or intracellular, but in certain situations the defensive reaction is excessive enough to cause inflammation. The classical tuberculin reaction is the prototype of this kind of response and results largely from the infiltrative and cytotoxic

side reactions of the tuberculoprotein–lymphocyte interactions. Typically, such reactions become apparent 24–72 hours after contact and are thus called delayed-hypersensitivity reactions to distinguish them from the IgE-mediated, immediate reactions. The main cellular components of the infiltrations characteristic of delayed hypersensitivity are lymphocytes and monocytes that localize around venules, and in severe reactions, necrosis may also occur.

Usually one considers T lymphocytes as the type of cell involved in cell-mediated reactions, but it is becoming increasingly likely that B cells may also be involved (Rocklin et al., 1979). Environmental agents that are most likely to induce cell-mediated immunity are low-molecular-weight, hydrophobic haptens, which are capable of becoming complete antigens by coupling to host carrier proteins in vivo. Cell-mediated sensitization to environmental agents seems to be favored by contact with small doses via the dermal route. There is much experimental evidence that the inhalation route can also induce cell-mediated immunity and may represent clinically important means of initiating pulmonary disease following inhalation exposure to such agents as beryllium (Marx and Burrell, 1973) and moldy hay (Richerson et al., 1978). It is unlikely that the gastrointestinal tract is involved in cell-mediated immune reactions to environmental agents.

Cell-mediated immune reactions involving the skin result in contact dermatitis (Fisher, 1973), which may result from contact with a wide variety of environmental agents and may be of plant, mineral, or synthetic origin. A few of the more common agents are given in Table 11-2. Occasionally chronic contact with one of these agents (e.g., beryllium or zirconium) will lead to more of a granulomatous response where fibroblasts, epitheloid cells, and giant cells arranged into granulomas predominate. Most people feel that this is a result of a chronic cell-mediated immune reaction, but others feel that it is a separate type of immune injury (Epstein, 1967).

Table 11–2. Common Contact Sensitins

Sensitin category	Examples
Plant	Poison ivy
	European primrose
Synthetic compounds	Benzocaine
	Epoxy resins
	Mercaptans
	Picric acid derivatives
	Chlorinated hydrocarbons
	Ethylenediamine
Minerals	Beryllium
	Nickel
	Cadmium
	Chromates

NONSPECIFIC COMPLEMENT ACTIVATION

It is now recognized that there are at least two major means of activating the complement cascade (Müller-Eberhard, 1975). Activation via the classical pathway is initiated primarily by antigen–antibody (IgG or IgM) complexes, whereas activation of the alternative pathway is antibody independent. Alternative-pathway activation is initiated by materials that tend to be colloidal or finely particulate in physical nature, or are highly polymerized substances in chemical nature (e.g., polysaccharides). This pathway is an immunochemical method by which the body differentiates self from nonself. Activation of the complement cascade by either method results in a number of biologic effects that are defensive and/or inflammatory. These effects range from chemotaxis of neutrophils and macrophages with subsequent enhancement of phagocytosis (opsonization), to the modulation of several inflammatory mediators and kinins. Because the complement activation system is intricately linked with the coagulation and kinin-generating systems, the resulting series of biologic reactions following stimulation may be quite complex. More than a potent stimulator is needed, however, and it is postulated that for an adverse reaction to occur by such a method, there also needs to be an intrinsic defect in the host, either an extralabile complement component or too little concentration of one of the control substances (Berrens et al., 1974). Initiation of complement activation via the classical pathway by environmental agents necessarily involves antibody and has been discussed previously. Knowledge is accumulating that contact with certain environmental agents may also activate the alternative pathway nonspecifically, that is, in the absence of antibody.

At least two iatrogenic reactions apparently involve nonspecific complement activation, namely, the anaphylactoid shock syndrome produced in certain people by injection of radiocontrast medium (Arroyave, Schatz, and Simon, 1979) or that which sometimes occurs immediately following initiation of extracorporeal renal dialysis (Craddock et al., 1977). Both syndromes involve complement alterations in the absence of specific antibody. The colloidal nature of the radiocontrast medium and the filter membranes or other synthetic components of the dialyzer are thought to be the responsible initiators. Peptidoglycan (Smith, Burrell, and Snyder, 1978) and lipopolysaccharide (Morrison and Ryan, 1979) cell wall components of bacteria and fungi have been shown to activate the alternative-complement pathway and to result in altered pulmonary function and circulating platelet levels when such organisms are inhaled in dense suspensions, such as might be produced in occupational settings. It has been suggested that the disease hypersensitivity pneumonitis may be initiated by complement activation leading to inflammation after inhalation of moldy vegetable dusts (Olenchock and Burrell, 1976; Burrell and Pokorney, 1977). Because complement is involved, but antibody is not, it is considered an immune-like reaction. A slightly different immune-like reaction may occur in byssinosis. A material associated with cotton bract dust (a tetrahydroxyflavan polymer) is known to react nonspecifically with the Fc portion of immunoglobulin molecules, that is, the non-antigen-reactive end (Edwards and Jones,

1973). The presence of this precipitated protein may possibly be inflammatory. In this case immunoglobulin is involved, but not in its usual well-known capacity.

Great care must be taken in interpreting results obtained from activating complement in vitro. Cotton dust (Kutz, Olenchock, Elliott, et al., 1979), chrysotile asbestos fibers (Saint-Remy and Cole, 1980), fungal extracts (Marx and Flaherty, 1976), pigeon dropping extracts (Berrens et al., 1974), and cereal grain extracts (Olenchock et al., 1980) are just a few of the substances known to activate complement in vitro, but there are far fewer studies available that have subjected test animals to in vivo inhalation testing to determine if these substances actually incite complement-dependent pulmonary reactions. Peripheral complement levels are not usually affected unless the challenge aerosol is very dense, yet exposures made on complement-deficient animals do not induce pulmonary responses (Burrell and Rylander, 1981).

Complement may be activated following ingestion of antigen, providing it is not digested. Aspirin and sodium salicylate may invoke bronchospasm in certain intolerant individuals, and depressed peripheral complement levels have been demonstrated in a portion of these (Arroyave et al., 1979). Adsorption of incompletely digested food across an immature gastrointestinal tract can depress serum complement in addition to inducing IgE (Strunk et al., 1978). An even more complicated pathogenesis involving complement and ingestants has been suggested in dermatitis herpetiformis. Patients with this disease also have elevated IgA, gluten sensitivity, and abnormalities of the jejunal mucosa. It has been postulated that undigested gluten antigen is adsorbed and reacts with non-complement-fixing IgA from prior sensitization, and that these complexes are deposited in the skin at this site; the deposited gluten is thought to activate complement nonspecifically and to induce inflammation (Massey et al., 1977).

HYPERPLASIA

The continued presence of antibodies or other immunologic effectors occasionally gives rise to a hyperplastic response. Chronic stimulation by IgE reactions may result in certain forms of cellular hyperplasia in chronic asthma, leading to the development of nasal polyps, bronchial smooth muscle hypertrophy, and mucous metaplasia in which the ciliated cells are often replaced by goblet cells. Basement membrane thickening or rupture may also occur in the bronchial tissues as a result of immune complexes (Callerame et al., 1971). Connective tissue autoantibodies are known to be produced in certain chronic pulmonary diseases (Burrell et al., 1964), and the continued presence of these antibodies over a long period of time results in interalveolar septal thickening (Burrell et al., 1974) and may possibly even contribute to fibrogenesis (Lewis and Burrell, 1976).

NONSPECIFIC MEDIATOR RELEASE

The inflammation that accompanies immune or immune-like reactions is brought about by the complex interplay of a number of biochemical mediators that have specific pharmacologic activities (Hubscher, 1977). Many of these mediators regulate the severity of allergic reactions and are in turn controlled by the hormones and neurotransmitters of the autonomic nervous system. With respect to bronchial smooth muscles, parasympathetic (cholinergic) stimulation results in constriction whereas sympathetic (adrenergic) stimulation results in relaxation. When these systems are balanced, the smooth muscles are in homeostatic control, but if either the system is preferentially stimulated one way or mediator release is excessive, then the organ receives unopposed stimulation (Szentivanyi, 1968). A number of artificial substances are known to cause the nonspecific release of histamine in vitro from eosinophils and neutrophils (Becker and Henson, 1973), so the possibility that natural exposure to environmental agents may do the same thing is very real. Such spontaneous histamine release is known to occur directly from stimulation by the cotton dust component methyl piperonylate (Hitchock et al., 1973). This material is one of several biologically active substances identified from cotton dust that may play a role in the disease byssinosis. Histamine release may also be stimulated by nonspecific complement activation affecting platelet target cells (Osler and Siraganian, 1972). In both of these instances, histamine release occurs through an IgE-independent pathway but resembles an allergic reaction.

β-Adrenergic Blockage

Rather than stimulating excessive mediator release, the possibility exists that environmental agents may upset the autonomic control balance by either preferentially stimulating the cholinergic pathway or blocking the adrenergic system. Cyclic adenosine monophosphate (cAMP) is synthesized in appropriate cells when the β-adrenergic receptor, the enzyme adenylate cyclase, is activated (Szentivanyi, 1968). Accumulation and release of cAMP stimulates adrenergic functions: in the mast cell there is an inhibition of mediator release, and in the smooth muscle a relaxation is effected. If the β-adrenergic receptors are blocked, cAMP synthesis is inhibited and there is no adrenergic stimulation to oppose the constricting effects of cholinergic stimulation. An environmental agent that appears to effect such β blockade is the industrial chemical toluene diisocyanate (TDI). Inhalation of this material leads to asthmatic reactions, and although some exposed workers develop IgE sensitivity to TDI (Butcher, Salvaggio, Weill, and Ziskind, 1976), the major effects seem due to this pharmacologic, immune-like mechanism (Butcher, Salvaggio, O'Neil, et al., 1977). The same signs and symptoms have also been reported in individuals exposed to certain organic insecticides that have anticholinesterase activity, which essentially results in excessive cholinergic stimulation (Corbett, 1974).

Potentiation of Immune Injury by Other Agents

The concurrent contact with an additional environmental agent(s) may modify the response to a single agent. The potentiating effect of many agents on infectious diseases (e.g., silica and tuberculosis) is due to agent interference of the immune system and will be discussed in the next section. The temporal relation of two or more contacts with the same or even different agents may bring about unique forms of immune-like injury quite apart from any immunologic interference. In such instances, contact with noninfectious but endotoxin-containing bacteria may enhance subsequent exposure to other agents. Translated in terms of environmental exposure, an individual under-going an allergic reaction due to ragweed pollen may be especially vulnerable if exposed to a dense aerosol of gram-negative bacteria, such as what might occur in an animal confinement facility. Although such an actual clinical relationship has not been studied, there is ample evidence to suggest that such might occur.

Bacterial endotoxin is ubiquitous and is capable of invoking a wide array of biologic effects. Profound effects of endotoxin occur on complement and coagulation system proteins, platelets, neutrophils, endothelial cells, and mononuclear cells (Morrison and Ulevitch, 1978). If such effects are temporally coupled with exposure to other agents discussed above, or even more endotoxin, the resulting inflammation may be more serious than with single contact with either agent alone. Such reactions resemble immune reactions, because immune accessory molecules and cells like complement and macrophages are involved, and there is a requirement for both sensitization and provocation contacts before the injury becomes manifest. Such reactions, however, do not require the agency of either antibody or specific lymphocyte responsiveness. The classical Shwartzman reaction is a case in point. To invoke the dermal manifestation of this reaction, a rabbit is first injected intradermally with endotoxin or endotoxin-containing toxin. After a critical period of time has elapsed (18–24 hours), the animal is subsequently given an intravenous dose of the same or unrelated endotoxin. This produces within hours at the site of the initial sensitizing injection, a large dermal reaction consisting of occlusive fibrin–neutrophil thrombi in the capillaries. The possibility of dual, spontaneous exposure to endotoxin as a cause of injury has been entertained for decades, but little study has been made on it.

If rabbits are exposed to an inhalation of an organism seemingly as innocuous as *Escherichia coli*, and then 24 hours later are given a small intravenous injection of the same organism, an immediate decline in pulmonary function is accompanied by a platelet-dependent hemorrhagic pneumonia (DeMaria and Burrell, 1980). This often lethal response is characterized by an extensive interstitial pneumonitis, hemorrhage, and focal accumulations of neutrophils and lymphocytes. Such a reaction was found to be modulated by prostaglandin action. Thus, an immune-like reaction is potentiated by repeated contact with the same noninfectious material and involves platelets, mediators, and probably complement. It is known that streptococcal toxins enhance the animal's response to endotoxin, which is antigenically unrelated to it (Schlievert and Watson, 1978). If an agricultural worker has a strep infection and then subsequently is exposed to an aerosol of gram-negative bacteria, injury to the lung is theoretically possible. Another ubiquitous cell wall component that might be capable of immune-like injury is peptidoglycan, the major cell wall component of gram-positive bacteria. This material is also able to activate complement (Smith et al., 1978) and is mitogenic for lymphocytes (Smith et al., 1980). In this latter fashion, it acts as its own immunologic adjuvant (Bice et al., 1977). In neither of these situations does infection play a role. Rather, the injury is due to unique biologic responses to environmental agents. Bacteria heretofore regarded as harmless are a major component of environmental dusts such as might be encountered in cotton mills (Cinkotai et al., 1977), animal confinement and slaughtering facilities (Dutkiewicz, 1978), barns or feedlots (Dutkiewicz, 1978), grain elevators (do Pico et al., 1977), and the like.

Interference with Immune Function

In addition to leading to immunologically induced injury or inflammation, contact with environmental agents can also induce aberrations in immune function. These aberrations can be stimulatory in the sense that either hyperactivity or increased levels of immune effectors are brought about. The aberrations can also result from inherent toxicity of the agents on various immunologic components. Although the field of toxicology has long recognized the effects of environmental agents on various organ systems, the concept of immunotoxicology is a rather new one (Vos, 1977; Sharma and Zeeman, 1980). The purpose of this section is to review how the normal components of the immunologic system are adversely affected by environmental agents. For this purpose, the immunologic systems considered will be macrophages, lymph nodes, lymphocytes, complement and other mediator systems, and the functional aspects of the various specific immunologic responses. The use of drugs to enhance or suppress the immune response purposefully is beyond the scope of this chapter, but the reader will find such information instructive (Webb and Winkelstein, 1984).

MACROPHAGES

The macrophage is considered to be one of the most important components of the immune response (Table 11-3). In addition to the well-known phagocytic role of these cells, the macrophage is essential in processing certain classes of antigens and presenting them to lymphoid cells. Concomitant with this function is the elaboration of mediators (monokines) that serve to stimulate

Table 11–3. Immunologic Functions of Macrophages

Phagocytosis
  Enhanced by Ig Fc receptor
  Enhanced by C3b receptor

Antigen presentation to lymphocytes
  Membrane-bound Ag; presentation to lymphocytes
  Expose unavailable determinants
  Antigen–RNA templates; processing of antigen
  Lymphocyte stimulation

Secretory products
  Enzymes
    Plasminogen activators
    Collagenase and elastase
    Lysosomal proteases
  Defense products
    Lysozyme
    C2, C3, C4, and C5
    Interferon
  Modulating factors (monokine production)
    T cell mitogen
    Differentiating factors
    Inflammatory mediators

Targets of T lymphocyte–Ag lymphokine production

Source: Modified from Burrell (1981).

lymphocytes (Rocklin et al., 1979). The macrophage itself is also an important source of inflammatory and defensive enzymes (P. Davies and Allison, 1976). Several complement components and the important defensive molecule, interferon, are produced in macrophages. Finally, the macrophage is a target cell for certain mediators or lymphocytes (Rocklin et al., 1979) that are produced by antigen–lymphocyte interaction. Thus, the macrophage is responsible for removal and uptake of antigen, production of key defensive products, and participation in the specific immune response in several ways. Any agent that can alter macrophage function is bound to have important immunologic consequences.

A number of environmental agents simply enhance or depress the phagocytic function of macrophages so as to interfere not only with the primary function but possibly also with the regulation of the specific immune responses. A number of environmental agents known to depress or enhance phagocytosis by macrophages are given in Table 11-4. For purposes of generalization, chemotaxis and engulfment of particles are both considered as phagocytic functions.

The most important environmental agent that affects macrophages is crystalline silicon dioxide or silica, which is a profound macrophage toxin (E. J. King et al., 1953; Kessel et al., 1963; Allison, Harrington, and Birbeck, 1966). Following ingestion of silica particles, macrophages undergo rapid morphologic changes leading to lysis. Silica alters the phospholipid structure of the plasma and lysosomal membranes in such a way that the integrity of the cell is lost (Allison, 1975). It is agreed that this event leads directly to fibrosis probably by the liberation of various intracellular factors

Table 11–4. Selected Environmental Agents That Affect Macrophages and Phagocytic Functions

Agent	Effect	Reference
Silica	In small quantities, depresses	Allison et al. (1966)
Asbestos	Enhances	K. Miller and Kagan (1977)
Fly ash	As particle size decreases, enhances, but is also cytotoxic	Aranyi et al. (1977)
Coal mine dust	Depression	Bingham et al. (1977)
Manganese dioxide	Depression and cytotoxicity	Bergström (1977)
Cigarette smoke	Depression	Haroz and Mattensberger-Kreber (1977)
Carbon monoxide	Enhanced	Snella and Rylander (1979)
SO_2	5–20 ppm, stimulates	G. V. Katz and Laskin (1972)
NO_2	25 ppm, depresses	G. V. Katz and Laskin (1972)
Formaldehyde	10 ppm, enhances; 20 ppm depresses	G. V. Katz and Laskin (1977)
Aflatoxin and other mycotoxins	Depression and cytotoxicity	Richard et al. (1978)

acting on fibroblasts (Heppleston, 1971), but by exactly what molecular pathway seems controversial at present (Reiser and Last, 1979).

Not only does the action of silica on macrophages lead to fibrosis; other immunologic functions are affected as well. When experimental animals are subjected to long-term silica inhalation exposures, both peripheral and pulmonary T lymphocyte function was altered, presumably because of indirect macrophage effects (D. S. Miller and Zarkower, 1974). However, when silica is given in an appropriate dose and route, it acts as an immunologic enhancer or adjuvant (Pernis and Paronetto, 1962), perhaps by enhancing phagocytosis (Spitznagel and Allison, 1970).

Certain forms of asbestos, which are mineralogic varieties of silicates, also lead to pulmonary fibrosis when inhaled, but their effect on macrophages is not as toxic; rather, the immunoregulatory role of macrophages is altered. Although alveolar macrophages exposed to asbestos do undergo morphologic alterations, they also increase the number of immunoglobulin receptor sites on their cell membranes (K. Miller and Kagan, 1976; K. Miller, Webster, Handfield, and Skikne, 1978). This property enables the macrophages to possess enhanced antigen adsorption powers (K. Miller and Kagan, 1977). Finally, asbestos also alters macrophage membranes in such ways as to promote lymphocyte binding to the macrophages (K. Miller, Weintraub, and Kagan, 1979). Thus, refined methods of examining the molecular and cellular actions of environmental agents on cells have revealed some rather intricate mechanisms by which immunologic functions may be ultimately altered.

ACCESSORY MOLECULES

Although a number of environmental agents are known to activate complement and presumably lead to inflammation (discussed above), a great void exists about how such complement depletion brought about by environmental agents may affect resistance to infection and immune responses. Complement is necessary to opsonize foreign particulate matter so that phagocytosis of such matter may be enhanced, and if the complement level were depressed, conceivably a depressed phagocytic function would occur as well. Although research is needed in this untouched area, it is known that a number of microbiologic components, particularly mycotoxins (Richard et al., 1978), may depress peripheral complement levels. The ubiquitous occurrence of aflatoxin suggests that this line of investigation should be pursued.

Interferon, a macrophage product, is an extremely important nonspecific defense mediator that is stimulated and released by certain viral and bacterial infections (Baron, 1973). This material confers passive protection on other cells not infected and serves to limit the spread of an infection in an individual and to prevent suprainfection by other agents, and its role in tumor therapy is currently of great interest. A number of environmental agents are known to depress interferon synthesis in in vitro culture systems and include coal dust, asbestos, nitrogen dioxide, arsenicals, and certain carcinogenic hydrocarbons (Hahon and Eckert, 1976). Some studies have been conducted in animal models, and such interferon inhibition has resulted in decreased resistance to subsequent challenge with an infectious agent (Coffin, 1972).

IMMUNOGLOBULIN SYNTHESIS AND B LYMPHOCYTES

Immunoglobulins are synthesized in bone marrow or B-dependent lymphocytes and plasma cells, differentiated to synthesize large amounts of protein. These antibodies may belong to one of five major classes depending on the biochemical and functional properties of the heavy polypeptide chains that make up a portion of the antibody molecule. Antibody synthesis may be purposefully enhanced or inhibited by drug therapy, but here we are concerned with the results of accidental contact with environmental agents on the antibody-producing systems. A number of environmental diseases are characterized by elevated immunoglobulin levels (very often IgA) in occupational diseases, including silicosis, complicated coal workers' pneumoconiosis, asbestosis, and berylliosis among others (Burrell, 1977). These findings suggest B lymphocyte stimulation by the responsible agents. A number of environmental agents seem to have a preferential enhancing effect on IgE synthesis; this group includes aluminum hydroxide, one form of silica, certain organic dyes, and a number of microbiologic components (Speirs and Speirs, 1979). Because IgE is the type of antibody that modulates immediate-type allergic reactions, the IgE-boosting effect of these agents might serve to influence inflammatory reactions at the expense of IgG production, and it has been suggested that the presence of allergic inflammation enhances the susceptibility to infection (Buckley et al., 1972).

It must not be inferred from these elevated immunoglobulin levels that natural dust exposure leads to enhanced immune responsiveness. When experimental animals are subjected to chronic silica or carbon dust inhalation in realistic concentrations, their specific antibody-producing cells are reduced following immunization compared to unexposed controls (Zarkower and Morges, 1972; D. S. Miller and Zarkower, 1974). Although short-term exposure produced enhancing effects, these were short-lived because long-term exposure readily reversed the immune responsiveness. Whether the effect of such agents is directly on B lymphocytes or indirectly via macrophages is unknown, but the maximum effect occurs at a time when the tissues are histologically normal in appearance (Burns, Zarkower, and Ferguson, 1980).

The previous studies have all measured immunoglobulin levels or numbers of specific, reactive B cells. More difficulty is encountered in trying to evaluate the effect of environmental agents on specific antibody responses, because of the conflicting reports, lack of adequate criteria, and poorly described test conditions encountered in the literature. Indeed, the new field of immunotoxicology requires the establishment of more adequate in vivo and in vitro methods of evaluating this aspect of environmental agents. The reader is referred to the review by Vos (1977), who has discussed the attributes of various procedures proposed for immunotoxicologic evaluation. Dose of agent, administration regimen, type of antigen selected for stimulus, timing of agent administration with respect to that of antigen sensitization, whether primary or secondary immunization is being evaluated, and time of evaluation after agent contact are just a few of the variables that will affect the evaluation of the test results. Depending on whose article one reads, DDT may have an enhancing, depressing, or no effect on antibody response (Sharma and Zeeman, 1980). Sometimes an environmental agent will be immunosuppressive only in high concentration or will be effective as measured against antigens that have no relevance to human disease, for example, sheep erythrocytes. The clinician needs to know whether a given agent may interfere with immune responses to clinically relevant antigens when encountered in environmentally realistic concentrations. Even when such a study is done properly, the results are startling. In spite of universal agreement about the immunologic consequences of silica, mice chronically exposed to realistic concentrations show no impairment to production of influenza virus antibody, nor do they show increased susceptibility to influenza infection (Zarkower et al., 1979). Clearly we need to establish sensible criteria and to use considerable judgment in evaluating immunosuppression data from environmental agents.

There are several steps of the immune response in which environmental agents might interfere with specific antibody responses. We have already discussed the effects on macrophages, which are essential for processing most antigens for lymphocyte action. The agent could be directly cytotoxic to lymphocytes, for example, beryllium salts (Marx and Burrell, 1973), and such a possibility must be considered when doing in

Table 11–5. Selected Environmental Agents That under Certain Experimental Conditions Interfere with Antibody Production

Agent category	Examples
Metals	Cadmium, lead
Organometals	Arsenicals, methyl mercury
Industrial organics	DDT, halogenated biphenyls (e.g., PCB)
Nonindustrial, environmental inhalants	Cigarette smoke, halothane anesthesia

vitro evaluation tests with such cells. Alternatively, the agent could interfere with lymphocyte proliferation, often by inhibiting protein or DNA synthesis, and a number of immunoregulatory drugs work in this fashion (Webb and Winkelstein, 1980). Finally, the agent could interfere with antibody synthesis, assembly, or release from plasma cells (Wei and McLaughlin, 1974). Sharma and Zeeman (1980) have discussed in greater detail additional ways in which environmental agents can affect immune responsiveness.

Keeping these limitations in mind, Table 11-5 lists some of the better defined environmental agents that affect antibody production. Missing from the table are common industrial air pollutants (ozone, nitrogen dioxide, and sulfur dioxide). Popular thought might ascribe inhibitory function to them, whereas in fact, well-controlled studies could find no antibody-suppressive effects following either inhalation or parental immunization (Matsumura, 1970). It is also apparent that industrial or occupational exposure are not the only avenues of contact with such agents; recreational (cigarette smoking) and even iatrogenic (anesthetic inhalants) contacts may lead to immunosuppression (Burrell, 1977).

Autoantibody Production

Concomitant with elevated immunoglobulin levels in these occupationally related diseases is the increased incidence in various autoantibodies. In addition to the cytotoxic connective tissue antibodies discussed previously, a greater incidence of elevated levels of antinuclear antibody (ANA) and rheumatoid factor (RF), itself an antibody for altered immunoglobulin, are known to occur in patients with asbestosis (Turner-Warwick, 1973), certain forms of coal workers' pneumoconiosis (Lippmann et al., 1973), and silicosis (Jones et al., 1975). In general, there is a greater incidence of ANA titers and there is a better correlation between presence of ANA and roentgenographic abnormality; that is, the more tissue involvement there is, the greater the chance for elevated ANA titer.

Cell-Mediated Immunity

The effect of environmental agents on T lymphocyte immunity has not received nearly as much emphasis as the effects on antibody production, primarily because it is technically more difficult to evaluate T cell responses than to determine serum titers. Most studies have focused on isolated T cells or obvious T cell functions such as graft rejection, but some of the antibody studies may in effect be reflections of altered T cell function if the immunization evaluation was made with a T-dependent antigen, that is, one requiring both T and B lymphocytes for the synergistic production of antibodies. Moreover, there are suppressor T cells that inhibit antibody production. If either helper or suppressor T cells are affected by an environmental agent, such would be reflected in inhibition of antibody production and would be erroneously interpreted as a B cell effect. Vos (1977) has stressed the importance of critical interpretation in such matters and has suggested the routine use of both T-dependent and T-independent (i.e., requiring only B cells for antibody production) antigens for immunotoxicology screening analysis.

Although many studies exist concerning the effects of certain agents when administered experimentally, too often these agents are used in unrealistically high concentrations or are given by unnatural routes. For instance, intravenous administration of silica will prolong graft acceptance, generally considered a T cell phenomenon, although in this case the effect is undoubtedly on the afferent limb (i.e., macrophages) of the immune response (Pearsall and Weiser, 1968). The bulk of the experimental work on silica points to the major effect being on macrophages (Burrell, 1981). Only minor differences in T cell responsiveness have been reported in human silicotic patients (Schuyler et al., 1977).

More definitive information exists about asbestos. Patients with radiographic evidence of asbestosis generally show a failure to produce delayed-type skin reactions to common antigens with which most normal controls react; also, their lymphocytes showed significantly lower responses to lymphocyte mitogens, and serum inhibitors of such lymphocyte transformation are often detected (Kagan et al., 1977; Haslam et al., 1978). Alteration of macrophage membranes of rats subjected to asbestos exposure results in long-term binding to lymphocytes (K. Miller et al., 1979), which could explain the depressed lymphocyte functions.

A few industrial chemicals have been studied immunotoxicologically (tetrachlorodibenzo-p-dioxin, di-n-octyltindichloride, certain polychlorinated biphenyls) with a view toward T cell immunity (Vos, 1977). Such chemicals exhibit a great deal of lymphocyte toxicity, but data related to immunologic function are scanty and conflicting.

In addition to performing standard immunologic tests for T cell number and function, it is imperative that these be backed up by histopathologic studies of thymus, spleen, and lymph nodes, as several agents previously mentioned may bring about atrophy or architectural impairment in these tissues. Care must be taken in interpretation of these changes, because they may be brought about in an indirect manner through the endocrine system, tumorigenic properties of the agent, impairment in utilization of nutrients, or presence of chronic pathogens (Vos, 1977).

Immuntoxicologic studies have been pri-

marily focused on industrial chemicals or occupationally related agents, but alteration of immune function can be induced by other types of agents as well. Although data on the effect of marijuana smoking on T cell function are conflicting (Nahas et al., 1974; Lau et al., 1976), significant alteration in T cell number and function is well documented in opiate addicts (McDonough et al., 1980).

Selected Agents

The discussion so far has been limited to specific kinds of immune injury and specific kinds of immune interference. The problem with such an approach is that the reaction to certain agents is exceedingly complex and more than one reaction is generated. More detailed discussion of selected environmental agents is therefore presented to illustrate the manifold nature such agents may have on the immune system, emphasizing how these immunologic changes contribute to functional and structural pathology.

Silica

The many effects silica has on the immunologic system have been recently reviewed, with the result that a unifying hypothesis of how these factors contribute to the pathogenesis of silicosis has been suggested (Burrell, 1981); it is summarized in Figure 11-1. Macrophage toxicity, lymphocyte stimulation, and autoantibody formation to connective tissue, altered immunoglobulin, and nucleoprotein have been discussed above. It is proposed that in sublytic doses, silica may stimulate macrophages to initiate immune responses to either altered proteins adsorbed to quartz particles (Scheel et al., 1954) or connective tissue previously damaged by macrophage enzymes. If serum globulins are adsorbed, rheumatoid factors and possibly immune complexes, composed of rheumatoid factor and immunoglobulin, are also produced. If the complement cascade is activated by these complexes, certain intermediates can activate macrophages to elaborate inflamma-

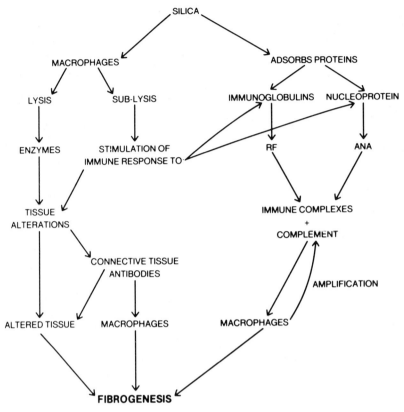

Figure 11–1. Proposed unifying hypothesis illustrating the various immunologic facets to the contribution to silicotic fibrosis. (From Burrell, 1981.)

tory mediators, at least one of which can in turn activate more complement (Schorlemmer and Allison, 1976). In this kind of amplification feedback, affected macrophages can exert their effect over a long time. Lung connective tissue antibodies also localize in situ (Vigliani and Pernis, 1963) and can lead directly to increased interalveolar septal thickening (Burrell et al., 1974) or indirectly to fibrosis by macrophage stimulation (Lewis and Burrell, 1976) All of these processes are fibrogenic, and because young fibroblasts produce the lung antibody-reactive antigen, more antigen is continuously being produced to react with antibody in the silicotic nodule.

MICROBIAL COMPONENTS

Considered here are structural cell wall components and metabolic by-products from microorganisms that are noninfectious under most conditions. Many of these agents are associated with the environmental inhalation disease, hypersensitivity pneumonitis (HP). Most forms of this disease are initiated with microorganisms associated with the decomposition of organic material, contaminated air humidifier systems, or animal excreta. A partial list of agents inciting HP is presented in Table 11-6. For more detailed information about such agents, see Lacey (1975).

Burrell and Rylander (1981) have recently presented a critique of the precipitin hypothesis and have attempted to pull together many of the known effects of the incitants into a unified hypothesis of pathogenicity. Initially, peptidoglycan cell wall components are postulated to activate the alternative-complement pathway (Smith et al., 1978), thereby inciting local inflamma-

Table 11–6. Representative Agents Associated with Hypersensitivity Pneumonitis

Active principle	Source	References
Thermophilic actinomycetes	Moldy hay, mushroom compost, bagasse, air conditioner systems	Cross (1968)
Aspergillus spp.	Moldy corn; moldy but uncomposted organic matter	Riddle et al. (1968)
Cryptostroma corticale	Moldy maple bark	Emanuel, Lawton, and Wenzel (1962)
Avian serum proteins; possibly fecal micro-organisms	Avian and rat droppings	Reed et al. (1965); Huis in 'T Veld and Berrens (1976)
Various amoebae	Contaminated air humidifiers	Edwards (1980)
Endotoxin?	Tap water	Muittari et al. (1979)

tion. This inflammation could alter the lung permeability in such a way as to permit macromolecular antigens to pass into the peripheral circulation and immunize the individual (Hill and Burrell, 1979). In addition, the cell wall components act as a built-in adjuvant (Bice et al., 1977; Smith et al., 1980) and enhance the induction of cell-mediated immunity. As these lymphocytes participate in the typical delayed-hypersensitivity reaction, lesions characteristic of HP are produced (Richerson et al., 1978). In addition, precipitins are produced to soluble antigens, and although immune-complex inflammation is a theoretical possibility, evidence to support this concept is lacking. Many microbial agents associated with HP also produce extracellular proteinases, the contribution of which to the pathogenesis of HP has yet to be evaluated; but such added toxicity is a distinct possibility.

The role of endotoxin in various forms of infectious diseases has long interested physicians, and a considerable body of knowledge exists about it (Morrison and Ulevitch, 1978; Morrison and Ryan, 1979). Nevertheless, its role in noninfectious diseases following inhalation of significant concentrations of gram-negative bacterial aerosols is attracting new interest. Following such inhalation, various nonspecific symptoms of malaise, chills, and fever have been reported (Rylander et al., 1977). In experimental situations, changes in various hematologic and pulmonary functions have

been noted (DeMaria and Burrell, 1980), as well as marked changes in inflammatory exudate cells in the lung (Rylander, Snella, and Garcia, 1975). Endotoxin is a B lymphocyte mitogen, activates complement and platelets, is chemotactic, and causes the release of many lysosomal and cytoplasmic enzymes from macrophages (Allison, Davies, and Page, 1973). Thus, significant inhalation from environmental sources represents a potential form of pulmonary injury.

The effects of mycotoxins on immunity, to say nothing about their relation to cancer induction, present formidable problems in the livestock industry and human health. Moreover, knowledge of these effects from spoilage fungi results in the costly quarantine of millions of dollars worth of agricultural products each year. Mycotoxins play roles in interfering with mechanisms of phagocytosis, damage complement components, affect antibody and cellular immune responses, and lower resistance to disease (Richard et al., 1978). These effects are produced from products from fungi not usually associated with primary infection, yet may be much more important in public health than infectious fungi.

COTTON DUST

Byssinosis is a disease confined to those who are exposed to various industrial processes of producing cotton. It is mainly a physiologic disease with little or no distinctive pathology attributable to the inhalation of

Table 11–7. Some Immunologic Effects induced by Cotton Components

Effect	Reference
Contains high concentration of endotoxin	Cavagna et al. (1969)
Contains histamine	Battigelli et al. (1977)
Nonspecific histamine release	Hitchock et al. (1973)
Nonspecific precipitation of immunoglobulins	J. H. Edwards and Jones (1973)
True antibodies can be produced against	Kutz et al. (1980)
Activates complement nonspecifically	Kutz et al. (1979)

Table 11–8. Representative Agents Causing Occupational Asthma

Agent	Occupation
Cereal grain and seed dust	Millers, grainery workers, bakers
Sawdusts and wood shavings	Carpenters
Gum arabic	Printers
Proteolytic enzymes	Formerly detergent manufacturers
Solder fluxes (aminoethyl ethanolamine)	Welders
Isocyanates (particularly toluene diisoscyanate, TDI)	Plastics workers
Platinum salts	Chemical workers, electroplaters
Trimellitic anhydrides	Plastics workers

Source: After Seaton (1984).

cotton dust alone (Pratt et al., 1980). Yet a number of immunologic facets connected with cotton particles are known and are summarized in Table 11-7. Epidemiologically, dust components are important in the pathogenetic sense, because it has been shown in several studies that dust levels are related to pulmonary impairment and that washing raw cotton fibers before milling appears to remove the bronchoconstrictive principle (Morgan, 1975).

MISCELLANEOUS INDUSTRIAL INHALANTS

Occupational or industrial asthma is another type of respiratory disease that is attributable to environmental agents and may involve immunologic responses. A number of agents have been incriminated, and they appear in Table 11-8. Formerly it was considered that bronchoconstrictive reactions were simply IgE mediated, but the reactions were occasionally seen in nonatopic individuals; further, the timing of the reaction (late), together with the presence of other symptoms (e.g., fever), with certain of these agents suggested other mechanisms were active as well. IgE-mediated mechanisms are indeed active against some of these agents, such as TDI (R. J. Davies et al., 1977), but additional mechanisms may also be operative. Some of the reactions can be explained by the nonspecific irritant effects of the agent in asthma-prone individuals. There has been

an overly liberal trend in ascribing immune-complex etiology to many of these agents on the basis of finding precipitating antibodies to the agents in patients' serum. Such antibody can be interpreted only as an indicator of intimate antigenic contact and not as evidence of a pathogenetic mechanism (Burrell and Rylander, 1981). Although IgE antibodies definitely appear in many workers exposed to toluene diisocyanate (TDI), such antibodies do not always compare with disease or response following bronchoprovocation. Following such bronchoprovocation testing, patients may exhibit early, late, or dual responses to testing, indicating complex or multiple etiologies. TDI also invokes a β-adrenergic blockade, which could lead to a pharmacologic asthmatic reaction that would mimic an immunologic reaction (R. J. Davies et al., 1977). In the late type of reaction to materials like trimellitic anhydrides, there is an association with elevated IgG levels, but the pathogenetic mechanism of such a finding, if any, is unclear (Zeiss et al., 1977).

The separate discussion of these few selected agents illustrates the danger in discussing mechanisms of injury or immune interference separately. Complex modalities of pathogenesis should always be kept in mind.

COMPLICATING FACTORS

Both of the above discussions on mechanisms of immune injury and environmental agents with immunotoxicologic properties are far too simplistic, because both ignore the contribution of two very important environmental factors that often coexist with each of these mechanisms or agents and that complicate the pathology tremendously: cigarette smoking and infection. Cigarette smoking by itself affects macrophage activity, secretory IgA production, and specific antibody induction, in addition to the more well-known effects on mucous membranes, ciliated epithelia, and other nonspecific defensive structures; however, its contribution to other environmental diseases is little known.

Heyden and Pratt (1980) have recently examined in detail the superimposed effects of cigarette smoking on various forms of occupational lung disease. It was learned that among men with high-risk exposure to byssinosis, only those who currently smoked developed the severe forms of the disease, including the chronic obstructive form, whereas only mild symptoms appeared in nonsmokers (Merchant et al., 1972). Moreover, those who quit smoking reported a disappearance of symptoms. In another study, autopsy results of cotton and non-cotton workers were compared with regard to smoking histories (Pratt et al., 1980). The rate of moderate to severe emphysema ranged from 16 to 19% in both categories of smokers, and it was negligible in non-smoking workers. Further analysis showed a highly significant ($p < 0.0001$) relationship of emphysema to cigarette smoking and an insignificant relation to cotton working. Other pathology studies have shown that only 37% of British patients receiving byssinosis compensation had any degree of emphysema at the time of death (C. Edwards et al., 1975).

Similarly, true respiratory impairment in coal workers' pneumoconiosis is due to the complicated or progressive massive fibrosis form of the disease, in which cigarette smoking plays a larger part than does exposure to coal dust (Morgan et al., 1980). Asbestos may be the most dangerous air pollutant known, in that exposure to the uncommon agent is definitely linked to an uncommon tumor, mesothelioma. When such dangerous exposure is coupled with cigarette smoking, mortality may be increased as much as a third (Selikoff and Hammond, 1979). The additive role of cigarette smoking to exposure to most of the other agents mentioned in this chapter is unknown but certainly worthy of inquiry.

An even more difficult complication in assessing the role of environmental effects on immune function is the role of concurrent secondary infections. Rylander (1974) focused attention on this when he compared the number and quantity of free lung cells in infection-controlled guinea pigs with those that were kept under ordinary conditions. Infection-controlled animals had significantly fewer macrophages and leukocytes in their pulmonary lavages. Because the alveolar lavage technique is very popular with those who study environmental toxicology, it is essential that these findings be kept in mind when interpreting such data from non-infection-controlled animals. Lindsey et al. (1971) called attention to the perils of using conventional rats for many types of experimental pathology purposes, in that the almost ubiquitous occurrence of chronic respiratory infection due to *Mycoplasma pulmonis* frequently contributes more to the results than the investigators' test materials. Indeed, some histologic results offered as evidence for various hypotheses were interpreted by Lindsey's group as typical mycoplasma histopathology. When a comparative immunologic and microbiologic study of experimental coal workers' pneumoconiosis was made in rats and mice, it was found that many of the parameters studied appeared earlier in the rodents chronically exposed to coal dust aerosols, but also eventually appeared in undusted controls months later, presumably as a result of uncontrolled secondary infections (Burrell, Flaherty, and Schreiber, 1977).

Such complicating factors as cigarette smoking and secondary infection are very difficult to assess experimentally and epidemiologically, but they must be taken into greater consideration in future studies.

REFERENCES

Allison, A. C. V. 1975. Effects of silica, asbestos and other pollutants on macrophages. In *Air pollution and the lung,* eds. J. D. Brain, D. F. Procter, and L. M. Reid, pp. 114–132. Jerusalem: Israel Universities Press.

Allison, A. C., Davies, P., and Page, R. C. 1973. Effects of endotoxin on macrophages and other lymphoreticular cells. *J. Infect. Dis.* 128:S 212–219.

Allison, A. C., Harington, J. S., and Birbeck, M. 1966. An examination of the cytotoxic effects of silica on macrophages. *J. Exp. Med.* 124:141–154.

Aranyi, C., Andres, S., Ehrlich, R., Fentens, J. D., Gardner, D. E., and Waters, M. D. 1977. Cytotoxicity to alveolar macrophages of mental oxides adsorbed on fly ash. In *Pulmonary macrophage and epithelial cells,* eds. C. L. Sanders, R. P. Schneider, G. E. Dagle, and H. A. Ragan, pp. 58–65. Springfield, Va.: ERDA, U.S. Dept. of Commerce.

Arroyave, C. M., Schatz, M., and Simon, R. A. 1979. Activation of complement system by radiographic contrast media: studies *in vivo* and *in vitro. J. Allergy Clin. Immunol.* 63:276–280.

Austen, K. F. 1978. The chemical mediators of immediate hypersensitivity reactions. In *Immunological diseases,* 3rd Ed., ed. M. Samter, pp. 183–209. Boston: Little, Brown.

Baer, R. L., and Gigli, I. 1979. Atopic dermatitis. In *Dermatology in general medicine,* 2nd Ed., eds. T. B. Fitzpatrick, A. Z. Eisen, K. Wolff, I. M. Freedberg, and K. F. Austen, pp. 520–528. New York: McGraw-Hill.

Baron, S. 1973. The defense and biological roles of the interferon system. In *Interferons,* ed. N. B. Finter, pp. 267–293. Amsterdam: North-Holland.

Barrowcliff, D. F., and Arblaster, P. G. 1968. Farmers lung: A study of an acute fatal disease. *Thorax* 23:490–500.

Battigelli, M. C., Craven, P. L., Fischer, J. J., Morey, P. R., and Sasser, P. E. 1977. The role of histamine in byssinosis. *J. Environ. Sci. Health* A12:327–339.

Becker, E. L., and Henson, P. M. 1973. *In vitro* studies of immunologically induced secretion of mediators from cells and related phenomena. *Adv. Immunol.* 17:93–193.

Bergström, R. 1977. Acute pulmonary toxicity of manganese dioxide. *Scand. J. Work Environ. Health* 3(S1):1–41.

Berrens, L., Guikers, C. L. H., and van Dijk, A. 1974. The antigens in pigeon-breeders disease and their interactions with human complement. *Ann. N.Y. Acad. Sci.* 221:153–162.

Bice, D. E., McCarron, K., Hoffman, E. O., and Salvaggio, J. 1977. Adjuvant properties of *Micropolyspora faeni. Int. Arch. Allergy Appl. Immunol.* 55:267–274.

Bingham, E., Barkley, W., Murthy, R., and Vassallo, C. 1977. Investigation of alveolar macrophages from rats exposed to coal dust. In *Inhaled particles IV,* ed. W. H. Walton, pp. 543–550. Oxford: Pergamon Press.

Buckley, R. H., Wray, B. B. and Belmaker, E. Z. 1972. Extreme hyperimmunoglobulinemia E and undue susceptibility of infection. *Pediatrics* 49:59–70.

Burns, C. A., Zarkower, A., and Ferguson, F. G. 1980. Murine immunological and histological changes in response to chronic silica exposure. *Environ. Res.* 21:298–307.

Burrell, R. 1977. Immunological reactions to inhaled physical and chemical agents. In *Handbook of physiology,* eds. D. H. K. Lee, H. L. Falk, S. D. Murphy, and S. R. Geiger, pp. 285–298. Bethesda, Md.: American Physiological Society.

Burrell, R. 1981. Immunological aspects of silica. In *Health effects of synthetic silica particulates,* ed. D. D. Dunnom. Philadelphia: American Society for Testing Materials.

Burrell, R., Flaherty, D. K., DeNee, P. B., Abraham, J. L., and Gelderman, A. H. 1974. The effects of lung antibody on normal lung structure and function. *Am. Rev. Respir. Dis.* 109:106–113.

Burrell, R., Flaherty, D. K., and Schreiber, J. E. 1977. Immunological studies of experimental coalworkers' pneumoconiosis. In *Inhaled particles IV,* ed. W. H. Walton, pp. 519–529. Oxford: Pergamon Press.

Burrell, R., and Pokorney, D. 1977. Mediators of experimental hypersensitivity pneumonitis. *Int. Arch. Allergy Appl. Immunol.* 55:161–169.

Burrell, R., and Rylander, R. 1981. The role of precipitins in hypersensitivity pneumonitis. *Eur. J. Respir. Dis.* 62:332–343.

Burrell, R., Wallace, J. P., and Andres, C. E. 1964. Lung antibodies in patients with pulmonary disease. *Am. Rev. Respir. Dis.* 89:697–706.

Butcher, B. T., Salvaggio, J. E., O'Neil, C. E., Weill, H., and Garg, O. 1977. Toluene diisocyanate pulmonary disease: Immunopharmacologic and mecholyl challenge studies. *J. Allergy Clin. Immunol.* 59:223–227.

Butcher, B. T., Salvaggio, J. E., Weill, H., and Ziskind, M. M. 1976. Toluene diisocyanate (TDI) pulmonary disease: Immunologic and inhalation challenge studies. *J. Allergy Clin. Immunol.* 58:89–100.

Callerame, M. L., Condemi, J. J., Bohrod, M. G., and Vaughn, J. H. 1971. Immunologic reactions of bronchial tissue in asthma. *N. Engl. J. Med.* 284:459–464.

Cavagna, G., Foa, V., and Vigliani, E. C. 1969. Effects in man and rabbits of inhalation of cotton dust or extracts and purified endotoxins. *Br. J. Ind. Med.* 26:314–321.

Cimo, P. L., Pisciotta, A. V., Rajendra, G. D., Pino, J. L., and Aster, R. H. 1977. Detection of drug-dependent antibodies by the [15]Cr lysis test: Documentation of immune thrombocytopenia induced by diphenylhydantoin, diazepam, and sulfisoxazole. *Am. J. Hematol.* 2:65–72.

Cinkotai, F. F., Lockwood, M. G., and Rylander, R. 1977. Airborne micro-organisms and prevalance of byssinotic symptoms in cotton mills. *Am. Ind. Hyg. Assoc. J.* 38:554–559.

Coffin, D. L. 1972. Interaction of infectious disease and air pollution. In *Environmental factors in respiratory disease*, ed. D. H. K. Lee, pp. 151–173. New York: Academic Press.

Corbett, J. A. 1974. *The biochemical mode of action of pesticides*. New York: Academic Press, pp. 107–164.

Craddock, R. P., Fehr, G., Brigham, K. L., Kronenberg, S. R., and Jacob, H. S. 1977. Complement and leukocyte-mediated pulmonary dysfunction in hemodialysis. *N. Engl. J. Med.* 296:769–774.

Cross, T. 1968. Thermophilic actinomycetes. *J. Appl. Bacteriol.* 31:36–53.

David, V. R. 1976. Lymphocyte mediators, activated macrophages and tumor immunity. In *Molecular and biological aspects of the acute allergic reaction*, eds. S. G. O. Johanson, K. Strandberg, and B. Uvniis, pp. 437–454. New York: Plenum Press.

Davies, P., and Allison, A. C. 1976. Secretion of macrophage enzymes in relation to the pathogenesis of chronic inflammation. In *Immunobiology of the macrophage*, ed. David S. Nelson, pp. 427–461. New York: Academic Press.

Davies, R. J., Butcher, B. T., O'Neill, C. E., and Salvaggio, J. E. 1977. The *in vitro* effect of TDI on lymphocyte cyclic adenosine monophosphate production by isoproterenol, prostaglandin, and histamine. *J. Allergy Clin. Immunol.* 60:223–229.

DeMaria, T. F., and Burrell, R. 1980. Effects of inhaled endotoxin-containing bacteria. *Environ. Res.* 23:87–97.

Dixon, F. J., Feldman, J. D., and Vazquez, J. J. 1961. Experimental glomerulonephritis. *J. Exp. Med.* 113:899–920.

doPico, G. A., Flaherty, W., Tsiatis, A., Peters, M. E., Rao, P., and Rankin, J. 1977. Respiratory abnormalities among grain handlers. *Am. Rev. Respir. Dis.* 115:915–927.

Dutkiewicz, J. 1978. Exposure to dust-borne bacteria in agriculture. I. environmental studies. *Arch. Environ. Health* 33:250–259.

Edwards, C., McCartney, J., Rooke, G., and Ward, F. 1975. The pathology of the lung in byssinosis. *Thorax* 30:612–623.

Edwards, J. H. 1980. Microbial and immunological investigations and remedial action after an outbreak of humidifier fever. *Br. J. Ind. Med.* 37:55–62.

Edwards, J. H., and Jones, B. M. 1973 Pseudoimmune precipitation by the isolated byssinosis "antigen." *J. Immunol.* 110:498–501.

Emanuel, D. A., Lawton, B. R., and Wenzel, F. J. 1962. Maple bark disease. *N. Engl. J. Med.* 266:333–337.

Emanuel, D. A., Wenzel, F. J., Bauerman, C. I., and Lawton, B. R. 1964. Farmers lung. *Am. J. Med.* 37:392–401.

Epstein, W. L. 1967. Granulomatous hypsersensitivity. *Prog. Allergy* 11:36–88.

Espinosa, E., Kushner, I., and Kaplan, H. M. 1969. Antigenic composition of heart tissue. *Am. J. Cardiol.* 24:508–513.

Fisher, A. A. 1973. *Contact dermatitis*, 2nd Ed. Philadelphia: Lea and Febiger, pp. 353–422.

Frank, M. M., Schreiber, A. D., Atkinson, J. P.,

and Jaffe, C. J. 1977. Pathophysiology of immune hemolytic anemia. *Ann. Intern. Med.* 87:210–222.

Frick, L. O. 1984. Immediate hypersensitivity. In *Basic and clinical immunology*, 5th Ed., pp. 241–270. Los Altos, Calif.: Lange.

Hahon, N., and Eckert, H. L. 1976. Depression of viral interferon induction in cell monolayers by asbestos fibers. *Environ. Res.* 11:52–65.

Haroz, R. K., and Mattensberger-Kreber, L. 1977. Effect of cigarette smoke on macrophage phagocytosis. In *Pulmonary macrophage and epithelial cells*, eds. C. L. Sanders, R. P. Schneider, G. E. Dagle, and H. A. Ragan, pp. 36–57. Springfield, Va.: ERDA—U.S. Department of Commerce.

Haslam, P. L., Lukoszek, A., Merchant, J. A., and Turner-Warwick, M. 1978. Lymphocyte responses to phytohemagglutinin in patients with asbestosis and pleural mesothelioma. *Clin. Exp. Immunol.* 31:178–188.

Hay, J. B. 1979. Delayed (cellular) hypersensitivity. In *Inflammation, immunity and hypersensitivity*, 2nd Ed., ed. H. Z. Movat, pp. 272–318. New York: Harper and Row.

Heppleston, A. G. 1971. Observations on the mechanism of silicotic fibrogenesis. In *Inhaled particles III*, vol. 1, ed. W. H. Walton, pp. 357–371. Old Woking Surrey, England: Unwin Bros.

Heyden, S., and Pratt, P. 1980. Exposure to cotton dust and respiratory disease. *J.A.M.A.* 244:1797–1798.

Hill, J. O., and Burrell, R. 1979. Cell-mediated immunity to soluble and particulate inhaled antigens. *Clin. Exp. Immunol.* 38:332–341.

Hitchock, M., Piscitelli, D. M., and Bouhuys, A. 1973. Histamine release from human lung by a component of cotton bracts. *Arch. Environ. Health* 26:177–182.

Hubscher, T. T. 1977. Immune and biochemical mechanisms in the allergic disease of the upper respiratory tract: Role of antibodies, target cells, mediators and eosinophils. *Ann. Allergy* 38:83–90.

Huis in 'T Veld, J. H. J., and Berrens, L. 1976. Inactivation of hemolytic complement in human serum by an acylated polysaccharide from a gram-positive rod: Possible significance in pigeon-breeder's disease. *Infect. Immun.* 13:1619–1625.

Ishizaka, K. 1971. Human reaginic antibodies. *Ann. Rev. Med.* 21:187–200.

Jones, R. N., Turner-Warwick, M., Ziskind, M.,

and Weill, H. 1975. High prevalence of antinuclear antibodies in sandblasters' silicosis. *Am. Rev. Respir. Dis.* 113:393–395.

Kagan, E., Solomon, A., Cochrane, J. C., Beissner, E. I., Gluckman, J., Rocks, P. H., and Webster, I. 1977. Immunological studies of patients with asbestosis. *Clin. Exp. Immunol.* 28:261–267.

Katz, G. V., and Laskin, S. 1977. Effect of irritant atmospheres on macrophage behavior. In *Pulmonary macrophages and epithelial cells*, eds. C. L. Sanders, R. P. Schneider, G. E. Dagle, and H. A. Ragan, pp. 58–65. Springfield, Va.: ERDA—U.S. Department of Commerce.

Katz, H. D., Bargatze, R. F., Bogowitz, A. C., and Katz, L. R. 1979. Regulation of IgE antibody production by serum molecules. *J. Immunol.* 122:2191–2197.

Kessel, R. W. I., Monaco, L., and Marchisio, M. A. 1963. The specificity of the cytotoxic action of silica: A study *in vitro*. *Br. J. Exp. Pathol.* 44:351–364.

King, E. J., Mohanty, G. P., Harrison, C. V., and Nagelschmidt, G. 1953. The action of different forms of pure silica on the lungs of rats. *Br. J. Ind. Med.* 10:9–17.

King, T. P., and Norman, P. S. 1978. Antigens that cause atopic disease. In *Immunological diseases*, 3rd ed., eds. M. Samter, D. W. Talmage, B. Rose, K. F. Austen, and J. H. Vaughn, pp. 787–803. New York: Little, Brown.

Kutz, S. A., Mentnech, M. S., Olenchock, S. A., and Major, P. C. 1980. Precipitation of serum proteins by extracts of cotton dust and stems. *Environ. Res.* 22:476–484.

Kutz, S. A., Olenchock, S. A., Elliott, J. A., Pearson, D. J., and Major, P. C. 1979. Antibody independent complement activation by cardroom cotton dust. *Environ. Res.* 19:405–414.

Lacey, L. 1975. Occupational and environmental factors in allergy. In *Allergy '74*, eds. M. A. Ganderton and A. W. Frankland, pp. 303–319. Kent: Pitman Medical.

Lau, R. J., Tubergen, D. G., Barr, M., Domino, E. F., Benowitz, N., and Jones, R. T. 1976. Phytohemagglutinin-induced lymphocyte transformation in humans receiving Δ^9-tetrahydrocannabinol. *Science* 192:805–807.

Lewis, D. M., and Burrell, R. 1976. Induction of fibrogenesis by lung antibody-treated macrophages. *Br. J. Ind. Med.* 33:25–28.

Lindsey, J. R., Baker, H. J., Overcash, R. G., Cassell, G. H., and Hunt, C. H. 1971. Murine chronic respiratory disease. *Am. J. Pathol.* 64:675–706.

Lippmann, M., Eckert, H. L. Hahon, N., and Morgan, W. K. C. 1973. Circulating antinuclear and rheumatoid factors in coal miners. *Ann. Intern. Med.* 79:807–811.

Marx, J. J., and Burrell, R. 1973. Delayed hypersensitivity to beryllium compounds. *J. Immunol.* 111:590–598.

Marx, J. J., Jr., and Flaherty, D. K. 1976. Activation of the complement sequence by extracts of bacteria and fungi associated with hypersensitivity pneumonitis. *J. Allergy Clin. Immunol.* 57:328–334.

Massey, A., Capner, P. M., and Mowbray, J. F. 1977. Activation of the alternative pathway by gluten. *Immunology* 33:339–342.

Matsumura, Y. 1970. The effects of ozone, nitrogen dioxide, and sulfur dioxide on the experimentally induced allergic respiratory disorder in guinea pigs. *Am. Rev. Respir. Dis.* 102:430–447.

McDonough, R. J., Madden, J. J., Falek, A., Shafer, D. A., Pline, M., Gordon, D., Bokos, P., Kuehnle, J. C., and Mendelson, J. 1980. Alteration of T and null lymphocyte frequencies in the peripheral blood of human opiate addicts: *In vivo* evidence for opiate receptor sites on T lymphocytes. *J. Immunol.* 125:2539–2543.

McMillan, R., and Gardner, F. H. 1977. The pathogenesis of immune thrombocytopenic purpura. *CRC Crit. Rev. Clin. Lab. Sci.* 8:303–332.

Merchant, J. A., Kilburn, K. H., O'Fallon, W. M., Hamilton, J. D., and Lumsden, J. C. 1972. Byssinosis and chronic bronchitis among cotton textile workers. *Ann. Intern. Med.* 76:423–433.

Miller, D. S., and Zarkower, A. 1974. Alterations of murine immunologic responses after silica dust inhalation. *J. Immunol.* 113:1533–1543.

Miller, K., and Kagan, E. 1976. The *in vivo* effects of asbestos on macrophages, membrane structures and population characteristics—a scanning electron microscope study. *J. Reticuloendothel. Soc.* 20:159–171.

Miller, K., and Kagan, E. 1977. Immune adherence reactivity of rat alveolar macrophages following inhalation of crocidolite asbestos. *Clin. Exp. Immunol.* 29:152–158.

Miller, K., Webster, I., Handfield, R. I. M. and Skikne, M. I. 1978. Ultrastructure of the lung in the rat following exposure to crocidolite asbestos and quartz. *J. Pathol.* 124:39–44.

Miller, K., Weintraub, Z., and Kagan, E. 1979. Manifestations of cellular immunity in the rat after prolonged asbestos inhalation. *J. Immunol.* 123:1029–1038.

Morgan, W. K. C. 1984. Byssinosis and related conditions. In *Occupational lung diseases*, 2nd Ed., eds. W. K. C. Morgan and A. Seaton, pp. 541–563. Philadelphia: W. B. Saunders.

Morgan, W. K. C., Lapp, N. L., and Seaton, D. 1980. Respiratory disability in coal miners. *J.A.M.A.* 243:2401–2427.

Morrison, D. C., and Ryan, J. L. 1979. Bacterial endotoxins and host immune responses. *Adv. Immunol.* 28:377–450.

Morrison, D. C., and Ulevitch, R. J. 1978. The effects of bacterial endotoxins on host mediation systems. *Am. J. Pathol.* 93:527–617.

Muittari, A., Kuusisto, P., Virtanen, P., Sovijarvi, A., Gronroos, P., Harmoninen, A., Antila, P., and Kellomaki, L. 1979. An epidemic of extrinsic allergic alveolitis caused by tap water. *Clin. Allergy* 9:53–66.

Müller-Eberhard, H. J. 1975. Complement. *Ann. Rev. Biochem.* 44:697–724.

Nahas, G. G., Suciu-Foca, N., Armand, J.-P, and Morishima, A. 1974. Inhibition of cellular mediated immunity in marijuana smokers. *Science* 183:419–420.

Olenchock, S., and Burrell, R. 1976. The role of precipitins and complement activation in the etiology of allergic lung disease. *J. Allergy Clin. Immunol.* 58:76–88.

Olenchock, S. A., Mull, J. C., and Major, P. C. 1980. Complement activation by commercial allergen extracts of cereal grains. *Clin. Allergy* 10:395–404.

Osler, A. G., and Siraganian, R. P. 1972. Immunologic mechanisms of platelet damage. *Prog. Allergy* 16:450–498.

Pearsall, N. N., and Weiser, R. S. 1968. The macrophage in allograft immunity. *Res. J. Reticuloendthel. Soc.* 5:107–120.

Pepys, J. 1969. Hypersensitivity diseases of the lungs due to fungi and organic dusts. In *Monographs in allergy*, vol. 4, pp. 1–147, eds. P. Kallós, M. Hašek, T. M. Inderbitzen, P. A. Miescher, and B. H. Waksman. Basel:S. Karger.

Pernis, B., and Paronetto, F. 1962. Adjuvant effect of silica (tridymite) on antibody production. *Proc. Soc. Exp. Biol. Med.* 110:390–392.

Petz, L. D., and Fudenberg, H. H. 1975. Immunological mechanisms in drug-induced cytopenias. *Prog. Hematol.* 9:185–206.

Pratt, P. C., Vollmer, R. T., and Miller, J. A. 1980. Epidemiology of pulmonary lesions in nontextile and cotton textile workers. *Arch. Environ. Health* 35:133–138.

Ranadive, N. S., and Movat, H. Z. 1979. Tissue injury and inflammation induced by immune complexes. In *Inflammation, immunity and hypersensitivity*, 2nd Ed., ed. H. Z. Movat, pp. 409–444. Hagerstown, Md.: Harper and Row.

Reed, C. E., Sosman, A., and Barber, R. A. 1965. Pigeon-breeders' lung. *J.A.M.A.* 193:81–85.

Reiser, K. M., and Last, J. A. 1979. Silicosis and fibrogenesis: Fact and artifact. *Toxicology* 13:51–72.

Richard, J. C., Thurston, J. R., and Pier, A. C. 1978. Effects of mycotoxins on immunity. In *Toxins: Animal, plant and microbial*, ed. P. Rosenberg, pp. 801–817. Oxford and New York: Pergamon Press.

Richerson, H. B., Seidenfeld, J. J., Ratajczak, H. V., and Richards, D. W. 1978. Chronic experimental interstitial pneumonitis in the rabbit. *Am. Rev. Respir. Dis.* 117:5–13.

Riddle, H. F. V., Channell, S., Blyth, W., Weir, D. M., Lloyd, M., Amos, W. M. G., and Grant, I. W. B. 1968. Allergic alveolitis in a maltworker. *Thorax* 23:271–280.

Rocklin, R. E., Bendtzen, K., and Greineder, D. 1979. Mediators of immunity: Lymphokines and monokines. *Adv. Immunol.* 29:55–136.

Roitt, I. M., Shen, L., and Greenberg, A. H. 1976. Antibody-dependent cell-mediated cytotoxicity. In *The role of immunologic factors in infectious, allergic, and autoimmune processes*, eds. R. F. Beers, Jr., and E. G. Bassett, pp. 281–288. New York: Raven Press.

Rylander, R. 1974. Influence of infection on pulmonary defense mechanisms. *Ann. N.Y. Acad. Sci.* 221:282–289.

Rylander, R., Andersson K., Belin, L., Berglund, G., Bergström, R., Hanson, L., Lundholm, M., and Mattsby, I. 1977. Studies on humans exposed to airborne sewage sludge. *Schweiz. Med. Wochenschr.* 107:182–184.

Rylander, R., Snella, M. C., and Garcia, I. 1975. Pulmonary cell response patterns after exposure to airborne bacteria. *Scand. J. Respir. Dis.* 56:195–200.

Saint-Remy, J.-M. R., and Cole, P. 1980. Interactions of chrysotile asbestos fibres with the complement system. *Immunology* 41:431–437.

Scheel, L. D., Smith, B., VanRiper, J., and Fleisher,

E. 1954. Toxicity of silica. *Arch. Ind. Hyg. Occup. Med.* 9:29–36.

Schlievert, P. M., and Watson, D. W. 1978. Group A streptococcal pyrogenic exotoxin: Pyrogenicity and enhancement of lethal endotoxin shock. *Infect. Immun.* 21:753:–763.

Schorlemmer, H. U., and Allison, A. C. 1976. Effects of activated complement components on enzyme secretion by macrophages. *Immunology* 31:781–788.

Schuyler, M., Ziskind, M., and Salvaggio, J. 1977. Cell mediated immunity in silicosis. *Am. Rev. Respir. Dis.* 116:147–151.

Seal, R. M. E. 1975. Pathology of extrinsic allergic bronchoalveolitis. In *Alveolar interstitium of the lung*. vol. 8, *Progress in respiration research*, eds. H. Herzog, F. Basset, and R. Georges. Basel: S. Karger.

Seaton, A. 1984. Occupational asthma. In *Occupational lung diseases*, 2nd Ed., eds. W. K. C. Morgan and A. Seaton, pp. 498–520. Philadelphia: W. B. Saunders.

Selikoff, I. J., and Hammond, E. C. 1979. Asbestos and smoking. *J.A.M.A.* 242:458–459.

Sharma, R. P., and Zeeman, M. G. 1980. Immunologic alterations by environmental chemicals: Relevance of studying mechanisms versus effects. *J. Immunopharmacol.* 2(3):285–307.

Smith, S. M., Burrell, R., and Snyder, I. S. 1978. Complement activation by cell wall fractions of *Micropolyspora faeni*. *Infect. Immun.* 22:568–574.

Smith, S. M., Snyder, I. S., and Burrell, R. 1980. Mitogen response to *Micropolyspora faeni* cell walls. *J. Allergy Clin. Immunol.* 65:298–304.

Snella, M.-C., and Rylander, R. 1979. Alteration in local and systemic immune capacity after exposure to bursts of CO. *Environ. Res.* 20:74–79.

Speirs, R. S., and Speirs, E. E. 1979. An *in vivo* model for assessing effects of drugs and toxicants on immunocompetence. *Drug Chem. Toxicol.* 2:19–33.

Spitznagel, J. D., and Allison, A. C. 1970. Mode of action of adjuvants: retinol and other lysosome-labilizing agents as adjuvants. *J. Immunol.* 104:119–127.

Strunk, R. C., Pinnas, J. L, John, T. J., Hansen, R. L., and Blazovick, J. L. 1978. Rice hypersensitivity associated with serum complement depression. *Clin. Allergy* 8:51–58.

Szentivanyi, A. 1968. The beta-adrenergic theory of the atopic abnormality in bronchial allergy. *J. Allergy* 42:203–232.

Turner-Warwick, M. 1973. Immunology and asbestosis. *Proc. R. Soc. Med.* 66:927–930.

Unanue, E. R., and Dixon, F. J. 1967. Experimental glomerulonephritis: Immunologic event and pathogenetic mechanisms. *Adv. Immunol.* 6:1–90.

Vigliani, E. C., and Pernis, B. 1963. Immunological aspects of silicosis. *Adv. Tuberc. Res.* 12:230–279.

Vos, J. G. 1977. Immune suppression as related to toxicology. *CRC Crit. Rev. Toxicol.* 5:67–101.

Webb, R., Jr., and Winkelstein, A. 1984. Immunosuppression, immunopotentiation, and anti-inflammatory drugs. In *Basic and clinical immunology*, 5th Ed., eds. D. P. Stites, J. D. Stobo, H. H. Fundenberg, and J. V. Wells, pp. 271–287. Los Altos, Calif.: Lange.

Wei, C.-M., and McLaughlin, S. 1974. Structure-function relationship in the 12, 13-epoxy trichothecenes novel inhibitors of protein synthesis. *Biochem. Biophys. Res. Commun.* 57:838–843.

Zarkower, A., and Morges, W. 1972. Alteration in antibody response induced by carbon inhalation: A model system. *Infect Immun.* 5:915–920.

Zarkower, A., Scheuchenzuber, W. J., and Burns, C. A. 1979. Effects of silica dust inhalation on the susceptibility of mice to influenza infection . *Arch. Environ. Health* 34:372–376.

Zeiss, C. R., Patterson, R., Pruzansky, J. J., Miller, M. M., Rosenberg, M., and Levitz, D. 1977. Trimellitic anhydride-induced airway syndromes: Clinical and immunologic studies. *J. Allergy Clin. Immunol.* 60:96–103.

12

Hematopoietic System

Brigid G. Leventhal and Atiya B. Khan

The hematopoietic system does not serve as a portal of entry for toxic materials and is thus spared injury in many situations; however, it is extremely sensitive to some environmental influences because of the requirement for rapid synthesis and destruction of cells with consequent heavy metabolic demands. The cellular elements arise within the bone marrow from pluripotent stem cells. Any materials toxic to stem cells or their microenvironment could therefore result in underproduction of all cellular elements. Once stem cells have differentiated, the component elements can be individually affected. Various types of injury may occur to the hematopoietic system, including (a) general suppression of hematopoiesis or of one of the more differentiated cellular elements, (b) abnormal hematopoiesis, as when a specific phase of the metabolic process is impaired, (c) interference with the functional capacity of specific blood elements without an actual decrease in cell numbers, (d) increased demand for formation of blood elements, and (e) changes leading to malignant transformation to leukemia and other blood cancers (e.g., chromosomal damage).

In the final analysis, toxicity to the hematopoietic system per se is really the primary effect only in patients who have failure of stem cell production or who develop hematopoietic malignancy. When toxic changes occur in the function of mature cellular elements—for example, the hypoxemia that accompanies carbon monoxide poisoning—the primary target organs are myocardium and brain; however, the blood serves an important role as the "window" to the diagnosis and is itself abnormal. We have therefore selected some of these conditions for discussion in the context of this chapter. It should also be mentioned that most of the conditions discussed in this chapter are relatively rare and do not have a significant impact on the health of the general population; however, again, because blood is a tissue that is relatively easy to assay, study of molecular mechanisms of disease in blood cells has often greatly advanced our general knowledge.

Suppression of Hematopoiesis

The term aplastic anemia is used to describe pancytopenia of varying degrees of severity with a hypocellular or truly aplastic bone marrow. Aplastic anemia may not be fully developed at the time of the initial examination, and each of the cellular elements may not decline at the same rate. The pathogenesis of aplastic anemia is often obscure, and the primary problem in any individual patient could be a result of a defect either in the microenvironment or in the pluripotent stem cell. The fact that there is damage to all major marrow cell lines suggests that the basic defect is situated prior to the committed compartments. The occurrence of aplastic anemia either in association with or followed by paroxysmal nocturnal hemoglobinuria has been considered to reflect stem cell injury with subsequent emergence of new abnormal clones. The success with marrow transplants from HL-A matched sibling donors is also taken as evidence that many cases of aplastic anemia are due to a persistent abnormality induced in the stem cell population. The average annual death rate from this disease in whites in the United States is quite low in individuals below the age of 50, although there may be a slight peak in adolescent males; after 50, however, it climbs with increasing age. It is estimated that the overall incidence is about 4.8 per million people in the United States (Szklo, 1980).

A number of environmental factors have been thought to be important in the etiology of aplastic anemia. Industrial solvents, particularly benzene, have been recognized since the turn of the century as having potential toxicity to the bone marrow. Benzene is extensively used as a solvent in industry, and definite limits for exposure have been established. Although benzene is highly volatile, with a boiling point of 80°C, the distillation process used in the preparation of many petroleum products such as paint removers, kerosene, degreasers, and Stoddard's solvent, is often incomplete, leaving uncertain quantities of benzene in these solvents, which may be used in the home as well as in industrial settings. At least single cases of aplastic anemia have been reported after the use of these other solvents, and it is not clear whether the anemia is due to the solvent itself or to the contaminating benzene (Erslev, 1972a; Zenz, 1980). Pancytopenia may occur years after actual exposure to benzene, but such delayed reactions should always be suspected of being coincidental. In most cases, the bone marrow depression appears shortly after exposure to the chemical, with a close relationship between amounts and duration of exposure, and degree of bone marrow suppression. Some individuals go on subsequently to develop leukemia, and leukemia has been induced in laboratory animals after exposure to benzene (Erslev, 1972a).

Industrial exposure to trinitrotoluene has also resulted in aplastic anemia, and exposure to toluene among glue sniffers is thought to be dangerous. A number of these organic solvents metabolize through epoxide formation. This transformation seems to occur in the metabolism of benzene, styrene, and trichlororethylene. Ring epoxidation also takes place to some degree in the metabolism of toluene and xylene, but these latter substances do not appear to induce as severe hematopoietic injury as benzene (Zenz, 1980).

Inhalation of another group of solvents, the chloroethanes, has also been associated with the development of blood dyscrasias. The National Institute for Occupational Safety and Health (NIOSH) estimates that several million workers each year are exposed to these solvents (Zenz, 1980). The insecticides lindane and DDT have also been shown to have potential bone marrow-toxic properties; in fact, widespread spraying with DDT was thought at one time to be possibly the single most important factor in the etiology of aplastic anemia in Mexico (Sanchez Medal et al., 1963).

In the United States, medication is thought to represent a highly significant etiologic factor in aplastic anemia. The drug most often discussed in this context is chloramphenicol. Chloramphenicol is a broad-spectrum antibiotic that has been available commercially in the United States since 1949. Reports of cases of aplastic anemia with a history of exposure to chloramphenicol began to appear in the medical literature shortly after it entered the antibiotic market. Szklo (1980) describes a study done by the California State Department of Health in which it was shown that when the number of grams of chloramphenicol sold per million population was correlated with mortality for aplastic anemia in the United

States 1 year later, a strikingly high correlation coefficient of $+.92$ ($p < 0.01$) was found. Concomitant with the realization that chloramphenicol can induce prolonged self-sustaining bone marrow hypoplasia, it was found that it also can cause brief reversible bone marrow suppression in many, if not all exposed patients. This drug-dependent bone marrow failure is associated with an increase in serum iron and with nuclear vacuolization of bone marrow cells. It may involve granulocytes and platelets as well as erythrocytes. It is not clear whether this is an early, still reversible manifestation of impending chloramphenicol-induced aplasia or whether the latter represents an unrelated and more idiosyncratic response (Erslev, 1972a).

Of the other drugs suspected of being associated with aplastic anemia, a good case seems to exist for phenylbutazone, and for quinacrine, which was widely used in malaria prophylaxis. A death rate of 20 per million was found in areas where quinacrine was routinely used for prevention of malaria, whereas a rate of only 2 per million was found in military installations not using quinacrine (Szklo, 1980). At least 50 other drugs have been associated with cases of aplastic anemia. In general, it is impossible to determine whether these associations are causal, because control data are lacking.

Inorganic and organic mercury, in micromolar concentrations in experimental situations, inhibits colony formation in primary cultures of mouse bone marrow (Strom et al., 1979). Chronic mercury poisoning in children, which is usually medication induced, may cause pancytopenia of the marrow (Anderson et al., 1975). Hematopoietic toxicity has also been reported from methyl mercury exposures. Chromosome analysis on lymphocytes from human subjects with increased concentrations of methyl mercury in their blood cells following the ingestion of contaminated fish show a significant correlation between the frequency of cells with chromosomal breaks and the methyl mercury concentration. In addition to the known neuropathology, methyl mer-

cury ingestion in humans is associated with hypoplasia of the bone marrow and lymph node atrophy, which one assumes, because of the known chromosomal damage, is related to stem cell injury (Takeuchi and Eto, 1977).

It is thought that ionizing radiation can also play an etiologic role in aplastic anemia, also presumably through direct killing of stem cells (Cronkite, 1967). In general, studies examining the relationship of radiation to aplastic anemia have not been able to quantify the degree of exposure. There are reports that aplastic anemia may occur months or years after a brief exposure to radiation such as that of patients treated with x rays for spondylitis (Court-Brown, 1957). Ichimaru et al. (1972) showed the atomic bomb survivors exposed to 1 rad or more had a 1.8 times greater incidence of aplastic anemia than survivors exposed to less than 1 rad, but this difference was not significant at the $p = 0.05$ level.

Aplastic anemia has also been reported to develop after long-term continuous exposure to small amounts of radiation as from internally deposited thorium (Duane, 1957). Matanoski et al. (1975) looked at the causes of death for radiologists and compared this with the death rate for internists. They found an excess of 43 times the risk of death from aplastic anemia in the cohort of radiologists joining their specialty society in 1920–1929, but not in later cohorts. One might infer from this that there were higher levels of exposure in the earliest years and that it is this higher level of exposure that is needed to induce aplastic anemia.

It is interesting that a study of Marshall Islanders who had survived an accidental exposure to radioactive fallout during the atomic bomb testing program showed that 16 years after the event, platelet and granulocyte levels were lower in the exposed than in a nonexposed age-matched control cohort, suggesting a sustained level of damage to the hematopoietic system (Conard et al., 1971).

Long-term low-dose microwave exposure of experimental animals has been reported to induce peripheral blood lymphocytosis, an increase in the number of DNA-synthesizing cells in lymph nodes, and a slight decrease in the red blood cell count (Czerski, 1975). There were no obvious morphologic changes in bone marrow, but ferrokinetic studies demonstrated that erythrocyte production as measured by ^{59}Fe incorporation was significantly decreased. All of these changes occurred as a result of intentional experimental exposure. There are no reported cases of human disease, to our knowledge, that have been caused by microwave exposure from environmental or industrial sources; however, it is of interest that the erythroid stem cell is the one most sensitive to the effects of ionizing radiation and the one that is universally affected by the administration of chloramphenicol. It therefore seems possible that at higher microwave dose exposure there might be a more dramatic effect on the bone marrow as a whole.

Another environmental factor that has been associated with the development of aplastic anemia is the relatively ubiquitous hepatitis virus. In general, in these cases pancytopenia begins within 1 year after the onset of hepatitis. Hagler et al. (1975) presented detailed clinical information for 153 patients of whom 137 developed aplastic anemia within 1 year after the episode of hepatitis. Of these 137 patients, 36 (26%) had been exposed to another potentially myelotoxic agent before developing hepatitis, such as chloramphenicol. They suggest that it is possible that some patients could have suffered idiosyncratic damage of the liver and bone marrow from the same drug exposure, or that they might have developed marrow toxicity as a consequence of faulty drug metabolism by an injured liver; however, it seems likely that in at least some cases there is direct marrow damage by the virus.

Other viral infections have been known to affect committed stem cells and inhibit their replication. Congenital rubella shows a particular predilection for growth in the megakaryocyte with resultant thrombocytopenia (Raksen et al., 1967), and other viral disease such as rubella and Thai hemorrhagic fever can be associated with a dramatic fall in platelet count and abnormal-appearing megakaryocytes (Aster, 1972).

Female hormones, either endogenous or exogenously administered, can result in cyclic changes in platelet count. Alcohol, which is a direct marrow toxin, may inhibit platelet production as well as lead to secondary nutritional disorders that disturb hematopoiesis (Aster, 1972).

The committed red cell precursor may also be the only cell whose replication is inhibited. Transient erythroblastopenia of childhood is a self-limited suppression of erythropoiesis that frequently follows viral infections. The associated anemia may be severe for a few weeks (Lipton and Nathan, 1980).

Abnormalities in Hematopoiesis

Certain toxic substances, rather than depressing the stem cell pool, can be envisioned as causing toxicity because they are incorporated into the developing cells and result in an abnormal end product. The best-known example of this in humans occurs as a result of lead poisoning. In lead intoxication, the synthesis of both globin and heme is impaired. The two most clearly demonstrated blocks in the heme-biosynthetic pathway are (1) impaired conversion of protoporphyrin to heme, probably because of a defect in heme synthetase activity and (2) impaired conversion of δ-aminolevulinic acid to porphyrobilinogen because of a defect in the activity of aminolevulinic acid dehydrogenase (Moore, 1972). There is some evidence for increased hemolysis and a decreased erythrocyte life span in lead poisoning as well as a direct effect in inhibition of red cell production. The anemia is usually relatively mild. Normocytic, slightly hypochromic red cells are seen, with some elevation in reticulocyte count (2–7%). The most striking feature is the basophilic stippling, which is most marked in the young polychromatophilic cells. These basophilic granules have been shown to be composed of altered ribosomes (Harris and Kellermeyer, 1973).

Lead poisoning occurs today in adults largely because of industrial exposure or accidents, and in children because of pica concomitant lead ingestion. Although it still occurs, lead poisoning due to improper storage and transport of water or other liquids (lead containers and pipes) or the burning of battery cases for fuel for household heating is infrequent. The distillation of illicit liquor through leaden worms or car radiators enhances the incidence of lead poisoning in certain areas. The important symptoms of lead poisoning are the acute encephalopathy, seen most often in children, and the peripheral neuropathies that are the usual presenting complaints of adults. The anemia is usually not clinically important; rather, when the combination of anemia and stippled erythrocytes is noted, the physician is alerted to the fact that the patient has been exposed to lead, and preventive measures may be taken before overt signs of toxicity become evident.

Functional Impairment of Normally Formed Cells

The toxic event that results in poor function of a particular organ system may not necessarily occur during formation of the cell, but rather may affect an already fully formed cell and, in some way, prevent optimal function.

ACQUIRED OR SECONDARY METHEMOGLOBINEMIA

This results when the rate of formation of methemoglobin exceeds the rate of reduction because of the action of chemical agents (Harris and Kellermeyer, 1973). Methemoglobin is formed when the iron of deoxyhemoglobin is oxidized from the ferrous to the ferric state. The symptoms are related to anoxemia, because methemoglobin cannot transport oxygen, and they range from mere alarm at the presence of cyanosis to headache, gastrointestinal disturbances, coma, and death. Symptoms usually develop in patients with more than 35–40% of hemoglobin in the met form.

Nitrites, sulfonamides, and aniline derivatives are the substances most commonly incriminated in the development of methemoglobinemia. Nitrites are usually absorbed from the gastrointestinal tract. This may follow the ingestion of food treated with sodium nitrite as a preservative. Nitrites may also be inhaled by chemical workers, arc welders, and cardiac patients receiving amyl nitrite, among others. Nitrates, which may be present in well water, may be reduced to nitrites by intestinal bacteria and absorbed as well. Numerous instances of methemoglobinemia and some fatalities (in infants) have been reported from the ingestion of well water high in nitrates, the use of bismuth subnitrate as an antidiarrheal agent, or the intake of food high in nitrates.

Aniline derivatives are probably the most potent formers of methemoglobin; inhalation of fumes or dust, oral ingestion, or dermal absorption of any of the aromatic nitro or amino compounds may result in profound pigment changes. Although most frequently seen because of industrial accidents or misuse, instances have also been described as caused by exposure to diaper labels, freshly dyed blankets or shoes, or ingestion of colored crayons. Acetophenetidin and acetanilid are two of the most commonly used compounds that may produce methemoglobinemia.

Sulfhemoglobinemia is of importance mainly because it must be ruled in or out when pigmentary causes of cyanosis are considered. The chemical nature of the compound is not known with certainty. The sulfur may substitute for one of the nitrogen atoms in the pyrrole ring or between the iron and its polypeptide bond. Sulfhemoglobinemia has been noted with methemoglobinemia and hemolytic anemia; usually this is thought to be secondary to a toxic chemical, but this is not always proven. Clinically it is seen in association with the habitual ingestion of an oxidizing drug (Bromo Seltzer, acetanilid, acetophenetidin, etc.) and not infrequently associated with chronic constipation, which may lead to excessive absorption of nitrites and sulfides after excessive intake of precursors of these chemicals (Harris and Kellermeyer, 1973).

CARBOXYHEMOGLOBINEMIA

Carboxyhemoglobin, which is incapable of carrying oxygen, is formed when the blood is exposed to carbon monoxide (CO). This results in the cherry-red color of the blood that is characteristically noted, particularly at post mortem in fatal cases of poisoning; however, the true site of CO poisoning is probably the blocking of cytochrome a_3 oxidase in the mitochondria (Zenz, 1980). This is the same enzyme that is affected in cyanide and hydrogen sulfide poisoning. However, the laboratory index for carbon monoxide poisoning is the blood level.

During 1968–1975, CO was listed on death certificates as the underlying cause of 8764 deaths in the United States; 5782 by motor vehicle exhaust, 1093 by incomplete combustion of domestic fuels, and 1889 through occupational exposure at blast furnaces and kilns or to partially combusted industrial fuels. CO is an occupational hazard for workers involved with internal combustion engines, foundries, petroleum refineries, pulp mills, and steel mills, and others who have intermittent acute exposures such as firefighters.

There is CO in the environment from automobile exhaust fumes, and in addition, smokers have chronically elevated carbxyhemoglobin levels. Again, it should be emphasized that although this is a toxicity that is discovered through monitoring the blood, the heart should probably be considered the major target organ of chronic carbon monoxide poisoning, in that CO at commonly found levels can clinically affect cardiac function and influence the occurrence and severity of coronary artery disease. Recommended safety standards may not provide the same degree of protection to individuals who smoke as to nonsmokers, and a higher risk from exposure is sustained by individuals at higher altitudes or with physical impairments that interfere with normal oxygen delivery to the tissues.

FUNCTIONAL STUDIES OF LEUKOCYTES

Neither the effects of the overall environment nor those of the local one on leukocyte function have been well studied. Exposure to ultraviolet light in experimental settings is known to be immunosuppressive in some animal systems, and this can be related to changes in the subpopulations of lymphoid cells present (Letvin et al., 1980). DuRuisseau (1977), in the course of performing normal physical examinations for regular and prospective hospital employees, found that their differential white count changed during a heat wave, with an increase in the percentage of lymphocytes and a decline in the percentage of granulocytes. A number of drugs that are classified as "anti-inflammatory" can be shown to inhibit the migration of leukocytes; these include steroids, indomethacin, and aspirin. It is interesting that Warne and West (1980) noted that during the summer months aspirin was relatively ineffective in suppressing leukocyte migration into areas of chemically induced inflammation in rats, whereas the same seasonal pattern was not seen with indomethacin; however, none of these rather poorly documented general effects is well understood.

One chemical substance that has been studied for its effect on the local environment of the functioning white cell is cigarette smoke. Cigarette tobacco is a complex mixture, and even its major chemical groups or the major fractions of tobacco smoke condensate are too complex to achieve the ideal of relating biologic effects to single chemical components. Polymorphonuclear leukocytes from the oral cavity cluster and fail to spread and migrate after exposure to cigarette smoke. This effect is related to the gas phase, in which acrolein and cyanide are present (Kilburn, 1974). Water-soluble fractions of whole cigarette smoke can act as a chemotactic agent themselves but can also inhibit leukocyte chemotaxis in response to other agents (Bridges et al., 1980). In high enough concentrations, these materials can also cause inhibition of adherence of polymorphonuclear leukocytes to nylon fiber columns (Bridges et al., 1980). In addition, alveolar macrophages of smokers have decreased activity of oxidoreductases and hydrolases by histochemical techniques. The migration rate of macrophages from nonsmokers is at least three times as fast as that for smokers, and the phagocytic competence of macrophages is also reduced in smokers (Kilburn, 1974). One assumes that some of the pulmonary toxicity that is reported from inhalation of a variety of noxious chemicals is preceded by similar effects in destroying the local defense of the blood-borne cells, but that this happens so completely and so quickly that what is noted is the end product of damage to lung rather than these preliminary steps.

QUALITATIVE DISORDERS IN PLATELET FUNCTION

Recently assays have been developed that allow the qualitative evaluation of platelet function in vitro. One of the most widely studied is the ability of the platelet to aggregate when it releases ADP after contact with collagen. Aspirin when present in the circulation results in a variety of platelet abnormalities, most of which can be attributed to its inhibitory effect on the release of intrinsic platelet ADP. As a result, platelet aggregation that is induced by collagen, connective tissue, or epinephrine is abnormal, and increased bleeding or bruising may result in individuals who ingest aspirin. A number of other drugs used in clinical medicine have also been shown to inhibit platelet function, although the real definition of a clinically important deleterious effect on hemostasis has not been as clearly established as for aspirin. These drugs include phenylbutazone, some antihistaminics, and a variety of psychotropic agents in the phenothiazine and dibenazepine classes (Weiss, 1972). It is of interest that there is a differential impact of certain agents on newborn platelets as compared with the impact of the same agents on maternal platelets. Membrane-active agents that prevent release of ADP from platelets and prevent platelet aggregation were found to cross the placental barrier, and, in general, the effect on fetal platelets was 5–10 times that on the maternal platelets (Brown, 1974).

In contrast, the effects of smoking on platelets appear to be to enhance platelet adhesiveness and reduce clotting time. These effects are thought to be mediated by nicotine-induced catecholamine release, in that catecholamines have been shown to enhance ATP- or ADP-induced platelet aggregation (Kilburn, 1974).

Environmental Factors Resulting in Increased Production of Normal Elements

ERYTHROCYTOSIS DUE TO LOW ATMOSPHERIC PRESSURE

Studies have been done comparing individuals living at sea level, in Lima, Peru, with those living at 14,900 feet above sea level in Morococha, Peru, at atmospheric pressures of about two-thirds the normal (Hurtado, 1960). These latter individuals appear to be healthy and have a normal life span. Adjustment to this environment includes polycythemia and a shift in the oxygen dissociation curve to the right, so that oxygen is more easily released into the tissues. There is also a concomitant expansion in total blood volume. These latter two factors are more practical adjustments than polycythemia, because unfortunately the polycythemia leads to an associated increase in blood viscosity, which tends to reduce blood flow and negates some of the advantage derived from the higher hemoglobin concentration. It may also lead to thrombotic complications (Erslev, 1972b).

HEMOLYTIC PROCESSES

Important hemolytic syndromes are often the results of the administration of a common agent to an individual with an underlying abnormality of the red cell that renders that individual susceptible to hemolysis. The best example is glucose 6-phosphate dehydrogenase deficiency, which is present in many racial groups throughout the world. Many drugs have been associated with hemolysis in these individuals, most notably primaquine and sulfa drugs. A number of drugs can cause hemolysis in otherwise normal individuals. Inhalation of arsine gas is a well-recognized cause of hemolytic anemia. Arsine arises in the course of many industrial processes. In most cases nascent hydrogen, generated by the action of acid on metal, reacts with arsenic compounds to form the gas. The arsenic is usually present as a contaminant of either the acid or the metal, so that a history of actually working with an arsenic compound is not always obtained. Intoxication with copper salts is also known to produce hemolysis in humans, although the mechanism is not known. Hemolytic anemia has also been observed in astronauts exposed to 100% oxygen and in at least one patient to whom hyperbaric oxygen was administered. Rarely bee stings and spider bites have been associated with severe hemolysis. Although snake venom is well known to cause hemolysis in vitro, hemolysis does not often occur in vivo (Beutler, 1972).

DISORDERS OF INCREASED GRANULOCYTE CONSUMPTION

The marrow reserve for granulocyte production is so enormous that a rise rather than a fall in circulating granulocyte count is the rule in situations where increased destruction occurs, as must be true in acute pyogenic infections. Thus, toxic causes of granulocyte destruction are not known at the present time.

INCREASED PLATELET CONSUMPTION

It is possible mechanically to remove platelets in the course of plateletpheresis at a rate that results in thrombocytopenia, because the platelets cannot be manufactured sufficiently rapidly to replace them. In addition, fall in circulating platelet count has been seen in divers during even "safe" decompression. A tentative explanation for these observations is that asymptomatic bubbles form during decompression and that platelets adhere to these. The platelet–bubble aggregates may then be filtered out through the pulmonary vascular bed. In a mountain environment, at 9800 and 17,600 feet, under conditions of both hypoxia and decompression, normal volunteers were found to have a transient fall in platelet count lasting a few days. This was also assumed to be related to sequestration in the pulmonary capillary bed (Gray et al., 1975). Although these effects of pressure changes at the moment are important only for a few individuals, with an increase in the accessibility of space travel, space shuttles, and the like, it seems that atmospheric effects on hematopoiesis will assume increasing importance.

Changes Leading to the Development of Malignancy (Including Injury to the Chromosomes)

The environment clearly plays an important role in the etiology of cancer in many organ systems. In the hematopoietic system a number of the same factors that result in aplastic anemia and chromosome damage can also be associated with the development of malignancy. Thus, groups heavily exposed to ionizing radiation as from atomic bombs, radiotherapy, and occupational contact have an increased incidence of leukemia, as do those exposed to chemicals such as benzene. However, the actual conversion of a normal cell to a malignant one is a complicated process, and not all cells exposed to the same environment undergo malignant degeneration simultaneously or at all. Although this chapter is not addressed to genetic factors in hematologic disease, it is important to note that although only a small portion of cancers are known to exhibit Mendelian patterns of inheritance, yet over 200 single-gene disorders have been linked to neoplasia (Mulvihill, 1977). In some situations the mutant gene is expressed directly as a hereditary neoplasm, but in others it results in a preneoplastic lesion that in turn carries a high risk of cancer. These disorders, although rare, are very important to recognize, because they may provide clues to genetic environmental interactions in carcinogenesis. The chromosome instability syndromes of Bloom and Fanconi predispose to cancer, particularly leukemia. Treatment of Fanconi's anemia with androgenic anabolic steroids may result in hepatomas, suggesting genetic susceptibility to chemical carcinogenesis (Meadows et al., 1974), and reports of excess cancer risk in presumed carriers of the genes for ataxia telangiectasia and Fanconi's anemia raise the possibility that heterozygosity for these traits may account for a sizable proportion of cancers in the population at large.

A more general example of genetic environmental interaction may be the metabolism of polycyclic hydrocarbons to epoxides by the aryl hydrocarbon hydroxylase (AHH) microsomal enzyme system. Some of the metabolites are carcinogenic. The expression of AHH induction is probably controlled by an autosomal trait in inbred mice (Gelboin et al., 1972). Kellerman et al. (1973) have studied the AHH system of lymphocytes from patients with lung cancer and controls. AHH was induced in lymphocytes by 3-methylcholanthrene. The system was more highly inducible in lymphocytes from patients with lung cancer than in normal individuals, suggesting that a genetic factor affecting the metabolism of possible carcinogens may be important in determining whether a particular individual develops cancer.

International variation in the incidence of some tumors may reflect genetic as well as environmental mechanisms. Such a mechanism, for example, may explain the deficits of chronic lymphocytic leukemia and other B cell tumors among Oriental populations (Fraumeni, 1977). In the same manner, black children have not shown the sharp peak of acute lymphocytic leukemia characteristically seen among white children in the United States, whereas they seem to have a disproportionate share of nonlymphocytic leukemia (Gordis et al., 1981).

In this discussion, however, it is also important to recognize that even those individuals who are genetically identical do not simultaneously develop cancer on exposure to environmental factors. There is, for example, approximately a 20% rate of concordance for the development of acute leukemia in identical twins when the first twin is diagnosed under the age of 6 (Miller, 1971). This might suggest an intrauterine environmental factor. However, the concordance diminishes dramatically as the age at diagnosis of the first twin increases, and there are many well-documented identical twin pairs discordant for the development of acute leukemia as well as Ph+ chronic myelogenous leukemia.

In the last few years, observations that have potential etiologic import in lymphomas have been made most consistently in the area of B cell tumors. It appears that there may well be a spectrum of disorders that range from polyclonal immunoblastic lymphadenopathy to monoclonal Burkitt's lymphoma. This concept forces us to place new emphasis, in explaining etiology, on the regulatory interactions within the immune system. The breakdown of the normal regulatory system could result either from the production of B cells that have a selective growth advantage, such as through transformation by EB virus, through the 14q+ translocation or the 8q− deletion, or from controller cells that have been inactivated, perhaps genetically or through the use of drugs or other environmental factors (Leventhal and Kaizer, 1981).

Chronic antigenic stimulation leading to unchecked lymphoid proliferation may be an environmental etiologic factor common to hereditary and acquired immunodeficiency disease as well as lymphoid malignancy. Chronic antigenic stimulation within the environment might be a particularly attractive hypothesis to explain the increasing incidence of multiple myeloma in the United States population, particularly in black males, because this is a tumor arising in mature antibody-forming cells (Fraumeni, 1977; Leventhal and Kaizer, 1981).

Viruses have been associated with the development of the non-Hodgkin's lymphomas and Burkitt's tumor, and recently antibodies against a human retrovirus HTLV were identified in a cluster of Japanese patients with adult T cell leukemia, which is endemic in southwest Japan, suggesting that this virus might be involved in the etiology of this subset of malignancy (Robert-Guroff et al., 1982). No viruses have been identified in Hodgkin's disease, but case clusters are frequently reported in communities, particularly in schools, which suggests the possibility of an infectious or environmental process.

One must consider that, in addition to genetic–environmental interactions, there may be interaction of several procarcinogens and carcinogens in the environment of particular individuals who develop cancer. An example of this type of phenomenon in vitro is the ability of caffeine to interfere with the postreplication repair of cells injured by other agents (Hansson, 1978). At present, we are aware of no clinical situation where an in vivo demonstration of this sort of synergism has been established.

Conclusions

It seems that a number of substances including chemicals, pesticides, drugs, heavy metals such as mercury, ionizing radiation, and viruses can result in severe damage to marrow stem cells, which may result in secondary failure of marrow production with aplastic anemia or may progress to the development of frank malignancy. The latter may indicate a defect in the efficiency of the repair process from these various injuries in the myeloid system and possibly may relate to other environmental influences such as antigen overload with disordered immune regulation in the lymphoid system. Other environmental influences may result in overproduction of certain blood elements or malfunction of fully formed elements. These conditions are better understood for the red cell than for the platelet or leukocyte. Emphasis has been placed on the complex multifactorial nature of most of these conditions. Coexistence of genetic or other acquired diseases may make a particular individual more susceptible to the influence of a particular noxious stimulus in the environment. The blood itself is not often the target for environmental toxicity; however, because of its easy accessibility as a tissue for study, it has often provided us with important diagnostic information and better understanding of the underlying mechanism of the diseases in question.

REFERENCES

Anderson, J. A., and Narsimhan, M. J., Jr. 1975. Chemical drug poisoning. In *Nelson textbook of pediatrics*, 10th Ed., eds. V. S. Vaughn III, R. J. McKay, and W. E. Nelson. Philadelphia: W. B. Saunders

Aster, R. H. 1972. Thrombocytopenia due to diminished or defective platelet production. In *Hematology*, eds. W. J. Williams, E. Beutler, A. J. Erslev, and R. W. Rundles, pp. 1124–1131. New York: McGraw-Hill.

Beutler, E. 1972. Hemolytic anemia due to chemical intoxication. In *Hematology*, eds. W. J. Williams, E. Beutler, A. J. Erslev, and R. W. Rundles. pp. 482–483. New York: McGraw-Hill.

Bridges, R. B., Hsieh, L., and Haack, D. G. 1980. Effects of cigarette smoke and its constituents on the adherence of polymorphonuclear leukocytes. *Infect. Immun.* 29:1096–1101.

Brown, A. K. 1974. Special susceptibility of the fetal and neonatal hematopoietic system to chemical pollutants including drugs administered to the mother. *Pediatrics* 53:816–817.

Conard, R. A., Demoise, C. F., Scott, W. A., and Makar, M. 1971. Immunohematological studies of Marshall Islanders sixteen years after fallout radiation exposure. *J. Gerontol.* 26:28–36.

Court-Brown, W. M., and Doll, R. 1957. *Leukemia and aplastic anemia in patients irradiated for ankylosing spondylitis*, Medical Research Council Special Report Series No. 295. London: Medical Research Council, pp. 1–135.

Cronkite, E. P. 1967. Radiation induced aplastic anemia. *Semin. Hemtol.* 4:273–277.

Czerski, P. 1975. Microwave effects on the blood forming system with particular reference to the lymphocyte. *Ann. N.Y. Acad. Sci.* 247:232–242.

Duane, G. W. 1957. Aplastic anemia fourteen years following administration of thorotrast. *Am. J. Med.* 23:499.

DuRuisseau, J. P. 1977. Effects de la canicule sur la formule leucocytaire dans une population de normaux. *Union Med. Can.* 106:888–890.

Erslev, A. J. 1972a. Aplastic anemia. In *Hematology*, eds. W. J. Williams, E. Beutler, A. J. Erslev, and R. W. Rundles, pp. 207–227. New York: McGraw-Hill.

Erslev, A. J. 1972b. Secondary polycythemia. In *Hematology*, eds. W. J. Williams, E. Beutler, A. J. Erslev, and R. W. Rundles, pp. 544–555, New York: McGraw-Hill.

Fraumeni, J. F., Jr. 1977. Environmental and genetic determinants of cancer. In *Proceedings of Conference on Carcinogenesis and Mutagenesis, J. Environ. Pathol. Toxicol.,* Park Forest, Ill.: Pathotox Publishers, pp. 19–30.

Gelboin, H. V., Wiebel, R. J., and Kinoshita, N. 1972. Microsomal aryl hydrocarbon hydroxylase: On their role in polycyclic hydrocarbon carcinogenesis and toxicity and the mechanism of enzyme induction. In *Biological hydroxylation mechanisms*, eds. G. S. Boyd and R. M. S. Semllie, Biochemical Society Symposia No. 34, pp. 103–133. London: Biochemical Society.

Gordis, L., Szklo, M., Thompson, B., Kaplan, E., and Tonascia, J. 1981. An apparent increase in the incidence of acute non-lymphocytic leukemia in black children. *Cancer* 47:2763–2768.

Gray, G. W., Bryan, A. C., Freedman, M. H., Houston, C. S., Lewis, W. F., McFadden, D. M., and Newell, G. 1975. Effect of altitude exposure on platelets. *J. Appl. Physiol.* 39:648–651.

Hagler, L., Pastore, R. A., and Bergin, J. J. 1975. Aplastic anemia following viral hepatitis: Report of two fatal cases and literature review. *Medicine* 54:139–164.

Hansson, K. 1978. Caffeine enhancement of chromosomal aberrations induced by thiotepa in bone marrow cells of mice. *Hereditas* 89:129–131.

Harris, J. W., and Kellermeyer, R. W. 1973. *The red cell,* rev. ed. Cambridge, Mass.: Harvard University Press.

Hurtado, A. 1960. Some clinical aspects of life at high altitudes. *Ann. Intern. Med.* 53:247.

Ichimaru, M., Ishimaru, T., Tsuchimoto, T., and Kirshbaum, J. D. 1972. Incidence of aplastic anemia in A bomb survivors in Hiroshima and Nagasaki, 1946–1967. *Radiat. Res.* 49:461–472.

Kellerman, G., Shaw, C. R., and Luyten-Kellerman, M. 1973. Aryl hydrocarbon hydroxylase inducibility and bronchogenic carcinoma. *N. Engl. J. Med.* 289:934–937.

Kilburn, K. H. 1974. Effects of tobacco smoke on biological systems. *Scand. J. Respir. Dis. (Suppl.)* 91:63–78.

Letvin, N. L., Green, M. I., Benacerraf, B., and Germain, R. N. 1980. Immunologic effects of whole body ultraviolet irradiation: Selective defect in splenic adherent cell function *in vitro. Proc. Natl. Acad. Sci.* (U.S.A.) 77:2881–2885.

Leventhal, B. G., and Kaizer, H. 1981. Etiologic factors in non-Hodgkin's lymphoma. In *Childhood non-Hodgkin's lymphoma,* ed. J. Graham-Pole, pp. 1–11. Progress in Pediatric Hematologic Oncology Series. Littleton, Mass. PSG Publishing Co.

Lipton, J. M., and Nathan, D. G. 1980. Aplastic and hypoplastic anemia. *Ped. Clin. North Am.* 27:217–236.

Matanoski, G. M., Seltser, R., Sartwell, P. E., Diamond, E. L., and Elliott, E. A. 1975. The current mortality rate of radiologists and other physician specialists: Specific causes of death. *Am. J. Epidemiol.* 101:199–201.

Meadows, A. T., Naiman, J. L., and Valdes Padena, M. 1974. Hepatoma associated with androgen therapy for aplastic anemia. *J. Pediatr.* 84:109–110.

Miller, R. W. 1971. Deaths from childhood leukemia and solid tumors among twins and other siblings in the United States, 1960–1967. *J. Natl. Cancer Inst.* 46:203–209.

Moore, C. V. 1972. Sideroblastic anemia. In *Hematology*, eds. W. J. Williams, E. Beutler, A. J. Erslev, and R. W. Rundles, pp. 349–357. New York: McGraw-Hill.

Mulvihill, J. J. 1977. Genetic repertory of human neoplasia. In *Genetics of human cancer,* eds. J. J. Mulvihill, R. W. Miller, and J. F. Fraumeni, pp. 137–143. New York: Raven Press.

Raksen, A. R., Richter, P., Tallal, L., and Cooper, L. Z. 1967. Hematologic effects of intrauterine rubella. *J.A.M.A.* 199:111.

Robert-Guroff, M., Nakao, Y., Notake, K., Ito, Y., Sliski, A., and Gallo, R. C. 1982. Natural antibodies to human retrovirus HTLV in a cluster of Japanese patients with adult T cell leukemia. *Science* 215:975–978.

Sanchez Medal, L., Castanedo, J. P., and Garcia Roja, F. 1963. Insecticides and aplastic anemia. *N. Engl. J. Med.* 269:1365.

Strom, S., Johnson, R. L., and Uyeki, E. M. 1979. Mercury toxicity to hemopoietic and tumor colony forming cells and its reversal by selenium *in vitro. Toxicol. Appl. Pharmacol.* 49:431–436.

Szklo, M. 1980. Aplastic anemia. In *Reviews in cancer epidemiology,* ed. A. H. Lilienfeld, pp. 218–224. Amsterdam, New York: Elsevier-North Holland.

Takeuchi, T., and Eto, K. 1977. Pathology and pathogenesis of Minamata disease. In *Minamata disease,* eds. T. Tsuhaki and K. Irukayama, pp. 103–142. Amsterdam, New York: Elsevier-North Holland.

Warne, P. J., and West, G. B. 1980. Seasonal variation in drug action and animal responses in models of inflammation. *Int. Arch. Allergy Appl. Immun.* 61:111–113.

Weiss, H. J. 1972. Acquired qualitative platelet disorders. In *Hematology,* eds. W. J. Williams, E. Beutler, A. J. Erslev, and R. W. Rundles, pp. 1171–1175. New York: McGraw-Hill.

Zenz, C. 1980. *Developments in occupational medicine.* Chicago: Year Book Medical Publishers.

13

Cardiovascular System

Dennis D. Reichenbach

The medical literature concerning environmentally related diseases of the cardiovascular system is quite limited. Whether this represents a lack of effect on the cardiovascular system or a lack of knowledge is not entirely clear. The medical profession does not appear to be as attuned to thinking of the possibility of environmental factors having a role in cardiovascular pathologic processes as it is in other organ systems. It may be that the relationship is not straightforward and that cardiovascular toxicity in response to a given agent requires interaction with some other agent before it can be expressed, as in experimental vitamin E deficiency and experimental alcoholic cardiomyopathy. The direct effects that agents may have on the myocardium range from effects on electrical activity and metabolic function to cell injury and necrosis, whereas effects on the vascular system may result in secondary changes of ischemia on the myocardium.

Myofibrillar Degeneration

The myocardium responds to injury in a relatively limited number of ways. Infarction associated with thrombotic coronary occlusion is one of the more commonly rec-ognized injury patterns. Another pattern arises when cardiac injury selectively involves myocardial cells and has been induced by a variety of stimuli, including environmental and toxic agents. Primarily because of the nonvascular nature of this injury, the morphology differs from that seen in infarction. When infarction occurs, not only do the cardiac muscle cells undergo irreversible change following coronary occlusion, but irreversible injury also occurs in the more resistant stromal connective tissue cells, capillaries, small blood vessels, nerves, and so on. After a period of 18–24 hours, the area of injury can be identified by light microscopy by loss of nuclear staining of all tissue elements; also, the necrotic myocardial cells in longitudinal section will have preserved striations at diastolic sarcomere length. Subsequent host response, with polymorphonuclear leukocyte infiltration, phagocytosis by macrophages, and fibrous replacement, is well described.

In those forms of myocardial injury that do not involve obstruction of coronary blood flow, as seen with some toxic and metabolic stimuli, only the myocardial cells may be affected, and there will be continued blood flow through the capillaries adjacent to the injured cells. The injured myocardial cells are no longer able to maintain cell membrane ionic gradients, and there is an influx of calcium into the injured myocardial cells. This results in marked disruption of internal architecture of the cytoplasm with loss of striations and the appearance of dense cytoplasmic bands composed of actin-myosin filaments associated with translocation of mitochondria. Although this can be identified with hematoxylin–eosin stain, Gomori trichrome staining allows the injury to be more readily identified. In contrast to the cytologic changes in infarction, the cytoplasmic disruption of architecture in selective myocardial cell necrosis is seen within minutes of injury stimuli

The general process, sequence, and dating of events in healing and repair have been described in experimental models as well as in human myocardium (Reichenbach and Benditt, 1970). With selective myocardial cell necrosis (myofibrillar degeneration), there is very little acute inflammatory response. The primary response is one of mononuclear infiltration, with phagocytosis of necrotic debris, and ultimately collapse and condensation of the reticulum stroma with a variable (usually slight) degree of interstitial fibrosis. There is evidence from experimental models that some myocardial cells exhibiting cytoplasmic injury and disruption of architecture may be associated with synthesis of the cytoplasmic constituents and restitution of cellular architecture. Because of the observations of potential reversibility in cells showing myofibrillar disarray, the term degeneration has been applied to this injury.

The distribution of the lesions may differ from that seen with vascular injury and may be helpful in trying to understand the mechanism of injury. Myocardial cell injury in the immediate subendocardial zone suggests injury directly affecting myocardial cells rather than a vascular mechanism, in that this zone of myocardial cells receives its nutrient supply directly from the ventricular lumen. Injury scattered throughout the ventricular wall and especially near the epicardium also suggests a nonischemic or nonvascular mode of injury, and is probably due to direct injurious effects on susceptible myocardial cells.

Although the morphologic changes are not specific for a given agent, it is possible to identify those cases in which there has been selective injury to myocardial cells and to separate them from infarction. In trying to ascertain the mechanism of such injury, toxic and metabolic causes need to be considered.

Cardiomyopathy

The cardiomyopathies primarily affect cardiac muscle and are usually diagnosed by excluding other causes of cardiac disease such as ischemic heart disease, hypertension, valvular heart disease, or congenital heart disease. Pathophysiologically, they have been classified as congestive, hypertrophic, restrictive, and obliterative. In the more common form, the major clinical manifestation is congestive heart failure and has been designated as a congestive cardiomyopathy. The pathologic changes are not specific for the underlying etiology, and this is generally ascertained by the association of relevant clinical information. Pathologically, the changes include biventricular hypertrophy and dilatation, interstitial fibrosis, focal endocardial thickening, and mural thrombi. Myocardial cell necrosis is usually not a prominent feature. In many cases the cause of the cardiomyopathy is unknown. In the United States in those cases where the association has been made, alcohol is the most common cause of congestive cardiomyopathy. The development of cardiomyopathy may be the result of interaction of more than one factor. This is evident not only in the cardiomyopathy attributed to cobalt in humans, but also in alcoholic cardiomyopathy.

Rats fed alcohol (35%) for 16 weeks, associated with adequate protein intake, minerals, and so on, continue to gain weight and do not show morphologic cardiac abnormalities. Rats fed alcohol with laboratory stock diet without supplemental minerals, vitamins, and so forth, develop poor weight gain and cardiac enlargement with evidence of cardiomyopathy. Microscopically, the myocardial cells show vacuolization and fragmentation of myofilament, and biochemically there is an increase in cardiac catecholamine levels.

ANTHRACYCLINES

Daunorubicin and doxorubicin (Adriamycin) are bacterium-derived anthracycline antibiotics used as cancer chemotherapeutic agents. Although they are not associated with environmental exposure, they do provide a model of chemical agents producing congestive cardiomyopathy (Mason, 1979; Van Vleet et al., 1980). Within minutes of administration of doxorubicin, nucleolar segregation occurs in myocytes as the drug penetrates the nuclei. Doxorubicin apparently intercalates itself within the DNA, inhibiting protein and nucleic acid synthesis. The acute effects of anthracyclines include hypotension, tachycardia, and arrhythmias. The latter are thought to be related to drug-induced release of histamine and catecholamines (Balazs and Ferrans, 1978). The chronic effects include cardiac dilatation, degeneration and atrophy of cardiac muscles with interstitial edema and fibrosis, and occasional mural thrombi.

One of the earliest histologic changes is formation of cytoplasmic vacuoles due to dilatation of the sarcoplasmic reticulum. Some myocytes appear pale because of loss of myofilaments and may be nonvacuolated. Ultrastructural changes include loss of myofilament register, dilatation of the sarcoplasmic reticulum, accumulation of lipid droplets, and mitochondrial changes. These latter changes include focal loss or dilatation of the outer mitochondrial membrane and formation of concentric membranous lamella and electron-dense matrix bodies. Altered cells may be seen throughout the myocardium and may have normal-appearing cells adjacent to them. The cardiomyopathy has been induced in the rabbit, rat, pig, monkey, and beagle dog.

The distribution of lesions varies somewhat with the species and has not been as well studied in humans as in animals. In dogs, the lesions are more severe in the left ventricular free wall and septum, less frequent in the right ventricle and left atrium, and least in the right atrium. Within the left ventricle, the changes are more severe in the subendocardial area, while they are generalized throughout the right ventricle. In the rabbit, the changes are least severe in the right ventricle. In both the rabbit and the rat, the lesions tend to concentrate around intramyocardial arteries, whereas no such distribution occurs in dogs.

The development of the cardiomyopathy is related to the total cumulative dose received. In humans, clinical evidence of cardiac injury is seen with a total dose greater than 550 mg/kg/m^2. Radiation treatment to the mediastinum (600–700 rad) from 6 months to 14 years before administration of the anthracyclines will enhance the cardiac damage. Also, administration of the drug to a patient over the age of 70 increases the risk of cardiac injury at a lower dose of Adriamycin.

OTHER CHEMICAL AGENTS

There are a number of reports of exposure to a chemical followed by the development of clinical evidence of cardiac injury. In such limited numbers of cases, it is difficult to establish a cause-and-effect relationship, as opposed to a merely coincidental association or the possible role of some other undefined contributing factor. In one report, a 24-year-old white male had a 5-year history of repeated inhalation of shoe-cleaning fluid containing trichloroethylene (67%), methylene chloride (18%), dipropylene glycol (10%), and methylene ketones (5%) (Mee and Wright, 1980). This was associated with the development of progressive heart failure and low voltage on the electrocardiogram. Autopsy findings described cardiac enlargement and focal endocardial thickening, which suggests a congestive cardiomyopathy.

The temporal relationship of exposure and the development of cardiac changes in the following case suggest a more clear cause-and-effect relationship. A 27-year-old plumber was painting in an unventilated room for several hours. He initially developed headache and nausea and subsequently developed shortness of breath and paroxysmal nocturnal dyspnea and orthopnea. He had no significant past cardiac history or other toxic exposure. He developed progressive heart failure that responded to digitalis and diuretics. The electrocardiogram showed tachycardia, low voltage, and T-wave inversion. Clinical manifestations of heart failure subsided after 10 days, and the electrocardiographic changes returned to normal after 6 months. All viral and bacterial studies were normal. The methyl cellulose-type paint contained mixed isomers of amylacetate and no evidence of benzene, toluene, or xylene (Weissberg and Green, 1979).

In another case report, a worker was massively exposed to methylenedianiline (MDA), an epoxy resin hardener used in the plastics and rubber industry (Brooks et al., 1979). There were pulmonary, cutaneous, and oral routes of entry of the agent into the body. The 20-year-old worker developed electrocardiographic changes of lateral wall injury with elevation of LDH isoenzyme. The electrocardiographic changes returned to normal after 1 year.

Isolated reports, particularly in Soviet literature, have raised suspicion regarding occupational exposure to benzene derivatives, pesticides, organosilicon monomer, methyl methacrylate, and butyl isocyanate, as inhaled substances that may produce adverse cardiovascular effects.

AEROSOL PROPELLENTS

The fluoroalkane gases used to propel aerosols are toxic in experimental animals (Taylor and Drew, 1975). Within seconds to minutes after inhalation of these substances there is a sinus node slowing, and the myocardium remains sensitized to asphyxially induced arrhythmias for several hours. The half-life of these propellents is 40–90 minutes. A 10-minute exposure of dogs to varying concentrations of dichlorodifluoromethane (Freon 12) or trichloro-

monofluoromethane (Freon 11) has demonstrated the relationship between concentration and induction of fatal arrhythmia. Exposure at concentrations below 15% has never caused death. At 15% (150,000 ppm), there was only minimal sinus slowing. At 15% to 17%, 7 of 16 (44%) animals died, and at concentrations of 17.5% to 21%, 12 of 19 (63%) animals died. At concentrations above 21.5% (215,000 ppm), there were no survivors. The mode of death was suppression of spontaneous pacemaker activity, resulting in profound bradycardia and asystole. Because death occurs within such a short period following exposure to the agent, no light-microscopic changes are evident.

With ordinary use of these agents, environmental levels are far below those associated with effects on the sinus node. Peak levels in beauty salons, for example, reach 310 ppm. However, the concentrations in a plastic bag comparable to a deliberate sniffer may be 350,000–400,000 ppm, a level that was uniformly fatal in dogs (Reinhart et al., 1977).

Other compounds have been demonstrated experimentally to sensitize the heart to epinephrine-induced arrhythmias. These compounds include isobutane, propane, dimethyl ether, and vinyl chloride. In experimental animals, benzene inhalation is associated with cardiac sensitization to epinephrine-induced arrhythmias, and there have been some clinical cases reported following exposure to benzene. Heptane causes cardiac sensitization in experimental animals, but no human cases have been reported. Chloroform induces arrhythmias in experimental animals and in 1 of 3500 human cases where it has been used as an anesthetic agent. Trichloroethylene has been associated with arrhythmias in experimental animals, and several human deaths have been associated with this agent. Acute exposure of anesthetized dogs to trichloroethylene results in a dose-dependent decrease in arterial pressure, vasodilatation, decrease in myocardial function as measured by heart rate and stroke output on contractility, and the production of arrhythmias. Ventricular ectopic beats and T-wave abnormalities have been described in asymptomatic workers with industrial exposure to trichloroethylene.

CARBON MONOXIDE

The possibility of occupational carbon monoxide poisoning is widespread, because most industrial items manufactured today involve some process of heat-fire combustion or oxidation. Other important sources of carbon monoxide are cigarette smoking and pollution from automobile exhaust. The effects of carbon monoxide on cardiovascular function and development of cell injury are largely a reflection of the concentration of carbon monoxide (Zenz, 1979).

Animal Studies

Exposure of cynomolgus monkeys (Eckardt et al., 1972) essentially continuously for 104 weeks to carbon monoxide concentrations of 65 ppm resulted in carboxyhemoglobin concentrations of 6% to 8%. No cardiac lesions were observed. In acute experiments with higher levels of carbon monoxide, focal myocardial necrosis, frequently distributed in the subendocardium, and myocardial lipid accumulation especially located in the interventricular septum and outer wall of the right ventricle, have been demonstrated in dogs. The most severe changes have been seen in animals exposed for 60 minutes or more, where blood carboxyhemoglobin levels reach 40–50%. These animals also exhibited marked right ventricular dilatation. Exposure to lower levels of carbon monoxide for a 6-week period of time resulted in electrocardiographic changes after 2 weeks of exposure. Pathologic signs included dilatation of the right ventricle and evidence of small older scars and fatty degeneration, but no acute myocardial necrosis was evident. Carboxyhemoglobin levels ranged between 2.6% and 12%. Exposure to carbon monoxide resulting in carboxyhemoglobin levels of 75% or greater for an hour result in subendocardial hemorrhage

and myocardial necrosis in all animals. Animals exposed to high levels of carbon monoxide for 7 days to 3 months developed scattered foci of injury showing early organization without acute inflammatory cells and frequent foci of calcification. The lack of acute lesions in the chronically exposed animals fits with the demonstrated acclimatization that occurs with chronic exposure to carbon monoxide, primarily in the form of increased red cell mass.

Two main biologic targets of activity of carbon monoxide are the hematin in blood and within the mitochondrial cytochrome a_3. When carbon monoxide combines to hemoglobin, the hemoglobin becomes inactive in oxygen transport, and cytochrome a_3 is bound by carbon monoxide and loses its reactivity with oxygen. Both of these effects ultimately affect mitochondrial function. The importance of the binding to cytochrome a_3 and the lesser damage of binding to hemoglobin was demonstrated by Goldbaum and co-workers (1975). Three groups of dogs were compared: Group I animals were exposed to 13% carbon monoxide, and their carboxyhemoglobin levels reached 54–90%; all animals died within 15 minutes to 1 hour. Group II animals were bled and the volume was replaced by infusion of lactate to make them anemic; all animals with a hemocrit of 12% survived. Group III animals were bled to the same anemic state as the animals in Group II, but were transfused with red cells exposed to carbon monoxide to replenish the total red cell mass. These animals had a carboxyhemoglobin level of 57% to 64%. All animals survived. These experiments indicate that even high levels of carboxyhemoglobin may be tolerated if the effect of carbon monoxide binding has the same effect as the reduced carrying capacity of hemoglobin for iron, and suggests that the toxic effects may be related to binding of other hematin molecules, particularly cytochrome a_3 oxidase.

Following exposure to carbon monoxide, the equilibration with hemoglobin is not an immediate reaction. In vitro, when whole blood is shaken with 100% carbon monoxide, only 26% of the hemoglobin is converted to carboxyhemoglobin in 5 minutes, and complete saturation occurs only after 20 minutes. The dissolving of carbon monoxide in blood after leaving the lungs allows it to reach other organs and tissues to interfere with mitochondrial function. Further demonstrations of the effect of carbon monoxide on nonhemoglobin components of myocardial function have demonstrated a decrease in cardiac function in an isolated perfused rabbit heart system using Krebs-Ringer and no hemoglobin. In control animals, the perfusate was equilibrated with 48% oxygen, 48% nitrogen, and 4% carbon dioxide. In the study animals, the perfusate was equilibrated with 48% oxygen, 50% carbon monoxide, and 2% carbon dioxide. During 90 minutes of perfusion, the left ventricular pressure and dP/dT were measured. There was a greater decline in function and in ATP levels with carbon monoxide than with nitrogen.

Human Disease

There is an association between carbon monoxide levels in the air and the fatality rate from acute myocardial infarction (Cohen et al., 1969). In an epidemiologic study of 35 hospitals in the Los Angeles area, the case fatality rate in patients admitted with acute myocardial infarction was higher in the high-pollution areas of Los Angeles County and was evident in those areas only during periods of relatively increased carbon monoxide pollution. Because oxygen extraction in the myocardium is greater than in any of the other organs, carboxyhemoglobin levels of 9% result in a decrease in the venous P_{O_2} in the coronary sinus. The normal individual adapts by increasing coronary blood flow. In patients with obstructive coronary disease this compensatory mechanism is limited, and the coronary sinus P_{O_2} level may reach almost zero; in addition, rather than lactate being extracted, lactate is produced. Carbon monoxide exposure in patients with obstructive coronary disease will result in impaired exercise performance with carboxyhemoglobin levels as low as 1.6%. Carbon monoxide in-

halation in angina patients is associated with a decrease in stroke index and an increase in left ventricular and diastolic pressure. In monkeys with experimentally induced acute myocardial infarction, carbon monoxide hemoglobin levels of 9% significantly lower the threshold for inducing ventricular fibrillation.

LEAD

Clinically, a form of cardiomyopathy has been observed in "moonshine" drinkers and attributed to lead. Myocardial alterations can be produced by administration of lead to experimental animals (Asokan, 1974; Khan et al., 1977; Shaper, 1979). Rats fed 1% lead acetate for 6 weeks showed ultrastructural changes with myofibrillar fragmentation and separation of myofilaments, dilatation of the sarcoplasmic reticulum, and swelling of the mitochondria. There were no changes in myocardial electrolytes (potassium, sodium, calcium, and magnesium) and there was no measurable myocardial lead. The significance of the changes is unclear, and this model apparently does not mimic the clinical form of cardiomyopathy in which there is alteration of electrolytes with decreased magnesium and potassium, and increased calcium and sodium. Mice fed lead acetate in distilled water for 2 weeks and sacrificed 7 days later showed microscopic changes that were related to blood lead levels. Blood lead levels below 20 μg/100 ml were associated with normal light- and electron-microscopic appearance. With blood lead levels above 20 μg/100 ml, there was peripheral condensation of the nuclear chromatin, some disorganization of the nucleolus with loss of reticular architecture, and loss of a distinct nucleolonema. With blood lead levels greater than 40 μg/100 ml, the mitochondria show enlargement and distortion of the crista with some vacuolization. The sarcoplasmic reticulum is mildly to moderately dilated. Blood lead levels greater than 60 μg/100 ml are associated with widening of the intercalated disk, some disruption of myofibrils with focal lysis, and cytoplasmic lipid vacuoles. No clear-cut cell necrosis, however, is described. The lead is primarily bound to mitochondria and lysosomes. The nuclear and nucleolar changes are thought to be related to disturbances of RNA metabolism. Other myocardial electrolytes were not measured, and it is unclear whether this model produced an alteration in cardiac function.

Administration of lead in chick embryos has been demonstrated to be associated with the development of congenital cardiac anomalies. These primarily involve the development of aortic stenosis, aortic valve malformation, and pulmonary valve malformations, and in a smaller number of cases, a thin dilated left ventricular wall.

Lead also alters the myocardial responsiveness to norepinephrine. Rats received lead via mother's milk from birth to weaning; after a 4-month, lead-free period when there were no overt signs of lead intoxication, the response to catecholamines was tested. Administration of norepinephrine resulted in more ventricular premature contractions than in controls.

COBALT

In the 1960s, several episodes of severe heart failure with death occurred in beer drinkers of several cities (Shaper, 1979). Cobalt, which had been added to beer after manufacture to maintain the head on tap beer that was dissipated by residual detergent on glasses, was suspected. It was discovered that the cobalt concentration in cardiac muscle of these individuals was 10 times higher than that of non-beer drinkers. It appears that the cardiotoxic effect is not straightforward and requires some other factors to develop. The concentration of 1 to 5 ppm used in the brewing process is quite low and would require considerable quantities of beer (25 pints/day) to supply about 8 mg of cobalt; this amount is less than that given for refractory anemias due to renal failure and is without evidence of cardiotoxic effect. As much as 30 mg of cobalt per day have been used therapeutically without evidence of cardiotoxic effect. It is suspected that a combination of cobalt plus myocardial injury related to chronic alcohol ingestion and/or nutritional deficiency are necessary for the toxic effects to become manifest. Ultrastructurally, the myocardial cells show increase in cytoplasmic glycogen, some fragmentation and degeneration of myofibers, and enlargement of mitochondria, which are also increased in number. Cobalt is present in mitochondria in experimental animals. Administration of cobalt (26 mg/kg for 8 weeks) to experimental animals results in myofibrillar degeneration, myocytolysis, and lipid droplet accumulation within myocardial cells. Cobalt plus ethanol does not increase the severity of the changes, but if the animals are maintained on beer for 36 days before administering cobalt, the cardiotoxic effects appear to be enhanced. The primary energy source of the myocardium is long-chain fatty acids, but in their absence, pyruvate becomes preferred substrate. Cobalt competes with magnesium and calcium ions in enzymatic functions and therefore interferes with the breakdown of metabolites in the Krebs cycle in the metabolism of pyruvate and fatty acids (Barborik and Dusek, 1972).

MERCURY

Both organic and inorganic mercury compounds have been demonstrated to have an effect on cardiac function. In male rhesus monkeys given methyl mercury daily for 6 months, mercury levels were 0.5 μg/g of blood in one group and 1–2 μg/g of blood in the other group. Both groups exhibited similar changes in the myocardium, but they were more striking with the higher level of mercury. The changes were scattered myocardial cells showing myofibrillar degeneration (Mottet, 1974).

The effect of methyl mercury on the isolated spontaneously beating rat heart and left atrial papillary muscle preparations showed that the frequency of contraction and development of tension increased with a low dose of methyl mercury hydroxide (0.5 ppm), reaching a maximum of 2 ppm and subsequently declining (Su and Chen, 1979).

High concentrations were depressive from the beginning. The stimulatory effect was not blocked by propranolol and therefore not related to catecholamine release. Ultrastructurally, the myocardial cells showed swelling of mitochondria with disruption of the cristae and dilatation of the sarcoplasmic reticulum and cytoplasmic band formation typical of myofibrillar degeneration. The depressant effects of methyl mercury on isolated cardiac tissue appear to be closely related to changes in membrane structure and myofibrillar organization. Because mercurials are sulfhydryl inhibitors, the depression due to methyl mercury may be a result of inhibition of sodium potassium ATPase, calcium magnesium ATPase, and calcium transport in the sarcoplasmic reticulum or inhibition of enzymes in oxidated metabolism in the mitochondrium.

OTHER TRACE METALS

Focal myocardial fibrosis has been demonstrated in experimental rats with feeding of niobium, zirconium, cadmium, and antimony (Schroeder, 1974). Selenium–vitamin E deficiency in experimental animals produces myofibrillar degeneration and an increased mortality. Selenium–vitamin E deficiency in ducklings can be induced by feeding them tellurium or silver, and it shows similar kinds of myocardial injury (Van Vleet and Ferrans, 1977). In addition to the cardiac changes, the ducklings showed degeneration in skeletal muscle as well as in smooth muscle in the gizzard and intestinal tract. There is experimental evidence indicating that selenium–vitamin E deficiency may be induced or enhanced by administration of silver, copper, zinc, tri-*ortho*-cresyl phosphate, or polychlorinated biphenyls (Van Vleet, 1977). Dietary silver induces selenium deficiency in rats, chicks, turkeys, and pigs. Protection against the lesions induced by silver can be thwarted by administration of vitamin E but not by administration of selenium. Tellurium-induced myocardial injury is prevented by administration of either selenium or vitamin E.

Selenium–vitamin E functions to protect cellular membranes from damage by lipid peroxidation. Vitamin E acts as an oxidant to minimize lipoperoxidation, and selenium is an integral part of the enzyme glutathione peroxidase, which destroys formed peroxides. Animals deficient in vitamin E or a combination of selenium and vitamin E show lability of membranes, especially mitochondria and endoplasmic reticulum, but also of plasma membrane with resulting cell necrosis. Such membrane lability may play a role in the induction of cardiac arrhythmias and may be a mechanism of myocardial irritability associated with the development of ventricular fibrillation and sudden death.

Because of the general availability of vitamin E in nature associated with lipids as an oxidant, deficient levels of selenium and vitamin E are generally somewhat difficult to attain in the absence of a very unusual diet, and deficiency probably rarely occurs in humans. However, demonstration that a state of selenium–vitamin E deficiency can be induced by administration of a variety of other agents needs further investigation and identification of other possible agents. The mechanisms by which these agents impair the selenium–vitamin E membrane protection system could be such that they act as peroxidants, resulting in excessive production of lipoperoxides, and increase the need for selenium–vitamin E to maintain cell membrane protection. Another more likely mechanism is that these compounds interfere with the metabolism of selenium and thus render it biologically unavailable. This is supported by the fact that rats fed silver or tri-*ortho*-cresyl phosphate show decreased hepatic glutathione peroxidase activity, but normal to increased hepatic selenium content.

Atherosclerosis

Atherosclerotic heart disease, which has reached epidemic proportions during the latter half of the twentieth century in technically developed countries of the world, is the major cause of cardiovascular mortality in the United States and is caused by obstructive atherosclerosis in the coronary arteries. Epidemiologic studies show an increased risk of development of coronary artery disease with a number of factors, some of which are environmentally related such as diet and cigarette smoking.

There are markedly differing death rates from cardiovascular disease throughout the world, ranging from a high in Finland (996 per 100,000 population) to a low in Japan (94.8 per 100,000 population). During the same year (1977), the rate was 715 per 100,000 population in the United States. Within the United States there are real geographic differences in cardiovascular death rate with a twofold increase from low death rate to high-incidence areas. The high cardiovascular death rate areas are near the East Coast and in the Great Lakes area. The low cardiovascular death rate areas are in the Plains and Middle South. The variation between countries as well as within the United States is thought due to environmental influences, although the specifics are not clear.

It is not clear what accounts for the current high rate of atherosclerotic heart disease. Is this merely a reflection of increased numbers of individuals living to an age at which atherosclerosis becomes a significant problem, or has there been a real change in the frequency of the disease that might allow one to speculate about a potential environmental role in its development? No collection of specimens exists to allow objective evaluation of the appearance and extent of atherosclerosis over the past century, so indirect evidence relating to clinical appearance and clinical manifestations of the disease will have to suffice. The data suggest that atherosclerosis has progressed from an uncommon disease to a frequently occurring one, and that change has occurred within the last 60–70 years (Michaels, 1966).

Heberden provided the first clinical description of angina pectoris in 1768; it was remarkably complete, and by 1782 he had encountered 100 cases. By 1800, angina pectoris was known to be related to coronary artery disease. During the 150 years following its first description, angina pectoris appears to have been an exceedingly uncommon, almost a rare process. Medical textbooks written during that time regarded angina pectoris as a rare or uncommon entity. William Osler had an interest in angina pectoris and in 1897 published a report of 60 cases. In 1910 he described his experiences with an additional 208 cases. It is of interest that in his observations, he stated that in 10 years not a single case of angina pectoris occurred in Montreal General Hospital. On the average, only one case per year of angina pectoris was seen on the wards of large general hospitals, and an active consultant might see 10–15 cases per year. He made no mention of acute myocardial infarction. The clinical manifestations of acute myocardial infarction and coronary thrombosis were described in 1912 by Herrick.

Another indication that the disease has changed markedly during this century is seen in the ratio of male to female death rates due to heart disease. In 1900 in the United States, England, and Wales, the ratio was approximately 1:1. By the mid-1920s, the ratio had begun to change because of an increase in male deaths. Similar changes occurred in Canada in the mid-1920s in the 45–64 age group. This change in ratio occurred only with heart disease deaths and was not seen in other cardiovascular or renal deaths (Anderson, 1973).

An examination of the prevalence of coronary disease from a historical perspective suggests that angina pectoris was a well-recognized and well-described entity from the late 1700s; however, it was regarded as a rare or uncommon event, and the clinical manifestations of myocardial infarction were not described until the early nineteenth century. In the mid-1920s, an increase in the male death rate due to heart disease began in several countries at about the same time and continued into the 1960s. These data strongly suggest the possibility that some environmental factor or factors may be operating to have caused the dramatic change in the frequency of what was once considered an uncommon disease.

Although the average life span is now

longer than it was in the 1800s, there were still significant numbers of individuals who lived to be 50 years of age and older, who would provide a significant reservoir of individuals at risk for coronary disease if it were prominent. Population data recorded from England and Wales indicate that in 1850, a time when angina pectoris was a rare disease and myocardial infarction was unrecognized, there were 1.204 million males who were 50 years and older, certainly a significant population at risk for disease. By 1900 this number was over 2.2 million.

Evaluation of Risk Factors to Account for These Changes

An increase in tobacco consumption in the eighteenth and nineteenth centuries and a change in smoking habits appear to account for only a small part of the increase in the male death rate due to heart disease. Tobacco consumption is not well correlated with male:female death rate ratios in a number of countries; however, there was a twofold difference in tobacco consumption between Canada and the United States and England at a time when the mortality rates in all countries were increasing similarly. The per capita consumption of meat, sugar, and butter fat did not change significantly during this time, and although the per capita consumption of meat and sugar both increased (in the United Kingdom) from 1880 to 1920, there were no similar changes in consumption that can be correlated with the appearance of a high cardiac death sex ratio. Although there was considerable poverty in England in the 1800s, a significant portion of the population ate well and had a diet that was as plentiful in animal fat, including butter, milk, and eggs, as are the diets of today. Per capita consumption of animal fats in the United Kingdom appears to have changed relatively little since the 1800s to the 1960s.

The historical observations as well as the epidemiologic data from male:female death rate ratios provide tantalizing data suggesting that atherosclerosis of the magnitude that we currently are experiencing in Western technologic societies is a result of a real change that occurred in this century, perhaps between 1910 and 1925. This strongly suggests that some environmental factor or factors were introduced into the environment in these technologically developed societies.

Atherosclerosis is a complex process and involves the interaction of a number of factors. These include blood and cellular components, hemodynamic factors, and arterial wall factors, which may therefore help to explain why there is no simple correlation between the apparent change in the disease and any changes in risk factors.

Epidemiologic data have demonstrated that there is an association with the development of atherosclerosis and accelerated development in the presence of risk factors. However, the absence of any of the known risk factors does not necessarily confirm immunity from the process, and many individuals have significant and fatal atherosclerotic heart disease without any of the known risk factors. An elevated serum cholesterol is associated with an increased risk of development of atherosclerosis and with acceleration of the process; however, the majority of individuals who have had fatal myocardial infarction have had normal serum cholesterol (Goldstein et al., 1973).

A possible mode of action of environmental agent(s) in the development of atherosclerosis is suggested with the demonstration that the smooth muscle cells in the plaque are monoclonal or monotypic. This observation, initially demonstrated by Benditt and Benditt (1973) and subsequently confirmed by others, used the technique that previously had demonstrated that smooth muscle cells in leiomyoma were monoclonal and were interpreted as being the progeny of a single transformed cell. Approximately one-third of black females are heterozygous for glucose 6-phosphate dehydrogenase enzyme, and their cells exhibit mixtures of types A and B enzymes in tissue extracts. Because of random inactivation of the X chromosome in female cells early in embryonic life, tissues contain a mixture of the two cell types, each having one or the other of the X chromosome pair active. Smooth muscle cells in the fibrous cap of the atherosclerotic plaque demonstrate either type A or type B. This is consistent with a monoclonal origin of the cells and is interpreted as being the progeny of a single transformed cell. The media demonstrate a mixture of type A and type B isoenzyme. The fatty streak demonstrates a polyclonal pattern.

This observation also suggests a mechanism by which some of the risk factors may be operable. Those things that increase cell proliferation in the arterial wall increase the potential risk of cell transformation from whatever the agent, be it chemical or viral. Hypercholesterolemia and hypertension increase the rate of proliferation of cells. Chemical mutagens such as benzpyrene have been demonstrated to be carried in the β lipoproteins; thus, the importance of cholesterol in relation to atherosclerosis may not be in the absolute level of cholesterol but rather in what is being carried in the cholesterol fraction.

Increased mortality from coronary artery disease has been documented by epidemiologic studies with the specific occupational inhalant exposure of viscose rayon workers exposed to carbon disulfide in a 10-year follow-up of 343 workers exposed for 5 years to carbon disulfide (Tolonen et al., 1979). When this group was compared with an age-matched, nonexposed group of males, there was found to be an excess of coronary deaths in the exposed individuals. Age, hypertension, and exposure to carbon disulfide were risk factors on multivariate analysis. The estimated risk of death from coronary heart disease for a 30-year span was 31.9% for those exposed to carbon disulfide and 13.3% for those not so exposed. No studies indicate any specific or different manifestation pathologically for these individuals that could be attributed to carbon disulfide.

An increased mortality is also demonstrated in workers exposed to glycerol nitric esters while engaged in explosives man-

ufacturing. Deaths in these workers characteristically have occurred following a few days off the job. The risk appears to be the greatest following cessation of exposure, and it is suggested that the mechanism may be related to the vasodilator effect of the exposure on coronary vessels, with possible rebound vasospasm following withdrawal.

Lathyrism

Lathyrism can occur in both humans and animals and results from eating quantities of certain kinds of peas. Human cases have been reported in many parts of the world in which people turn to pea diets during times of famine. An upper motor neuron spastic type of paraplegia has been described in human cases. Experimental lathyrism in the rat results in dissecting aneurysm and may be produced by feeding the animal sweet peas (*Lathyrus odoratus* seeds) or diets containing β-aminopropionitrile. In addition to the dissecting aneurysm, bony deformity (limbs and vertebrae) and hindlimb paresis are also produced. The toxic factor in the flowering sweet pea that induces this change is β-(n-λ-glutamyl)aminopropionitrile. It has been found that a simpler compound, β-aminopropionitrile, will also produce lathyrism. Experimental animals show aortic histologic changes at 2 to 4 weeks, consisting of an increase in ground substance that stains metachromatically, and degeneration and disorientation of smooth muscle cells of the media. At 8 to 18 weeks there is loss of elastic lamella in the aortic media. The following have been demonstrated to be lathyrogenic agents in experimental animals: sweet pea seeds, β-aminopropionitrile (BAPN), propylamine, γ-aminobutyronitrile sulfate, aminoacetamide hydrochloride, α-(glutamyl)aminobutyronitrile, aminodipropionitrile aminoacetonitrile sulfate, glutamyl aminoacetonitrile, β-mercaptoethylamine hydrochloride, semicarbazide, ethanolamine, and sodium propionate. β-Sodium nitrile inhibits lysine oxidase and blocks cross-linkage of collagen and elastic fibers, thus impairing their tensile strength.

REFERENCES

Anderson, T. W. 1973. Nutritional muscular dystrophy and human myocardial infarction. *Lancet* 2:298–302.

Asokan, S. K. 1974. Experimental lead cardiomyopathy: Myocardial structural changes in rats given small amounts of lead. *J. Lab. Clin. Med.* 84:20–25.

Balazs, T., and Ferrans, V. J. 1978. Cardiac lesions induced by chemicals. *Environ. Health Perspect.* 26:181–191.

Barborik, M., and Dusek, J. 1972. Cardiomyopathy accompanying industrial cobalt exposure. *Br. Heart J.* 34:113–116.

Benditt, E. P., and Benditt, J. M. 1973. Evidence for a monoclonal origin of human atherosclerotic plaques. *Proc. Natl. Acad. Sci. (U.S.A.)* 70:1753–1756.

Brooks, L. J., Neale, J. M., and Pieroni, D. R. 1979. Acute myocardiopathy following tripathway exposure to methylenedianiline. *J.A.M.A.* 242:1527–1528.

Cohen, S. I., Deane, M., and Goldsmith, J. R. 1969. Carbon monoxide and survival from myocardial infarction. *Arch. Environ. Med.* 19:510–517.

Eckardt, R. E., MacFarland, H. N., Alarie, Y. C. E., and Busey, W. M. 1972. The biologic effect from long term exposure of primates to carbon monoxide. *Arch. Environ. Health* 25:381–387.

Goldbaum, L. R., Ramirez, R. G., and Absalon, K. B. 1975. What is the mechanism of carbon monoxide toxicity? *Aviat. Space Environ. Med.* 46:1289–1291.

Goldstein, J. L., Hazzard, W. R., Schrott, H. G., Bierman, E. L., and Motulsky, A. G. 1973. Hyperlipidemia in coronary heart disease. 1. Lipid levels in 500 survivors of myocardial infarction. *J. Clin. Invest.* 52:1543–1553.

Khan, M. Y., Buse, M., and Louria, D. B. 1977. Lead cardiomyopathy in mice. *Lab. Med.* 101:89–94.

Mason, J. W. 1979. Anthrycycline cardiotoxicity: Recognition, management and avoidance. *Compr. Ther.* 5:64.

Mee, A. S., and Wright, P. L. 1980. Congestive (dilated) cardiomyopathy in association with solvent abuse. *J. R. Soc. Med.* 73:671–672.

Michaels, L. 1966. Etiology of coronary artery disease: An historical approach. *Br. Heart J.* 28:258–264.

Mottet, N. K. 1974. Some subtle lesions of methyl mercury intoxication. *Lab. Invest.* 30:384–385.

Reichenbach, D. D., and Benditt, E. P. 1970. Catecholamines and cardiomyopathy. The pathogenesis and potential importance of myofibrillar degeneration. *Hum. Pathol.* 1:125–150.

Reinhart, C. E., Azar, A., Maxfield, M., Smith, P. E., Jr., and Mullin, L. S. 1977. Cardiac arrhythmias and aerosol "sniffing." *Arch. Environ. Health* 22:265–279.

Schroeder, H. A. 1974. The role of trace elements in cardiovascular disease. *Med. Clin. North Am.* 58:381.

Shaper, A. G. 1979. Cardiovascular disease and trace metals. *Proc. R. Soc. Lond.* 205:135–143.

Su, J. Y., and Chen, W. 1979. The effects of methyl mercury on isolated cardiac tissues. *Am. J. Pathol.* 95:753–761.

Taylor, G. J., and Drew, R. T. 1975. Cardiovascular effects of acute and chronic inhalation of fluorocarbon 12 in rabbits. *J. Pharmacol. Exp. Ther.* 192:129–135.

Tolonen, M., Nurminen, M., and Hemberg, S. 1979. Ten year coronary mortality of workers exposed to carbon disulfide. *Scand. J. Work Environ. Health* 5:109–114.

Van Vleet, J. F. 1977. Protection by various nutritional supplements against lesions of Selenium-Vitamin E deficiency induced in duckling by Tellurium or silver. *Am. J. Vet. Res.* 38:1393–1398.

Van Vleet, J. F., and Ferrans, V. J. 1977. Ultrastructural alterations in skeletal muscle of ducklings fed Selenium-Vitamin E deficient diets. *Am. J. Vet. Res.* 38:1399–1405.

Van Vleet, J. F., Ferrans, V. J., and Weirich, W. E. 1980. Cardiac disease induced by chronic adriamycin administration in dogs and evaluation of vitamin E and selenium as cardiac protectants. *Am. J. Pathol.* 99:13–42.

Weissberg, P. L., and Green, I. D. 1979. Methylcellulose paint possibly causing heart failure. *Br. Med. J.* 2:1113–1114.

Zenz, C. 1979. The epidemiology of carbon monoxide in cardiovascular disease in industrial environments: A review. *Prev. Med.* 8:279–288.

14

Nervous System Injury

Cheng-Mei Shaw and Ellsworth C. Alvord, Jr.

The nervous system is the one organ that is designed to monitor, pass on information to other parts of the body, and store information about its environment, leading the organism in responding and adjusting to changes in the environment. The perpetually changing interaction between an organism and its environment is a part of life itself.

Industry and technology have rapidly changed our environment and our life-style. The advantages of progress have been well recognized and serve as incentives for further advancement. However, the negative aspects of modern industry have yet to be accurately assessed. At certain times society tends to overreact to the deleterious effects of certain agents or industrial by-products, and at other times the chronic cumulative harmful effects of some agents are ignored or even intentionally or politically suppressed. The former occurs especially in affluent industrial states, whereas the latter tends to be found in less affluent, developing third-world countries.

It is not within the scope of this chapter to review all the experimental data available on neurotoxicology. The discussion here will be limited to the known human neuropathology caused by toxic agents and to closely related experimental data.

THE PROBLEM OF SELECTIVE VULNERABILITY

The nervous system is not a single organ but is composed of dozens, perhaps hundreds, of different structural and functional units that are interconnected to form a complicated supercomputer. The nervous system not only controls voluntary somatic and involuntary visceral functions of different parts of the body through its many segmental components but also governs the mental and physical activities of the whole organism through the integrated activities of its suprasegmental components.

The major problem for neuropathology is to define the precise localization and type of reaction and to correlate their abnormalities with the clinical observations. Thus, neuropathology is strongly based on clinical neurology, neuroanatomy, and neurohistology, as well as on general pathology.

Lesions in the nervous system produced by toxic agents are as a rule degenerative in nature; that is, they are regressive cellular changes usually without inflammation in those parts of the nervous system showing functional loss. While they are not so selective as many other types of neurologic diseases, *they rarely affect the whole nervous system indiscriminately.* Diffuse involvement of the nervous system may occur with a high dose of a toxic substance, or at the end stage of the disease process when the primary lesions may be mixed with various secondary changes. Many known toxic agents have a tendency to affect more than one anatomic site depending on the dose, but with a relatively low dose a certain cellular structure is apt to be involved by a particular agent at an early stage.

A specific affinity between a toxic agent and a certain cellular element at a certain location is an expression of the combined effects of several factors: (1) the toxicologic action of the agent, (2) the metabolic characteristics of the cellular element, and (3) the anatomic and physiologic properties peculiar to the site affected.

Studies of these phenomena are important, since they can be used as diagnostic criteria to isolate the cause of the disease, and they also can eventually expand our knowledge in understanding the mechanism of intoxication, thereby leading to successful treatment and prevention.

THE BLOOD–BRAIN BARRIER (BBB)

Capillaries in the central nervous system (CNS) are structurally different from those in other organs in that they have no intercellular pores or fenestrae between endothelial cells to allow passage of small molecules in plasma solutes. Endothelial cells in the CNS are sealed by tight junctions. In addition, pinocytosis in CNS capillary endothelial cells is virtually absent. The passage of plasma solutes into the CNS is very selective and independent of molecular size. It is transcellular and is mediated via either lipids or proteins. Lipid-soluble materials pass through the endothelial cell membrane readily and rapidly. Some lipid-insoluble materials, such as glucose and amino acids, pass through endothelial cells with the aid of specific carrier proteins that are present within the endothelial cells. The endothelial cells are wrapped by a sheet of basement membrane externally. In turn, astrocytic feet surround the basement membrane wrap-

ping capillaries. Cellular processes of oligodendroglia may also extend to the perivascular space, but neuronal processes do so only in a few very special sites such as the neurohypophysis and area postrema. Neurons and their processes are separated and presumably protected from circulating plasma solutes by the tight junctions of the capillary endothelium and by the glial processes. This selective impermeability of the cerebral vasculature is known as the blood–brain barrier (BBB). Similar structural characteristics are less well defined in the peripheral nervous system (PNS), but there is a blood–nerve barrier.

Many toxic agents are prevented from entering into the CNS parenchyma by the BBB. These agents may damage the PNS, since there is a different barrier in the PNS. Lipid-soluble materials, however, usually pass easily through the BBB to enter the CNS. Some toxic agents injure the vascular endothelial cells to break the BBB and then gain access into the CNS. In this case, the CNS lesion is actually a secondary effect.

Once a toxic agent enters into the CNS parenchyma, it may show an affinity for a particular type of cell or a particular type of cell organelle, thus causing a selective injury, or it may injure any cellular element indiscriminately, thus causing a widespread injury. Observations accumulate slowly from relatively small numbers of known poisonings in human beings and considerably more rapidly from animal experiments. Animal experiments are designed to clarify some of these complications but are themselves subject to many difficulties in interpretation, since species-specific susceptibilities and variations frequently occur. Thus, the results obtained in experimental animals are often difficult to translate into human situations.

The selective damage within the nervous system by certain toxic agents can usually only be observed within a certain dose range, which also depends on the mode of intake of the agent. The tendency of selective damage is lost when acute intoxication with a large dose occurs. Damage to other organs than the nervous system can also take place with acute high-dose intoxication resulting in secondary CNS damage due to cardiac arrest, respiratory arrest, hepatic failure, renal failure, or combinations of these. The separation of these pathogenetic processes is extremely difficult. The specific diagnosis of acute intoxication in these cases is ascertained only by toxicologic assay, and morphologic studies are often only ancillary.

At the other end of the spectrum, there is another type of intoxication that probably includes the majority of clinical cases, in which a low-dose exposure of toxic agents takes place causing no clinical symptoms or only vague generalized symptoms or transient neurologic symptoms, leaving no or very subtle, nonspecific morphologic changes in the nervous system.

FUNCTIONAL LOSS WITHOUT SPECIFIC STRUCTURAL CHANGES

Drug Effect

Drugs used for therapeutic purposes, especially those that are classified as tranquilizers, narcotics, hypnotics, sedatives, and anesthetics, are intended to modify consciousness, behavior, and perception to pain by affecting the CNS. With optimal doses the intended therapeutic purposes are achieved; the functional loss of the nervous system is only transient and reversible, leaving no specific structural changes in the nervous system. In a strict sense, the effect of these drugs can be categorized as a type of intoxication, but in practice they are not so regarded except in cases of lethal or sublethal overdose and drug dependency (addiction).

The drug overdose—whether accidental or the result of intended suicide—of CNS stimulants, depressants, and neuropsychotropic drugs induces hallucination, stupor, delirium, and coma, which may be followed by death. A possible idiosyncratic reaction directly attributable to the drug may occur, but this is rare. The majority of patients develop respiratory depression because of brain stem failure. As a result, hypoxia complicates the clinical course and

pathologic outcome. Depending on the duration of survival, cerebral edema, venous congestion, petechial hemorrhages, cortical necrosis, and leukoencephalopathy may be found in the brains of these patients. These neuropathologic lesions are, however, secondary manifestations and should not be mistaken as direct effects of drugs.

Drug Dependency (Drug Addiction)

Opium addiction is typical of the group of drug dependency disorders that also includes involvement with cocaine, barbiturates, and many newly discovered hallucinogenic agents and CNS stimulants. In most societies habitual use of these agents is illegal, and many addicts use more than one agent, so that the true clinical, epidemiologic, and pathologic data are difficult to obtain.

The general consensus at present is that there are no neuropathologic changes characteristic of drug dependency, at least at the light-histologic level.

Drug addicts may die of an overdose as well as of other neurologic complications, including septic cerebral emboli secondary to bacterial endocarditis, phycomycosis, hypoxic encephalopathy, nutritional deficiency such as subacute combined degeneration of the spinal cord (Pentchew, 1958), and polyneuropathy, hepatic encephalopathy secondary to infectious hepatitis, and necrotizing arteritis (L. S. Adelman and Aronson, 1969; Roizin et al., 1972).

NONSPECIFIC AND SECONDARY STRUCTURAL CHANGES

Many toxic agents have depressive effects on respiratory and cardiovascular centers resulting in cerebral anoxia (hypoxidosis) and cerebral ischemia, which may induce irreversible changes in the CNS. Some agents damage capillary walls and induce changes in vascular permeability, which may cause cerebral edema. Other agents tend to injure the liver or kidney primarily and more severely than the CNS, and the neurologic effects may be complications of hepatic coma or uremia. Thus, many CNS lesions are not specific for the toxic agent.

Cerebral Edema (CE)

INTRODUCTION, CLASSIFICATION, AND PATHOGENESIS

Brain edema and brain swelling were once considered to be different conditions, one with an increase in the water content, and the other with an increase also in proteins and electrolytes. The two terms and their differences are of historical interest only.

Cerebral edema is extremely common. It may be associated with practically any acute or prolonged CNS damage, including trauma, tumor, infection, vascular disease, radiation effects, and metabolic disease, as well as intoxications by many different types of agents. It can produce a spectrum of changes:

1. It can subside, leaving very little trace of functional or structural damage.

2. It can persist with the primary pathologic process, such as tumor or hematoma, for a long period.

3. It can induce irreversible structural damage to the tissue, especially the cerebral white matter, leaving foci of degeneration, necrosis, or liquefaction.

Recent electron-microscopic, physiologic, and neurochemical techniques have shown that it is possible to quantitate the degree of edema and to distinguish pathogenetically different types of experimental edema, but these techniques are too complicated to be performed routinely in diagnostic human neuropathology. Because of inevitable postmortem artifacts in the human, light-microscopic studies of cerebral edema are usually equivocal, frequently not dramatic, and sometimes difficult to correlate with or to confirm the gross impression of cerebral edema. Even though cerebral edema has been recognized for centuries and its clinical and pathologic importance has been well known, the pathogenesis of cere-

bral edema has only recently been worked out.

There are three types of cerebral edema: vasogenic, cytotoxic, and interstitial or hydrocephalic (Klatzo, 1967; Klatzo and Seitelberger, 1967; Fishman, 1975).

Vasogenic Edema

Characterized by an increased permeability of the BBB, the vasogenic form of cerebral edema is the commonest and affects the cerebral white matter especially. The functional and structural integrity of capillary endothelial cells is altered. The extracellular fluid, including proteins, is increased. Radiation, cerebral contusion, hemorrhage, infarct, tumor, abscess, leptomeningitis, and lead encephalopathy are known to produce this type of cerebral edema.

Cytotoxic Edema

Cytotoxic edema is known to occur in cerebral hypoxia secondary to cardiac arrest and acute water intoxication. The BBB is not affected, so that there is no leakage of proteins. The cellular elements, including neurons, glia, and vascular endothelial cells, swell, and the extracellular fluid space concomitantly decreases. Both gray and white matter may be involved. Intoxication by triethyltin classically affects the white matter, and hypoxia the gray matter.

Interstitial (Hydrocephalic) Edema

Interstitial edema is seen in obstructive hydrocephalus, when an increase of water and sodium occurs within the periventricular cerebral white matter as a result of the absorption of ventricular fluid through the ependymal wall. The BBB is intact, and there is no protein leakage. The volume of the periventricular white matter is actually reduced despite the increase in the extracellular fluid volume.

CEREBRAL EDEMA IN INTOXICATION

It is probably not too much of an exaggeration to say that practically all cases of acute fatal intoxication show at least some degree of cerebral edema regardless of the type of causative toxic agent, even though the cause of death cannot be shown to be the cerebral edema. Surviving patients also commonly exhibit clinical manifestations that strongly suggest the presence of cerebral edema during the acute stage of an intoxication. The pathogenetic and pathophysiologic mechanisms of cerebral edema may vary considerably with different types of toxic agents, but the results seem to be quite similar and consistent.

The major problem is whether the cerebral edema is induced primarily by a toxic agent or is a secondary phenomenon due to cardiorespiratory, hepatic, or renal complications. Unfortunately, no clear distinction can be made in the majority of cases, since cerebral edema is so nonspecific, can be either primary or secondary, and can either be a result or serve as a cause within a vicious cycle commonly seen in these patients. The most probable answer is that it is a combination of both in most human patients.

Acute ethanol intoxication, acute methanol intoxication, acute carbon monoxide (CO) poisoning, ethylene glycol poisoning, drug overdoses due to various types of narcotics, sedatives, and tranquilizers, and acute intoxications from such heavy metals as lead, mercury, bismuth, tin, and arsenic are just a few well-known examples of intoxications inducing cerebral edema.

Lead, arsenic, triethyltin, methanol, and carbon monoxide poisoning effects are the best examples of a relatively pure, primary cerebral edema.

CLINICAL MANIFESTATIONS OF CEREBRAL EDEMA

Cerebral edema can be either focal or generalized. Focal edema usually surrounds focal pathologic processes, such as tumor, hemorrhage, infarct, or abscess, and it increases the focal neurologic deficit. In cases of intoxication, cerebral edema is usually generalized, so that its clinical symptoms are nonlocalizing and are identical with those of increased intracranial pressure (or intra-cranial hypertension): headache, vomiting, papilledema, and alterations of consciousness ranging from lethargy to deep coma.

In acute intracranial hypertension, the arterial blood pressure rises, the pulse rate slows, and slow, deep, stertorous respirations develop. A lumbar spinal puncture is usually contraindicated, but ventricular puncture is safe and shows the cerebrospinal fluid (CSF) pressure to be elevated (above 200 mm H_2O in the horizontal position).

In the advanced stage of generalized cerebral edema with transtentorial, cerebellar tonsillar, and/or axial herniation, the patient becomes deeply comatose, with decerebrate rigidity of the extremities as well as loss of pupillary, corneal, and vestibular reflexes due to the rostral brain stem compression. Cheyne-Stokes respiration, a fall in arterial blood pressure, an increase in pulse rate, and apnea may follow because of compression of the medulla oblongata.

In acute cerebral edema, plain skull X-ray films are usually unremarkable. In chronic increased intracranial pressure, however, decalcification of the sella turcica in adults and separation of the cranial sutures in children may be found.

The old techniques of pneumoencephalography and ventriculography show small ventricles (except in interstitial edema) and obliteration of the cerebral sulci. Computerized tomography (CT) is probably the best in vivo diagnostic tool currently available, in demonstrating compressed small ventricles and obliterated cerebral sulci and basal cisterns, as well as decreased density of the cerebral white matter in generalized cerebral edema. Herniations and displacement of the diencephalon, medial temporal lobes, and cerebellar tonsils can also be clearly visualized when they are present. Arteriography reveals very little displacement in vascular structures, except for transtentorial and tonsillar herniations, but transcerebral blood circulation is markedly slowed. Brain scans with radioactive isotopes show diffuse leakage of isotopes in cerebral white matter in vasogenic edema, no leaks in cytotoxic edema, and leaks in the periventricular region in interstitial edema.

GROSS PATHOLOGIC APPEARANCE OF GENERALIZED CEREBRAL EDEMA AND SECONDARY HERNIATIONS

The gross appearance of generalized cerebral edema depends on the extent and severity of the edema itself. A focal cerebral edema is much easier to detect because of the presence of an unaffected area serving as a built-in control in a given individual. In cases of diffuse edema in which no control area is available in a given brain, one has to compare the particular case with other unaffected brains. These comparisons are quite subjective depending on the experience of the observer. Mild diffuse edema can easily go unnoticed, especially when a considerable degree of cerebral atrophy was present before the development of a diffuse cerebral edema. The assessment of cerebral edema, even up to moderate or marked degrees, can be quite unreliable because of the absence of knowledge of the pre-existing state of cerebral atrophy.

The diffusely edematous brain is revealed externally by flattening of the normally rounded gyri and obliteration of the subarachnoid spaces in the sulci and basal cisterns. On sections of the brain the cerebral ventricles are reduced in size and sometimes completely obliterated. The bulk of the cerebral white matter is usually increased more than is the gray matter. In marked diffuse cerebral edema, the following secondary structural displacements can be found to confirm the gross diagnosis of diffuse cerebral edema: axial herniation, transtentorial herniation, and cerebellar tonsillar herniation.

Axial Herniation

Symmetrically increased bulk of tissue in the supratentorial cavity displaces the diencephalon and mesencephalon down through the tentorial notch into the subtentorial chamber. In the vasogenic type, the edema occurs selectively in the white matter. Since the largest bulk of the white matter is in the cerebrum, the degree of swelling between the supratentorial and subtentorial structures is disproportionate, with the increase of mass much greater in the supratentorial chamber.

The best way to evaluate axial herniation is to make a coronal section of the cerebrum at the level of the red nuclei. Normally, the red nucleus is situated above (dorsal to) the most dorsal limit of the hippocampus, as defined by drawing a line connecting the dorsal aspects of the hippocampus on both sides. The downward displacement of the red nucleus completely or partially below this line is an indication of axial herniation. The rest of the mesencephalon is similarly displaced caudally, the space constituting the cisterna ambiens is obliterated, and the medial tips of the temporal lobes are closely approximated against the sides of the midbrain.

Transtentorial Herniation

Unilateral transtentorial herniation accompanied by asymmetric mesencephalic deformity, and hemorrhagic necrosis of the msencephalic and rostral pontine tegmentum and Kernohan's notch in the contralateral cerebral peduncle is commonly seen in unilateral supratentorial masses with focal edema and is not a complication of generalized cerebral edema. Instead, bilateral symmetric transtentorial herniation of the uncus and variable amounts of the parahippocampal gyrus may accompany axial herniation. The extent of transtentorial herniation depends on individual variations in the size and shape of the tentorial notch. Transtentorial herniation and axial herniation in generalized edema are usually not so pronounced as those in focal edema associated with brain tumor or hematoma, since concomitant swelling of the subtentorial structures prevents a severe degree of displacement.

Cerebellar Tonsillar Herniation

In some cases the cerebellum may swell selectively or more severely than the cerebrum, but in most cases cerebellar and cerebral edema go together. Cerebellar tonsillar herniation is not always pathologic (De la Pava and Pickren, 1962) and can be either an expression of anatomic variation in the shape and size of the foramen magnum or a postmortem change. Downward herniation of the cerebellar tonsils into the foramen magnum and cervical spinal canal with compression of the medulla oblongata is a serious complication of increased intracranial pressure with diffuse edema or other mass lesions. One should keep in mind that cerebellar tonsillar herniation occurs in 18% of normal brains examined at autopsy (De la Pava and Pickren, 1962), and that increased intracranial pressure can be present without producing cerebellar tonsillar herniation. The significance is not in the degree of cerebellar tonsillar herniation per se but in the medullary compression that often occurs with cerebellar tonsillar herniation and that may cause death.

The medulla oblongata shows no significant morphologic changes in patients who die suddenly or shortly after cerebellar herniation, since time is needed for such changes to develop.

When patients survive longer by themselves or are kept alive by respirators, morphologic changes may be present, such as swelling, necrosis, petechial hemorrhages in the medulla, petechial hemorrhages, or hemorrhagic necrosis of cerebellar folia indented by the ridge of the foramen magnum. Autolysis and liquefaction followed by the disappearance of herniated cerebellar tonsils and displacement of autolyzed cerebellar tissue into the spinal subarachnoid space may be seen in patients who have been kept on a respirator for several days.

Microscopic Findings in Cerebral Edema

Controversy, skepticism, and disagreement have crowded the literature concerning the specificity and validity of light-histologic findings of cerebral edema, characterized by vacuolation of brain tissue and dilatation of perivascular and pericellular spaces. The reason for the controversy is that these changes are also common postmortem artifacts of paraffin-embedding of blocks from autopsied brains. The degree of spongy appearance in the brain tissue depends on the rate of postmortem autolytic changes, the interval between the time of death and the time of autopsy, the rate of fixation, and the rate of dehydration of the tissue at the time of preparation. As far as cerebral edema is concerned, a definitive interpretation of sections from paraffin blocks of "respirator brains" is almost impossible. Indeed, even in better prepared cases the differential diagnosis between vasogenic edema affecting the white matter and cytotoxic edema affecting both gray and white matter can often not be made by light-histologic techniques alone. One must remember that the classification of vasogenic, cytotoxic, and interstitial types of cerebral edema depends on electron-microscopic findings, on brain scans demonstrating various degrees of vascular permeability and diffusion of tracer materials into the periventricular white matter, and on chemical analysis of extracellular fluid. These techniques are not routinely performed on human autopsy material. Besides, human autopsied material usually shows such severe postmortem artifacts, especially rupture of cell membranes, that it is almost impossible to elucidate whether the fluid is extracellular or intracellular unless protein-rich fluid can be seen as evidence of breakdown of the BBB.

Despite these difficulties, and with some skepticism, the following findings are generally accepted as evidence of cerebral edema:

1. The white matter is much more vulnerable to edema formation, but the corpus callosum, internal capsule, subcortical arcuate or U fibers, and optic radiations frequently escape cerebral edema.

2. Edematous white matter appears loose, pale, and spongy, with pallor of myelin staining, swollen splaying of myelin sheaths, and diffusion of PAS-positive fluid into the parenchyma (Greenfield, 1939).

3. In acute edema, venous and capillary congestion with occasional extravasation of red blood cells, mild perivascular infiltration of lymphocytes, and swollen and vacuolated endothelium may be seen.

4. Oligodendroglia are markedly swollen.

5. Astrocytes may also show acute swelling and clasmatodendrosis.

6. The gray matter is usually spared in vasogenic edema, but may show mild grades of similar changes as seen in the white matter, especially in cases of acute necrosis, when perineuronal vacuolation with shrunken neurons may be quite marked.

7. In cytotoxic edema, the vascular permeability is usually preserved, so that PAS-positive fluid is not seen in the parenchyma, but the capillary endothelium is swollen and the capillary lumen obliterated rather than congested and distended as in vasogenic edema.

ELECTRON-MICROSCOPIC FINDINGS OF CEREBRAL EDEMA

Research on cerebral edema by electron microscopy (EM) was extremely active in the 1950s and 1960s. The EM findings of cerebral edema have been summarized by Hirano (1969).

In the cerebral white matter the fluid accumulation is in the extracellular space, although there is still some disagreement as to whether these spaces represent the enlargement of pre-existing extracellular spaces or pseudoextracellular spaces created by the rupture of swollen astrocytic processes. The capillary endothelium shows increased pinocytosis.

In the cerebral gray matter the effect of edema is milder and is represented by the expansion of glial cells and processes. A peculiar form of cerebral edema was produced by triethyltin, in which accumulation of fluid was found to be between myelin lamellae as well as within astrocytes and neurons (Aleu et al., 1963).

POSTEDEMATOUS LEUKOENCEPHALOPATHY

Edema may last for as long as the cause of the edema exists. The condition may worsen with the growth or extension of the lesion and with additional complications of hypoxia or ischemia. The condition may improve when the cause of edema is no longer present. The leaked fluid may be absorbed, the extracellular spaces may close, and the swelling cellular processes may subside. If the edema is mild, separation and tearing of white matter are minimal, and the lesion may heal with practically no trace or may leave only diffuse, mild, nonspecific gliosis in the cerebral white matter.

However, irreversible damage such as necrosis may remain in the white matter if the edema is severe. Various degrees of demyelination, degeneration, and gliosis can be found between the above extremes in the brain with subsiding of the edema. The subcortical arcuate fibers are usually spared, since they are compressed, not stretched by the deeper edema.

When white matter degeneration is present in the brains of hypertensive patients in which thickened and hyalinized small blood vessels are also present, the neuropathologic findings are essentially those of "Binswanger's encephalopathy" (Feigin and Popoff, 1963).

QUANTITATIVE DETERMINATION OF CEREBRAL EDEMA

Cerebral edema can be documented by macroscopic, light-microscopic, and electron-microscopic examinations of biopsied and autopsied specimens. The brain weight alone cannot be used as an indicator of cerebral edema, since there is such a wide range of normal variation (1300 ± 300 g). It is essentially irrelevant to compare the brain weight of an individual with the average brain weight of the general population even of the same age and sex.

Relative Morphometry

Obtaining the ratio of the weight of the brain stem and cerebellum to the weight of the whole brain may be useful in some cases. The weight of the brain stem and cerebellum is normally 0.15 × (whole brain weight − 200 g) (Dennis et al., 1961; Shaw, 1978). In vasogenic edema, the white matter is selectively swollen and, since the cerebral hemispheres have the greatest proportion of white matter, the whole-brain weight is disproportionately increased for the weight of brain stem and cerebellum. This deviation of the ratio can occur in numerous conditions, such as tumor or hemorrhage in the cerebrum or atrophy of the cerebellum, so that a rough estimate by this formula can only be used to supplement examination of the gross brain. This estimate is best done before fixation, since the postmortem water-binding capacity of edematous brain tissue and nonedematous brain tissue is different.

Ratio of Skull Capacity to Brain Volume

The oldest technique to determine the presence and degree of cerebral edema was to compute the ratio of the capacity of the skull to the volume and weight of the brain. Reichardt (1919) considered that cerebral edema was present when the gap was less than 8%. Alexander and Looney (1938) found that the normal differential ratio of skull capacity to brain volume ranged from 4% to 9%. They suggested that any ratio below 4% indicated edema and above 9% indicated atrophy. The drawback of this method was its awkwardness in measuring the skull capacity, which might result in errors, but Davis and Wright (1977) have developed simple methods of measuring intracranial volume with a balloon filled with water. Future advances in the technology of CT scan may make this measurement possible in the living subject.

Determination of Water Content

The most obviously straightforward method of determining the extent of CE, but inherently the most difficult to interpret, is to measure the water content of tissue samples. Stewart-Wallace, as early as 1939, used tissue samples of 1 to 10 g, cut and weighed as soon as possible, and put in dry heat at 110° C for 18 hours to attain a constant dry weight. The average water content of the normal cerebral cortex was 84.3% (Stewart-Wallace, 1939) or 84–86% (Alexander

and Looney, 1938), and of the normal centrum semiovale 70.7% (Stewart-Wallace, 1939) or 67–72% (Alexander and Looney, 1938), but considerable variation was noted in different areas of the white matter (e.g., 75.7% in the corpus callosum). In focal edema, one can offset this shortcoming by comparing the water content of the same area in the opposite cerebral hemisphere. In cases of cerebral edema associated with cerebral tumor or hemorrhage, Stewart-Wallace found a significant increase of water content in edematous white matter of up to 86% without significant increase of water content in the gray matter. Such comparisons are impossible in generalized edema, where Alexander and Looney (1938) found no correlation between water content in either white or gray matter in either edema or atrophy.

Specific Gravity

Measurements by Alexander and Looney showed the specific gravity of brain tissue to range from 1.030 to 1.070, with most edematous brain tissue being below 1.040. S. R. Nelson, Mantz, and Maxwell (1971) have developed a technique using a liquid gradient system of organic solvents to measure the tissue's specific gravity, which is determined by the depth to which the tissue sample sinks in the gradient column, but from a practical point of view it must be difficult to maintain the gradient with repeated use. The simplest way would be to use a graduated cylinder with water to determine the volume, and a good balance to determine the weight. Specific gravity is equal to the weight divided by volume. Such nondestructive measurements of fresh tissue, if rapidly performed to prevent overhydration of the tissue, then permit fixation and microscopic examination. If exposure to water is objectionable, one could use a cylinder filled with fixative, since the measurement of differences in height of the liquid can be made so rapidly that there would be no change in volume or damage to the tissue.

Radioiodinated Serum Albumin and Computerized Tomography

Clinically, intravenously injected radioiodinated serum albumin (RISA) uptake can be demonstrated by scintigraphic techniques to show abnormalities in permeability of the BBB and its localization. Computerized tomography (CT) with enhancement is even better and is widely used in the diagnosis of cerebral edema as well as of other pathologic processes in the brain of a living subject. Brain tissue has an absorption coefficient 3% more than water. An increase of water content in the brain tissue results in a decreased density that can be visualized and calibrated.

Vital staining techniques such as trypan blue (Klatzo, 1967), Evans' blue (Clasen, Cooke, Pandolfi, et al., 1962) or sodium fluorescein (Manz, 1974) have been commonly used in experimental animals to demonstrate BBB permeability in cerebral edema at the gross level. For electron microscopy, horseradish peroxidase is the most commonly used tracer.

INTOXICATIONS PREDOMINANTLY CHARACTERIZED BY DIFFUSE CEREBRAL EDEMA

Lead (Plumbism)

Susceptibility to lead intoxication and the clinical and pathologic manifestations of plumbism differ in adults and children. Adults tend to develop chronic lead poisoning characterized by peripheral neuropathy and dementia with or without convulsions, whereas children tend to develop acute signs of increased intracranial pressure (pseudotumor cerebri or lead encephalitis), which takes a short and rapid clinical course. Both show gastrointestinal tract disorders, including anorexia, constipation, abdominal colic, and vomiting, with or without microcytic hypochromic anemia, for weeks or months preceding the appearance of nervous system symptoms.

Numerous clinical reports on lead poisoning in children as well as in adults were made in the first half of this century. The sources of lead, mostly in inorganic form, were painted furniture, painted toys, nipple shields, drinking water from lead pipes or tanks, and fumes from burning battery casings. In Japan, lead-containing face powder of nursing mothers was said to be a common source. The incidence of lead poisoning was highest in infants and small children between 1 and 3 years of age, in whom teeth are erupting and in whom there is a great tendency to put anything into the mouth (McKhann and Vogt, 1933). Perversions of appetite, known as pica, were frequently observed in retarded or neurotic children, as well as in children with anemia or intestinal parasitosis, and have been considered to be a predisposing factor for lead poisoning (Mancleff et al., 1964). Lead is readily absorbed from the gastrointestinal tract and lungs, and occasionally through the skin.

Public education and legislation have almost completely removed lead from the household environment, so that these sources of acute plumbism in children are rare today.

Airborne lead is produced by automobile emissions and is probably the major source of lead in the environment today, but even this is decreasing as lead-free gasoline is replacing gasoline containing tetraethyl lead. Some industrial processes, such as smelting and coal combustion, still persist, and burning lead-containing car batteries as fuel is still practiced in poverty-stricken communities (Harris, 1976).

The onset of encephalopathy in children is evidenced by a change in mental state, persistent vomiting, clumsiness, and ataxia. Delirium, stupor, coma, seizures, and respiratory arrest may follow. Papilledema, meningismus, slow pulse, and elevated blood pressure are often found. X-ray films of the skull frequently show separation of the cranial sutures. A lead line in the metaphysis of long bones may be found by X-ray examination, but this is uncommon in young children. Laboratory tests showing blood lead levels greater than 60 μg/100 ml, urinary excretion of lead in amounts over 80 μg/24 hours (Byers, 1959), erythrocyte protoporphyrin greater than 50 μg/100 ml, basophilic stippling of erythrocytes, leukocytosis, and increases of pressure, and globulin and cells in the CSF are diagnostic criteria for lead encephalopathy.

Death occurs within a few days if victims go untreated. If treated with chelating agents the patient may survive, but permanent mental and neurologic sequelae, including seizures and mental retardation, may persist (Berg and Zapella, 1964; Perlstein and Attala, 1966).

In the general autopsy, intranuclear eosinophilic inclusion bodies are frequently found in epithelial cells of the proximal tubules of the kidney and in hepatic cells in acute lead intoxication (Blackman, 1936). In chronic stages these inclusion bodies are uncommon, but liver cirrhosis may be present.

In the CNS, acute lead encephalopathy in children is manifest essentially as cerebral edema with increase in water content (J. F. Smith et al., 1960). It was observed by Tanquerel des Planches in 1839 (cited by Wells et al., 1976) and has been repeatedly observed since. Detailed descriptions of the gross and microscopic changes have been reported by Blackman (1937) and Hassin (1921) in the 1920s to 1930s, and more recently by Popoff et al. (1963), Pentchew (1965), and J. F. Smith et al. (1960). The brains of patients who died during the acute stage are diffusely and markedly swollen, with flattening of the cerebral gyri and obliteration of the sulci, and with various degrees of transtentorial, axial, and cerebellar tonsillar herniations. On cut sections increased volume of the cerebral and cerebellar white matter is noted with compression of the ventricles. In some cases yellowish discoloration, decreased consistency, and even minute hemorrhages may be noted. Characteristic microscopic findings include (1) dilatation and distention of the perivascular spaces with PAS-positive exudate, (2) separation of nerve fibers by interstitial fluid and myelin breakdown in the white matter, (3) vascular changes, such as endothelial swelling, endothelial proliferation, capillary obliteration, capillary hypertrophy, petechial hemorrhages, and adventitial fibrosis, and (4) ischemic necrosis of neurons. These changes are found in the brains of patients who die following a short clinical course.

Amorphous eosinophilic and basophilic droplets in the perivascular spaces have been repeatedly observed since the first description by Blackman in 1937. Clasen, Hartman, Coogan, et al., (1974) found these droplets to be cytoplasmic inclusions of perivascular astrocytes and considered this finding to be quite pathognomonic for lead encephalopathy.

The morphologic findings in the brains of patients who survive for weeks or months, or of patients who manifest chronic lead encephalopathy, are somewhat different. Depending on whether the lead exposure was repeated, the brains of these patients may show changes of old necrosis and atrophy mixed with acute cerebral edema or simply long-standing leukoencephalopathy. Marked mesodermal reactions can be found, including proliferation of vascular walls, endothelial proliferation, adventitial fibrosis, and calcium deposits in the media, as well as astrocytic proliferation. Chronic demyelination and degeneration of the white matter, representing the late stages of edematous leukoencephalopathy, may mimic some of the diffuse sclerosis sometimes known as Schilder's disease (Verhaart, 1941).

Despite innumerable attempts, the production of lead encephalopathy in experimental animals failed repeatedly until 1966, when Pentchew and Garro produced multiple spotty hemorrhages in the cerebellum and serous transudates in the white matter in suckling rats, the nursing dams being fed lead carbonate. From 85% to 90% of the suckling rats developed clinical and pathologic lead encephalomyelopathy by 23 to 29 days after birth, and died within 2 weeks. Abnormal capillary permeability in the cerebral white matter, the rostral half of the striatum, the occipital lobe, and the thoracolumbosacral cord was demonstrated by intravenous injection of trypan blue.

This experiment has been confirmed and reproduced by many other investigators in young rats (J. A. Thomas Dallenbach, and Thomas, 1973; Press, 1977), chick embryos (Hirano and Kochen, 1973), hatched chicks (J. S. Nelson, Dahlgren, and Fischer, 1975) and juvenile rhesus monkeys (Clasen et al., 1974).

Pentchew and Garro (1966) concluded that the primary effect of lead was on the capillaries, with increased permeability. They termed this condition "dysoric encephalopathy" and considered it to be not specific for lead encephalopathy but typical of many other conditions, including Wernicke's encephalopathy in humans.

Subsequent investigators (Hirano and Kochen, 1973; J. A. Thomas et al., 1973; Clasen et al., 1974; J. S. Nelson et al., 1975; Press, 1977) have agreed that the primary site of lead poisoning is in the capillaries, and lead deposits have actually been found in endothelial cells. Changes in perivascular astrocytes and brain edema are secondary effects of the increased permeability of the capillaries. Press (1977) concluded that the primary target of lead is the endothelial bud (or angioblast) in growing capillaries in the CNS. This certainly correlates with the phenomenon of selective susceptibility of human infants and young experimental animals to lead encephalopathy.

Tin

Metallic tin has long been used for food containers, tin plating, soldering alloys, and collapsible tubes, all very common around the household. Tin in powder form or as tin oxide had been used as a medicine for parasitic infestations and furunculosis, and had been found to be relatively nontoxic, at least non-neurotoxic. In contrast, organic compounds of tin are extremely neurotoxic. Among various alkyltin compounds, triethyltin and diethyltin are the most toxic when given intraperitoneally to rats. When taken orally, triethyltin is 10 times more toxic than diethyltin (Magee et al., 1957).

Organic tin neurotoxicity in humans is rare. Only a few sporadic case reports have been recorded, chiefly as occupational hazards involving chemists working with organic tin compounds (Fortemps et al., 1978). Organic tin is absorbed through the gastrointestinal tract and respiratory epithelium. Two patients with organic tin poisoning reported by Fortemps et al. (1978) were exposed to a mixture of dimethyltin and trimethyltin.

An epidemic of organic tin poisoning involving 290 patients occurred in France in 1953–1954 and has been summarized by Foncin and Gruner (1979). The source of intoxication was found to be a preparation known under the trade name "Stalinon," which was intended to treat furunculosis and which contained diethyltin diiodide according to the labels, but was suspected to contain variable amounts of triethyltin (Foncin and Gruner, 1979).

The clinical symptoms are nonspecific, but intense headache is a constant initial symptom, followed by varying degrees of mental symptoms, such as confusion, disorientation, loss of memory, and alterations of consciousness, including lethargy, drowsiness, and terminal coma. During the epidemic in France (Foncin and Gruner, 1979), convulsions occurred in about 10% of the patients, papilledema in about 30%, flaccid paraplegia with sensory loss indicative of spinal cord involvement in about 15%. In over 30% of the cases death occurred 4–10 days after the acute onset. The cause of death in most cases was brain stem compression, secondary to intracranial hypertension. About one third of the patients recovered completely, but others survived with permanent sequelae, such as paraplegia, blindness, hemianopsia, sixth cranial nerve palsy, and various types of psychic symptoms and intellectual impairments.

The only autopsy reports on human organic tin encephalomyelopathy concern 10 fatal cases during the French epidemic (Foncin and Gruner, 1979), in whom the diagnosis of triethyltin poisoning was established retrospectively. The brain showed extensive and diffuse edema of the cerebral white matter, most marked in the centrum semiovale, with the subcortical fibers less involved. Gross and light-microscopic findings of cerebral white matter edema were not specifically different from those of cerebral edema due to other causes. The gray matter and blood vessels showed no primary lesions. The spinal cord in one case showed irreversible necrosis.

Although human cases of tin poisoning are uncommon, the experimental data on tin neurotoxicity are numerous. In the late nineteenth and early twentieth centuries, the possible toxicity of tin was extensively studied because of the development and popularization of food preservation in tin cans. Interest in tin toxicity subsided when it was concluded that metallic tin was not toxic and that tin cans were safe, although organic tin compounds were recognized to be toxic. Interest was renewed in the 1950s when fungicidal properties of certain organic tin compounds were suggested and when alkyltin compounds were being increasingly used in the plastics industry. The earlier reports of the neurotoxicity of alkyltin compounds, especially of triethyltin (TET), were reconfirmed (Stoner et al., 1955; Magee et al., 1957). Detailed neuropathologic and biochemical reports by Magee et al. (1957) on experimental brain edema produced by TET were followed by a wave of experimental studies using TET encephalopathy as an experimental model of brain edema. Triethyltin and diethyltin compounds were found to be the most toxic, the target site being almost exclusively in the CNS (Stoner et al., 1955; Magee et al., 1957). The interstitial edema of the cerebral white matter and the spinal cord was reversible. Electron-microscopic studies showed that the fluid accumulation was not in the extracellular spaces, as in the vasogenic edema seen in lead encephalopathy, but was intracellular and confined to the myelin sheaths, which showed splitting and vacuolization of myelin lamellae. The intramyelin vacuoles occurred in the region of the interperiod line. The accumulated fluid resembled a protein-poor plasma ultrafiltrate, as would be expected in extracellular fluid, but the extracellular spaces were not dilated and the BBB was intact (Aleu et al., 1963; Lee and Bakay, 1965).

The pathogenesis of triethyltin neurotoxicity, more specifically its myelotoxicity, is still elusive. The ultrastructural findings of TET edema in experimental animals appears to be almost specific and completely different from most of the known types of edema. Kolkman and Ule (1967) observed morphologic similarities between disseminated spongy degeneration of the white matter in funicular myelopathy, maple syrup disease, and hyperglycinemia in human children, and TET edema in experimental animals at light-histologic levels, and suggested that similar ultrastructural findings may be found in these human conditions.

In contrast to the marked edema discussed above for TET, A. W. Brown et al. (1979) showed that trimethyltin (TMT) did not produce edema in the rat brain but rather neuronal degeneration in the hippocampus, pyriform cortex, amygdaloid nucleus, and neocortex. These neurons showed selective chromatolysis, clumping of nuclear chromatin, fragmentation of nuclear material, and eosinophilic cytoplasm. Although these changes resemble ischemic changes of neurons, the authors thought that they were different because they showed a slower time course of development.

Alcohol

Acute alcoholic intoxication is a widespread phenomenon throughout the world. A mild-to-moderate acute intoxication with hyperactivity, hypomaniac symptoms, incoherence, dysarthria, ataxia, lethargy, and even stupor are frequently considered socially acceptable unless these symptoms cause injuries to oneself or to others.

The lethal amount of ingested alcohol is extremely variable because of enormous differences in individual tolerance. However, it is usually considered that a blood alcohol level and a brain alcohol level in excess of 0.5% is lethal.

The brains of patients who die of acute alcohol intoxication show no specific pathologic alteration, but diffuse edema and some congestion or petechiae are usually present. Microscopically, alterations are neither specific nor characteristic. Acute swelling with central chromatolysis or condensed and shrunken cytoplasm of nerve cells, acute swelling of oligodendroglia, engorged capillaries, and dilatation of perivascular spaces have been described. Increase in size of the cytoplasm, which contains vacuoles, and small droplets in epithelial cells of the ependyma and choroid plexus have been described by Courville (1955).

Acutely fatal alcohol intoxication is relatively rare with ethyl alcohol but is quite common with methyl alcohol, which is much more toxic. The brains of patients who die of acute methanol intoxication show variable degrees of cerebral edema with meningeal and subarachnoid petechial hemorrhages (Keeney and Mellinkoff, 1951). In addition, methanol affects ganglion cells in the retina and produces blindness, but this deficit may not be apparent in patients who die early of acute methanol intoxication.

One should be careful before ascribing the immediate cause of death to alcohol until all other possible causes such as pneumonia, trauma, hypothermia, aspiration, and suffocation are ruled out, and the blood and brain assays show a lethal concentration of alcohol.

Experimentally, by injecting various concentrations of alcohol into the internal carotid arteries of rabbits, Lee (1955) demonstrated increased permeability of the BBB due to endothelial cell damage. The damage was greater in the gray matter with lower doses, but became diffuse with increased doses.

Arsenic

Although the incidence was relatively low, acute arsenic poisoning occurred as arsphenamine encephalopathy, one of the major complications of the treatment for syphilis during the decades preceding penicillin. The condition was also known as hemorrhagic encephalitis, brain purpura, precapillary encephalorrhagia, toxic myelopathy, or serous apoplexy, and was considered to be a relatively well-defined clinical and pathologic entity. With the introduction of penicillin, arsphenamine was

no longer used for the treatment of syphilis, and acute or subacute arsphenamine encephalopathy has disappeared. Arsenic intoxication still occurs today, but the sources of arsenic are usually insecticides, industrial accidents, and contaminated drinking water, wine, bread, and beer. The doses are usually much lower, and the clinical neurologic manifestations are usually in the form of a peripheral neuropathy.

Because of such a drastic change in incidence, acute hemorrhagic encephalopathy (brain purpura) has even been considered to be unique to arsphenamine (Salvarsan) and not seen in intoxication by other arsenic compounds (Pentchew, 1958). Other investigators (Ecker and Kernochan, 1941) see no qualitative difference in the pathogenetic mechanism between arsphenamine poisoning and other arsenical intoxications.

Thirteen cases reported by Ecker and Kernohan (1941) did not receive arsphenamine and did not have syphilis. Four of them were known to have ingested large amounts of inorganic arsenic, but the remainder were not suspected to have arsenic poisoning clinically, although appreciable amounts of arsenic were found in the brain (more than 0.1 mg/100 g tissue). The gross and microscopic findings in these brains were not different from those of acute or subacute arsphenamine encephalopathy.

Unlike arsphenamine intoxication, accidental or sporadic arsenical encephalopathy in its acute form is not only rare because the doses of arsenic are lower and the intakes slower through the gastrointestinal tract or skin. It is also difficult to identify, because the source is not suspected and the causal relationship is not so clear as arsphenamine encephalopathy. Thus, most of our knowledge concerning acute arsenical encephalopathy has been obtained through studies of arsphenamine encephalopathy.

The incidence of arsphenamine reaction was 1 in 63,000 injections according to Stokes (1934), and 1 in 28,768 injections with 1 death for every 5398 patients according to Glaser et al. (1935). The incidence was higher in patients receiving injections twice a week than in those receiving injections once a week, in those who had malaria during or before the treatments, in those who were malnourished (Krainer et al., 1947), and in women who were pregnant (R.B. Nelson, MacGibbon, and Glyn-Hughes, 1943).

Clinical signs and symptoms of headache, irritability, and confusion most frequently appeared about 48 hours after the second or third injection in the first course of injections of Salvarsan. Nausea, vomiting, convulsions, and hyperpyrexia followed or were accompanied by progressive stupor that led into coma, and 54–75% of patients succumbed within 3 to 5 days after the onset of symptoms. Mental and neurologic sequelae persisted in patients who recovered.

At autopsy, the brains showed varying degrees of cerebral edema, numerous petechiae and perivascular effusions (mostly of ring type), swelling of endothelial cells, capillary thrombosis, focal necrosis, and demyelination preferentially in the white matter, especially of the corpus callosum, internal capsule, and centrum semiovale. Petechiae and ring hemorrhages were also frequently observed in the long tracts of the cerebral peduncle, basis pontis, and medulla.

For those who had emphasized the hemorrhagic nature of the lesions, the terms hemorrhagic encephalitis, brain purpura, or precapillary encephalorrhagia seem justified. The term serous apoplexy was used by those who were impressed with flooding with edema fluid (Milian, 1928). Nonhemorrhagic lesions with necrosis and softening have been recorded by Schmorl (1913) and Busse and Merian (1912), and demyelinating lesions were discussed by Russell (1937).

Many theories were suggested, including direct toxic effects on blood vessels, secondary toxic effects on blood vessels, central vasoparalysis, allergy, and thrombocytopenia, but the pathogenesis of arsenical encephalopathy remains elusive. Regardless of its pathogenesis, the lesions seem to be initiated by vascular damage, which leads to injury of the BBB and to edema of the white matter. Subsequent degeneration of capillary endothelium leads to the formation of thrombi, perivascular diapedesis, demyelination, necrosis, and gliosis. Varying degrees of severity of vascular damage appear to determine the different manifestations of perivascular hemorrhage, demyelination, and necrosis.

Reye's and Reye's-like Syndrome

A clinicopathologic condition known as Reye's syndrome has attracted a great deal of attention from both clinical and research investigators ever since the publication of Reye, Morgan, and Baral in 1963 concerning a group of children, most of whom died after becoming comatose following a mild infection. The children ranged in age from 5 months to 8½ years and were first seen because of an acute onset of persistent vomiting several days after prodromal symptoms of an upper respiratory infection, varicella, or otitis media. Deterioration of consciousness progressed from lethargy to coma with or without convulsions, decortication, and decerebration. Of the 21 patients, 17 died. At autopsy there were two common features, namely acute cerebral edema and fatty degeneration of viscera, including liver, kidney, and heart. The authors considered this syndrome to be a distinct clinicopathologic entity.

Many investigations have centered around epidemiologic, biochemical, electron-microscopic, toxicologic, virologic, and clinical aspects, and some animal experiments have also been reported. For more details, readers are referred to the following reviews and proceedings of symposia: *Symposium on Reye's Syndrome,* Columbus, Ohio, 1974 (Pollack, 1975); Delvito and Keating (Advances in Pediatrics, vol. 22, 1975); Pediatric Clinics of North America, vol. 28, No. 2; and *First International Conference on Reye's Syndrome,* Halifax, Nova Scotia, Canada, 1978 (Crocker, 1979).

The acute symptoms and signs of cerebral edema in children and adolescents consist of recurrent or persistent vomiting and progressive alteration in the level of consciousness occurring several days after a specific or nonspecific viral illness, and are associated with abnormal laboratory findings indicating liver dysfunction.

The presence of cerebral edema can be shown by a tight, or bulging anterior fontanelle, papilledema, headache, intractable vomiting, and signs of axial, transtentorial, or cerebellar tonsillar herniation. CT scans, ventricular (or more dangerously, lumbar) punctures, intracranial monitoring devices, and autopsy studies confirm these clinical signs. Cerebral edema due to focal space-occupying masses, encephalitis, meningitis, or acute obstructive hydrocephalus can usually easily be ruled out.

The preceding viral illnesses vary. They may be specific diseases, such as chicken pox (varicella), herpes zoster, herpes simplex, rubeola, rubella, polio, vaccinia, adenovirus, Epstein-Barr virus, reovirus, influenza A and B, parainfluenza, coxsackie A and B, or ECHO virus; or they may be nonspecific and poorly defined illnesses, flulike respiratory syndromes (sore throat, bronchitis, rhinorrhea), or gastrointestinal symptoms (diarrhea).

Pertinent abnormal laboratory findings include hypoglycemia, elevated serum transaminase (SGOT, SGPT), hyperammonemia, prolongation of prothrombin time, and elevated blood urea nitrogen (BUN).

Characteristic findings in the liver are microvesicular lipid droplets within the cytoplasm of periportal hepatocytes with very little necrosis or inflammation. Electron-microscopic abnormalities in the liver have been considered to be unique by some investigators who regard liver biopsies to be diagnostic of Reye's syndrome: mitochondrial injuries including matrix disorganization and swelling with outer membrane rupture. In addition, lipid droplets, glycogen depletion, and increase of peroxisomes may be noted.

A case of Reye's syndrome is defined by the U.S. Center for Disease Control (CDC) as one with an acute onset of a noninflammatory encephalopathy with (1) microvesicular fatty metamorphosis of the liver diagnosed by biopsy or autopsy or (2) a threefold or greater rise in SGOT, SGPT, or serum ammonia. If CSF is obtained, it must have no more than 8 leukocytes/mm^3.

The brain characteristically shows diffuse cerebral edema with or without evidence of transtentorial or axial herniation at autopsy. Light-histologic findings are not specific. Ultrastructural changes in the brains of three patients in the acute stage of Reye's syndrome, as described by Partin et al. (1975), include neuronal mitochondrial injuries, swelling of astrocytic cytoplasm and processes with partial glycogen depletion, and myelin bleb formation resembling triethyltin intoxication.

Similar conditions had been reported in the literature before the 1963 report of Reye et al. "Acute meningoencephalitis of childhood" (Brain et al., 1929) resembles Reye's syndrome in all aspects except for the ring hemorrhages in the brain that can be found in cerebral edema with arsenic and lead intoxication. Some cases of "pseudotumor cerebri," postinfectious or parainfectious encephalomyelitis, acute toxic encephalitis in childhood (Grinker and Stone, 1928), toxic encephalopathy (Eiben, 1967), would be classified as Reye's syndrome today if lipid degeneration of the viscera had been recorded or if liver dysfunction had been demonstrated by appropriate laboratory tests, most of which were not available in the earlier studies or were not reported in the later studies. Barr et al. (1968) reviewed the autopsy files of Ottawa Civic Hospital from 1952 to 1967 and were able to find six cases that fit the definition of Reye's syndrome.

Epidemiologic studies have confirmed the important association between viral infections and Reye's syndrome, but viruses are rarely isolated from these patients. The incidence of Reye's syndrome appeared to be correlated with epidemics of influenza B (Reynolds et al., 1972; Corey et al., 1976), but sporadic cases are most commonly associated with chicken pox (Turel et al., 1975).

An endemic condition, widely known as "Ekiri syndrome," has occurred in Japan and shows similarities both clinically and pathologically to Reye's syndrome. It was implicated with bacillary dysentery but is rarely seen today.

Many toxins have also been nominated as possible agents causing Reye's syndrome. An unusually high incidence of Reye's syndrome during the rainy season in northeastern Thailand led groups of investigators to conclude that aflatoxins might be the agent responsible for Reye's syndrome in that locality. Aflatoxins are heat-stable metabolites of certain strains of *Aspergillus flavus* that may contaminate food-stuffs and that have been found in the tissues of patients dying of Reye's syndrome in Thailand. Aflatoxin B_1 is the most potent toxin in the group (Bourgeois et al., 1971; Olsen et al., 1971). Acute aflatoxin B_1 intoxication has been experimentally produced in macaque monkeys, and its similarities to Reye's syndrome in human children have been noted (Bourgeois et al., 1971). Dhiensiri et al. (1979), however, challenged the above argument and counterclaimed that pesticides, not aflatoxins, were responsible for Reye's syndrome in northeastern Thailand. Similarities have been noted between Reye's syndrome and "Jamaican vomiting sickness," which has been shown to be due to an intoxication with hypoglycins derived from the seed of the unripe ackee fruit (Colon et al., 1974; Lowry, 1975).

Salicylates and phenothiazine intoxications have been found in a few cases of Reye's syndrome (Mortimer and Lepow, 1962; Makela et al., 1980).

An association between Reye's syndrome and various medications has been suspected for some time. Based on recent case-controlled studies from Arizona, Ohio, and Michigan, the CDC issued a statement and advised physicians and parents of the possible increased risk of Reye's syndrome associated with the use of aspirin or other salicylate-containing drugs in children with chicken pox or influenza-like illness in the February 12, 1982 issue of its *Morbidity and Mortality Weekly Report* (31:55–61).

The position of the CDC was endorsed by the American Academy of Pediatrics' Committee on Infectious Diseases in June 1982 (*Pediatrics* 69:810–812) and by the Food and Drug Administration (FDA) in August 1982 (*FDA Drug Bulletin* 12:9–10).

The results obtained by four state epidemiologic study groups were purely statistical, and all parties that endorsed a possible aspirin–Reye's syndrome association admitted that there was no proof of a causal relationship between salicylates and Reye's syndrome. Since the specific pathogenetic mechanisms for development of Reye's syndrome are completely unknown, their position and the data have been criticized and challenged (Hoekelman, 1982; J. T. Wilson and Brown, 1982). While a verification or nullification of the possibility by scientific researchers may take years, a compliance to the recommendation of CDC, FDA, and the American Academy of Pediatrics should result in a decline in cases of Reye's syndrome if a causal relationship does exist (Glezen, 1982).

We must remember that Reye's syndrome is a clinical syndrome that could easily include a wide range of heterogeneous conditions. Cerebral edema and fatty degeneration of the viscera are neither pathognomonic nor specific for any etiopathogenetic entity. Both conditions can be induced by numerous poisons and can be caused by many other factors, including trauma, hypersensitivity, physical agents, and deranged metabolism. The combination of two nonspecific pathologic findings may select a smaller group out of a huge pool of heterogeneous conditions but does not necessarily transform it into a specific disease entity. Moreover, cases that are compiled by the aforementioned criteria could include at least three theoretically possible variants: (1) those with independent encephalopathy and hepatopathy, (2) those with encephalopathy caused by hepatopathy, and (3) those with hepatopathy due to encephalopathy. Although the third possibility is quite unlikely, the first and second remain very difficult to separate.

The most recent attempt to unify all these divergent claims is the concept of a synergistic interaction between two etiologic factors, specifically a virus–toxin interaction.

It is extremely difficult to obtain direct evidence of such an interaction in human patients, but numerous examples have been proven in animal experiments. Friend and Trainer (1970) demonstrated that young mallard ducks that had been exposed to PCB, (polychlorinated biphenyls) developed a fatty visceromegaly and nonspecific encephalopathy following exposure to duck hepatitis virus. Crocker and Ozere (1979), who had suspected forest sprays in the development of Reye's syndrome, have demonstrated that young mice pre-exposed to pesticides were killed by an otherwise benign dose of encephalomyocarditis virus. These authors analyzed the ingredients of pesticides and found the emulsifying agents used as carriers of the pesticides to be responsible for altering the host response to a sublethal dose of virus. Similarly, Dhiensiri et al. (1979) argued that herbicide and virus interaction were responsible for the high incidence of Reye's syndrome in northeastern Thailand.

Other Toxins

Cerebral edema may be seen in acute intoxications with many other agents, including metals, gases, organic solvents, drugs, animal toxins, and plant toxins. Reported autopsy cases are sporadic, and it is often not clear whether cerebral edema is a primary phenomenon or is secondary to hypoxic-ischemic encephalopathy due to shock or cardiorespiratory arrest. We must remember that cerebral edema is generally a nonspecific manifestation that can be seen very frequently in acute intoxications with a high dose of virtually any toxin.

Intoxications Manifested as Hypoxic-Ischemic Encephalopathy

The CNS requires a constant supply of a large amount of oxygen to oxidize glucose in order to maintain its well-being and to function. The oxygen consumption of the brain, which accounts for only 2% of the body weight, is 20–25% of the total oxygen consumption in adults and about 50% in infants.

In order to maintain an uninterrupted energy supply, since neither storage nor substitutes of energy occurs in the CNS, the CNS depends on the cardiovascular system and on the environment for adequate supplies of oxygen and glucose.

The supply of oxygen may be insufficient (hypoxia) or completely interrupted (anoxia) due to many conditions including the following:

- Insufficient air or oxygen in the air
- Insufficient number of available red blood cells to carry oxygen, as in anemia or CO poisoning
- Obstruction of the airways or insufficient alveolar surface to absorb oxygen in various pulmonary diseases
- Anomalous circulation between the lungs and the heart
- Cardiac failure
- Cardiovascular collapse
- Occlusion or narrowing of the blood vessels
- Failure of oxygen consumption in the brain because of inhibition of respiratory enzymes by poisons
- Lack or insufficiency of the substrate (glucose) that is necessary for oxidation
- Increased demand for oxygen beyond the available supply
- Any combination of the above

The terminology has become somewhat complicated because anoxia, hypoxia, ischemia, oligemia, or hypoxemia have been used loosely, often interchangeably, without maintaining clear distinctions. Theoretically these terms can be clearly defined, and in some well-designed experimental conditions they may be distinguished from each other. In practice, however, especially in human cases, it is almost impossible to distinguish them accurately. Ischemia and oligemia almost always result not only in anoxia or hypoxia and hypoglycemia but also in hypercarbia, but anoxia or hypoxia are not always combined with ischemia, oligemia, hypercarbia, or hypoglycemia. Hypoglycemia typically does not occur with hypoxia.

Barcroft (1925) recognized four main types of anoxia:

1. *Stagnant anoxia* results from arrest or decrease in blood flow (ischemia, oligemia). In this condition, the supply of all types of energy, including not only oxygen but also other substrates (e.g., glucose), is interrupted. Simultaneously the evacuation of metabolic waste products is inadequate, resulting in acidosis due to the accumulation of lactic acid, one of the most important causes of edema.

2. *Anemic anoxia* is due to decreased numbers of circulating red blood cells (as in anemia or blood loss), or to the binding of hemoglobulin by CO, resulting in insufficient number of oxygen carriers to the brain.

3. *Anoxic anoxia* occurs when there is an inadequate oxygen intake in cases of respiratory insufficiency or a low content of oxygen in the air (e.g., high altitudes).

4. *Metabolic or toxic anoxia* refers to conditions in which oxygen consumption is interfered with, as in hypoglycemia or cyanide poisoning, even though the oxygen supply is sufficient.

Other classification schemes have agreed on the first three types but disagree on the fourth type. Pentchew (1971) divided the fourth type into "Wirkstoffmangel" and "substrate dysergosis," while Brierley (1976) separated it into "histotoxic anoxia" and "hypoglycemia."

Regardless of the type of etiopathogenesis, the effect of anoxia-hypoxia is relatively stereotyped, with death of some cells and tissues, and reaction of the surviving cells and adjacent tissues. The morphologic appearances vary depending on the severity and the duration of the insult.

The CNS undergoes a series of structural changes when oxygen is cut off. These changes take many hours to become visible on gross and light-histologic examination, but subcellular changes can be detected within minutes by electron microscopy. Once the structural changes begin, the chain of events does not stop until the affected cells and tissues are dead and dissolved. Experimentally the sequence can be traced by studying animals at different stages, beginning with normal tissue and ending with no tissue. The death of cells and tissues is known as necrosis, and the process of dying is known as necrobiosis; however, the two are not always distinguished. In studies of pathologic specimens of humans and experimental animals, one can visualize only a random phase of the process that is terminated by the death of the individual and not necessarily at the end of the chain of events. As a result, structural changes appear quite different among patients who suffered apparently similar conditions. Furthermore, the length, severity, and type of hypoxia, as well as the difference in susceptibility to hypoxia among different cellular elements and among different anatomic sites, make the manifestations of structural damages extremely protean.

SELECTIVE VULNERABILITY OF THE CNS TO HYPOXIA

Except for the extremely severe case, all elements in every part of the CNS are not uniformly damaged by hypoxia. The cellular elements and the topographic areas involved show characteristic patterns that are determined by the order of different degrees of tolerance to oxygen deprivation among these structural units. This phenomenon is known as selective vulnerability to hypoxia and has been extensively studied (Schade and McMenemey, 1963).

Two major theories have been put forward to explain this selective vulnerability. Vogt and Vogt (1922) developed the concept of "Pathoklisis," assuming that differences in basic metabolism and chemistry of different parts of the CNS would account for the selective vulnerability to injury. By contrast, Spielmeyer (1925) proposed the vascular theory, that is, that the selective vulnerability was due to differences in distribution and disposition of blood vessels that supply the affected areas. Many variations on the vascular theory have been suggested.

1. Vascular spasm (Spielmeyer, 1925)
2. Anatomic and morphologic peculiarities of blood vessels in vulnerable areas (Uchimura, 1928)
3. Hemodynamic (or hydrodynamic) factors (Zülch and Behrend, 1961; Lindenberg, 1963; Meldrum and Brierley, 1971)
4. Vascular compression by tissue edema caused by focal accumulation of lactic acid (Lindenberg, 1955, 1963; Myers, 1979)
5. No reflow phenomenon (Ames et al., 1968)

Scholz (1953) suggested that a combination of pathoclitic and vascular factors determined selective vulnerability, and Lindenberg (1963) suggested that a local accumulation of lactic acid in the tissue is the key factor determining the type of tissue injury. The amount of lactic acid accumulation depends on the amount of glucose metabolism, which in turn depends on the amount of blood and the amount of glucose in the blood infused into the brain. Myers and Yamaguchi (1977) showed the first direct in vivo evidence of the harmful effects of glycolysis: lactate in ischemic brains of monkeys. A high concentration of lactic acid (greater than 20 μmol/g tissue) alters cell membrane structure and function, and breaks the BBB resulting in brain edema followed by tissue injury (Myers, 1979). Plum (1983) elaborated further that the accumulation of lactate primarily damages astrocytes resulting in necrosis of all cellular elements, whereas cerebral ischemia with milder glycolysis causes selective neuronal damage.

The controversy is still far from settled. The major problem may be in the heterogeneity of just what constitutes "selective vulnerability" of the brain to hypoxia, as well as just what is "vascular." Selective vulnerability implies unequal damage within an organ or tissue to a particular insult and does not necessarily define any specific pattern of unequal damage of a tissue by all types of hypoxia. Similarly, the terms *vascular* and *hypoxia* imply anything related to cardiovascular-pulmonary structures and functions and their disturbances. There are just too many variables to be included under such a large umbrella.

One should make a clear distinction between "vascular anatomy," which is more or less static with some individual variations, and "circulatory physiology and chemistry," which are dynamic and fluctuating.

Similarly, one should distinguish differences in susceptibility at a cellular level from those at a topographic level. Differences of susceptibility at cellular levels may be influenced more by the inherent metabolic requirements of the cells (Pathoclisis), whereas the vascular anatomy and the type of injury may determine the specific location of the damage within the same tissue. In addition, the types and modes of hypoxia and the ages of patients may play some role in determining the patterns of selective lesions.

At the Cellular Level

In general, neurons are known to be most susceptible to hypoxia, followed by oligodendroglia, astrocytes, microglia, and blood vessels. Hypoxic and ischemic changes of neurons, especially large pyramidal cells, have been extensively studied and found to be more specific than other cellular elements. Different types of neurons also have different degrees of susceptibility to hypoxia. For example, in the cerebellar cortex, Purkinje cells are the most vulnerable, granule cells next, and Golgi cells least (Scholz, 1953).

ISCHEMIC CHANGES OF NEURONS. The process begins with subtle alterations that can only be elucidated by careful and controlled fixation of brains in experimental animals (A. W. Brown and Brierley, 1968) and ends with the disappearance of the neurons.

According to A. W. Brown and Brierley (1968) and Brierley, Brown, and Meldrum (1971), the earliest changes in neurons are microvacuolation in the cytoplasm, characterized by expanded mitochondria. The stage of microvacuolation is transient and is followed by the stage of ischemic cell change, in which neurons and their proximal neurites are shrunken, the cytoplasm staining a vivid pink with eosin, and the nucleus staining dark and having practically no discernible nucleolus. This stage can be identified in the well-perfused brains of experimental primates from 30 minutes to 4 hours after a hypoxic episode. The stage of ischemic cell change progresses, with encrustations characterized by spherical or irregular bodies on the surface or close to the surface of cell bodies. These encrustation bodies are shrunken, dense perikarya and dendrites as visualized by electron microscopy. In the stage of "ischemic neurons" or "homogenizing cell change," the cell body shrinks and becomes more angular. The cytoplasm loses Nissl bodies and becomes diffusely acidophilic, staining diffusely pink with eosin. The nucleus also shrinks, becoming irregular or angular, and stains darkly so that the nucleolus becomes inconspicuous. These changes are quite distinct and different from all other changes, such as those of postmortem autolytic changes or fixation artifacts, and have been considered as relatively reliable criteria for making a diagnosis of early hypoxic-ischemic changes even in the human at autopsy. These changes can be seen in patients who die as early as 30 minutes after an anoxic episode, but unequivocal alterations are usually seen from 10 hours after the event to a few days (Jacob, 1963). Although there is no complete agreement regarding whether these changes are reversible, most investigators believe that the neurons will proceed to disappear by progressive loss of staining affinity.

ISCHEMIC NECROSIS OF NERVE FIBERS AND MYELIN. Damage of myelin sheaths does not become apparent until 18 to 24 hours after an ischemic episode. There is progressive failure of staining of the affected myelin without obvious structural disintegration. However, the tissue undergoes progressive granular breakdown for the following few days, and sudanophilic lipids (mostly cholesterol esters) appear within progressively enlarging macrophages within about 1 week.

Increasing production of large, plump, lipid-filled macrophages (gitter cells or compound granule cells) begins at the edge of the necrotic area.

REGRESSIVE AND REACTIVE CHANGES OF GLIAL CELLS AND BLOOD VESSELS. The necrobiosis of glial cells following hypoxia-ischemia is less specific and has not been studied as extensively as the changes in neurons. Astrocytes show swelling of cell bodies with concomitant loss of processes (clasmatodendrosis) within the first few days after an ischemic episode. The astrocyte may die, the nuclei becoming first pyknotic and irregular and then disappearing, and the cytoplasm undergoing dissolution. These swollen, irregularly shaped astrocytes are also known as ameboid neuroglial cells, but the term is quite misleading because the cells are dying, not moving. Alternatively, presumably following less severe hypoxia-ischemia, the astrocyte may recover, swelling and accumulating small lipid granules in the swollen cytoplasm. Petito et al. (1982) showed different reactions of astrocytes between those in areas of ischemic neuronal damage and in areas of infarction in a rat model of temporary four-vessel occlusion. Severe swelling with disrupted plasma membrane of astrocytes leading to tissue edema was observed in the infarcted areas but not in the regions of ischemic neuronal damage. Plum (1983) hypothesized that the astrocytic damage is due to increased regional lactate, which is the by-product of glycolysis.

Astrocytes that are not destroyed by hypoxia-ischemia, and astrocytes that are located in the periphery of a necrotic lesion undergo hypertrophic changes of the cell body and processes, and proliferation by amitotic and mitotic division to fill the partially damaged area or to cover the edge of the liquefied necrotic area. This process is known as gliosis, astrogliosis, or astrocytosis.

The reaction of oligodendroglia to hypoxia-ischemia is relatively inconspicuous. Acute swelling of oligodendroglia, characterized by swelling and vacuolation of the cell body with or without the accumulation of mucinous fluid, may progress so that the cell undergoes dissolution, or it may recover and return to normal. These changes are almost always present to a certain extent in autopsy specimens and are considered to be due to postmortem changes. Antemortem acute swelling of oligodendroglia is difficult, if not impossible, to distinguish from these postmortem changes, except possibly by degree.

Microglia proliferate by mitotic division and phagocytose dead neurons (neuronophagy), cell processes (dendrophagocytosis), and myelin debris (myelophagy) beginning a few hours after anoxia-ischemia and extending over weeks to months as they invade the necrotic area from the small blood vessels, usually at the edge of the lesion, less commonly within the lesion.

When the hypoxic damage is restricted to neurons, the blood vessels may appear entirely normal; however, when the hypoxic change attains the level of tissue necrosis, the capillaries proliferate and branch extensively within the necrotic lesion, if small, or in the periphery, if the lesion is large. The blood vessel walls are thickened, the endothelial cells swollen, and the perivascular adventitial (Virchow-Robin) spaces become filled with lipid-rich phagocytes.

Selective Topographic Lesions (Topistic Lesions of Vogt)

There are several topographic lesions of the CNS that are characteristically produced by vascular insufficiency, circulatory failure, or both. Not all of these lesions occur simultaneously in every patient who suffers from some type of anoxic-ischemic event. Some patients may show one type and distribution of lesion, whereas other patients show similar lesions in other topographic distributions, even though all the patients appeared to suffer from essentially similar types of anoxic-ischemic insults. The reasons for such variations are not clear but may relate to minor variations in the functional state of the microcirculation.

The extent of the lesions and of their macroscopic and microscopic findings depend on the severity and duration of the insult as well as on the length of survival after the insult. Although there are no perfect correlates between the topography of the lesions and the type of anoxic-ischemic insult, there are some statistical tendencies for a certain type of anoxic-ischemic event to produce lesions in relatively constant locations; for example pallidal necrosis is seen in CO poisoning, watershed zone necrosis with systemic hypotension.

LAMINAR OR PSEUDOLAMINAR NECROSIS. This condition was originally recognized in cases of cortical atrophy associated with dementia paralytica, as well as in cases of sclerosing cortical atrophy associated with cerebral palsy, idiocy, and epilepsy. Subsequently, it was found in many other disease conditions, including CO poisoning, arteriosclerotic vascular disease, cerebral embolism, cardiac arrest under anesthesia, and hypotension from shock and asphyxia. The accumulating evidence eventually led to the conclusion that laminar necrosis is most likely related to an impaired cerebral cortical circulation.

According to Courville (1971), laminar necrosis in the cerebral cortex results from a fusion of multiple focal necroses. When nerve cells of only one layer of the cerebral cortex are destroyed, the lesion is called laminar necrosis; and when more than one layer of nerve cells becomes necrotic, the lesion is called pseudolaminar necrosis. In practice, however, the former is so rare that the two terms are used interchangeably. Grossly, pseudolaminar necrosis can be seen as an intracortical band of dark discoloration or granular necrosis if the patient survives longer than 36 hours after the anoxic-ischemic event. A linear cystic space may be present with concomitant reduction of the cortical thickness if the patient survives weeks or months. Variable degrees of neuronal loss, spongy degeneration, capillary proliferation, gitter cell accumulation, neuroglial proliferation, and cystic degeneration can be seen depending on the duration of the necrosis. Pseudolaminar necrosis is most commonly found in the parieto-occipital region, which corresponds with a watershed zone between the anterior, middle, and posterior cerebral arteries, and at the depths of sulci; however, practically the whole cerebral cortex may be involved in cases of severe ischemia. The third layer of the cerebral cortex is the most vulnerable, followed by the fifth and sixth layers. The second and fourth layers are relatively resistant, and the first or molecular layer is the most resistant layer. Astrogliosis is usually present in the first layer no matter how extensive the cortical necrosis. According to Pfeifer (1928), the intermediate portion of the cortex (layers III and IV) has the richest capillary bed and demands the most abundant blood supply, and thus would be the portion most sensitive to a lack of oxygen.

WATERSHED INFARCT (ARTERIAL BOUNDARY ZONE LESION). In this condition, ischemic alterations or necrosis are concentrated along the watershed between major anastomoses of large arteries or in terminal areas of the major arterial distributions in the cerebral cortex and cerebellum. The distinction between watershed and terminal distribution is essentially irrelevant, since this type of lesion is most commonly due to stagnant anoxia secondary to cardiac arrest or systemic arterial hypotension severe enough to allow the linear resistance to arterial flow to become the major factor defining the failure of perfusion. The lesion is most severe and frequent in the parieto-occipital region, which corresponds to the watershed area between the territories of the anterior, middle, and posterior cerebral arteries. Depending on the size of the lesion, it extends anteriorly along the intraparietal and superior frontal sulci in the watershed between the anterior and middle cerebral arteries, and toward the temporal pole along the inferior temporal gyrus in the watershed between the middle and posterior cerebral arteries. This anatomic distribution of the lesions also corresponds to granular atrophy of the cerebral cortex (Pentchew, 1971), which is produced by intermittent episodes of transient cardiac in-

sufficiency with significant drops in blood pressure, these episodes recurring over many months or years so that vascular fibrosis and perivascular gliosis lead to minute meningocerebral scars that produce small pits ("granular atrophy") that are best seen when the leptomeninges are stripped off postmortem. The extent of the lesion varies from one individual to another, is usually at least slightly asymmetric, and may even be unilateral. The lesion may be part of a large wedge-shaped infarct, involving both cerebral cortex and subcortical white matter, or it may consist of only pseudolaminar necrosis. In the cerebellum, the watershed area between the territories of the superior and inferior cerebellar arteries lies in the horizontal sulcus or the inferior semilunar lobule and usually includes the dentate nucleus. The watershed areas in the basal ganglia are less conspicuous and inconsistent except for the boundary zone between the anterior and middle cerebral arteries, which runs through the head of caudate nucleus and the anterior limb of the internal capsule.

HIPPOCAMPAL NECROSIS [HIPPOCAMPAL SCLEROSIS, SOMMER'S SECTOR, SOMMER'S LESION, AMMON'S HORN (CORNU AMMONIS) SCLEROSIS, INCISURAL SCLEROSIS]. Hippocampal necrosis is probably the most famous lesion in neuropathology—famous not only because of its frequency and the long history of disputes centering around the pathogenesis of this lesion, but also because of confusions in terminology. To begin with this last point, it should be noted that Sommer (1880) described the lesion, not the normal cytoarchitectural variations, in the hippocampus; and that Ammon was an Egyptian deity represented with ram's horns, not an investigator of anything. Thus, the original Latin *cornu ammonis* is a better anatomic term, less misleading than its English translation, "Ammon's horn."

The hippocampus was so named because of its resemblance to a seahorse, except that its "tail," the parahippocampal gyrus, curves behind its "belly," the subiculum, rather than in front, when viewed on cut coronal sections. The same region was named cornu ammonis or Ammon's horn because of its resemblance to a pair of ram's horns when viewed from behind through the lateral ventricles. This region is a part of the limbic cortex and has a highly distinct anatomic architecture. It consists of two C-shaped interlocking convolutions: the dentate gyrus or dentate fascia, which consists of a band of densely packed granule cells, and the hippocampus proper, which consists of a layer of densely packed large pyramidal cells.

Sommer (1880) described the first histologic lesion and demonstrated the special vulnerability of a segment of the hippocampus that became known as Sommer's sector. Unfortunately, Sommer's lesion approximately corresponds to the field H_1 of Rose (1935), who divided the hippocampus into five segments, from H_1 to H_5. The H_1 field is the most inferior-lateral segment and merges medially into the subiculum, the beginning of the parahippocampal gyrus. Segments H_3 to H_5 are most superior and medial, enclosed by the dentate gyrus, and are also known as the end or foot plate. The H_2 segment lies superiorly, lateral to H_3, superior and medial to H_1.

The order of vulnerability to hypoxia-ischemia is generally considered to be H_1, end plate (H_3 to H_5), and dentate gyrus, and H_2; however, the lesions frequently do not correspond exactly to the anatomy. The H_2 field is known as the resistant segment, but this is only relative because total infarction of the hippocampus may occur with severe hypoxic-ischemic events. In the initial stage of hypoxia-ischemia the affected neurons undergo ischemic changes, followed by the disappearance of the neurons and concomitant gliosis.

These were the selective lesions that Vogt and Vogt (1922) attributed to Pathoclisis and that Spielmeyer (1925) attributed to a vascular factor. R. L. Friede (1966) demonstrated certain chemical and histochemical differences between H_1 and H_2 sectors, and supported the concept of Pathoclisis, whereas Uchimura (1928) showed a particularly long course and a very fine caliber of the vessels

in the vulnerable sector, and Scharrer (1940) further stressed the rakelike pattern of the capillaries supplying Sommer's sector. Lindenberg (1955) also studied the vascular pattern supplying these areas and concluded that the vulnerability of the cornu ammonis is not a vulnerability to O_2 deficiency but a topographic vulnerability of its arteries to accentuated pressure related to the edge (incisura) of the tentorium in cases of transtentorial herniation, hence the term *incisural sclerosis*. Our bias is toward the vascular, emphasizing Uchimura's branch of the posterior cerebral artery through the obliterated hippocampal fissure to the susceptible region, different from the branch to the less susceptible dentate gyrus through the choroidal fissure.

Sommer's lesion has been found in about 50% of epileptic patients and in patients who suffered from all kinds of hypoxic and ischemic events, the lesion appearing of varying durations from very acute to very chronic. Speculations have been raised concerning the possibility of a vicious cycle being established, with epileptic seizures producing hypoxia, hypoxia producing the lesion, the lesion becoming gliotic, and the edges of the gliotic lesion irritating the remaining neurons and becoming epileptogenic.

BASAL GANGLIA. Pallidal necrosis, formerly considered to be a specific lesion of CO poisoning, has been found in all types of hypoxia. When the lesion occurs in infancy, it may leave a scar that will later be known as "status dysmyelinisatus" because of the simultaneous damage to the myelinated fibers. This lesion can also be produced by kernicterus, in which damage to certain nuclei, such as the subthalamic, commonly occurs and provides evidence of differential diagnostic significance.

According to Lindenberg (1971), the lateral nuclei of the thalamus are more vulnerable, whereas Brierley (1976) considers the anterior nuclear complex to be the most vulnerable. In the newborn the lateral geniculate nuclei are very frequently involved, and "status marmoratus" affects many of the main thalamic nuclei.

CEREBELLUM. Purkinje cells are particularly vulnerable in O_2 deficiency. Basket cells are less vulnerable, so that "empty baskets" can frequently be demonstrated with silver stain for axons. Granule cells are relatively resistant, and Golgi cells the most resistant to hypoxia.

CEREBRAL WHITE MATTER. Selective necrosis of the cerebral white matter with very little or no involvement of the gray matter occurs in infants, especially premature infants, but it is relatively uncommon in adults. Necrosis of the cerebral white matter in infants tends to occur in the centrum semiovale, more especially around the trigone of the lateral ventricles, where the lesion is known as periventricular leukomalacia. This distribution is thought to represent the watershed between the middle and posterior cerebralarteries, which penetrate relatively straight through the developing cortex and white matter. The lesions also occur more rostrally, at the lateral edge of the body of the ventricle, in the watershed between the anterior and middle cerebral arteries.

In adults, diffuse degeneration of the cerebral white matter was considered to be characteristic of CO poisoning with delayed neurologic deterioration. However, Plum et al. (1962) found the similar condition to be a sequela of anoxic anoxia, anesthesia, and cardiac arrest.

DIFFERENT TYPES OF ANOXIA-HYPOXIA

Stagnant Anoxia

Stagnant anoxia is also known as ischemia or oligemia, and is characterized by arrest or insufficiency of the blood circulation. The most common causes of circulatory arrest are acute heart failure, myocardial infarct, and complications of cardiac surgery and anesthesia. Acute poisoning with methanol, ethanol, morphine, barbiturates and other narcotics, snake venom, and poisonous mushrooms may also cause cardiac arrest or cardiovascular collapse, but most of these conditions are preceded by some type of respiratory failure, so that a pure stagnant anoxia is rarely seen.

In the human, cardiac arrest usually occurs suddenly and unexpectedly, so that its exact duration is usually not known. The duration of cerebral ischemia required for permanent brain damage has not been critically defined in humans, and the results obtained from animal experiments vary widely, ranging from 15 to 60 minutes. However, it is generally considered that complete clinical recovery is unlikely if the period of cardiac arrest lasts more than 5 minutes at normal body temperature.

If death occurs within 6 hours of the arrest, the brain usually shows no gross abnormality. Microscopic findings are so subtle that they are almost impossible to distinguish from the usual postmortem artifactual changes.

Swelling of the brain, with or without congestion or hyperemia, may appear and become maximal 48–72 hours after the arrest, with evidence of compression of the ventricular cavities and axial herniation. Congestion and granular appearance of the cortex may be recognized as early as 48 hours but usually remain equivocal until several days after the arrest. However, microscopic findings, characterized by ischemic neuronal changes and neuronal necrosis, are visible within 6 to 12 hours; moreover, capillary proliferation, edema, and glial proliferation are quite evident at 48 hours and progressively proceed to cystic laminar necrosis of cerebral cortex. With increasing duration of survival, necrosis becomes more pronounced with concomitant atrophy and gliosis. Involvement of the basal ganglia and thalamus is quite common but less constant, and the pattern of involvement is less predictable. With long survival up to 1 year or longer, secondary degenerations, both Wallerian and retrograde, may occur in descending tracts (e.g., pyramidal) and thalamic nuclei.

Oligemic brain damage due to systemic hypotension tends to localize in the boundary zones between major arterial territories in both the cerebral cortex and the cerebellum. When cardiac insufficiency is intermittent and repetitive, granular atrophy of the cerebral cortex results along these arterial border zones.

J. H. Adams, Brierley, Connor, and Treip (1966) summarized the neuropathology of stagnant hypoxia and stated that oligemic brain damage due to systemic arterial hypotension conforms to one of the following three patterns, of which the first two are the most common:

1. Watershed (arterial boundary zones) infarcts in the cerebral and cerebellar cortices with variable involvement of the basal ganglia
2. Generalized ischemic changes of cerebral and cerebellar cortices, frequently with thalamic damage
3. Generalized ischemic changes of the cerebral and cerebellar cortices with variable accentuation along the arterial boundary zones

In all instances, the hippocampi are spared or are only mildly involved. According to these authors and confirmed experimentally in primates (Brierley, Brown, Excell, and Meldrum, 1969), the first type of brain damage appears to be caused by a major and abrupt episode of hypotension followed by a rapid recovery, while the second type is usually associated with hypotension of a relatively slow onset but of long duration, and the third type appears to be associated with hypotension of an abrupt onset followed by a sustained period of a partial recovery.

Anemic Anoxia

Anemic anoxia is induced by severe anemia or hemorrhage that causes a decrease in the number of erythrocytes or a diminished production of hemoglobin, which in turn fails to transport sufficient amounts of oxygen to the CNS. Since CO has an affinity for hemoglobin that is 200–250 times greater than that of oxygen, carboxyhemoglobin prevents the transport of oxygen to the CNS and causes anemic anoxia.

CARBON MONOXIDE POISONING. Common both at home and in industries, both accidental and suicidal, CO results from the incomplete combustion of carbon during fires, explosion, coal mine accidents, internal combustion engines, and household gases.

The concentration of CO in the atmosphere normally is below 1/100,000. Nausea occasionally appears at a concentration of 1/5000, headache and asthenia at 1/3000. A concentration of 1/1000 may cause severe and even fatal poisoning, a concentration of 1/500 causes death within 4 to 5 hours, and a concentration of CO of 1/20 in air causes death within 15 minutes (Bour et al., 1967).

In humans, expressed in terms of the amounts of CO in the blood, dyspnea on exertion and slight headache appear when the level of carboxyhemoglobin exceeds 20%. Severe headache, fatigue, and impaired judgment appear at levels of 30%. Consciousness is lost at a level of 60% to 70%, and death rapidly occurs at a concentration of 70% or higher (Brierley, 1976). Three different clinical types of CO poisoning have been recognized:

1. *Acute poisoning.* Symptoms of nausea, light-headedness, headache, vertigo, and weakness appear promptly after the exposure. If the exposure is sustained, the patient becomes progressively drowsy, unconscious, and incontinent, and may develop muscular twitchings or convulsions leading to death. The skin and mucous membranes may be cyanotic, occasionally with erythematous rashes. Confusion, hallucinations, and choreic movements may precede convulsions and coma.

2. *Chronic poisoning.* Individuals who are chronically exposed to nonlethal but toxic levels of CO may develop chronic headache, nausea, vomiting, general weakness, memory deficit, and impairment of intellectual activity.

3. *Relapsing CO poisoning.* Relapse is frequently seen in individuals who apparently recover from the acute effect of CO poisoning but develop a recurrence of

symptoms leading to prolonged mental and neurologic sequelae followed by death after an interval ranging from days to weeks in duration. This pattern had been considered to be unique for CO poisoning, but Plum et al. (1962) showed that delayed neurologic deterioration occurs in other types of hypoxia as well.

Brierley (1976) classified the clinical symptomatology of CO poisoning into monophasic and biphasic types. The former includes acute and chronic poisoning, and the latter is equivalent to the relapsing type of poisoning. The neurologic complications of CO poisoning have been reviewed by Garland and Pearce (1967), who called attention to the rarity of clinical evidence of permanent brain damage among the survivors. They also pointed out that there is not a combination of neurologic and psychiatric symptoms that can be regarded as the specific consequence of CO poisoning, since similar signs and symptoms can be found following other types of hypoxia and hypoglycemia.

The neuropathologic aspects of CO poisoning have been extensively discussed and reviewed but appear to be far from being resolved (Lapresle and Fardeau, 1967).

For some time, pallidal necrosis and leukoencephalopathy have been considered unique neuropathologic findings, but the general consensus today is that CO encephalopathy does not present any lesions fundamentally different from those caused by other anoxic conditions.

If there is any finding that can be considered characteristic of CO poisoning, that would be the cherry or pinkish red color of all viscera including the brain, due to the presence of carboxyhemoglobin. Unfortunately, this finding can only be seen in patients who die from an acute intoxication. Diffuse and widespread necrotic lesions have been found in various topographic regions of the CNS, including the basal ganglia (particularly the globus pallidus), cerebral white matter, Ammon's horn, and other brain structures. Among all these lesions, pallidal necrosis and leukoencephalopathy

are most frequent, even though they are not specific in CO poisoning.

Lesions of the Globus Pallidus. Necrotic lesions of the globus pallidus are the most frequent, found in 16 of 22 cases of CO poisoning (Lapresle and Fardeau, 1967). They are usually bilateral, involving the anteromedial portion, and may extend into the adjacent internal capsule. The lesion may be quite small and can be missed without serial or multiple-step sections. Diapedetic hemorrhages, and later, hemosiderin-laden macrophages and frequent deposits of pseudocalcium in the wall of blood vessels, are found in cases of long survival.

CO Leukoencephalopathy, Diffuse Myelinopathy of Grinker (1925). Some investigators discussed its resemblance to diffuse and multiple sclerosis (Grinker, 1925; Meyer, 1932; Courville, 1957; Brucher, 1962). Jacob (1939) emphasized the relationship between the relapsing type of CO poisoning and the development of leukoencephalopathy, but such a correlation has not been proven by other investigators. Similar leukoencephalopathy has been reported in many other conditions, including complications of anesthesia (Steegmann, 1939; Pentchew, 1958; Brucher and Laterre, 1962), cardiac arrest (J. C. Richardson et al., 1959; Plum et al., 1962), carbon disulfide poisoning (Arend et al., 1964), morphine poisoning (Lindenberg, 1963), hypoglycemia (Lawrence et al., 1942; J. E. Richardson and Russell, 1952), and strangulation (Jacob et al., 1962).

The demyelination is predominant in the centrum semiovale of the cerebrum with preservation of the U fibers. The cerebellar white matter may be involved occasionally. Many authors emphasize characteristic patterns of demyelination, which have been described as "moth-eaten," "speckled," "striped," or "checkered" with persistence of myelin patches in the perivascular regions (Courville, 1957; Schwedenberg, 1959; Wender, 1963).

Brucker (1967) described three successive stages of demyelination: a speckled zone of a "checkered appearance," a microcystic zone, and a zone of necrosis with confluent small cavities to illustrate the range of myelin and axon destruction in the cerebral white matter. Lapresele and Fardeau (1967) classified the lesions of the centrum semiovale and commissural structures into four types: (1) multifocal necrotic lesions with partial coalescence, (2) massive necrosis, (3) confluent areas of demyelination, and (4) rare necrotic lesions in the white matter. These authors found lesions in the white matter in 16 of 22 cases: 3 cases of type 1, 4 cases of type 2, 6 cases of type 3, and 3 cases of type 4.

Hippocampal Lesions. Although all the neuropathologic changes seen in CO poisoning have the appearance and typical localization of anoxia-ischemia, the incidence of Ammon's horn lesions is not constant. Lapresle and Fardeau (1967) found Ammon's horn lesions of variable severity ranging from Sommer's sector lesions to complete hippocampal necrosis, in 10 of 22 cases.

Lesions of Cerebral Cortex. According to Osetowska (1971a,b), cerebral cortical lesions are a constant feature in almost all cases, ranging from selective neuronal loss to pseudolaminar cortical necrosis. Lapresle and Fardeau (1967), however, found cortical lesions in only 12 of 22 cases, admitting that the low incidence may have been due to insufficient sampling of cortical areas.

Cerebellar Lesions. Since the damage to the CNS in CO poisoning is basically not different from those of other types of anoxia-ischemia, one would assume that homogenizing changes of Purkinje cells would be the most common cerebellar lesion in CO poisoning. In fact such a statement is frequently found in textbooks, even though the frequency of such findings is usually not clearly stated. Therefore, one may be surprised to find the statement of Lapresle and Fardeau (1967) contradicting such a general belief of rather obscure origin. These authors contended that the Purkinje cells are

generally uninvolved, and instead observed parenchymatous necrosis (five cases), white matter pallor (five cases), and partial or complete lysis of the granular layer, this last condition becoming such a commonly seen state, known as état glace, that opinions differ widely, some regarding it as a significant lesion that Friede (1963) has almost reproduced by allowing anerobic glycolysis to continue.

Lesions in Other Parts of the CNS. Necrotic lesions have been observed in other sites of the CNS, including the reticular zone of the substantia nigra, putamen, hypothalamus, thalamus, and subthalamic nucleus. These lesions are, however, infrequent and inconstant.

Experimental CO Poisoning. Hemorrhagic necrosis of basal ganglia has been produced in mice, guinea pigs, rabbits, and dogs with CO by Photakis (1921), and softening of the globus pallidus with occasional extension into the putamen or internal capsule was observed in dogs and cats by Meyer (1932). Nonselective gray matter damage such as neuronal necrosis was seen by Ferraro and Morrison (1928) and Lewey and Drabkin (1944) in rabbits and dogs. Lund (1956) reported changes in the Ammon's horn neurons and Purkinje cells in monkeys. Cerebral white matter demyelination and necrosis have been produced in dogs and cats by Meyer (1932), Lewey and Drabkin (1944), and Preziosi et al. (1970). Van Bogaert et al. (1938) were unable to produce definite neuropathologic lesions by CO intoxication in rhesus monkeys, but Ginsberg and Myers (1974) produced CO leukoencephalopathy with relatively infrequent pallidal necrosis in juvenile rhesus monkeys. The latter authors evaluated possible correlations between the physiologic data of individual animals and the degree of neuropathologic changes in the white matter, but found no relationship between the extent or duration of the hypoxic period and the severity of the leukoencephalopathy. Instead they found that the size of the lesion was related to both the extent of systolic hypotension and the magnitude of systemic metabolic acidosis.

Anoxic Anoxia or Hypoxic Hypoxia

Anoxic anoxia or hypoxic hypoxia implies that the blood leaving the lungs is either devoid of or deficient in oxygen. This condition occurs with decreased availability of O_2 (as in the atmosphere at high altitudes), when O_2 is replaced by other gases (as in anesthetic or industrial accidents or by smoke), and with various respiratory problems (when the lungs or cervical spinal cord are injured or when the trachea is obstructed). Asphyxia following hanging and drowning also belongs to this type of anoxia. At sea level, hemoglobin is normally 95–98% saturated with O_2. O_2 does not begin to fall below 90% until altitudes of 10,000 feet or higher are attained, when dyspnea appears and mental concentration becomes difficult. Consciousness cannot be retained for more than a few minutes above 18,000 feet (Cohen, 1966).

It has been generally believed that brain damage can result from a simple reduction in the O_2 content of arterial blood. Scholz (1953) and Brucher (1967) contended that ischemia-oligemia caused cerebral and cerebellar cortical and Ammon's horn necrosis, whereas hypoxemia produced necrosis in the globus pallidus, striatum, and subthalamic nucleus. Brierley (1976) argued that critical physiologic data were lacking in human cases to support such a contention. Exposing rhesus monkeys and baboons to subatmospheric decompression in a decompression chamber, Brierley and associates (Brierley and Nicholson, 1969; Nicholson et al., 1970) were able to produce lesions in the arterial boundary zones of the cerebrum and cerebellum. Damage to the basal ganglia was inconstant and variable. These investigators also observed bradycardia and decreased respiratory rate toward the end of the decompression. They considered that the brain damage could not be attributed to an uncomplicated hypoxemia but was most likely due to a secondary oligemia-ischemia as the result of myocar-

dial depression. Thus, they believe that a neuropathology of hypoxic hypoxia is the same as that of anemic hypoxia.

Histotoxic and Metabolic Hypoxia

CYANIDE POISONING. Cyanide combines with neuronal cytochrome oxidase and catalase to block hydrogen and electron transport, which utilizes the oxygen derived from the dissociation of oxyhemoglobin. Hemoglobin remains saturated with oxygen, because the metabolic block is in the tissue rather than in the blood.

Cyanides are the most rapidly acting poisons known. Absorption on inhalation is so rapid that death may be almost instantaneous. No significant neuropathologic alterations are found except for some hyperemia or petechial subarachnoid and subdural hemorrhages. When taken orally, cyanides act more slowly, and patients develop headache, nausea, dyspnea, circulatory collapse, and convulsions, and they progress to coma and death within minutes or hours. Only a few human cases of relatively longer survival have been reported (Lambert, 1919; Schmorl, 1920; Edelmann, 1921). The case of Lambert (1919) survived 16 days and showed small hemorrhages in the cerebral and cerebellar white matter, loss of Purkinje cells, and cerebral cortical lesions. The case of Edelmann (1921) died 36 hours after the accident and showed diffuse hyperemia and hemorrhagic necrosis of the globus pallidus. Cyanide poisoning from ingestion of a large amount of apricot or other fruit seeds containing amygdalin has been reported (Sayre and Kaymakealan, 1964). Amygdalin itself is harmless but may release a toxic level of cyanide following mild acid hydrolysis or the action of enzymes. A case of acute cyanide poisoning after taking Laetrile (containing amygdalin) for cancer therapy has been reported by Shragg et al. (1982). This patient developed pulmonary edema and lactic acidosis. No neuropathologic findings have been reported.

Despite the paucity of neuropathologic data on human intoxications from cyanogenic glycoside poisonings, there are many experimental data that have been summarized by Brierley (1976). Meyer's experiments (1933) on dogs and rabbits showed neuropathologic findings that were not different from those of CO poisoning. Ferraro (1933) produced demyelinating lesions in the cerebral white matter of cats and monkeys, and called attention to the morphologic resemblance to multiple sclerosis. Hurst (1940, 1942) produced two basic types of white matter lesions in rhesus monkeys by repeated intramuscular injection of potassium cyanide: (1) poorly demarcated partial demyelination and (2) sharply demarcated white matter necrosis that resembled Schilder's disease rather than multiple schlerosis. The globus pallidus, caudate nucleus, putamen, and substantia nigra were also affected in this order of frequency. Ammon's horn was not involved in any animal. Necrosis of the cerebral and cerebellar cortex was produced only with repeated massive doses of potassium cyanide, which required resuscitation of the animals.

Hicks (1950) described damage ranging from necrosis of scattered neurons to complete dissolution of a region not unlike that seen in infarction in cats given intraperitoneal sodium cyanide (NaCN). Haymaker et al. (1952) administered cyanogen chloride (CNCl), hydrocyanic acid (HCN), or NaCN into dogs via different routes. The pathologic changes in the CNS were essentially the same regardless of the type of cyanide administered and the route of its administration. Cytoplasmic eosinophilia (acute ischemic change) of neurons was observed in the cerebral cortex and Purkinje cells 2–3 hours after the administration. Neuronal loss with glial reaction increased with length of survival and was found in the cerebral cortex, striatum, pallidum, substantia nigra, thalamus, and cerebellum. Ammon's horn lesion and demyelination were uncommon.

Levine and Stypulkowski (1959a) and Levine and Wenk (1959) produced lesions of both gray and white matter in rats by a single dose of hydrogen cyanide and potassium cyanide. The production of selective white matter lesions did not depend on repeated exposures but rather on maintenance of optimal depth and duration of intoxication. In a subsequent experiment, Levine and Stypulkowski (1959b) ligated the common carotid artery on one side of rats preceeding an exposure to cyanide and found localization of gray matter lesions on the side of the carotid ligation and bilateral selective lesions of the white matter. They concluded that the gray matter involvement was most probably due to the accompanying ischemic and/or hypoxic hypoxia, while the white matter lesions were due to direct cyanide effect. Hirano et al. (1967) showed that the earliest EM alteration in the white matter was swelling of the axons, within which the mitochondria were expanded and their cristae more or less disorganized. Demyelination appeared to be secondary to axonal damage.

Brierley, Brown, and Calverley, (1976) employed physiologic monitoring of lightly anesthetized rats during intravenous NcCN infusion at a rate that would avert apnea. Six animals developed white matter lesions, but only one had lesions of the gray matter, which were attributed to that animal's marked hypotension, cardiac arrhythmias, and apnea. It was concluded that, in the absence of secondary respiratory or circulatory complications, the damage produced by cyanide was confined to the cerebral white matter. The authors questioned whether the entity of pure histotoxic brain damage really exists.

AZIDE POISONING. Sodium azide (NaN$_3$) is a widely produced industrial chemical product and has been used in rocket fuels and as a herbicide, insecticide, and molluscicide. Organic azides and diazides have been used in the treatment of hypertension. The effect of NaN$_3$ is similar to that of cyanides, inhibiting the action of cytochrome oxidase and causing cell asphyxia. Accidental intoxication by azides may produce transient hypotension, but there have been no neuropathologic reports on human intoxications.

Experimentally Hurst (1942) produced necrosis or demyelination in the optic nerves and tracts in monkeys by repeated administration of NaN_3. The basal ganglia were frequently involved, with the striatum suffering more than the pallidum. Unlike experimental KCN poisoning, lesions in the centrum semiovale were rare, and cortical lesions were frequent but mild. Hicks (1950) and Környey (1963) observed necrosis of the corpus callosum, optic chiasm, and head of the caudate nucleus in rats with experimental intoxication of NaN_3. The results obtained by Mettler and Sax (1972) with an intravenous injection of NaN_3 in rhesus monkeys were quite different. A single intravenous injection of NaN_3 induced convulsions associated with apnea and a fall in blood pressure. Some recovered animals showed ataxia. Autopsy 1–55 weeks after the experiment showed various degrees of cerebellar damage, ranging from Purkinje cell loss in the depths of sulci through semilunar lobular necrosis to almost complete decortication. These lesions could not be produced in control animals that had convulsions and apnea induced by oil of wormwood, or that were preanesthetized before the administration of NaN_3 and showed no convulsions. These authors concluded that the cerebellar lesions were due to the cumulative effects of impaired ventilation, hypotension, and impairment of oxidative enzymatic activity.

HYPOGLYCEMIA. The CNS is almost totally dependent on the oxidation of glucose for its energy source. When the blood glucose level falls, muscles, liver, and kidneys oxidize other substrates to maintain their functions, but the brain has only a limited ability to do so. Thus, cerebral functions fail when blood glucose falls. Hypoglycemia may lead to damage in the brain when the associated coma becomes irreversible. Whereas the onset of symptoms in cerebral anoxia is rapid, the onset of symptoms in hypoglycemia is delayed for 30 to 45 minutes, because there are some glucose stores in the brain.

Hypoglycemia is an important cause of seizures, mental confusion, and coma in adults, and of mental retardation and sei-

zure disorders in infants. There are numerous diseases that cause hypoglycemia: starvation, intestinal malabsorption syndrome, liver diseases, insulin-producing pancreatic tumor, insulin overdose, and alcohol intoxication. The most common cause in adults is probably insulin overdose for the treatment of diabetes mellitus. Accidental insulin overdose was common during the days of insulin shock therapy for schizophrenia or other psychoses, but within the past few decades insulin shock therapy has been gradually replaced by various other antipsychotic agents. Hypoglycemia in childhood is most often caused by a different set of disease conditions, including disturbances of glycogen metabolism, galactosemia, hepatic diseases, and other endocrine disturbances.

The neuropathologic findings show some variations, but there is no doubt that they closely resemble those that occur in other types of anoxia (Meyer, 1963). Depending on the length of survival and severity, the brain damage following irreversible hypoglycemia includes ischemic changes of neurons, pseudolaminar cortical necrosis, diffuse demyelination of cerebral white matter, loss of Purkinje cells, focal necrosis of basal ganglia, and diffuse cortical atrophy in cases of prolonged survival. In other words, lesions of variable locations occurring in all types of anoxia can be found in the brains of patients who die of irreversible hypoglycemia. Among all these lesions, cerebral cortical necrosis, Ammon's horn lesions, and diffuse demyelination of the cerebral white matter are relatively constant, whereas lesions in the basal ganglia and Purkinje cell damage are relatively uncommon.

Experimental Hypoglycemia. Reports on experimental hypoglycemia in animals are numerous. In uncomplicated insulin-induced hypoglycemia, Brierley et al. (1971) demonstrated diffuse ischemic neuronal changes in the neocortex with some concentration in the occipital and parietal regions in 7 of 15 rhesus monkeys. Ischemic neuronal changes in the hippocampus, striatum, and cerebellar Purkinje cells were infrequent. In longer-surviving rhesus monkeys, Myers and Kahn (1971) found neuronal loss and gliomesodermal reaction in the striatum, neocortex, and hippocampus in decreasing order of frequency. These experiments showed that brain damage occurred when the blood glucose level fell to about 1 mmol/liter (20 mg/100ml) or below if hypoglycemia was uncomplicated with hypotension, hypoxia, or convulsions. Similar brain damages were produced with a higher blood glucose level if the hypoglycemia was complicated with hypotension, hypoxia, or convulsions.

If Plum's glycolysis–lactate hypothesis (1983) is correct, one would expect to see more or less pure ischemic neuronal damages in the brains with untreated hypoglycemia. Rapid restoration of blood glucose levels without concurrent oxygenation may be more harmful than hypoglycemia alone.

Cerebral Lesions Associated and Complicated with Liver Failure

The history of liver–brain relationships goes back to antiquity (I. A. Brown, 1957; Cumings, 1959). The association of "changes in mind" with jaundice was well known to Hippocrates, Celcius, and Galen. The last even considered the liver to be the seat of the mind. In the Chinese language, "heart and liver" are still used to designate the mind.

COPPER INTOXICATION

Wilson's disease (hepatolenticular degeneration) is considered to be a type of copper intoxication in which exogenous Cu absorbed from the intestines fails to bind to α-globulin to become ceruloplasmin because of an endogenous metabolic failure. As a result, an excessive amount of free Cu or Cu loosely bound to albumin is absorbed into tissues, such as the brain and liver, and causes damage to these organs. The source of Cu is exogenous—the normal diet—but it requires a heredofamilial endogenous metabolic defect to be deleterious.

In contrast to Wilson's disease, the effect of simple intoxication due to exogenous Cu overdose without an auxiliary endogenous factor is less well known.

Copper is an essential element for human and animal nutrition. It is an essential constituent of several proteins, enzymes, and some naturally occurring pigments, including ceruloplasmin, cytochrome c-oxidase, tyrosinase, and many others. In the majority of Cu-containing enzymes, the Cu acts as a cofactor.

Copper-deficient diets hinder normal structural and functional development of many organs. Cu-deficient syndromes occur in many different animal species and include "swayback," anemia, brittle bones, skin disorders, hair pigmentation, vascular defects, and myocardial fibrosis. Of these, "swayback" in lambs is mainly neurologic, manifesting with ataxia and characterized by diffuse demyelination and degeneration of the cerebral white matter.

As far as simple Cu toxicity is concerned, the first pathologic description in humans and animals was by Mallory (1925), who produced pigmentary cirrhosis of the liver in rabbits by giving Cu acetate and Cu powder orally, intratracheally, and subcutaneously. Rabbits and sheep, the latter extremely sensitive to poisoning with Cu, died from occlusion of the renal tubules by hemoglobin casts. Mallory discussed 10 human cases of hemochromatosis, most of them exposed to alcohol or copper or both, all of whom showed pigmentary cirrhosis of the liver, similar to that of the rabbits poisoned with Cu. Even though the Cu level of the liver in those patients was found not to be elevated, Mallory considered that chronic poisoning with Cu was the cause of the hemochromatosis.

The first neuropathologic study of Cu poisoning in humans was probably that of Courville (1964), who reported a 60-year-old chronic diabetic who ingested three quarters of a bottle of Clinitest tablets, containing copper sulfate. The patient developed hypertension, enlarged liver, edema of the legs and periorbital region, and left hemiplegia, and died of massive gastrointestinal bleeding 10 days after the ingestion of the tablets. The brain showed fragmented white matter, pale neurons in the basal ganglia, and a focus of ischemic cell changes, but the specificity of these changes was doubted.

Acute Cu poisoning may manifest as nausea, vomiting, and diarrhea (Nicholas, 1968). Cu poisoning is particularly likely to occur when highly acidic food, such as pickled foodstuffs, is stored in copper vessels or tanks (Ross, 1955). Its occurrence has been reported in persons drinking cocktails that were shaken in a copper cocktail shaker from which the inner silver lining had worn off (Wyllie, 1957). Chronic Cu poisoning in human newborn babies was reported by Blomfield (1969) due to Cu contamination from a stopcock used in exchange transfusion, causing intravascular hemolysis, enhanced agglutination of red blood cells, and increased bilirubin, because Cu competes with bilirubin for albumin binding. No neurologic symptoms have been implicated in any of these reported cases.

Relative Cu intolerance in sheep compared to cattle and piglets has been well known to stock farmers in Britain and Australia for many decades. Spontaneous acute and chronic Cu poisoning in sheep, characterized by hemolytic jaundice, has been observed. Autopsy studies showed central necrosis and fatty damages of the liver with some fibrosis, as well as increased Cu level in the liver (Pearson, 1956). Pathologic changes in the CNS of these sheep were reported by Doherty et al. (1969), who described spongy degeneration of the white matter in the midbrain, pons, medulla, and cerebellum. The cerebrum was spared except for mild spongy degeneration in the internal capsule.

According to Todd (1969), there are two distinct phases in chronic Cu poisoning of ruminants: the initial latent phase in which Cu accumulates in the tissue over weeks or months without clinical symptoms, and the later toxic phase, which is manifested by an acutely fatal course of jaundice and hemoglobinuria due to "hemolytic crises." The accumulation of Cu is almost entirely located in the liver, and other organs including the brain show virtually no elevation of Cu, findings in contrast with Wilson's disease.

In experimentally produced Cu poisoning, Ishmael et al. (1971) found spongy degeneration in the cerebral white matter in six of eight sheep, and in the spinal cord in three. Large, pale astrocytic nuclei suggestive of Alzheimer's type II glia were found within the spongy white matter, even though Cu was not elevated in the CNS. Electron-microscopically, vacuoles in the white matter were found to be in the outer tongue of oligodendroglial cytoplasm or expanded endoplasmic reticulum (Howell et al., 1974).

Other experiments include those of Vogel (1959), who found Cu in neurons that showed degenerative changes in fish kept in water containing copper sulfate. Intraventricular injection of minute amounts of Cu (52–208 μg) into the brains of cats promptly produced persistent quadriplegia. Autopsy showed hydropic swelling of myelin sheaths in the early stages, progressing rapidly to focal necrosis in the peripheral margins of the spinal cord, brain stem, and cerebrum (Vogel and Evans, 1961).

MANGANESE INTOXICATION

Although Cu plays an important role in Wilson's hepatolenticular degeneration, simple exogenous Cu intoxication does not produce clinical features or pathologic alterations of organs akin to Wilson's disease. A long exposure to inhalation of manganese (Mn) dust, however, is associated with production of liver cirrhosis and neurologic syndromes that may be mistaken for Wilson's disease, parkinsonism (paralysis agitans), or multiple sclerosis.

Chronic human Mn intoxication was first described by Couper (1837), who reported on five Mn ore crushers who developed a series of neurologic syndromes manifesting muscular weakness, paraplegia, tremor, speech difficulty, salivation, and a tendency to lean forward while walking. More than half a century elapsed before chronic Mn poisoning was rediscovered by two German authors. Embden (1901) described two patients who engaged in grinding MnO_2 and who developed extrapyramidal syndromes that he correctly disgnosed as chronic Mn poisoning. Von Jaksh described three men who worked in the same factory for drying MnO_2 slime and who developed neurologic syndromes initially diagnosed as atypical multiple sclerosis in 1901, and only later as chronic Mn poisoning (von Jaksh, 1907).

Casamajor (1913) described chronic Mn intoxication in nine patients who worked in the separating mill connected with a large mine that produced 85 different ores, including zinc, Mn, and iron, but not lead and arsenic. Mn was considered the most likely toxic agent. Edsall et al. (1919) reviewed cases reported in Europe and America, added several cases found in the same mill reported by Casamajor (1913), concluded that the symptoms of chronic Mn poisoning are quite definite, and listed the following findings in the order of appearance:

1. History of work in Mn dust for at least 3 months
2. Languor and sleepiness
3. Stolid, masklike faces
4. Low, monotonous voice, economical speech
5. Muscular twitching, varying from tremor to myoclonus
6. Muscle cramps at night and stiffness of legs
7. Slight increase in tendon reflexes
8. Ankle and patellar clonus
9. Retropulsion and propulsion
10. Wide-based, slapping gait
11. Uncontrollable laughter, less frequently crying
12. No sensory change

Since then, many more cases of chronic Mn poisoning have been reported from Mn mines in Spain, Morocco, Egypt, Chile, Cuba, India, and Japan.

Chronic Mn intoxication has been essentially an industrial and occupational disease occurring principally via inhalation of Mn dust. It is common not only among miners and ore crushers in Mn mines, but also in dry-cell battery workers, electric welders, steel mill workers, nickel mill workers, and aluminum factory workers.

The replacement of lead by Mn as the antiknocking agent in gasoline may result in the pollution of the air by Mn, but its effects on our health cannot be foreseen at this time (Mena, 1979).

Clinical Manifestations

The clinical signs of Mn poisoning are quite characteristic and include a variety of extrapyramidal syndromes. Most older reports emphasized the similarities to Parkinson's and Wilson's diseases. Mena (1979), however, observed initial psychoneurotic syndromes, which have been known as "locura mangania" (manganic madness), and which are more characteristic, even constant findings. This stage lasts for about 1 to 3 months and includes emotional instability, such as easy laughter, ready crying, irritability, nervousness, insomnia, compulsive singing and dancing, uncontrollable violence, and hallucinations.

Barbeau et al. (1976) stressed the dissimilarities to the clinical findings in parkinsonism, noting some manifestation of dystonia in all victims of Mn intoxication, whereas dystonia is not a common feature of Parkinson's disease.

Laboratory findings, including liver function tests, have been within normal limits (Mena, 1979). Chronic Mn intoxication is not fatal, but the prognosis is usually poor (Cook et al., 1974). Improvement or disappearance of the neurologic syndromes has been noted in some patients (Mena, 1979; Cook et al., 1974) when the patients are removed from exposure, but in many others the neurologic sequelae have remained stationary.

PATHOLOGY. Since chronic Mn intoxication is usually not fatal, pathologic studies of this condition have been scarce. The first autopsy report was made by Casamajor (1913), who described biliary cirrhosis of the liver and some tract degeneration in the pons. The first detailed pathologic report was that of Ashizawa (1927), who described diffuse degenerative changes in the CNS with accentuated neuronal loss in the pallidum, putamen, and caudate nucleus, with only a mild gliovascular proliferation 3 years after onset. The degeneration of the large ganglion cells was more pronounced than that of the small.

The patient reported by Canavan et al. (1934) had been followed for 13 years before his death at age 69. The abdominal and thoracic viscera were not examined. The brain showed diffuse cerebral cortical atrophy with dilatation of the lateral ventricles and marked shrinkage of the basal ganglia. Significant microscopic changes included degeneration of nerve cells, satellitosis, and gliosis practically uniformly in the caudate nucleus, putamen, globus pallidus, and thalamus.

The cases of Stadler (1936) and Parnitzke and Peiffer (1954) showed similar findings in the lenticulostriate nuclei, but Voss (1939) described degenerative changes in the anterior horn cells and corticospinal tracts characteristic of amyotrophic lateral sclerosis, but occurring unilaterally in his case. The case reported by Bernheimer et al. (1973) showed marked spotty degeneration in the zona compacta of the substantia nigra in addition to mild pallidal atrophy and generalized astroglial proliferation in certain cortical areas, putamen, pallidum, and red nucleus.

Animal Experiments

Mella (1924) injected intraperitoneally 1 mg of manganese chloride into rhesus monkeys every other day for 18 months and produced choreic or choreoathetoid movements followed by rigidity and then fine tremors and contractures of the hands. Autopsy revealed markedly elevated Mn concentrations in many organs, especially the liver (15-fold) and the brain (10-fold). The liver showed acute hepatitis with necrosis, small hemorrhages, and fibrosis. The brain showed degenerative changes, most pronounced in the striatum and pallidum. Findlay (1924) found that rabbits were most susceptible to the poison, dying 22–48 hours

after a subcutaneous injection of 10 to 60 mg of $MnCl_2$, from severe parenchymal degeneration of the liver and kidneys. Repeated injection of smaller doses led to the development of liver cirrhosis in rabbits, rats, and guinea pigs. Hurst and Hurst (1928) also produced liver cirrhosis with subcutaneous injections of $MnCl_2$ but failed to produce degenerative changes in the CNS in rabbits and guinea pigs.

Grünstein and Popowa (1929) produced severe lesions, mainly in the small neurons in the striatum of rabbits, by chronic exposure of Mn. Van Bogaert and Dellemagne (1943) observed alternate extension and flexion of the upper limbs with spreading of the fingers and toes in monkeys receiving MnO_2 through inhalation. Pathologic changes were confined to the spinal cord and the cerebellum.

Pentchew et al. (1963) used intramuscular injections of MnO_2 suspended in olive oil. The monkeys developed clumsiness, excitement, falling, and dystonic postures about 9 months after the first injection. The autopsy of a monkey 14½ months after the first injection showed almost total neuronal loss of the subthalamic nucleus and the medial pallidum with proliferation of bizarre glial cells. The glial proliferation extended into other areas but was most dense in the habenular nucleus and field H of Forel. These lesions were almost identical to those reported in humans by Ashizawa (1927), Stadler (1936), and Parmitzke and Peiffer (1954), but no reference was made to the cases of Canavan et al. (1934) and Voss (1939).

Some similarities (or rather dissimilarities) of clinical manifestations among parkinsonian humans, chronic Mn intoxication in humans and experimental animals, and the side effects of L-dopa (a dopamine precursor widely used to treat parkinsonism) have led to extensive studies on the relationship between Mn and catecholamine metabolism. Dopamine has been found to be diminished in the striate nuclei of patients with parkinsonism (Hornykiewicz, 1966) and chronic Mn intoxication (Bernheimer et al., 1973). Although there were some differences in the results of other catecholamine levels, experimental chronic Mn intoxication in squirrel monkeys (Neff et al., 1969), rabbits (Mustafa and Chandra, 1971), and rats (Chandra and Srivastava, 1970; Bonilla and Diez-Ewald, 1974) consistently showed diminished dopamine and homovanillic acid levels in the striatum or in the whole brain.

Manganese in human tissues has been found to be elevated with L-dopa toxicity (Cotzias et al., 1971; Bonilla and Diez-Ewald, 1974). Weiner et al. (1978) found increased Mn and decreased Cu in the brains of guinea pigs following chronic administration of L-dopa and the direct-acting dopamine agonists, bromocriptine and lergotrile.

Barbeau et al. (1976) hypothesized that Mn blocks dopaminergic pathways at the presynaptic level, causing cytoplasmic accumulation of dopamine and extrapyramidal syndromes, and that repeated administration of Mn causes permanent presynaptic damage of dopaminergic pathways resulting in a decreased level of tissue dopamine. Some neuroleptic drugs, such as phenothiazines, butyrophenones, and raserpines, block dopamine receptors or diminish dopamine in the basal ganglia and produce catalepsy and/or parkinsonism. Mn concentration is increased after potent phenothiazines (Borg and Cotzias, 1962), and decreased with reserpine in the striatum of rats (Donaldson et al., 1974). Such interaction of trace metals, especially of Mn, with neurotransmitters during the course of neuroleptic drug treatment has opened up a new field of neurochemical and neurophysiologic research.

OTHER TOXIC AND DRUG-INDUCED LIVER DISEASES

Necrosis and degenerative changes of the liver can be induced by innumerable exogenous toxins, including large groups of industrial poisons and medicinal agents. Notable among these poisons are phosphorus, carbon tetrachloride, chloroform, ether, organic arsenicals, quinacrine, sulfonamides, urethane, 6-mercaptopurine, tetracycline, and paracetamol. Massive hepatic necrosis following halothane anesthesia has been especially studied since the 1960s. The incidence was probably less than 1 in 10,000 administrations of anesthesia, but the "National Halothane Study" (1969), a large retrospective investigation, failed to demonstrate a direct relationship between halothane and hepatotoxicity. Hypersensitivity, latent viral hepatitis, idiosyncrasy, and a multifactorial pathogenesis have been considered. The last has been supported by animal experiments requiring hypoxia and phenobarbital stimulation of the hepatic drug-metabolizing enzyme system to produce helothane hepatic necrosis (McLain, Sipes, and Brown, 1979; Ross et al., 1979).

Indirect liver injury as a result of hypersensitivity can be seen with numerous drugs, including tranquilizers, sedatives, anticonvulsants, antibiotics, antiarthritic agents, hormones, and metabolic agents. In cases of hepatitis due to drug hypersensitivity, there is no correlation between the amount of the drug consumed and the degree of the hepatic injury.

The CNS complication of toxic hepatitis is a single event of acute coma, characterized by delirium, convulsions, and occasionally decerebrate rigidity, often ending fatally. Both clinical and pathologic findings are similar regardless of the specific agent or drug.

In contrast to acute toxic hepatitis, there is a large group of cases of chronic liver cirrhosis of unknown etiology. Hunt et al. (1963) found seven cases of arsenical cirrhosis, seven cases of hemochromatosis, two cases of Wilson's disease, and two cases of gold cirrhosis by assaying the concentrations of iron, zinc, cobalt, copper, gold, and arsenic in the livers of 450 cases of various liver diseases, including ordinary alcoholic cirrhosis.

Encephalopathy and Neuropathy Associated with Renal Failure

Mercury bichloride ($HgCl_2$), carbon tetrachloride (CCl_4), potassium bichromate

(KCr_2), uranium nitrate (UNO_3), ethylene glycol, and diethylene glycol are well-known nephrotoxins. They primarily affect the kidney, causing renal failure and uremia. Neurologic complications, such as uremic encephalopathy and neuropathy, were formerly common consequences of poisoning caused by these agents. However, the introduction of hemodialysis and peritoneal dialysis for the treatment of renal failure has successfully eliminated or reduced the incidence of uremia and its complications following poisonings. But, in turn, a new set of neurological complications arising from such treatments, known as dialysis encephalopathy and dialysis dementia, has developed.

The former is a transient neurologic syndrome and the latter is characterized by a progressive course of relentlessly increasing neuropsychiatric syndromes. No known neuropathologic lesions have been found in either disorders, but dialysis dementia has been found to result from chronic aluminum intoxication.

DIALYSIS DEMENTIA, PROGRESSIVE DIALYTIC ENCEPHALOPATHY, DEMENTIA DIALYTICA

In 1972, Alfrey et al. reported a neurologic syndrome that occurred in five patients from the Denver area receiving chronic hemodialysis; it was clearly different from those of uremic and dialysis encephalopathies.

The condition was characterized by intermittent speech difficulty, dysnomia, and multifocal bursts of slow-wave discharges on EEG, followed by a progressive and unrelenting course of tremor, myoclonus, asterixis, motor dyspraxia, memory loss, personality changes, psychosis, seizures, and ataxia. These patients had received hemodialysis for 38 to 75 months before the onset of the syndrome. The clinical symptoms could be aggravated by dialysis. All patients died within 6 to 7 months after the onset and the autopsy disclosed no gross or microscopic abnormalities of the brain. Intoxication was suspected and the brains of these patients were assayed for various metals. Chromium, strontium, cobalt, iron, molybdenum, manganese, zinc, lead, magnesium, bromide, nickel, and phosphate levels were found to be not different from those of controls. However, the brain potassium and rubidium were found to be lower and tin and calcium were found to be higher. Similar experiences were reported from Chicago (Mahurker et al., 1973), Great Britain (Wardle, 1973), and Australia (Barrett and Lawrence, 1975). Wardle (1973) speculated that a deficiency of dopamine may be the cause, whereas Barrett and Lawrence (1975) suggested a slow virus infection.

Alfrey et al. (1972, 1976) noticed that aluminum-containing, phosphate-binding gels had been widely given orally as a method of controlling serum phosphorus levels in uremic patients on dialysis, and that all dialysis dementia patients had routinely received these gels for at least 2 years before the onset of progressive encephalopathy. The first patient in the Denver area was found in 1971, approximately 2½ years after phosphate-binding aluminum had been routinely prescribed. These authors reported a higher than normal aluminum level in muscle, bone, and gray matter of the brain in patients who had died with dialysis dementia and suggested that this syndrome might result from aluminum intoxication. Complete autopsy in 12 patients revealed only slight microscopic neuropathologic abnormalities. The brain tissue from the patients was inoculated into the brains of primates without showing evidence of slow virus infection during the following 3½ years (Alfrey et al., 1976). Flendrig et al. (1976) in Holland, Elliot et al. (1978) in Scotland, Parkinson et al. (1979) in Newcastle, Rozas et al. (1978, 1979) in Michigan, and Poisson et al. (1978, 1979) in Paris reported their epidemiologic observations, including serum aluminum levels and aluminum concentrations in the water used for dialysis. These authors concluded that progressive dialysis dementia is caused by aluminum intoxication. The source of the aluminum may not be limited to the aluminum-containing medication; another possibility is the water used for dialysis. The aluminum level is 10 to 20 times higher in the gray matter of dialysis dementia patients than of control subjects and 4 to 5 times higher than that of uremic patients on dialysis but without clinical evidence of dementia. Clinical neurologic expression of dialysis dementia is not specific; it is essentially similar to the case of industrial aluminum intoxication reported by McLaughlin et al. (1962). Poisson et al. (1979) reported a permanent clinical remission in six patients with dialysis dementia after they corrected the oral intake of aluminum compound and used deionized dialysate.

The problem of dialysis dementia seems to have been solved in the late 1970s, but the relationship of aluminum and clinical dementia has intrigued many investigators and has led to widespread and controversial studies of the role of aluminum in Alzheimer's disease.

Aluminum is one of the most abundant elements in the earth's crust. Just a few examples of the myriad aluminum products that are indispensable in our daily life are cooking utensils, window frames, window shades, wrappers, baking powder, drugs, containers, cosmetics, and ornaments. Traditionally, aluminum has not been regarded as an important toxicant when it is taken orally, because the gastrointestinal tract is considered a formidable barrier to aluminum absorption (Campbell et al., 1957) and because aluminum has been regarded to be physiologically inert (Deobold and Elvehjem, 1935). However, recent investigators have shown that some aluminum can be absorbed through the gastrointestinal tract mucosa if a large enough quantity is taken orally (Kaehny et al., 1977). Furthermore, aluminum absorption from the gastrointestinal tract can be accelerated with the administration of parathyroid hormone in both humans and animals (Mayor et al., 1980), especially in individuals with impaired renal function. Aluminum toxicity involves not only the CNS but also red blood cells (Elliott et al., 1978), heart, lung, and bone. Only one human case of industrial aluminum intoxication has been reported (McLaughlin et al., 1962): a 49-year-old man who had worked 13½ years in the ball mill room of an aluminum factory and who developed mental deterioration, speech difficulties, Jacksonian seizures, left hemiparesis, muscle twitching, clonic jerking—progressing to coma and death about 9 months after the onset. The clinical presentation resembled very much that of Creutzfeldt-Jakob disease and dialysis dementia. The autopsy showed bronchopneumonia and pulmonary fibrosis containing aluminum particles. Aluminum level was 20-fold increased in the brain and lungs and 122-fold in the liver. No Alzheimer neurofibrillary degeneration was found in the brain.

In 1942 Kopeloff et al. found that aluminum hydroxide paste placed in the monkey brain was epileptogenic. Experimental seizures produced with aluminum hydroxide were nonprogressive, chronic, and recurrent, and have been widely studied as a model in epilepsy research.

Klatzo et al. (1965) injected various antigens that were suspended in Holt's adjuvant, the basic ingredient of which was alum phosphate, into the brains of rabbits. These rabbits developed weakness and ataxia followed by convulsions, nystagmus, and opisthotonus 7–10 days after the injection, and died 3–8 days later. This was the clinical syndrome that had been observed by Scherp and Church 26 years earlier (1937), when they injected herpesvirus suspended in aluminum salts. Klatzo et al. found vacuoles in neurons of the affected animals and reported this as a method of inducing edema in neurons.

Terry and Peña (1965) applied Klatzo's technique to rabbits in order to produce vacuolated neurons, but to his surprise the clear area of neuronal cytoplasm was found by EM not to be vacuolated but to consist of filaments. For the following 15 years aluminum compounds have been used to induce neurofibrillary changes in neurons in various species of animals. Although Alzheimer's neurofibrillary tangles differ by showing helical twisting of tubules, aluminum-induced neurofibrillary tangles in animals have been extensively studied as an experimental model of Alzheimer's neurofibrillary tangles.

In conjunction with the observation that dementia dialytica was most likely due to an aluminum intoxication, and that aluminum injected intracerebrally could induct neurofibrillary tangles in animals resembling human Alzheimer's neurofibrillary tangles, Crapper et al. (1976) found elevated aluminum levels in the brains from patients who suffered from Alzheimer's disease. The question whether aluminum plays a significant role in the causation of Alzheimer's disease or senile dementia has evoked controversy for the last few years and has not been answered definitely.

In favor of the theory are the following findings: (1) Aluminum intoxication induces dementia in humans (McLaughlin et al., 1962; Alfrey et al., 1976); (2) cats that receive intracerebral injections of aluminum manifest deficits in short-term retention of newly learned tasks before manifesting neurologic signs and neurofibrillary tangles in the brain, the number and distribution of which correlate with the aluminum concentration (Crapper and Dalton, 1973); (3) the aluminum level is elevated in the brains of Alzheimer's patients (Crapper et al., 1976); (4) the number of neurofibrillary tangles correlates with the aluminum concentration in human brains (Crapper et al., 1976); and (5) aluminum was demonstrated by scanning EM with X-ray spectrometry within the nuclear region of tangle-bearing neurons (Perl and Brody, 1980).

Opposed to the theory are the following findings: (1) No neurofibrillary tangles have been found in the brains of aluminum-intoxicated patients (McLaughlin et al., 1962; Alfrey et al., 1976); (2) the human neurofibrillary tangles are morphologically different from those of aluminum-induced tangles in animals by EM (Kidd, 1964; Terry and Peña, 1965; Wisniewski et al., 1970); (3) there is a difference in the anatomic localization of the human tangles and the experimentally induced tangles; (4) there is a lack of elevated aluminum concentration in the brains of some human cases of Alzheimer's disease; and (5) there is a lack of as-sociated anomalies, such as senile plaques or granulovacuolar degeneration, which are common in patients with Alzheimer's disease, but are absent in animal brains receiving aluminum injections.

In summary, while aluminum may not be an inducer, it may be a promoter or an accelerator of Alzheimer's disease.

Neurologic Complications of Deficiency Diseases Secondary to Intoxication

Because of many scientific achievements and the extensive education of the public over the last few decades, the nutritional deficiency diseases due to simple malnutrition, unbalanced diets, or abnormal eating habits have become relatively rare in modern communities. They still exist in the third world, however, and even in developed countries. They still occur secondary to various diseases, including malabsorption syndromes, hyperemesis, chronic gastritis and esophagitis, and chronic diarrhea. These are usually prevented or corrected with adequate nutritional supplements. Other nutritional deficiency diseases still exist, although in a somewhat disguised form.

Most of the nutritional deficiency diseases today are due to or associated with chronic alcoholic intoxication or alcohol abuse. This is probably more of a social or cultural problem than a medical problem. In fact, most abusers pose no serious medical problem and do not commonly seek medical attention. Most people do not drink alcoholic beverages under close medical supervision. Instead, they neglect to maintain their own health and are simultaneously neglected by their families and friends. As a result, simple and easily preventable deficiency diseases continue to erupt among chronic habitual drinkers.

The most renowned complication of chronic alcoholics is Wernicke's encephalopathy, which has been generally considered to be due to vitamin B_1 (thiamine) deficiency. Because most patients with Wernicke's encephalopathy are found among chronic alcoholics, and because most chronic alcoholics are found within Western societies, a false impression has been given that Wernicke's encephalopathy is due to alcohol intoxication per se. Indeed, even though Wernicke himself reported a nonalcoholic case, Wernicke's encephalopathy has been discussed under the section on alcoholism or alcohol intoxication in most textbooks.

WERNICKE-KORSAKOFF ENCEPHALONEUROPATHY

In 1881, Carl Wernicke described a new clinicopathologic entity that he termed "acute hemorrhagic superior polioencephalitis." Clinical manifestations included ophthalmoplegia, ataxia, inflamed optic disks, and a disturbance of consciousness varying from confusion to delirium and stupor. He described three patients: Two were chronic alcoholics and one was a 20-year-old nonalcoholic seamstress who developed the syndrome following 4 weeks of persistent vomiting due to pyloric stenosis as the result of sulfuric acid poisoning. Death occurred 10–12 days after the onset of the syndrome, and the neuropathologic findings described by Wernicke as "hemorrhagic encaphalitis" were characterized by multiple punctate hemorrhages in the massa intermedia, wall of the third ventricle, and gray substance of the floor of the fourth ventricle. Although the original concept of Wernicke that this syndrome was caused by an acute inflammatory process has been disproven, the anatomic localization of the lesions and the types of neuropathologic changes are still valid today. The involvement of the mammillary bodies was the only subsequent addition to his original description (Gamper, 1928).

In 1887, Korsakoff described 20 cases of an amnestic psychosis accompanying alcoholic polyneuropathy; he pointed out that the psychic symptoms and the polyneuropathy were two different manifestations of the same disease and termed the syndrome "psychosis polyneuritica." Two years later, Korsakoff (1889) reported additional examples of this disorder in patients without alcoholism but with puerperal sepsis, typhoid fever, hyperemesis gravidarum,

and persistent vomiting in intestinal obstruction. He postulated that the psychic symptoms were due to a toxemia, "cerebropathia psychica toxaemica." A close relationship between Wernicke's encephalopathy and Korsakoff's psychosis was never appreciated by either Wernicke or Korsakoff, but since then numerous resports on the clinical and pathologic findings of both Wernicke's encephalopathy and Korsakoff's syndrome have demonstrated beyond any doubt that the two frequently share similar and overlapping clinical and pathologic changes.

The association of Korsakoff's psychosis with Wernicke's encephalopathy is so common that the two conditions are now generally regarded as one syndrome. In a series of 245 patients, including 82 autopsies, Victor, Adams, and Collins (1971) found that more than 90% of patients with Wernicke's encephalopathy showed mental symptoms, and that over 80% showed signs of polyneuropathy as well. The pathogenesis of the Wernicke-Korsakoff syndrome was not settled until the 1930s, when the possibility of avitaminosis was brought up by a series of observations showing close similarities in the neuropatholigic findings in experimental thiamine deficiency in animals (Prickett, 1934; Alexander, 1940), in a human infant (Tanaka, 1934), and in human Wernicke's encephalopathy. The therapeutic effects of thiamine were shown on Korsakoff's psychosis by Bowman et al. (1939), and on Wernicke's encephalopathy by Joliffe et al. (1941). Since then numerous reports have confirmed the effectiveness of thiamine on most of the components of these syndromes, and acute thiamine deficiency has been established as the major etiology of these disorders.

Clinical Features

The triad of Wernicke's encephalopathy consists of ophthalmoplegia, ataxia, and mental changes. The onset is usually abrupt, but the eye signs and ataxia may precede the mental symptoms by several days. The most common eye signs are horizontal and vertical nystagmus followed by lateral rectus paralysis, which is usually bilateral. The patient complains of diplopia and shows internal strabismus, but the eye problem may progress to complete external ophthalmoplegia. A unilateral third-nerve palsy may occur as a prominent variant. The gait is wide-based, and the ataxia tends to involve the trunk and lower extremities more than the upper extremities. The mental symptoms undergo a series of characteristic changes: Initially there are delirium, global confusion, dullness, and apathy; these progress into a stage of amnesic-confabulatory psychosis (as originally described by Korsakoff); the end stage is a state of permanent dementia (Victor et al., 1971). Hypothermia may result from lesions in the hypothalamus. Death may occur in 10 to 14 days in the absence of treatment and may be surprisingly sudden. The ocular palsies, if treated promptly, disappear rapidly in a matter of minutes to hours following treatment with large doses of parenteral thiamine, but the nystagmus and ataxia regress more slowly, and the amnesia rarely regresses to any great degree, being incomplete in about 80% of cases. However, the mental symptoms, including the amnestic-confabulatory psychosis, can be prevented if the treatment is begun early, that is, before the mental symptoms appear. Treating severely vitamin-depleted alcoholic patients—who may appear dehydrated—with a large amount of glucose without accompanying thiamine may precipitate Wernicke's encephalopathy.

The blood pyruvate levels are usually elevated, and the transketolase activity of erythrocytes is reduced.

Pathologic Findings

The pathologic lesions in the CNS are confined to the walls of the third ventricle, aqueduct, and fourth ventricle: the mammillary bodies, hypothalamus, dorsomedial thalamus, periaqueductal gray matter, and superficial tegmentum of the pons and medulla. The pathologic changes consist of vacuolation, demyelination, and necrosis of the parenchyma in these areas with marked gliovascular proliferation and relative preservation of neurons. Petechial hemorrhages are found in patients who die during the acute stage of the disease, but according to Victor et al. (1971) only 20% of their cases showed petechial hemorrhages. In neuropathologic practice today, patients with acute Wernicke-Korsakoff disease rarely come to autopsy, because most of them have been promptly recognized and treated with large doses of thiamine. However, atrophy of the mammillary bodies with hemosiderin pigment and usually with marked gliosis of the periaqueductal region and the wall and floor of the third and fourth ventricles are frequently found in the brains of alcoholic patients who die of other diseases and who may or may not have had recorded episodes of Wernicke-Koraskoff syndrome in the past. The gliosis of the hypothalamus and the tegmentum of the brain stem are not specific and cannot be diagnostic for old Wernicke-Korsakoff syndrome, but the atrophy and old hemorrhage in the mammillary bodies are diagnostic of healed Wernicke-Korsakoff syndrome.

Clinicopathoanatomic correlations in Korsakoff's psychosis have incited the interest of many investigators. Concomitant lesions in the cerebral cortex and in the mammillary bodies have been considered to be responsible for the amnesia, but Victor et al. (1971) placed the responsible lesions for the amnesia in the diencephalon, more specifically in the medial dorsal nucleus and perhaps the medial pulvinar of the thalamus.

In the PNS, the peripheral neuropathy may appear independent of Korsakoff's psychosis or Wernicke's encephalopathy, and is generally known as alcoholic neuropathy.

Victor et al. (1971) found that 92% of their 230 alcoholic patients showed evidence of peripheral neuropathy, although only two thirds of them showed tenderness, pain, weakness, sensory deficits, and absent or diminished deep tendon reflexes, predominantly involving the distal portions of the extremities. No case of cranial nerve involvement was found in their series, 70% involved only the lower extremities, and 30% showed involvement of both lower and upper extremities.

The histopathologic findings of alcoholic neuropathy vary from case to case depending on the severity and on the stage of the pathologic process. There are no significant clinical or pathologic differences between beriberi neuropathy and alcoholic neuropathy. For this reason, alcoholic neuropathy has been considered to be due to thiamine deficiency, just as in beriberi neuropathy (Shattuck, 1928). A direct toxic effect of alcohol as the etiology of alcohol neuropathy was ruled out by the early human experiments of Strauss (1935), who demonstrated clinical improvement in 10 patients with alcohol neuropathy who received thiamine but were allowed to drink whiskey continuously. However, thiamine deficiency as the sole cause of alcoholic neuropathy has been questioned, because the neuropathy has been quite difficult to produce in mammals by thiamine deficiency and because the clinical recovery from the neuropathy following thiamine treatment is very slow.

Some investigators consider that both toxic effects of alcohol and thiamine deficiency are responsible. Victor et al. (1971) consider that thiamine may not be the only vitamin responsible, and that other B vitamins, such as pyridoxine (vitamin B_6) and pantothenic acid, or a combination of several B vitamins, may be deficient in alcohol neuropathy.

SUBACUTE NECROTIZING ENCEPHALOPATHY, LEIGH'S ENCEPHALOPATHY

This entity, with many similarities to Wernicke's encephalopathy, has been considered to be associated with an inherited abnormality of thiamine metabolism. Leigh's encephalopathy (1951) occurs in infants and children, is recessively inherited, and therefore is frequently familial; however, treatment with thiamine is practically ineffective. The onset is more gradual and the clinical course is longer than in Wernicke's

encephalopathy, usually lasting for months or years, frequently with partial remissions. Like those in Wernicke's encephalopathy, the lesions of Leigh's consist of parenchymatous necrosis with capillary proliferation and relative preservation of neurons in the wall of the third ventricle, periaqueductal region, and the floor of the fourth ventricle. Unlike Wernicke's encephalopathy, however, other lesions occur in Leigh's encephalopathy and are usually much more extensive, often extending into more laterally situated thalamic nuclei, lenticular nuclei, optic nerves, and even cerebellum and spinal cord; in addition, the mammillary bodies—almost universally affected in Wernicke's encephalopathy—are rarely affected.

Cooper et al. (1970) and Murphy et al. (1974) showed that there is an inhibitor of ATP–thiamine pyrophosphate phosphotransferase in the brains of patients with Leigh's encephalopathy. However, this hypothesis has to be further tested before an effective treatment is developed.

BERIBERI

Beriberi is caused by a dietary deficiency of thiamine and is characterized by cardiac and peripheral nerve lesions. The cardiac lesion tends to occur in the acute form and consists of acute dilatation of the right heart. The peripheral nerve lesion is found more frequently in the chronic form of thiamine deficiency (refer to section on Wernicke-Korsakoff syndrome). The clinical symptoms of beriberi polyneuropathy begin distally in the lower extremities with burning pain and numbness, progressing to motor weakness, sensory deficit, and loss of deep tendon reflexes, even becoming widespread to include the lower cranial nerves.

Beriberi polyneuropathy is primarily demyelinative, followed by degeneration of the axis cylinders (Pekelharing and Winkler, 1893). The lesions have been confirmed in humans and birds (Bertrand et al., 1934; Zimmerman, 1943), but Bertrand et al. (1934) contend that there is no stage of degeneration of myelin without an accompanying lesion of the axon in vitamin B–deprived pigeons. In patients with atrophy of nerves due to long-standing neuropathy, Wallerian degeneration may extend proximally into the nerve roots or even into the dorsal columns of the spinal cord, but nerve degeneration is usually more severe in the distal portions. Central chromatolysis of ventral horn cells and dorsal root ganglia can be found in the early stages and in the more acutely progressive cases.

Central Pontine Myelinolysis

In 1959 Adams, Victor, and Mancall described a new neuropathologic entity called central pontine myelinolysis (CPM). Numerous case reports and reviews have followed. CPM is a relatively uncommon condition that is characterized by a symmetric, centrally located, demyelinating lesion in the basis pontis.

Clinical Manifestations

CPM has been reported in both sexes, without racial preference and in persons ranging in age from 3 to 72 years. The condition is almost always a terminal and fatal complication of some pre-existing disease, which includes both neurologic (such as brain tumors, dementia, Wernicke's encephalopathy, Wilson's disease, and transverse myelitis) and non-neurologic conditions (such as uremia, scleroderma, leukemia, liver cirrhosis, pneumonia, viral and fungal infections, severe vomiting in pregnancy, and carcinomas in other organs). The duration of these pre-existing diseases ranges from a few weeks to several years. Dehydration, malnutrition, and metabolic and electrolytic abnormalities are the most common abnormalities found, and the most common denominator has been a too-rapid correction of hyponatremia.

The clinical manifestations of CPM depend on the size and extent of the lesion. CPM may be found incidentally at autopsy in patients showing no clinical neurologic findings in life; in full-blown cases with a large lesion in the pons, however, quadri-plegia, pseudobulbar palsy, and coma are common features. McCormick and Danneel (1967) reviewed 69 cases, including 3 of their own, and listed the following neurologic symptoms and signs in order of frequency: (1) reflex changes, (2) pathologic reflexes, (3) quadriparesis or quadriplegia, (4) extraocular muscle palsies and pupillary disturbances, (5) convulsions, (6) tremors, (7) dysarthria, (8) dysphagia, (9) incontinence, and (10) mutism. A large number of patients were comatose for varying periods of time preceding death, and the coma was usually preceded by confusion, disorientation, delirium, and obtundation.

The majority of reported cases and our own experiences (six cases) were diagnosed at autopsy. The diagnsis of CPM in life is very difficult but not impossible. The history of pre-existing chronic illness, alcoholism, malnutrition, cachexia, persistent vomiting associated with inappropriate antidiuretic hormone secretion, and the finding of hyponatremia or hypernatremia and neurologic findings and signs suggesting bilateral upper brain stem involvement should suggest the diagnosis. The condition of most patients worsens while they are being treated in the hospital. Death usually occurs in the third and fourth weeks after the clinical onset. Arrested or healed cases have been documented, with CT evidence of pontine lesions.

Pathologic Findings

The principal and characteristic lesion of CPM is in the center of the basis pontis and is primarily demyelinative. The rostral pons is more constantly and extensively involved than the caudal pons. The lesion is triangular or diamond-shaped in the midline of the dorsal basis pontis when it is small, but it may extend centrifugally to involve practically the whole basis pontis except for the peripheral rim and the ventral portion of the pontine tegmentum. Islands of longitudinal tracts in the basis pontis are frequently preserved. Small lesions may be grossly inconspicuous, poorly defined granular areas or areas of brown-gray discoloration, but large and older lesions may show softening and partially liquefactive necrosis. Microscopically, the lesions show destruction of myelin sheaths with relative preservation of neurons and axons. Gitter cells are abundant and often contain myelin breakdown products. Cavitation with loss of axons can be found, especially in the center. Oligodendroglia have been found to be markedly reduced in numbers. Astrocytic reaction is present but modest. The lesions are well demarcated but have irregular borders. No significant degree of inflammation or vascular changes is present. The crossing fibers are usually more extensively destroyed than the longitudinal tracts.

Minor pathologic changes have been reported in other parts of the CNS. Adams et al. (1959) described pallor of the dorsal columns of the spinal cord, and petechial hemorrhages in the medulla in one patient, as well as neuronal changes similar to those seen in pellagra in another case. Necrosis of the striate body and demyelination of the cerebellar white matter were reported by Mathieson and Olszewski (1960). Kepes et al. (1965) reported neuronal degeneration and microglial reaction in the right putamen. The case of Klavins (1963) showed multiple foci of demyelination in the cerebellum, cerebral peduncle, and optic radiation, which were morphologically similar to those of the pontine lesions. We have also found randomly localized focal demyelinating lesions in the hippocampal white matter, lateral thalamus, and geniculate nucleus, as well as pseudolaminar necrosis of cerebral cortex. Lesions suggesting anoxic changes have been found (Mathieson and Olszewski, 1960; Paguirigan and Lefken, 1969). These associated lesions in the CNS have not been emphasized because they are inconstant and variable, both in frequency of appearance and in their anatomic location. They are relatively nonspecific morphologically, resembling lesions of anoxic origin. Mathieson and Olszewski (1960) accepted that some lesions seen in their cases were anoxic in nature, but they offered no explanation for others, such as necrosis of

the striate body and demyelination of the cerebellar white matter. Adams (1962) accepted that the neuronal loss in the cerebellum, hippocampus, and basal nuclei in case number 2 was due to anoxia but contended that the cortical necrosis and demyelination of the subcortical white matter in the cerebrum of case number 1 were probably due to the same mechanism that causes CPM. We agree with Adams (1962) that these associated focal lesions in the cerebrum and cerebellum are parts of the manifestations of the pathologic process that also causes CPM, and they deserve further investigation.

Etiology and Pathogenesis

Many hypotheses have been proposed during the last two decades in an attempt to explain the cause and pathogenesis of CPM: alcoholism (Adams et al., 1959), malnutrition, (Victor et al., 1971), vascular insufficiency, chronic edema (McCormick and Danneel, 1967), drug intoxication, and electrolyte abnormalities (Berry and Olszewski, 1963; Conger et al., 1969).

The role of alcoholism has been denied because of reports of a large number of nonalcoholic patients. Nutritional deficiency as the etiology is nebulous, and no case has been shown to respond to large does of vitamins. Salt depletion or hyponatremia has been frequently reported in patients who showed CPM (Adams, 1962; Kepes et al, 1965; Conger et al., 1969), but replacement therapy and correction of electrolytes have only rarely reversed the clinical course of patients. Indeed, too-rapid correction may aggravate the condition, with continued deterioration despite prompt parenteral therapy for electrolyte abnormalities. Norenberg et al. (1982) contend that it is not the hyponatremia itself that causes CPM but the rate of correction of the hyponatremia, which is the factor causing the development of CPM. They compared a group of hyponatremic patients who developed CPM with a group who did not and found that the former showed a more rapid and more marked rise of serum sodium concentration. This hypothesis is the best current explanation of the paradox that patients typically develop neurologic findings of CPM a few days after admission to the hospital and continue to deteriorate in spite of improved electrolyte balance.

DIRECT EFFECTS OF INTOXICANTS

In previous sections we have discussed varieties of neuropathologic lesions that are induced by intoxicants but that are not specific for the intoxication. These lesions cannot be distinguished from those of other etiologies, such as vascular diseases, physical trauma, metabolic disturbances, or hypersensitivity states. Indeed, some of them are obviously secondary effects of cardiopulmonary collapse, liver failure, or renal failure, rather than a direct effect of the intoxicant.

The CNS is separated from the external and internal environments by the blood–brain barrier. Most toxins cannot pass this barrier and cannot gain access to the CNS parenchyma unless the barrier is damaged, either directly by the toxin or indirectly through effects on other organs. A few intoxicants, such as anesthetic agents, pass this barrier without damaging effects, and some other toxins may do so with very little detectable damage to the barrier.

Pathologic lesions that have been proven to be directly produced by intoxicants are few. Most such intoxicants lack firm proof and remain controversial.

Intoxications Causing Predominantly Neuronal Degeneration

There are few intoxicants that produce selective neuronal damage in the cerebral cortex, cerebellar cortex, basal ganglia, brain stem, and spinal cord with very little or no damage to the myelin, neuroglia, and Schwann cells. In part this reflects the different sensitivities of our techniques for assessing damage to neuroglia, Schwann cells, and myelin, which are not so refined as those for assessing neuronal changes.

ORGANIC MERCURY, MINAMATA DISEASE

The neurotoxicity of metallic mercury has been known for many centuries, but its neuropathologic features have not been well documented. Diffuse cerebral edema, congestion, and cerebral purpura have been observed in sporadic human autopsied cases and in experimental animals (Osetowska, 1971b).

Our knowledge of the toxic effects of organic mercury on the nervous system is relatively new. Hunter et al. (1940) described the clinical findings in four patients suffering neurologic disturbances following industrial exposure to methyl mercury and confirmed the neurotoxicity of methyl mercury in rats and a monkey. One of their patients died 15 years later, and the pathologic findings were reported by Hunter and Russell (1954). The CNS of this patient showed degeneration of the cerebral and cerebellar cortices, widespread but most marked in the calcarine cortex and granular cell layer of the neocerebellum. These lesions correlated well with the clinical manifestations of ataxia, dysarthria, and constriction of the visual fields. When an epidemic of a "strange neurologic disease" appeared in fishing villages along Minamata Bay in southern Japan in the 1950s, Japanese investigators at Kumamoto University struggled several years before finding the etiology of this new disease. Four autopsy cases were reported by Takeuchi, Tanoue, Kambara, et al. (1957), who pointed out that the disease consisted of a toxic encephalopathy with very close similarities to the case reported by Hunter and Russell (1954). Eventually they were able to identify the causative toxic agent to be organic alkylmercury compounds found in the effluent from the nearby fertilizer and plastic factory.

This condition has become known as Minamata disease and was the forerunner of many massive environmental health disasters induced by contemporary industrialization. Despite the sensational publicity from the standpoint of public health, medical research, and humanistic and legal aspects, the lessons have not been well learned. Similar disasters, some on a much larger scale involving thousands of patients, have been reported not only in Niigata, Japan but also in Iraq, Afghanistan, and South America. Organic mercury is probably one of the best investigated poisons both in humans and in experimental animals.

Human Intoxication by Organic Mercury Compounds: Source and Route of Entry

Sporadic occurrences in small groups of patients were reported among workers in a laboratory dealing with di-methyl mercury (Edwards, 1865) and in industries manufacturing fungicides and insecticides containing organic mercury compounds (Hunter et al., 1940; Herner, 1945; Ahlmark, 1948; I. A. Brown, 1954; Hay et al., 1963). The organic mercury in these accidents was in the form of powder or dusts, and it gained access to the body mostly by inhalation, but perhaps also by absorption through the skin. Indeed, the three patients reported by Okinaka et al. (1964) were poisoned following skin application of an ointment containing methyl mercury thioacetamide as a treatment for fungal infection.

Most cases, coming from several major and minor outbreaks, by now totaling several thousands of patients, have been poisoned following oral consumption of contaminated foodstuffs:

1. Fish and shellfish that were contaminated by industrial effluents containing alkylmercury in Minamata and Niigata, Japan (Tsubaki, Sato, Kondo, et al., 1967; Kumamoto University Study Group of Minamata Disease, 1968)
2. Breads or porridge made from seed grains that were coated with fungicides in Sweden (Engleson and Herner, 1952), Iraq (Jalili and Abbasi, 1961; Bakir et al., 1973), Pakistan (Haq, 1963), Guatemala (Ordonez et al. 1966), and Ghana (Derban, 1974)
3. Pork from hogs that were fed with seed grain coated with fungicides in New Mexico (Pierce et al., 1972)

Clinical Manifestations and Diagnosis

Evidence of methyl mercury poisoning typically appears several weeks, months, or even years after the continuous ingestion or absorption of a toxic dose, and consists predominantly of signs and symptoms of CNS involvement. Ataxia, dysarthria, and constriction of visual fields is the classic triad reported by Hunter et al. (1940) and observed in advanced cases of Minamata disease with moderate poisoning. In addition, sensory disturbances and difficulty in hearing were frequently found among patients in Minamata.

As increasing numbers of patients were described in Minamata, Niigata, Sweden, and Iraq, it has been found that the clinical manifestations of methyl mercury poisoning vary so widely that the clinical diagnosis of methyl mercury poisoning can be extremely difficult, if not impossible. Constriction of visual fields was considered to be relatively pathognomonic for methyl mercury poisoning, providing that retinal diseases were ruled out. Tsutsui and Okamura (1974) found a high incidence of disturbance of ocular pursuit movements and ocular dysmetria, and considered these signs to be quite characteristic of Minamata disease. However, these signs were found only in moderately severely affected patients in whom areas 18 and 19 of the paravisual cortex as well as the cerebellar cortex were involved.

Severe cases showed marked and generalized mental and neurologic deterioration progressing to spastic quadriparesis and coma, terminating in death within 100 days. Those who survived from severe methyl mercury encephalopathy were left with permanent disability with apallic syndrome and idiotic disorders (Takeuchi and Eto, 1976). At the other end of the spectrum, minor symptoms and signs may be few and subtle, including numerous nonspecific neurotic and psychiatric symptoms, such as fatigue, inability to concentrate, memory impairment, paresthesias, pain, and headache (Hook et al., 1954; Tsubaki, 1968; Tatetsu et al., 1969).

The clinical manifestations of methyl mercury encephalopathy are extremely variable, depending on the amount and duration of methyl mercury ingested and on the individual susceptibility. Similar syndromes and signs can be found in numerous other diseases, including toxic encephalopathy due to substances other than methyl mercury, chronic leptomeningitis, chronic encephalitis, many types of degenerative diseases of the CNS (including Alzheimer's disease), various slow-virus diseases, and cerebrovascular diseases. In mild cases, in which only subjective complaints are present, the diagnosis of methyl mercury intoxication is especially elusive, since these symptoms cannot be distinguished from those of cervical spondylosis, diabetic neuropathy, cerebral vascular disorders, hysteria, psychoneurosis, or even malingering (Tsubaki, 1974).

Ever since the several outbreaks of methyl mercury poisoning that have occurred throughout the world—most of which were the result of direct industrial hazards—extreme efforts have been made to prevent pollution of water and contamination of foodstuffs by mercury. Originally aimed at organic mercury, these efforts are now being directed also at inorganic mercury, which can be methylated by microorganisms in river and lake sediments (Jensen and Jernelov, 1969). Methyl mercury contamination of fish and wild fowl has been found to be alarmingly serious. A cat on northwestern Ontario reserves was shown by pathologic examination to have methyl mercury encephalopathy (Takeuchi, D'Itri, Fisher, et al., 1977*b*). Sixty-one Canadian Indians living in northwestern Quebec were found to have elevated mercury levels of more than 200 ng/ml, which has been considered by the WHO to be the lowest blood concentration associated with adverse health effects. Shepard (1976) has expressed difficulties in making a definite diagnosis of mild methyl mercury intoxication. Even with adquate knowledge of blood and brain mercury levels

over a 3-year period, including the autopsy, extensive brain assay, and neurohistologic evidence in a 71-year-old patient who had a blood mercury level of 551 μg/ml, tremor, hearing loss, and elevated brain tissue level of mercury, Wheatley et al. (1979) found the definitive diagnosis elusive.

PATHOLOGIC FINDINGS. The first autopsy report of methyl mercury intoxication was the human case reported by Hunter and Russell (1954). The patient died 15 years after the onset of paresthesias of the limbs and mouth followed by concentric constriction of the visual fields, speech difficulty, mild deafness, ataxia, nystagmus, and incoordination. These followed exposure to dusts of methyl mercury phosphate and nitrate. He was markedly incapacitated and remained relatively unchanged for 15 years, but his mental state was unaffected. The patient developed hypertension during the last years of his life and died of heart failure attributed to myocardial infarction at age 38.

The pathologic lesions in the CNS were multifocal atrophy of the cerebral cortex and cerebellum, most pronounced in the anterior calcarine cortex and the cerebellar folia in the depths of sulci in both lateral lobes posterior to the primary fissure and declive and culmen in the vermis. The topographic distribution of the atrophy in the cerebellum was highly suggestive of severe hypoxia, but the selective destruction of granule cells with relative sparing of Purkinje cells was the opposite of what one would expect in hypoxia. Hunter and Russell (1954) concluded that the changes were directly referable to the toxic action of organic mercury compounds, but they were unable to offer a better explanation for the localized nature of the degeneration than to suggest that the affected areas were, for some reason, more susceptible.

The epidemic of the strange disease *(Kibyo)* that appeared in the Minamata district of Kyushu, Japan, beginning in 1953 puzzled the Japanese and world medical communities for several years. Takeuchi et al. (1957) first described the pathologic lesions in four autopsied cases and concluded that it was a toxic encephalopathy. They added more observations on two subacute cases and four chronic cases; in 1959 they finally concluded that the neuropathologic picture was very similar to that reported by Hunter and Russell in 1954 and urged that organic mercury be investigated as the possible causative agent. During the ensuing years, the etiology of the strange disease now known as Minamata disease was finally established, and the diagnosis of methyl mercury intoxication has been made on increasing numbers of patients. As the number of patients increased, the extent of the clinical spectrum was expanded to include many patients who did not show the classical neurologic syndromes of methyl mercury encephalopathy but showed milder and less specific neurologic signs or subjective neuropsychiatric complaints. A suit was brought against the company that had polluted the bay, and the court ruled that the company was responsible for causing the disease in March 1973. As the patients were compensated for the damage, the number of applications to be certified as a patient with Minamata disease increased, and, as of November 1972, 1255 individuals were officially certified as patients, but several thousand more applications were pending verification (Harada, 1978). Among these patients were many who showed atypical clinical manifestations, formes frustes, mild cases, latent forms, and clinical symptoms of delayed onset. The problem concerning the diagnosis of Minamata disease thus became not only medical and scientific but also social, political, and economic. A Minamata disease verification committee was set up to certify patients with Minamata disease to qualify for receiving indemnity both in Minamata and Niigata. Patients were classified into six different categories: (1) Minamata disease, (2) effects of organic mercury toxicity present, (3) effects of organic mercury toxicity cannot be denied, (4) unknown, (5) not Minamata disease, and (6) re-examination necessary. The first three categories were qualified for compensation. This type of policy may be acceptable as a compromise for residents who lived within known polluted geographic areas, such as Minamata. However, such criteria and classification cannot be used for patients who reside in other areas where exposure to organic mercury compounds is not known or who have mild symptoms that are generally not specific (Tsubaki, 1974).

Similar difficulties and frustrations have occurred in the pathologic diagnosis of methylmercury poisoning. The neuropathologic findings reported during the early days of the epidemic in Minamata by Takeuchi et al. (1957) and Shiraki and Takeuchi (1971) were based on the autopsy of patients who died of fulminating methyl mercury encephalopathy, as in the case of Hunter and Russell (1954). Therefore, the findings were relatively constant, uniform, and severe, showing marked cerebellar degeneration (predominantly of the granular cell layer), spongy degeneration of the middle layers of the calcarine cortex, less severe and focal degeneration of the precentral and postcentral cortices, and frequent involvement of the putamen. Definitive pathologic changes were not found in peripheral nerves even though sensory symptoms indicating some type of sensory neuropathy were present in practically all of the patients. With more cases coming to autopsy, it was found that the anatomic distribution of the pathologic lesions in the CNS was much less selective in young children and infants (Matsumoto et al., 1965; Takeuchi and Eto, 1977), and in severe cases.

Takeuchi, Eto, Okabe, et al. (1977a) reviewed their 72 autopsied and 6 biopsied cases and classified them into six grades according to the severity and extensiveness of lesions. The basic pathologic change was that of single-cell necrosis with no or very little phagocytic reaction but with marked neuroglial reaction. As years went by, more patients with mild intoxication or with late onset of symptoms came to autopsy at old ages; the pathologic changes became not only less characteristic but also less clear and superimposed on other nonspecific degenerative changes of the CNS and cerebral blood vessels associated with senescence.

Takeuchi and Eto (1977), Eto et al. (1974), and Ikuta et al. (1974) were still able to separate those histopathologic lesions in the CNS characteristic of methyl mercury poisoning from nonspecific aging changes and changes due to cerebrovascular diseases in patients who showed chronic and mild clinical symptoms and who died at old ages.

However, it is inevitable that neuropathologists will face many frustrations, similar to those of the clinical neurologists (Tsubaki, 1974), when patients with mild or questionable exposure showing equivocal symptoms are presented for definitive diagnosis. Wheatley et al. (1979) reported on a 79-year-old Cree Indian who lived in a contaminated area and ate contaminated fish, and who showed toxic levels of Hg in his blood and hair 2 years before death. He showed tremors in his hands on several occasions and had diminished hearing of unknown duration. Higher, but not yet toxic levels of mercury were found in the brain, liver, and kidneys, but his CNS showed no histopathologic evidence of methyl mercury intoxication.

The case reported by I. A. Brown (1954) showed lesions in the ventral horns and pyramidal tracts of the spinal cord, resembling amyotrophic lateral sclerosis both clinically and neuropathologically. In the case of Hay et al. (1963), lesions in the white matter included the corpus callosum, anterior commissure, and subcortical white matter, as well as the cerebellar and cerebral cortex. In Brown's case phenyl mercury acetate was the cause of the poisoning and in the case of Hay et al., ethyl mercury chloride. Both ethyl and phenyl mercury are known to be less toxic as compared to methyl mercury. Whether the destructive lesions in different anatomic locations will be found to be characteristic of these two compounds must await more reports.

Experimental data on organic mercury poisoning in animals is voluminous. The lesions vary in anatomic sites with each species: The cerebellum seems to be the primary target in cats, the peripheral nerves and nerve roots in rats and mice, and the cerebral cortex in nonhuman primates. There is also a dose-specific effect, with maximal changes occurring in the dentate nucleus of the cerebellum, basal ganglia, and brain stem following a large dose of methyl mercury over a short period of time in monkeys (Shaw et al., 1975).

There are several excellent reviews and books, including "Methylmercury in Fish: A Toxicological and Epidemiological Evaluation of Risks" by Berglund et al. (1971), *Mercury in the Environment,* edited by Friberg and Vostal (1972), *Mercury, Mercurials and Mercaptans,* edited by Miller and Clarkson (1973), *Minamata Disease,* compiled by the Kumamoto University Study Group of Minamata Disease (1968), *Methylmercury Poisoning in Minamata and Niigata,* Japan, edited by Tsubaki and Irukayama (1975), and "Neuropathological Aspects of Organic Mercury Intoxication, Including Minamata Disease," by Shiraki (1979).

METHANOL INTOXICATION

As discussed previously, ethyl alcohol (ethanol) is our oldest and most popular social beverage; it has been legalized in most societies worldwide, although its hazards to life and health are well known and notorious. It affects the tissues and organs of the whole body, but the health hazards are seldom due to the direct effect of the ethanol. The health hazards are mostly secondary to the chronic and excessive consumption of ethanol, which predisposes to accidents, violence, and a number of diseases, and exaggerates pre-existing diseases.

On the contrary, methanol (wood alcohol or methyl alcohol) is much more toxic and has been known to cause either death or blindness in a large percentage of cases. Wood and Buller (1904) collected 275 cases of blindness and death related to methanol poisoning. It has been estimated that 6% of blindness in the U.S. Armed Forces during World War II was due to methanol poisoning (Cooper and Kini, 1962).

Source, Routes of Entry, and Doses

Methanol has been widely used as an organic solvent contained in varnish and shellac, and is used in the manufacture of paint, shoes, rubber, synthetic textiles, linoleum, dyes, and perfumes. It was used as an ingredient of patent medicine and tonics in the past and is still contained in denatured alcohol to prevent the oral consumption of rubbing alcohol.

Methanol is absorbed via the respiratory and gastrointestinal tracts as well as the skin. Poisoning among industrial workers by inhaling methanol fumes has been reported, and 200 ppm of methanol in the air is the maximum limit of safety in industry (Bennett et al., 1953). Methanol-containing skin rubs, hand lotions, and hair tonics may also be sources of poisoning. However, the most common form of methanol intoxication is the oral consumption of beverages in which a high proportion of methanol was included, accidentally or knowingly.

When ethanol was prohibited during the era of prohibition, privately distilled "moonshine" or "bootleg" whisky was produced and consumed. Methanol is much cheaper than ethanol because of its lower manufacturing cost and because it is not taxed, so that it was consumed straight or mixed in ethanolic drinks. A drink known as "heads" is a diluted shellac thinner, which usually contains 2.3–2.8% methanol and 51.4–61.5% ethanol. When one manufacturer changed the proportion of methanol and ethanol, 18 people were poisoned and 8 died in Kentucky (Kane et al., 1968). Methanol intoxication of this form tends to occur in clusters or in epidemics. An outbreak of 323 cases in Atlanta occurred in 1951 as a result of the ingestion of adulterated liquor (Bennett et al., 1953). Reports on epidemics involving small numbers of patients are numerous.

There is an extremely wide range of individual variation in tolerance to the ingestion of methanol without developing toxic signs. Ingestion of from 70 to 100 ml of methanol is usually fatal (Cooper and Kini, 1962), but as little as 10 ml of methanol has been fatal (Thienes, 1940). Blindness has resulted from an intake of as little as 4 ml of methanol (Bennett et al., 1953), but six Russians were known to drink 4 liters of 40% methanol without developing sequelae of methanol toxicity (Roe, 1946), and one man drank 1 pint of a 10% mixture daily without producing ill effects (Burhans, 1930). It appears that methanol is potentially toxic in any amount to anyone, but some individuals can tolerate more than others. However, there is no test known to determine the degree of tolerance or the risk of each individual until he or she tries.

Clinical Manifestations

Unlike ethanol intoxication, in which symptoms and signs of toxicity appear during the course of at the end of heavy drinking, methanol intoxication is characterized by an asymptomatic latent period between the ingestion of methanol and the onset of symptoms and signs. There is a wide range of individual variation in the length of this asymptomatic latent period, just as there is in tolerance. The symptoms of intoxication may appear as soon as an hour or as late as 72 hours after the ingestion (Cooper and Kini, 1962), but the latent period is usually between 12 and 24 hours. The initial symptoms are fatigue, headache, dizziness, vomiting, and abdominal cramps, followed by visual disturbances, which consist of yellow vision, photophobia, blurring or indistinct vision, and a diminished sensation of light. Blindness, partial or complete, may develop within hours or over days or weeks. In more severe cases, intense abdominal cramps, weakness, convulsions, and coma appear. Respirations may be rapid and shallow or of the Kussmaul type.

Examination typically shows dilated pupils with sluggish or no light reaction, with or without evidence of visual loss. The optic nerves are markedly hyperemic with mild to severe edema of the optic disk and the adjacent retina. Focal retinal hemorrhages and decreased intraocular tension have been found in some patients. The correlation of the funduscopic findings and the severity of the visual symptoms and signs is generally poor. Mental confusion, memory loss, maniacal behavior, and delirium may occur before stupor and coma. There is no good correlation between the severity of the symptoms and the dose of methanol consumed. The progression of the clinical symptoms can be so rapid that some patients will not reach the hospital alive.

Laboratory Data and Pathogenesis

The most significant laboratory finding in patients with methanol intoxication is severe metabolic acidosis as determined by the CO_2-combining power of the blood, which falls to below 20 mEq/liter. The blood pH is low, as is that of the urine. Moderate ketonemia, albuminuria, and acetonuria may also occur. Serum sodium and potassium are generally normal, except in those who are overtreated with alkali for acidosis and develop hypokalemia or hypernatremia. Bennett et al. (1953) observed consistently higher methanol levels in the CSF than in the blood. Roe (1943) reported elevated lactic acid levels in blood.

The metabolism of ingested methanol in humans is about five times slower than that of ethanol. Up to 50% of ingested methanol is eliminated unchanged through the lungs, and 2–10% through the kidneys. Methanol is also secreted into the gastric juices in concentrations 5–12 times greater than those in the blood even 10 days after poisoning (Bennett et al., 1953).

A large part of the ingested methanol is oxidized to formaldehyde and then to formic acid by an alcohol dehydrogenase in the liver and kidney. Formic acid is 6 times and formaldehyde 33 times as toxic as methanol (Keeney and Mellinkoff, 1951). It is likely that the asymptomatic latent period represents the time required for methanol to break down into significant levels of formaldehyde and formic acid, which then cause the toxic syndrome. Formic acid is excreted in the urine, reaching a maximum value in 1 to 2 days after ingestion but continuing for 4 to 10 days. Formic acid is considered to be the major cause of the fall in pH and CO_2-combining power of the blood (Roe, 1943), and formaldehyde is thought to be the major agent responsible for the retinal injury in that it is concentrated in the vitreous, which is right next to the ganglion cells of the retina.

Pathologic Findings

The findings at autopsy in fatal cases of methanol poisoning include variable degrees of cerebral edema and hyperemia, pulmonary edema with patchy atelectasis, and petechial hemorrhages and minor hemorrhages in many organs (Menne, 1938; Branch and Tonning, 1945; Chew et al., 1946; Keeney and Mellinkoff, 1951; Bennett et al., 1953). Petechiae have been especially numerous in the walls of the third ventricle, the periaqueductal region, and the floor of the fourth ventricle (Schneck, 1979). Necrosis of the putamina with cystic changes has been found and regarded as a specific finding for methanol poisoning by some (Orthner, 1953). McLean et al (1980) reported extensive cystic necrosis of the putamina and frontal while matter as well as widespread neuronal damage throughout the cerebrum, cerebellum, brain stem, and spinal cord in a patient who had been blind with a parkinsonian syndrome and mild dementia following acute methanol poisoning 11 months earlier. Their second patient was alive at the time of the report, showed similar clinical findings and CT-lucent areas in prefrontal white matter and putamina 9 months after acute methanol poisoning.

The significance of the pathologic changes in the eyes has been the subject of some conflict, as some patients died rapidly before unequivocal histologic changes appeared in the retina and because of difficulties in fixation and preparation of eyes for histologic examination. Most authors, however, agree on the presence of antemortem degeneration of all neuronal elements, the ganglion cells, internal and outer granular cells. MacDonald (1929) described cystic spaces in the layer of ganglion cells, irregular external nuclear layer, irregular rod and cone nuclei, migration of pigment granules, and congestion of choroidal vessels. Edema and hyperemia and later associated gliosis have been observed in the optic nerves and have been considered as secondary degeneration.

Ingested methanol is distributed throughout tissues in relation to their water content (Cooper and Kini, 1962). The aqueous and vitreous humors of the eye and the CSF thus acquire the highest concentration of methanol (Benton and Calhoun, 1952). This partly explains the predilection for injury to the retina and to the CNS, even though formaldehyde, one of the degradation products of methanol, is the accepted cause of the retinal injury and not methanol itself. The retina has a greater oxygen consumption via aerobic glycolysis in proportion to its iron content than any other tissue. Formaldehyde disturbs retinal glycolysis and respiration by interfering with ATP generation, and uncouples oxidative phosphorylation (Potts and Johnson, 1952; Cooper and Kini, 1962).

Prognosis

Although the narcotic effect of very high methanol levels may be the cause of death in some cases, most patients die of severe metabolic acidosis. Thus, the prognosis depends on the degree of severity of the acidosis and the effectiveness of the treatment of acidosis. Those who die are almost always blind or nearly so. All patients with severe retinal edema are left with variable degrees of visual loss. Many patients have some recovery of vision, especially those who are treated early in the course of the poisoning. Primary optic atrophy appears in 1 to 2 months in cases of permanent retinal damage.

Treatment

The treatment should consist of three parts: (1) Administer ethanol to saturate the alcohol dehydrogenase to prevent degradation of methanol; (2) treat the metabolic acidosis by administering intravenous bicarbonate; and (3) remove methanol and its toxic by-products by dialysis (Chew et al., 1946; Roe, 1969). Needless to say, the earlier the treatment is begun, the better the prognosis.

Animal Experiments

Since it was not known that there are marked species differences in the metabolism of methanol, the data obtained from animal experiments in the early days were controversial and there were discrepancies as compared with human cases. It was primarily Roe (1946) and subsequently Gilger and Potts (1955) who showed that the toxic effects of methanol on nonprimates were due to the narcotic effect seen with overdoses of various alcohols and were completely different from the effects seen in humans. Metabolic acidosis (due to the metabolism of methanol into formic acid) and marked toxicity to the retina (due to another metabolic product, formaldehyde) are observed only in humans and monkeys. In spite of this, no significant differences in retinal glycolysis and respiration, and their disturbances by formaldehyde, were found between nonprimate and primate retinas in vitro (Potts and Johnson 1952; Cooper and Kini, 1962). Cooper and Kini (1962) postulated three explanations for these species differences: (1) slow metabolism of methanol but rapid breakdown of formaldehyde in nonprimates, (2) poorly vascularized retinas in rabbits and guinea pigs, and (3) differences in the sensitivity of retinal cells to formaldehyde.

ALCOHOLIC CEREBELLAR DEGENERATION (RESTRICTED DEGENERATION OF THE CEREBELLAR CORTEX IN ALCOHOLIC PATIENTS)

A distinct cerebellar syndrome has been recognized in patients with chronic alcoholism. The clinical manifestations are practically constant, characterized by wide-based ataxic gait, incoordination of the legs, and truncal ataxia with mild or no involvement of the arms or speech. Nystagmus is infrequent. The syndrome is most common in middle-aged males with a long history of chronic alcohol abuse, but a history of abstinence may be present in some patients.

Following an extensive analysis of 50 cases and a review of the medical literature concerning "restricted degeneration of the cerebellar cortex in alcoholic patients," Victor, Adams, and Mancall (1959) concluded that the majority of these patients showed a characteristic biphasic clinical course in which the initial progressive phase developed over a short period of time, reaching a point of maximum intensity in weeks or months, and followed by the second phase of neurologic stability that lasted for many years.

The neuropathologic change in these patients is also remarkably stereotypic. The lesion is almost always localized in the anterior vermis with varying degress of extension into the most anterior and superior portions of the cerebellar hemispheres. Earlier investigators stressed a selective involvement of Purkinje cells but, based on meticulous pathologic studies of 11 autopsied cases, Victor et al. (1959) concluded that all elements of the cerebellar cortex are involved. They refuted the idea of primary involvement of any single cell type in the cerebellar cortex but admitted that Purkinje cells, being the most sensitive element, may be the only cells to show pathologic alteration in cases with only mild involvement. The inferior olives are also almost always involved, but the involvement of the deep cerebellar nuclei is less constant and the dentate nuclei, cerebellar white matter, and brain stem nuclei are usually spared.

Many etiologic factors had been implicated by earlier investigators, including syphilis, tuberculosis and other infectious diseases, cancer, diabetes mellitus and other metabolic diseases, as well as cerebrovascular diseases. Alcohol as an etiologic factor was first suggested by A. Thomas (1905), subsequently supported by Stender and Lüthy (1931), and now recognized as the only factor common to all these patients (Romano et al., 1940; Victor et al., 1959). However, as in other forms of chronic alcoholic complications, such as Wernicke-Korsakoff encephaloneuropathy and alcoholic neuropathy, the same argument has persisted regarding whether the cerebellar degeneration is due to repeated direct narcotic effects of alcohol, to the associated malnutritional states in chronic alcoholism, or to both. Cerebellar syndromes have been reported in patients with severe vitamin deficiencies, such as pellagra, but we are not aware of any pathologic report verifying cerebellar degeneration similar to that of alcoholic cerebellar degeneration. Furthermore, dramatic recovery or clinical improvement by vitamin treatments is the general rule in Wernicke-Korsakoff encephaloneuropathy but not in alcoholic cerebellar degeneration.

PHENYTOIN (DIPHENYLHYDANTOIN, DILANTIN)

Since its introduction as an anticonvulsive drug by Merritt and Putnam in 1938, phenytoin (DPH) has been the drug of choice in the treatment of many forms of epilepsy, especially grand mal and psychomotor seizures. Because of the nature of the conditions for which it is given, DPH is administered daily for many years in order to maintain an effective plasma level, which is generally considered to be 10–20 μg/ml. DPH may be prescribed alone but usually is administered with other anticonvulsive drugs, such as phenobarbital.

The pharmacodynamics and pharmacokinetics of DPH have been intensively investigated. The therapeutic effects and toxicity of DPH depend on its plasma levels, which do not necessarily correlate with the administered dose. Since DPH has to be taken by epileptic patients for an extended period of time, many of these patients contract other diseases, including injuries or pregnancy, for which the patient will be treated with other appropriate medications or procedures. Pregnancy has been known to lower the plasma DPH level, presumably by extension of its distribution to the fetus. DPH is also known to lower the effects of some steroids, contraceptives, anticoagulants, and antibiotics.

In contrast, simultaneous administration of some other drugs may increase the plasma levels of DPH. Isoniazid and disulfiram are well known for such effects, and DPH toxicity may appear as the result of adding these drugs without increasing the dose of DPH itself (Houghton and Richens, 1974). Some other antiepileptic drugs, especially sulthiame, are known to act similarly.

Toxic symptoms may appear when the

plasma DPH level exceeds 20 μg/ml. Severe intoxications with DPH are rare, but mild side effects are relatively common, and transient if the dose is decreased. The incidence of side effects ranges from 12% to 38% of DPH-treated patients (Schmidt, 1982).

The anticonvulsant activity of DPH is due to its action on the basic properties of membranes, synapses, and metabolic processes by elevating membrane potentials, raising thresholds, reducing conduction velocity and spike amplitude, and reducing or abolishing repetitive firing of nerve cells and processes.

Three major neurologic syndromes are induced by DPH: encephalopathy, cerebellar degeneration, and peripheral neuropathy. These syndromes are generally accepted to result from DPH toxicity, since the appearance of symptoms and signs correlates with an increase in the DPH plasma levels, and since the symptoms disappear when the DPH plasma level is lowered by reducing or discontinuing DPH administration.

Encephalopathy (Anticonvulsant Encephalopathy)

The clinical features of DPH-induced encephalopathy are quite variable, usually mild but proportional to the increasing plasma concentrations of DPH: irritability, headache, tremor, vertigo, ataxia, dysarthria, nystagmus, delirium, psychosis, depression, deterioration of intellectual function, choreoathetosis, asterixis, dystonia, orofacial dyskinesias, spasticity, increased deep tendon reflexes, and others. These are all reversible and disappear after reduction in dose or discontinuation of DPH therapy, providing that these symptoms are not due to other anticonvulsive drugs, such as carbamazepine or primidone, or to other neuroleptic drugs such as phenothiazine, diazepam, or mitrazepam. A reversible syndrome including progressive mental deterioration, brain stem and cerebellar signs, EEG changes, and an increase in seizure frequency during treatment with DPH has been denoted as anticonvulsant encephalopathy or phenytoin encephalopathy (Levy and Fenichel, 1965). Increased seizure frequency without other signs of clinical toxicity but with high DPH concentration has been observed in some patients and considered as "paradoxic intoxication" (Troupin and Ojemann, 1975). No specific neuropathology is known for these conditions.

Cerebellar Degeneration

Nystagmus and ataxia indicative of cerebellar malfunction are well-known clinical manifestations of DPH toxicity. The symptoms are clearly related to the plasma DPH levels. Nystagmus can appear at a serum DPH level of about 20 μg/ml, ataxia at 30 μg/ml, and mental changes at 40 μg/ml (Kutt et al., 1964).

Cerebellar atrophy or degeneration with diffuse loss of Purkinje and granule cells has been reported in many epileptic patients with DPH (Hoffmann, 1958; Selhorst et al., 1972; Ghatak et al., 1976; Rapport and Shaw, 1977; Koller et al., 1980; McLain et al., 1980). Purkinje cell loss and Bergmann's gliosis have been produced in experimental animals with high plasma DPH levels (Kokenge et al., 1965).

With this experimental evidence and clinical, pharmacologic, and pathologic correlations observed in human patients, it is generally agreed that DPH can cause selective degeneration of the cerebellum, especially of Purkinje cells, in humans. For example, cerebellar degeneration has been observed in a patient receiving DPH but without seizures (Rapport and Shaw, 1977). However, the reverse is not always true; that is to say, cerebellar atrophy or degeneration in epileptic patients treated with DPH is not always caused by DPH. Cerebellar degeneration, selective or associated with other lesions in the CNS, is a relatively common type of pathologic process that can be caused by a large number of etiologic agents. One of the most common causes of cerebellar degeneration, especially of selective degeneration and death of Purkinje cells, is hypoxia-ischemia, which is a frequent complication of major motor seizures and status epilepticus, and which was observed in epileptic patients by Spielmeyer (1930) long before the introduction of DPH.

Although there are no generally accepted criteria to separate a cerebellar degeneration induced by DPH toxicity from that caused by hypoxia-ischemia, we believe that DPH toxicity produces more generalized lesions and hypoxia-ischemia more focalized lesions. This difference in the distribution of lesions in some cases is striking, in that vascular lesions tend to localize at the depths of fissures and sulci or to be lobular in arterial boundary zones, whereas toxic lesions are more diffuse and show no preference for watershed areas. However, the difference is relative, and often no difference can be seen, because many patients show cerebellar degeneration due to a mixture of both effects. In early and mild stages, Purkinje cells are selectively destroyed and Bergmann's gliosis follows. In more advanced or severe cases, granule cells are involved and their number is reduced. Almost total destruction of both Purkinje and granule cells may be seen in patients with severe and prolonged DPH intoxication, but these are usually combined with a history of frequent status epilepticus.

Peripheral Neuropathy

Weakness and dysesthesia with loss of deep tendon reflexes in the lower extremities have been noted in 8% to 18% of epileptic patients receiving long-term DPH treatments, often in combination with other anticonvulsants (Lovelace and Horwitz, 1968; Dobkin, 1977). These findings are more likely to occur in patients who have been on therapy for more than 10 years. Nerve conduction is impaired. Vitamin B_{12} and folic acid deficiency have been suspected as pathogenic factors, but their levels have been found to be normal, and treatment with folic acid does not produce any improvement in the polyneuropathy (Horwitz et al., 1968). The primary pathologic changes are thought to be axonal degeneration, but there have been no histologic studies to prove this.

VINCRISTINE (VCR) TOXICITY

Vincristine sulfate (Oncovin R) is a vinca alkaloid that has been in use as an antineoplastic chemotherapeutic agent since the 1960s. The mechanism of the antineoplastic activity is considered to be inhibition of microtubule formation in the mitotic spindle, resulting in an arrest of cell division at metaphase. It has been found to be most effective in the treatment of acute lymphoblastic leukemia in children, but its use has been extended to treat lymphomas and other solid tumors. VCR is usually administered intravenously and orally, but occasionally it may be given intrathecally for leptomeningeal leukemia, since VCR does not cross the BBB. VCR may be given singly as an antineoplastic drug but more commonly is used in combination with other antineoplastic chemotherapeutic agents in so-called MOPP (VCR, nitrogen mustard, procarbazine, and prednisone) or eight-in-one cocktails.

Unfortunately, VCR is highly neurotoxic. The most common toxic manifestation is a peripheral neuropathy, which occurs in almost every patient who receives VCR (Rosenthal and Kaufman, 1974). Both sensory and motor components are involved. Spinal nerves are most commonly involved, but cranial and autonomic nerves may also be affected. VCR polyneuropathy is usually symmetric. The earliest and most consistent objective sign is suppression of the ankle jerk (Sandler et al., 1969; Holland et al., 1973). Loss of ankle jerk alone was noted in 60% of patients, and 48% eventually manifested depression of other deep tendon reflexes. Paresthesias involving the feet or hands or both may appear simultaneously or be followed by loss of deep tendon reflexes; this was found in 57% of 392 patients (Holland et al., 1973), but serious objective sensory loss was relatively uncommon, occurring in only 4%. These symptoms may last for several weeks before the appearance of motor involvement, which is characterized by impaired dorsiflexion of the toes and feet and of the extensors of the fingers and wrists, eventually progressing to foot drop, wrist drop, and slapping gait. Bilateral ptosis, diplopia, abducens nerve palsies, and facial palsies have been observed in 4% to 10% of patients (Sandler et al., 1969). Bilateral vocal cord palsies were found in 5 of 392 patients (Holland et al., 1973). These symptoms are partially or completely reversible when the drug is withdrawn. Paresthesias are the most readily reversible, followed by motor and sensory loss. Deep tendon reflexes return slowly, if at all.

VCR polyneuropathy is usually related to the total dose of VCR and to the duration of treatment, but there are some exceptions. Severe VCR neurotoxicity manifested by quadriplegia, quadriparesis, or paraplegia, and bulbar palsy have been reported in patients who received relatively small doses of VCR. The case of Weiden and Wright (1972) had pre-existing Charcot-Marie-Tooth syndrome, but the cases of Mubashir and Bart (1972) and Wheeler and Votaw (1974) neither had a pre-existing neurologic disorder nor received other neurotoxic drugs. Weiden and Wright (1972) emphasized that the pre-existing neurologic disorder predisposed the patient to a severe VCR neurotoxicity, whereas Casey et al. (1973) reported no signs of excessive susceptibility to VCR neurotoxicity in a patient with a pre-existing severe diabetic neuropathy. Mubashir and Bart (1972) and Wheeler and Votaw (1974) considered these manifestations to be "idiosyncrasy" of VCR. An interesting phenomenon was reported by Hildebrand and Kenis (1971), who observed three patients developing severe neuropathy after discontinuing VCR administration but after receiving different drugs, isoniazid in two and L-asparaginase in one. The authors suggested that a cumulative toxicity of VCR and isoniazid or L-asparaginase might be responsible for the pathogenesis of the late appearance of severe polyneuritis.

Pathologic observations by Moress et al. (1967) on three autopsied patients with acute lymphoblastic leukemia who had been treated with VCR and who developed severe and irreversible peripheral neuropathy showed a varying degree of myelin loss and axonal degeneration. The majority of evidence, however, suggests that VCR is toxic primarily to the neurons and its processes rather than to myelin or Schwann cells.

In addition to the polyneuropathy, seizures and mental changes suggestive of CNS involvement have been reported during VCR therapy. VCR toxicity has been suggested in many of these reports. However, a clear causal relationship between VCR administration and CNS symptoms has not been established. In most cases, underlying neuropathologic conditions, such as leptomeningeal leukemia, infectious diseases, or cerebral hemorrages, could not be ruled out. In some cases the seizures were shown to be related to VCR-induced hyponatremia and not to the drug itself (Fine et al., 1966).

Neuropathologic reports of VCR toxicity are relatively few compared to the many clinical reports. Most neuropathologic reports have focused on the peripheral nervous system (Moress et al., 1967; McLeod and Penny, 1969), but a fatal encephalopathy in a 2½-year-old child who died 3 days after receiving 3 mg intrathecal VCR was reported by Schochet et al (1968). The autopsy showed striking changes characterized by clumped Nissl bodies separated by clear areas and acidophilic rhombohedral crystals in the cytoplasm of the ventral horn cells of the spinal cord and motor nuclei of the medulla. The clear areas of the cytoplasm were argentophilic and consisted of skeins of interwoven neurofilaments. The crystals appeared as either parallel rows of punctate osmophilic densities or arrays of circular profiles, depending on the plane of section. Schochet et al. (1968) also studied rabbits that showed neuronal changes that closely resembled those found in the human case in the reticular formation, hypoglossal nucleus, and dorsal motor nucleus of the vagus in the medulla, as well as in neurons in the pons and ventral horns of cervical cord. Shelanski and Wisniewski (1969) reported autopsy findings in three children who had been treated with VCR for leukemia, only one of whom showed clinical VCR neurotoxicity before death in the following year. Diffuse or patchy tigrolysis by light histology and neurofibrillary degeneration by electron microscopy were similar to those observed by Schochet et al. (1968) in neurons of spinal ganglia, spinal cord, medulla, pons, and cerebellum. These changes are essentially similar to those seen in experimentally produced neurofibrillary degeneration in animals or HeLa cells by colchicine and vinblastine (Robbins and Gonatas, 1964). All of these agents have been considered to be mitotic spindle inhibitors. Colchicine has been shown to exert its antimitotic action by binding to the subunit protein of the mitotic spindle tubule (Shelanski and Taylor, 1967). This binding has been shown to occur also with other cytoplasmic microtubules, including those in the nervous system (Adelman et al., 1968). As a result, microtubules are broken down with concomitant proliferation of neurofilaments, axoplasmic flow is disrupted, and eventually axonal degeneration occurs.

Intoxications Causing Predominantly White Matter Damge

Damage to white matter may be spongy in appearance microscopically or not.

Spongy Degenerations

Spongy Degeneration of the Cerebral and Cerebellar White Matter in Infancy (van Bogaert-Bertrand Type, Canavan's Disease)

Many investigators consider this disorder to be a chronic edema in infants of unknown etiology. This is a rare condition characterized by diffuse spongy degeneration or vacuolation of the cerebral and cerebellar white matter occurring in young infants. Clinically, it is difficult to distinguish this disorder from Tay-Sachs' disease or various leukodystrophies, such as Krabbe's or Schilder's diseases. The onset of the disease is noted within the first few months of life; indeed, some of the cases show signs of abnormality at birth. Clinical manifestations include arrest of psychomotor development, spasticity or flaccidity, enlarging head, blindness, and deafness, progressing to death at 2 or 3 years of age. A few cases have been designated as juvenile forms because of a later onset and survival up to late adolescence.

Megalencephaly has been considered to be one of the most characteristic macroscopic features. The brain of Canavan's case (1931) weighed 1890 g at age 16 months. However, enlargement of the brain is not a constant feature throughout the whole duration of clinical course. Adachi and Aronson (1967) found that the brain at autopsy may be swollen, normal, or atrophic. Coronal sections of the cerebrum show soft, pale, and gelatinous white matter with poor gray-white demarcation. The ventricles may be normal, compressed, or dilated depending on the stage of the illness.

The histologic features are relatively constant and unique in showing spongy appearance of the subcortical white matter, often extending into the deeper layers of the cerebral cortex. The spongy appearance is due to multiple small vacuoles ranging from 50 to 100μm in diameter. Concomitant paucity of myelin is invariably present. Electron-microscopically, the vacuoles represent swollen astrocytic cytoplasm and interlaminar blebs of myelin. Most authors have found the spongy degeneration to be most striking in the cerebrum, often involving the centrum semiovale, but some (Zu Rhein et al., 1960; Sachs et al., 1965) found it to be more striking in the cerebellar white matter. The internal capsule, corpus callosum, and fornix are relatively well preserved in the early stages. Vacuolation of the optic nerves, optic tracts, basal ganglia, and spinal cord is frequently found, as well as vacuolation of the ganglion cell layer of the retina (Zu Rhein et al., 1960). Astrocytic type II astrocytes are found throughout the cortex.

Originally, this condition was thought to be a type of diffuse sclerosis or leukodystrophy, a variant of Krabbe's disease (Globus and Strauss, 1928; Canavan, 1931; Jervis, 1942). Earlier cases were found mostly in Jewish children and siblings were frequently affected, so that it was considered to be a genetically determined metabolic disorder. Decreased ATPase activity has been found in abnormal mitochondria of the astrocytes, but no enzyme defect has been demonstrated. Blackwood and Cumings (1954) considered the condition to be due to arrest of myelination at an early stage of fetal life. van Bogaert and Bertrand (1949) suggested that the basic process is consistent with chronic edema. The water content in apparently normal white matter was increased to 92.2% and in demyelinated white matter 91.5% in case A, who was 23 months of age at the time of autopsy (Blackwood and Cumings, 1954). The water content in the fresh white matter was 86.9% in the case of Zu Rhein et al. (1960), biopsied at age 8 months. Zu Rhein et al. (1960) and Sachs et al. (1965) agreed with van Bogaert and Bertrand (1949), and considered the poor myelination of the white matter to be secondary to cerebral edema.

Sachs et al. (1965) raised the possibility of a toxic encephalopathy. They considered the case of Globus and Strauss (1928) to be more suggestive of intoxication than of endogenous metabolic or degenerative diseases because the 7-month-old infant became suddenly ill and died in 4 days. They also noted electron-microscopic similarities with triethyltin poisoning in animals. Assays of metals have been performed in two cases: the case of Zu Rhein et al. (1960) showed increased urinary zinc and copper, and the case of Sachs et al. (1965) showed a 10-fold increase of calcium in the liver and white matter. Sachs et al. thought that a metal-dependent enzyme system might be specifically involved. Evidence supporting metal intoxication remains insufficient.

Fatty degeneration of the liver has been occasionally recorded (Blackwood and Cummings, 1854; Sachs et al., 1965). Thus, spongy degeneration of the white matter may be a special form of Reye's syndrome occurring in young infants who are more tolerant to cerebral edema because of their expansible skull, resulting in a protracted clinical course and early megalencephaly. The strikingly spongy appearance of the af-

fected white matter may be due to a slightly different pattern of fluid distribution in the developing white matter compared to the more mature myelinated white matter.

Isonicotinic Acid Hydrazine (INH)

Spongy degeneration of the white matter, myelin destruction, and gliosis have been produced with INH in the dog brain by Palmer and Noel (1965) and in the cerebellar white matter of Peking ducks by Carlton and Kreutzberg (1966). Palmer and Noel (1965) produced similar lesions in dogs with methanolsulfonate derivatives of INH.

Cuprizone

Cuprizone, a chelator used as a reagent for copper analysis, has been found by Carlton (1967) to be toxic, producing hydrocephalus, edema, demyelination, and astrogliosis of the cerebellar white matter in mice. Suzuki and Kikkawa (1969) produced spongy degeneration of the brain stem, cerebrum and cerebellum, and Alzheimer's type II astrocytes by feeding mice cuprizone. Johnson and Ludwin (1981) demonstrated a "dying back" phenomenon of oligodendroglia by EM, with recurrent demyelination and remyelination of axons in the CNS of mice, produced by oral cuprizone.

Hexachlorophene

Hexachlorophene (HCP), 2,2'-methylene-bis(3,4,6-trichlorophenol), was patented in 1941 by Gump, and was used extensively as an antimicrobial agent for more than three decades. It was incorporated into many cosmetics, toilet soaps, and antiseptic solutions, and was sold over the counter, probably most commonly as a 3% emulsion known as pHisoHex. It also has anthelmintic effects and was used to treat clonorchis sinensis (Liu et al., 1963). Until the mid-1970s, it was common practice to bathe newborn babies and burned patients with pHisoHex to prevent and control the spread of staphylococcal skin infection. By this time, because of a proposal to use HCP as a broad-spectrum fungicide and bactericide on food crops, the FDA had become interested in the potential toxicology of HCP, not only through the GI tract but also through the skin. HCP is absorbed only slightly through intact skin, but is easily absorbed through premature or damaged skin. Curley et al. (1971) demonstrated that the mean HCP concentration was 0.02 μg/g in cord blood at birth but rose to 0.11 μg/g in blood at the time of discharge 1–11 days later from hospitals where newborn babies were regularly bathed with pHisoHex.

The neurotoxicity of HCP has been shown to be age dependent, and the pattern of lesions in the brain in human patients varies widely depending not only on the age of the patient but also on the dose and route of administration.

The first clinical case of HCP toxicity in humans was reported by Herter (1959) in a baby who received application of 3% HCP daily for 4 days, developed peeling of the skin and generalized convulsions, but recovered 6 days later. Wear et al. (1962) reported 10 patients who accidentally ingested HCP and who developed symptoms of toxicity, which were mainly gastrointestinal and not neurologic. Liu et al. (1963) used oral HCP, 20 mg/kg/day for 3 days, to treat clonchris sinensis in 150 patients, and found gastrointestinal symptoms, including diarrhea, abdominal pain, and vomiting, to be very common, involving over half of the patients. Mild neurologic symptoms were also common, but were severe in only one patient, who became comatose during the fourth day but recovered completely. Fatal cases of HCP toxicity were reported by Lustig (1963), Mullick (1973), Martinez et al. (1974), Henry and diMaio (1974), and Lockhart (1972). Lockhart (1972) reported seizures, disorientation, irrational behavior, and coma in patients with extensive burns following applications of HCP, and seizures and respiratory failure in four women who left vaginal packs with 3% HCP in situ for several days. Two of these women died.

Larson (1968) found the serum HCP concentration to be elevated to 4 to 78 μg/ml serum in eight patients who developed "burn encephalopathy," and suggested that HCP treatment was the most likely etiologic agent for "burn encephalopathy."

According to Mullick (1973), two adult patients who ingested a large amount of HCP and died within 48 hours did not show either cerebral edema or vacuolation of the white matter, but four children who developed clinical symptoms 6 hours to 10 days after topical application of HCP showed severe vacuolation of the cerebral white matter. A 46-year-old woman who died 44 hours after ingestion of 200 ml pHisoHex showed no abnormality in the brain (Henry and DiMaio, 1974).

The case of Martinez et al. (1974) was a 7-year-old boy who ingested 45 ml of pHisoHex in a 3-day period and died about 5 days later. The brain showed edema and extensive white matter vacuolation, especially predominant in the optic pathways.

Premature infants are especially susceptible to HCP toxicity. Powell et al. (1973) reported spongy vacuolation of the brain stem in seven premature infants who were topically exposed more than three times to HCP. Extensive epidemiologic and clinico-neuropathologic studies by Shuman et al. (1974, 1975) of 248 children and 46 premature infants from the University of Washington Hospital and Children's Orthopedic Hospital from 1966 to 1974 showed that the vacuolar degeneration of the reticular formation in the caudal brain stem, the site of vasomotor and respiratory centers, was related to whole-body bathing with HCP. Indeed, it was the preliminary report of these findings in 1972 that led to a controversy between the CDC, which did not want to lose a potentially beneficial drug, and the FDA, which had banned over-the-counter sales of HCP.

The severity of the neuropathologic lesions is age and dose dependent. It is found predominantly in the reticular formation of the caudal brain stem (medulla) in premature infants weighing less than 1400 g and when undiluted pHisoHex was used. It can occur in older infants or even adults when their skin is abnormal (e.g., with burns or dermatitis), but the lesions tend to affect the central tegmental tract in the rostral brain stem (midbrain).

The type of lesion induced by HCP is quite characteristic. The central tegmentum of the medulla and/or caudal pons shows clusters of small vacuoles. Similar lesions were produced in young rats by topical and parenteral administration of hexachlorophene; indeed, 1-week-old rats can be killed by two daily baths in pHisoHex (Shuman, Leech, and Alvord, 1975).

Cerebral edema and spongy degeneration of the cerebral and cerebellar white matter were produced by HCP in rats by Kimbrough and Gaines (1971). Electron-microscopic studies showed accumulation of fluid within myelin sheaths, the features resembling those of triethyltin and INH intoxication (Lampert et al., 1973).

OTHER DAMAGE TO WHITE MATTER

Damage to white matter need not produce a spongy appearance. Several examples are discussed in the following paragraphs.

Marchiafava-Bignami Disease *

In 1903 two Italian pathologists, Marchiafava and Bignami, described a peculiar neuropathologic entity that occurred in three Italian peasants who were heavily addicted to cheap red wine. The pathologic lesions described were sharply circumscribed areas of gray degeneration, sometimes cystic, localized to the central portion of the corpus callosum and other commissural bundles. The condition was considered for decades to be indigenous to adult Italian males of lower socioeconomic class who were addicted to local crude red wine (Lolli, 1941). This presumption was gradually refuted as other cases were reported involving other ethnic groups in other countries in Europe and in North and South America, and in persons who habitually drank beer, whis-

key, white wine, or other spirits than the crude Italian red wine. Ironside et al. (1961) reviewed 88 documented cases in the medical literature including 60 Italians, 8 Frenchmen, 2 Frenchwomen, and 18 others, and added the second English patient who drank beer and stout. By 1971 Castaigne et al. (1971) found the total number of acceptable cases in the literature to have increased to 105, to which they added 10 more cases from France. Although the patients are no longer exclusively of Italian extraction, the incidence in Latins, especially Italians, is still remarkably high; and there have been no cases reported from Scandinavia, where alcohol consumption is usually considered to be high. No cases have been reported from the Far East, and only two Asians, including a Thai (Ishizaki et al., 1970) and an Indian (Leong, 1979).

Almost all the patients have been adult males except for the two Frenchwomen; almost all have been chronic alcoholics except for two patients reported in the United States and one in Malaysia, in whom the history of alcoholism could not be obtained (King and Meehan, 1936; Merritt and Weisman, 1945). The condition is rare and the clinical manifestations are not clear-cut as the distinct neuropathologic findings; hence, the antemortem diagnosis is almost impossible.

Marchiafava (1933) attempted to distinguish this rare syndrome (which he called dementia alcoholica progressiva) from the usual and less specific form of alcoholic dementia and emphasized its fairly sudden onset with convulsions, stupor, rigidity of the limbs, dysphasia, and dyspraxia. Lolli (1941) stressed the prominent mental and psychic manifestations, such as excitability, irritability, fits of rage, acts of violence, changes in affection, moral and sexual perversions, confusion, dementia, and epileptic seizures as contrasted with patients with Wernicke's encephalopathy in whom neurologic symptoms and signs predominate. Ironside et al. (1961) also observed hallucinations, amnesia, and symptoms similar to those of delirium tremens. However, Castaigne et al. (1971) distinguished acute

* Marchiafava's Disease, Dementia Alcoholica Progressiva of Marchiafava, Postcoholic Commissural and Central Necrosis.

and chronic forms, the chronic form showing progressive dementia with or without subacute phase. The duration of the illness varies from a few days to several months, with an average of 3 to 6 weeks.

The pathologic features are constant, even diagnostic, characterized by sharply outlined demyelination or necrosis in the central portion of the corpus callosum, the anterior commissure, and occasionally the optic chiasm and brachium pontis. The lesion in the corpus callosum is best seen on coronal sections of the brain. The lesion does not involve the whole dorsoventral extent of the corpus callosum but preserves the dorsal and ventral lamellae, although it may extend laterally and dorsally into the centrum semiovale.

The internal capsules and subcortical arcuate fibers are always spared. The lesion is usually most marked in the anterior third of the corpus callosum and in the midline, but two symmetric lesions on each side of the midline may be seen in the posterior corpus callosum. The less common lesions in the brachium pontis are bilateral and symmetric.

Microscopically, the lesion has been considered to be primarily demyelinative with relative preservation of axons in the early stage or in mild cases, but necrosis and cyst formation are frequently seen. Inflammatory reaction is absent or mild. Lipid-laden gitter cells are abundant, but astrocytic proliferation or gliosis is minimal.

Because of the peculiar anatomic distribution involving commissural tracts symmetrically and the lack of gliosis, this condition can easily be distinguished from demyelinative plaques of multiple sclerosis. The resemblance to the lesions of experimental cyanide leukoencephalopathy, posthypoxic leukoencephalopathy, and chronic relapsing carbon monoxide poisoning has been frequently cited; and the possibilities of poisoning due to an impurity in the beverage or an adulterating substance such as hematoxylin, ethnic predisposition factors, vascular factors, edema, and nutritional factors have been discussed, but the etiology and pathogenesis remain entirely speculative. The condition may rarely be associated with polyneuritis and Wernicke-Korsakoff encephaloneuropathy. A state of malnutrition is often lacking, and no apparent response to thaimine treatment has been noted.

Experimentally, an area of degeneration in the corpus callosum similar to the lesions observed in humans has been produced in dogs fed heavy doses of alcohol over a long period (Testa, 1929).

Methotrexate (MTX) Toxicity

MTX is a folic acid antagonist and has been one of the most popular antineoplastic agents in the management of childhood leukemia, especially acute lymphoblastic leukemia, since the late 1950s. It is also widely used in the treatment of other primary intracranial tumors in children. It may be administered alone but more commonly is used in conjunction with other chemotherapeutic agents and/or X-irradiation. For leukemia, MTX may be given orally or intravenously, but for CNS tumors, especially for leukemic leptomeningeal infiltrates, intrathecal or intraventricular routes with or without an indwelling reservoir have been the choice of treatment, since MTX does not normally cross the BBB.

Following several large-scale controlled clinical trials, prophylactic CNS therapy and intensive systemic chemotherapy have been shown to be very effective in preventing CNS relapse and prolonging the duration of complete remission in leukemic patients. About 50% of patients are currently being cured with presymptomatic CNS therapies, usually including 2400 rad cranial X-irradiation and various doses of intrathecal MTX according to the age of the patient (Pochedly, 1979; Bleyer and Griffin, 1980).

The price to be paid for this "truly sensational breakthrough" is frequent MTX neurotoxicity, especially in cases of intrathecal and intraventricular administrations, where 4–61% of patients show evidence of neurotoxicity (Gagliano and Costanzi, 1976). According to Bleyer (1977), the risk of clinical leukoencephalopathy is the highest (estimated to be 45%) when all three modalities are used, and 2–15% with two modalities. The clinical manifestations of MTX toxicity occur with greater frequency as the survival time of the patient increases.

ACUTE MTX REACTIONS. About 30% of patients receiving intrathecal MTX show some combination of headache, fever, nausea, vomiting, nuchal rigidity, and CSF pleocytosis within several days after the injection. These syndromes are the result of chemical arachnoiditis, which is self-limited and disappears within 72 hours.

Transient or permanent paraparesis or paraplegia accompanied by sensory deficits and sphincter disturbance may follow lumbar intrathecal injection of MTX. A focal elevation of MTX concentration because of abnormal CSF dynamics related to the presence of leptomeningeal leukemia or epidural CSF leakage, and the possible presence of a neurotoxic preservative in commercial MTX and diluents have been considered as etiologic factors for these complications (Gagliano and Costanzi, 1976). Focal seizures and hemiplegia after a course of chemotherapy have also been observed (Allen, 1978).

In one patient, paraplegia persisted for 7 months until death (Sullivan and Windmiller, 1966). The autopsy showed demyelination of anterior, lateral, and posterior funiculi of a segment of the thoracic cord, as well as perivascular leukemic infiltrate in the same region. This patient had also received radiation to the spinal cord 6 months before death, so that factors other than MTX may have played a role in producing the lesion.

The case reported by Back (1969) died 30 minutes after developing paraplegia and showed no anatomic lesions. This was considered to be due to a hypersensitivity reaction.

CHRONIC MTX ENCEPHALOPATHY. Kay et al. (1972) reported a group of seven patients who developed insidious onset of tremor, confusion, ataxia, irritability, somnolence,

and dementia during prolonged treatment with systemic and intrathecal MTX. The condition did not respond to whole-brain irradiation of 500 to 1300 rad, but six cases improved following discontinuation of MTX and administration of folinic and folic acid. One patient progressed to coma and death. The autopsy showed multiple necrotic lesions in the temporal and parietal lobes. The authors interpreted these lesions to be of vascular origin. Three years later, "disseminated necrotizing leukoencephalopathy" (Rubinstein et al., 1975) and "subacute leukoencephalopathy" (Price and Jamieson, 1975) were reported as complications of treatment of leukemia and lymphoma. Rubinstein et al. (1975) reported detailed neuropathologic findings in four children with acute lymphoblastic leukemia (ALL) and one child with Burkitt's lymphoma. All children had received triple intrathecal therapy including MTX, cytosine arabinoside, and hydrocortisone as well as whole-brain X-irradiation before or during intrathecal chemotherapy. Characteristic neuropathologic findings were discrete foci of noninflammatory coagulative necrosis in the cerebral white matter with relative paucity of phagocytosis, but conspicuous axonal swellings, spongy degeneration of the white matter, and a moderate astrocytic response in the adjacent regions. Price and Jamieson (1975) described similar lesions in the cerebrum in 10 autopsied and 3 biopsied patients among 231 patients who had ALL and were treated with whole-brain X-irradiation and chemotherapy. Comparison of the clinical data between the two groups of patients with and without leukoencephalopathy revealed the common denominator to be cranial X-irradiation of 2000 rad or more followed by intrathecal MTX. Neuropathologic findings were characterized by noninflammatory multifocal white matter necroses containing various amounts of mineralized cellular debris and diffuse reactive gliosis. In the more severe cases the necrotic foci were confluent, and extensive areas of demyelination were present. The authors interpreted these lesions to have been caused by MTX that diffused into the cerebral parenchyma by damage of the BBB induced by the X-irradiation.

Similar pathologic changes have been reported as a complication of the treatment of other brain tumors (Shapiro et al., 1973) with intraventricular MTX and brain X-irradiation.

Leukoencephalopathy has not been reported with CNS irradiation in the 1800- to 2400-rad range, the dose recommended for the treatment of ALL. It rarely occurs with high-dose intravenous MTX alone (Rosen et al., 1979), or with intrathecal MTX alone (Fusner et al., 1977).

Irradiation

The effects of irradiation are discussed in Chapter 3 and will not be discussed in detail here. The CNS lesions induced by irradiation include demyelination, coagulative necrosis with paucity of phagocytic reaction in the white matter, focal and diffuse vascular proliferation, fibrinoid necrosis, and excessive mesenchymal proliferation including adventitial fibrosis of blood vessels. The lesions resemble those induced by intrathecal MTX except for the vascular and mesenchymal reactions that can be seen in MTX leukoencephalopathy infrequently. The separation of MTX-induced and irradiation-induced leukoencephalopthy is virtually impossible.

Subacute Myelo-Optic Neuropathy (SMON): Clioquinol Intoxication

In the mid-1950s, about the same time that "a strange disease" appearing locally in Minamata was gaining publicity, another strange neurologic disease appeared in the central and northern parts of Japan (Kusui and Kamide, 1958). The disease was characterized by the subacute onset of ascending dysthesia and paresthesia of the lower extremities following prodromal gastrointestinal disorders, such as abdominal pain or diarrhea for days to weeks. The symptoms frequently progressed to include motor impairments (paraparesis or paraplegia,

urinary and fecal incontinence) and visual impairment. The condition was called transverse myelopathy or disseminated encephalomyelopathy or polyneuritic syndromes associated with enterocolitis until 1965, when Tsubaki, Toyokura, and Tsukagoshi concluded that this was a distinct clinicopathologic entity and proposed a term, "subacute myelo-optic neuropathy," following their studies of 20 clinical and 6 autopsied cases. All 6 autopsied cases showed a characteristic clinical syndrome of sensory, motor, and visual impairments for a period of 1 month and 2½ years preceding death and showed symmetric bilateral degeneration of the posterior and lateral columns most marked in the thoracolumbar spinal cord, diffuse and patchy demyelination and degeneration of peripheral nerves and lumbar dorsal roots, and diffuse demyelination of the optic nerves.

Since then the condition has been well known by its abbreviated name, SMON. Initially the condition was sporadic, but the number of new patients suddenly increased in 1963 until 1000 to 2000 new patients were being reported annually (Kono, 1975). The Japanese Ministry of Health and Welfare formed a special SMON Research Commission in 1969 to combat this newly appearing and rapidly spreading disease of unknown etiology until it was finally traced to a drug, clioquinol, which had been prescribed widely for gastrointestinal disorders in 1970. The sale of clioquinol was suspended by the Japanese government on September 8, 1970. The incidence of new cases of SMON disease declined rapidly to 36 in 1971, 3 in 1972, 1 in 1973, and none since, but the total claimed was more than 10,000 patients during this period (Shigematsu, 1975). In 1972, the SMON Research Commission was terminated, and the SMON Research Committee took over and continued their investigation until 1975.

The disease was uncommon in children younger than 10 years old and was more prevalent in women than in men. All microbiologic, epidemiologic, metabolic, and biochemical studies yielded no clues until 1970, when Takasu et al. noted that the tongue of some SMON patients was coated with greenish fur and Igata et al. found two SMON patients excreting greenish urine and feces. The chemical analysis of urinary sediment from these patients yielded iron chelate of clioquinol (5-chloro-7-iodo-8-hydroxyquinoline), as well as a large amount of clioquinol crystals (Yoshioka and Tamura, 1970). Subsequently, clioquinol was also found in the green fur from tongues of SMON patients by gas chromatography (Imanari and Tamura, 1970).

Retrospective studies of the patients' histories revealed that there was a strong association between clioquinol and SMON disease, and the appearance and number of SMON patients correlated with the increased annual production, import, and consumption of clioquinol between 1950 and 1970 (Kono, 1975). Tsubaki et al. (1971) reported that from a survey of public hospital charts, 16.7% of 263 patients who received clioquinol for their various gastrointestinal disorders developed SMON disease, whereas none of 706 patients who did not receive clioquinol for digestive diseases developed SMON disease. They also found that the incidence of SMON was 35.4% among 110 patients who took the drug for more than 2 weeks, but only 2.6% among 153 patients who took it for less than 13 days.

Experimental production of SMON or SMON-like diseases in various species of animals was carried out. Susceptibility and toxic doses varied among different species and strains of animals. Rats and hamsters were said to be less sensitive (Kono, 1975). Peripheral neuropathy was produced in rabbits by injecting a suspension of clioquinol (Igata and Toyokura, 1971). Myelooptic neuropathy similar to that of human SMON disease was produced in mongrel and beagle dogs and cats (Tateishi et al., 1973) and monkeys (Kodama et al., 1973) by the chronic oral administration of clioquinol, but negative results were also reported (Brückner et al., 1970; Hess et al., 1972).

NEUROPATHOLOGIC FEATURES OF SMON. Autopsy reports with neuropathologic de-

scriptions of SMON disease (so designated later) first appeared in 1962 and flourished in the Japanese literature for the next few years under various diagnostic terms, such as myelitis, myelopathy, recently prevailed spinal disease, paralytic patients following abdominal symptoms, nonspecific encephalomyelitis, and dorsolateral funiculomyelitis, but finally unified under the term SMON (Shiraki, 1979).

One hundred thirty-two autopsied cases from 62 institutions were registered in the pathology section of the SMON Research Comittee. Of these 132 cases, 113 cases were designated as typical SMON and 7 as atypical SMON. Six cases were diagnosed as other diseases than SMON, and another 6 were discarded because no spinal cord was included in the specimen (Egashira, 1975).

Peripheral Nerves and Nerve Roots. Severely disrupted axons manifesting vacuolation, swelling, fragmentation, tortuosity, and separation from the myelin sheath were observed in the acute stage, whereas demyelination was more marked in chronic cases. Changes were more marked in the posterior roots than in the anterior roots, and were randomly focal in peripheral nerves. The changes in the nerve roots were most conspicuous in the cauda equina. In general, nerve roots and nerves in the distribution of the lower half of the body were involved and those in the upper half of the body were spared. Vagus nerve rootlets near the medulla frequently showed similar changes.

Dorsal Root Ganglia. Neuronophagia preceded by vacuolation and accompanied by periganglionic spheroid bodies were found most at the lumbosacral level, moderately at the thoracic and mildly at the cervical level.

Spinal Cord. One of the most consistent neuropathologic features was symmetric degeneration of the dorsal and lateral columns. Most frequently, the whole dorsal column was affected in the lumbar cord, but only the fasciculus gracilis was involved in the thoracic and cervical segments. Degeneration of the lateral corticospinal tracts was not apparent in the cervical level, became apparent at the midthoracic cord, and was most pronounced at the lumbar level.

Optic Nerve and Retina. Diffuse symmetric or randomly focal degeneration of the optic nerves, chiasm, and tracts was present. The changes were generally more severe in the distal portions near the lateral geniculate nuclei, but the neurons in this nucleus were preserved. When the retina was involved, degeneration of the inner ganglion cell layer in the papillomacular region was noted.

Other Lesions in the Nervous System. Hypertrophy of inferior olives and glomerular dendritic hypertrophy of olivary neurons were found in 3 among 30 autopsied cases by Tsutsumi (1976). Cytoplasmic vacuolation in the neurons of olivary and paraolivary nuclei were frequent. Central chromatolysis was found in the ventral horn cells of the spinal cord, brain stem, and Betz cells.

Practically no new case of SMON disease has been reported in Japan since 1973, following the removal of clioquinol from the market in 1970, but there are still some problems remaining unsolved. Clioquinol (enterovioform) has been widely used in Europe and in the United States. A large number of American tourists used to take enterovioform with them when they went abroad for "tourist's diarrhea." SMON or SMON-like syndrome or optic neuritis or "unusual gait" associated with clioquinol was not unknown in Europe, Australia, and the United States, but the incidence had been far less than that in Japan (Gholz and Arons, 1964; Kaeser and Wüthrich, 1970; Kean, 1972; Selby, 1972).

Several speculations have been offered to explain why the epidemic of SMON disease involving more than 10,000 patients between 1950 and 1970 occurred only in Japan, even though the drug was available worldwide. These speculations include the following:

1. The Japanese may have an ethnic specificity or genetic predisposition to the drug.
2. Dose and duration of treatment may have been a factor. It was common practice for Japanese patients to receive a larger quantity of clioquinol or clioquinol-containing drugs for a long period for various vague intestinal ailments. Selby (1972) estimated that patients in Australia represented less than 1% of the more than 10 million Japanese who received clioquinol during the same period.
3. Synergistic effects may have occurred with other factors, such as pre-existing gastrointestinal disorders, other drugs, other toxins, or microorganisms.

Another factor that has been favored by those defending clioquinol was the fact that there was no history of clioquinol ingestion in 5% to 15% of Japanese patients with SMON. However, the same 5–15% of the patients that should remain even after the removal of clioquinol from the market appeared to vanish with those who took clioquinol. Paresthesias or painful dysesthesias preceded by intestinal ailments is not a specific syndrome. Unless evidence of optic nerve and corticospinal tract degeneration appeared in more advanced cases, the clinical diagnosis of SMON disease based on peripheral neuropathy following gastrointestinal disorders cannot be expected to be 100% correct. Other conditions due to vitamin deficiencies or celiac disease (Cooke and Smith, 1966) can easily be diagnosed as SMON during an epidemic, and conversely a diagnosis of toxic disease manifesting relatively nonspecific clinical symptoms is extremely difficult to diagnose correctly when the condition is neither epidemic nor endemic.

The prognosis of SMON disease was relatively unfavorable. Sobue et al. (1971) followed 684 patients for 6 months to 10 years and found 7% cured, 54% improved, 25% unchanged, and 19% showing recurrent symptoms. Ninety-three percent of patients suffered from persistent dysesthesia. The mortality ranged from 3% to 5%, and permanent blindness was seen in 2% to 3% of the patients.

Intoxications Causing Predominantly Peripheral Neuropathies

Peripheral neuropathy can be induced by innumerable toxic agents. Practically all neurotoxic agents may be deleterious to peripheral nerves in one way or another. The number of organic and inorganic substances known or suspected to produce peripheral neuropathy is still increasing because of the growing use of chemicals in medicine, industry, and agriculture. New chemicals are being manufactured purposefully or introduced into our environment accidentally as side-products of other products every year. In theory, these chemicals are tested for their safety before they are permitted to be used as drugs, insecticides, or pesticides, and their disposal is carefully controlled. However, species differences in toxicity are well known, so that the results of safety tests obtained in experimental animals are not always perfect, and poisonous chemicals may be inadvertently introduced into the environment, causing a health hazard.

Peripheral neuropathy may be only a regional phenomenon among a wide spectrum of neurotoxicity involving many other parts of the CNS (e.g., alcohol, methyl mercury) or may be the sole clinicopathologic manifestation of deleterious effects in some poisons, such as diphtheria toxin or nitrofuran.

Peripheral neuropathy caused by toxic agents is generally called toxic neuropathy. However, toxic neuropathy shares clinical and pathologic features of neuropathy caused by other metabolic diseases, such as vitamin deficiency, diabetic neuropathy, and uremic neuropathy. In other words, peripheral neuropathy is a very common clinical and pathologic entity that is very heterogeneous in terms of etiopathogenesis, is moderately heterogeneous in terms of topistic involvement, but is remarkably homogeneous in terms of the clinical symptoms and pathologic findings. Because similar pathologic changes are produced by many toxic materials, no causative diagnosis can be made by studying the tissue alone. Clinical history of exposure, epidemiologic data, environmental studies, and chemical assays of blood, urine, tissue, and hair at crucial times are necessary for a causative diagnosis.

Since peripheral nerves conduct three major functions, clinical symptoms of neuropathy may be manifested by disturbance of sensory, motor, and autonomic functions singly or combined, involving one or more portions of the body. Neuropathies may be classified by their cardinal clinical features into sensory, motor, autonomic, or mixed types.

Peripheral nerves form an extensive network throughout the body, interconnecting each other and with the spinal cord and the brain stem. Although a neuropathy involving the whole peripheral nervous system simultaneously is theoretically possible, especially in the advanced stage of the disease, the common clinical manifestation begins a focal involvement of one or a few nerves. Depending on the site(s) of involvement, neuropathies can also be classified into distal or proximal, mononeuropathy or polyneuropathy, mononeuropathy multiplex, radiculopathy, or bilateral symmetric neuropathy.

In addition, depending on the mode of onset and clinical course of the disease, one can designate the condition as an acute, subacute, chronic, progressive, or relapsing neuropathy.

If the etiology of a neuropathy is known, it is probably most proper to make a diagnosis with the name of the causative agent preceding the term neuropathy, as in the cases of lead or arsenic neuropathy. Even though the etiology and pathogenesis are not completely known, a peripheral neuropathy is frequently named with the systemic disease it associates with, as in cases of uremic or diabetic neuropathy. The classification of toxic neuropathy has been made under different types of exogenous toxins (Walton, 1968; Bradley, 1974; Weller and Cervós-Navarro, 1977), including metals (lead, arsenic, thallium, gold, mercury), drugs (anticonvulsants, chemotherapeutic, antimetabolities, sedatives), industrial organic chemicals (solvents, insecticides, herbicides), and foods and beverages.

Obviously one can combine all or some of the above classifications and make a diagnosis quite descriptive but not necessarily distinctive—for example, chronic distal sensorimotor polyneuropathy.

Pathologic classification is relatively simple, since the major constituents of the PNS are limited to three, and their histologic arrangement is stereotyped. Since the nerve consists of axon, myelin (and its parental Schwann cell), and interstitial connective tissue, the respective primary histopathologic types are axonopathy, myelinopathy, and interstitial neuritis or their combinations. Since myelin is formed by Schwann cells, myelinopathy in a way implies Schwann cell damage. Interstitial neuritis includes acute and chronic inflammation of perineurial and endoneurial connective tissue and blood vessels, hereditary hypertrophic neuritis of Dejerine-Sottas, as well as neuropathy in amyloidosis with secondary axonal or myelin injury; these are at most only remotely related to toxic neuropathy and will not be discussed further.

The distinction between axonopathy and myelinopathy in practice is not so clear-cut as their names imply. Because the axon and the myelin are so closely related and depend on each other for their integrity, damage to one results in secondary but rapid injury to the other. Only in the early stage can one observe a predominant involvement of the one with a relative preservation of the other to make that distinction.

The literature on peripheral neuropathy is immense. Recent books on this subject include *Peripheral Neuropathy* by Dyck et al. (1975), *Pathology of Peripheral Nerves* by Weller and Cervós-Navarro (1977), and *Disorders of Peripheral Nerves* by Bradley (1974).

AXONAL DEGENERATIONS

With a few notorious exceptions, neuropathy due to most toxic agents is primarily an axonopathy, especially a "dying back" neuropathy (Prineas, 1969; Cavanagh, 1979) or central-peripheral distal axonopathy (Spencer and Schaumburg, 1976).

The primary lesion is in the distal axons, and the degenerative process progresses centrally (centripetal degeneration). The longest fibers tend to be affected first. Initial symptoms tend to be sensory disturbances, such as tingling, burning, numbness, and pain (paresthesia, dysesthesia, hypesthesia, painful dysesthesia) beginning in the toes or fingers bilaterally and symmetrically with progression toward the trunk. Sensory loss is characteristically in "stocking-glove" distribution, since nerve fibers are affected according to length of axons without regard to nerve roots or to lumbar or brachial plexus distribution. Damage to the motor components of the nerve results in weakness of dorsiflexion of the feet and hands. Extensor muscles are usually more severely involved than flexor muscles. Loss of deep tendon reflexes may occur with or without objective motor or sensory loss. Gait disturbances may appear as a result of both motor weakness and loss of proprioceptive senses.

Pathologic changes are more marked in the distal portions of the nerves and are characterized by swelling of random axons, usually large myelinated fibers, followed by fragmentation of the axons. At a slightly later stage, phagocytosis of myelin and axonal debris by Schwann cells can be observed. Phagocytosis by macrophages is also present when the axonal destruction is marked. Axonal necrosis and phagocytosis of debris extend centripetally with concomitant Schwann cell proliferation. The changes eventually terminate in a complete dissolution and disappearance of nerve fibers. Endoneurial fibrosis, characterized by an increase in interstitial connective tissue, occurs in proportion to the loss of nerve fibers.

Cavanagh (1979) divided toxic "dying back" axonopathy into three groups that were based on hypothetical pathogenetic mechanisms: Group 1 (energy dependent), Group 2 (pyridoxal phosphate dependent), and Group 3 (filamentous and vacuolomembranous). Group 1 neuropathy includes arsenical, thallium, or nitrofuran poisoning, where the changes are basically similar to that of thiamine deficiency. In this group pyruvate metabolism is impaired, resulting in a deficit of energy production to maintain the structural and functional integrity of axons, expecially in their distal portion. The actual metabolic level of impairment of pyruvate metabolism differs among these agents. Group 2 includes isoniazid, hydralazine, ethionamide, and porphyria, which interfere at various levels with pyridoxine metabolism. Group 3 is a heterogeneous group containing two distinct types; one with filamentous accumulation as seen in *n*-hexane, methyl butyl ketone (MBK), carbon disulfide, acrylamide, and vincristine intoxications, and another with vacuolar and membranous changes as seen in triorthocresyl phosphate (TOCP) poisoning. Clioquinol intoxication (SMON) and Dapsone poisoning are included in this group as unclassified. In Group 3, the long spinal pathways as well as the peripheral nerves also show degeneration.

This type of classification is quite comprehensive and intriguing. As the pathogenesis of the neuropathy due to many other toxins is elucidated, this type of classification will be modified and refined, but eventually it will gain more popular support as the relationship becomes clearer between these neuropathies and other human degenerative disease, such as amyotrophic lateral sclerosis, Friedreich's ataxia, and Werdnig-Hoffmann's disease, which also show evidence of a "dying back axonopathy." We have discussed SMON in the section on intoxications predominantly causing white matter damage, even though Cavanagh (1979) classified SMON (clioquinol intoxication) in his Group 3 as a "dying back" neuropathy in which spinal tracts degenerate. There are some similarities in the anatomic distribution of lesions among SMON, TOCP, and thallium poisoning, but the data on the chronic CNS lesions in TOCP and thallium poisoning are still too scanty.

Some outbreaks of toxic neuropathies should be noted:

1. There have been several outbreaks of tri-*ortho*-cresyl phosphate (TOCP) intoxication:

a. Ginger paralysis (ginger jake), 1930–1931: More than 20,000 human cases of toxic neuropathy occurred in the midwestern and southwestern United States during prohibition days in 1930 and 1931. This was shown to be a result of consumption of an adulterated alcoholic beverage known as "Jamaica ginger" or "jake," which contained about 2% TOCP (M. I. Smith and Elvove, 1930). The reason for including TOCP as one of the adulterants was never known.

The clinical picture developed over three stages and was quite uniform. The first stage was represented by gastrointestinal symptoms, including nausea, vomiting, diarrhea, and abdominal pain, which lasted for a few days. Following a symptom-free interval of about 10 days, the second stage was characterized by soreness of leg muscles and numbness of toes and fingers. These developed for several days and were followed by weakness of the toes and bilateral foot drop. Following another interval of about 10 days, weakness of the fingers and wrist drop appeared. Sensory deficits were absent. Early pathologic studies showed that the neuropathy was primarily that of myelin degeneration (M. I. Smith and Lillie, 1931). However, more recent studies revealed that TOCP neuropathy is an axonopathy affecting the largest, longest fibers first, especially their most distal portion (Cavanagh, 1964; Prineas, 1969). Although degeneration of anterior horn cells in the spinal cord was described earlier (M. I. Smith and Lillie, 1931), TOCP poisoning is now considered to be predominantly a peripheral neuropathy.

The follow-up of patients with jake paralysis and animal experiments have revealed that the process of "dying back" from distal axon extends into the spinal cord to involve the posterior columns and the spinocerebellar tracts, as well as the ventral horn cells and the corticospinal tracts (Cavanagh, 1964).

b. Swiss outbreak, 1940 (Jordi, 1952): Eighty officers and soldiers came down with paralysis following a transient gastrointestinal disorder after eating cheese sandwiches grilled with TOCP, a cooling fluid for machine guns, which was placed in olive oil cans by mistake. Most patients recovered, but 25% were left permanently disabled.

c. Morocco outbreak, 1959 (H. V. Smith and Spalding, 1959): More than 10,000 human patients were affected with TOCP poisoning when a lubricating oil for jet engines containing TOCP was mixed with olive oil for cooking use.

d. Bombay outbreak, 1960 (Vora et al., 1962): Fifty-eight cases of toxic polyneuropathy were encountered in Bombay in 1960 from consumption of mustard oil contaminated with *ortho*-cresyl phosphate. Some patients used the contaminated mustard oil for both cooking and massaging the body, but one patient used it only for massaging the body.

2. Outbreak of thallium poisoning, 1932, California (Bunch et al., 1933): "Thal-grain" containing 1% thallium sulfate to control ground squirrels was ground with the barley flour in the preparation of tortillas for human consumption. Thirty-one persons were affected, 14 were hospitalized, and 6 died. Clinical symptoms appeared 1–2 days after consumption, with acute gastrointestinal disorders and painful paresthesia of the extremities. Alopecia and stomatitis were common symptoms. Evidence of CNS involvement, such as myoclonic twitching, convulsions, psychosis, delirium, and coma, appeared in severe cases.

3. An industrial outbreak of MBK polyneuropathy, Ohio, 1973 (N. Allen et al., 1975): Eighty-six patients with a toxic neuropathy were found among 1157 employees in a factory producing plastic-coated and color-painted fabrics. The causative agent was traced to methyl *n*-butyl ketone (MBK), a solvent used as an ink thinner and as a cleaner. Methyl ethyl ketone (MEK) and methyl isobutyl ketone had been used as solvents until August 1972, when they began to be replaced by MBK. This reached maximal usage by December 1972. The first case of polyneuropathy appeared in June 1973. No new cases of toxic polyneuropathy appeared after MBK was completely removed from the manufacturing process and improvements made in ventilation.

4. Outbreak of *n*-hexane polyneuropathy, Japan, 1967 (Yamamura, 1969): Ninety-three cases of toxic polyneuropathy were found among 1662 workers in a small town near Nagoya, where slippers and sandals were manufactured in poorly ventilated households. The toxic agent was found to be *n*-hexane, which was used as a solvent in the pasting process. The air in the factory was found to contain 500–2500 ppm of *n*-hexane vapor, a level exceeding the maximum allowable atmospheric concentration of *n*-hexane of 100 ppm in Japan.

GIANT AXONAL NEUROPATHY

The giant axonal neuropathies have been classified under Group 3 (dying-back neuropathy with filamentous accumulation) by Cavanagh (1979), but because of its distinct histopathologic features it has been commonly known as "giant axonal neuropathy." This type of neuropathy has been found in *n*-hexane (Asbury et al., 1974; Korobkin et al., 1975), methyl *n*-butyl ketone (MBK) (Allen et al., 1975; Spencer et al., 1975), and acrylamide poisonings (Davenport et al., 1976), and is characterized by segmental distention of axons by packed neurofilaments.

SEGMENTAL DEMYELINATION IN TOXIC NEUROPATHIES

There are only a few known exceptions to the common dying-back axonopathy induced by the majority of intoxicants, and they produce selective damage of Schwann cells, producing a primary segmental demyelinating neuropathy.

Diphtheric Neuropathy

Diphtheric paralysis of the palate, respiratory muscles, and extremities following a latent period of weeks or months after acute faucial diphtheria is due to a demyelinating process involving nerves and nerve roots (Fisher and Adams, 1956). Demyelination occurs in the spinal nerve roots, particularly in the dorsal roots, dorsal root ganglia, and spinal nerves just distal to the dorsal root ganglia. Very few changes have been found in the peripheral nerves themselves. Diphtheria has been extinguished in modern societies because of the widespread use of immunizations, but the uniqueness of the properties of diphtheria toxin has prompted extensive investigative studies on segmental demyelination using diphtheria toxin as an experimental tool.

Lead Neuropathy

Lead is another poison that has been considered to produce segmental demyelination, largely on the basis of animal experiments (Fullerton, 1966). The type of lesion in human lead neuropathy is still unknown. Lead neuropathy is somewhat unique in another aspect compared to other toxic neuropathies in that it is almost purely motor, involves the arms more than the legs, and is not necessarily distal. Classic lead neuropathy involves the radial nerve in the working arm and causes wrist drop in painters.

REFERENCES

Adachi, M., and Aronson, S. M. 1967. Studies on spongy degeneration of the central nervous system (van Bogaert-Bertland type). In *Inborn disorders of sphingolipid metabolism*, eds. S. M. Aronson and B. W. Volk, p. 129. Oxford: Pergamon Press.

Adams, J. H. 1962. Central pontine myelinolysis. In *Fourth International Congress of Neuropathology proceedings*, ed. H. Jacob,

vol. 3, pp. 303–308. Stuttgart: George Thieme Verlag.

Adams, J. H., Brierley, J. B., Connor, R. C. R., and Treip, C. S. 1966. The effects of systemic hypotension upon the human brain. Clinical and neuropathological observations in 11 cases. *Brain* 89:235.

Adams, R. D., Victor, M., and Mancall, E. L. 1959. Central pontine myelinolysis. *Arch. Neurol. Psychiatry* 81:154.

Adelman, L. S., and Aronson, S. M. 1969. The neuropathologic complications of narcotics addiction. *Bull. N. Y. Acad. Med.* 45:225.

Adelman, M. R., Borisy, G. G., Shelanski, M. L., Weisenberg, R. C., and Taylor, E. W. 1968. Cytoplasmic filaments and tubules. *Fed. Proc.* 27:1186.

Ahlmark, A. 1948. Poisoning by methylmercury compounds. *Br. J. Ind. Med.* 5:117.

Aleu, F. P., Katzman, R., and Terry, R. D. 1963. Fine structure and electrolyte analyses of cerebral edema induced by alkyltin intoxication. *J. Neuropathol. Exp. Neurol.* 22:403.

Alexander, L. 1940. Wernicke's disease. Identity of lesions produced experimentally by B_1 avitaminosis in pigeons with hemorrhagic polioencephalitis occurring in chronic alcoholism in man. *Am. J. Pathol.* 16:61.

Alexander, L., and Looney, J. M. 1938. Physiological properties of brain, especially in senile dementia and cerebral edema. *Arch. Neurol. Psychiatry* 40:877.

Alfrey, A. K., LeGendre, G. R., and Kaehney, W. D. 1976. The dialysis encephalopathy syndrome. *N. Engl. J. Med.* 294:184.

Allen, J. C. 1978. The effects of cancer therapy on the nervous system. *J. Pediatr.* 93:903.

Allen, N., Mendell, J. R., Billmaier, D. J., Fontaine, R. E., and O'Neill, J. 1975. Toxic polyneuropathy due to methyl *n*-butyl ketone. *Arch. Neurol.* 32:209.

American Academy of Pediatrics' Committee on Infectious Disease 1982. Aspirin and Reye syndrome. *Pediatrics* 69:810.

Ames, A. III, Wright, R. L., Kowada, M., Thurston, J. M., and Majno, G. 1968. Cerebral ischemia: II. The no-flow phenomenon. *Am. J. Pathol.* 52:437.

Arend, R., Ferens, Z., Mizera, E., and Weiss, B. 1964. Étude anatomo-clinique d'un cas d'intoxication chronique par le sulfure de carbone (CS_2). *Rev. Neurol.* 110:21.

Asbury, A. K., Nielsen, S. L., and Telfer, R. 1974. Glue sniffing neuropathy, *J. Neuropathol. Exp. Neurol.* 33:191.

Ashizawa, R. 1927. Über einen Sektionsfall von chronischer Manganvergiftung. *Jpn. J. Med. Sci. Trans. Sect. VIII.* 1:173.

Back, E. H. 1969. Death after intrathecal methotrexate. *Lancet* 2:1005.

Bakir, F. Damluji, S. F., Amin-Zaki, L., Murtadha, M., Khalidi, A., Al-Rawi, N. Y., Tikriti, S., Dhahir, H. L., Clarkson, T. W., Smith, G. C., and Doherty, R. A. 1973. Methylmercury poisoning in Iraq. *Science* 181:230.

Barbeau, A. Inoue, N., and Cloutier, T. 1976. Role of manganese in dystonia. In *Advances in neurology*, eds. R. Eldridge and S. Fahn, pp. 339–352. New York: Raven Press.

Barcroft, J. 1925. The respiratory functions of the blood, Cambridge: Cambridge University Press.

Barr, R., Glass, I. H. J., and Chawla, G. S. 1968. Reye's syndrome: Massive fatty metamorphosis of the liver with acute encephalopathy. *Can. Med. Assoc. J.*, 98:1038.

Barratt, L. J., and Lawrence, J. R. 1975. Dialysis-associated dementia. *Aust. N. Z. J. Med.* 5:62.

Bennett, I. L., Jr., Cary, F. H., Mitchell, G. L., and Cooper, M. N. 1953. Acute methylalcohol poisoning: A review based on experiences in an outbreak of 323 cases. *Medicine* 32:431.

Benton, C. D., Jr., and Calhoun, F. P., Jr. 1952. The ocular effects of methyl alcohol poisoning: Report of a catastrophe involving three hundred and twenty persons. *Trans. Am. Acad. Ophthalmol. Otolaryngol.* 56:875.

Berg, J., and Zapella, H. 1964. Lead poisoning in childhood with particular reference to PICA and mental sequelae. *J. Ment. Defic. Res.* 8:44.

Berglund, F., Berlin, M., Birke, G., von Euler, U., Friberg, L., Holmstedt, B., Jonsson, E., Ramel, C., Skerfving, S., Swensson, A., and Tejning, S. 1971. Methylmercury in fish: A toxicological and epidemiological evaluation of risks, report from an expert group. *Nord. Hyg. T.* (Suppl. 4).

Bernheimer, H., Birkmeyer, W., Hornykiewicz, O., Jellinger, K., and Seitelberger, F. 1973. Brain dopamine and the syndromes of Parkinson and Huntington—clinical, morphological and neurochemical correlations. *J. Neurol. Sci.* 20:415.

Berry, K., and Olszewski, J. 1963. Central pontine myelinolysis. *Neurology* 13:531.

Bertrand, I., Liber, A. F., and Randoin, L. 1934. Altérations anatomiques du système nerveux au cours de l'avitaminose B expérimentale. *Arch. Anat. Microsc.* 30:297.

Blackman, S. S., Jr. 1936. Intranuclear inclusion bodies in kidney and liver caused by lead poisoning. *Bull. Johns Hopkins Hosp.* 58:384.

Blackman, S. S., Jr. 1937. The lesions in lead encephalitis in children. *Bull. Johns Hopkins Hosp.* 61:1.

Blackwood, W., and Cumings, J. N. 1954. A histological and chemical study of 3 cases of diffuse cerebral sclerosis. *J. Neurol. Neurosurg. Psychiatry* 17:33.

Blomfield, J. 1969. Copper contamination in exchange transfusion. *Lancet* 1:731.

Bleyer, W. A. 1977. Current status of intrathecal chemotherapy for human meningeal neoplasms. *Natl. Cancer Inst. Monogr.* 46:171.

Bleyer, W. A., and Griffin, T. W. 1980. White matter necrosis, mineralizing microangiopathy, and intellectual abilities in survivors of childhood leukemia: Associations with central nervous system irradiation and methotrexate therapy. In *Radiation damage to the nervous system*, eds. H. A. Gilbert and A. K. Kagan, pp. 155–173. New York: Raven Press.

Bonilla, E., and Diez-Ewald, M. 1974. Effect of L-DOPA on brain concentration of dopamine and homovanillic acid in rats after chronic manganese chloride administration. *J. Neurochem.* 22:297

Borg, D. C., and Cotzias, G. C. 1962. Interaction of trace elements with phenothiazine drug derivatives. *Proc. Natl. Acad. Sci. U.S.A.* 48:617.

Bour, H., Tutin, N., and Pasquier, P. 1967. The central nervous system and carbon monoxide poisoning. I. Clinical data with reference to 20 fatal cases. In *Carbon monoxide poisoning*, vol. 24, *Progress in brain research*, eds. H. Bour and I. McA. Ledingham, pp. 1–30. Amsterdam: Elsevier-North Holland.

Bourgeois, C. H., Shank, R. C., Grossman, R. J., John, D. C., Wooding, W. P., and Chandhavimol, P. 1971. Acute aflatoxin B_1 toxicity in the macaque and its similarities to Reye's syndrome. *Lab. Invest.* 24:206.

Bowman, K. M., Goodhart, R., and Jolliffe, N. 1939. Observations on role of vitamin B_1 in the etiology and treatment of Korsakoff psychosis. *J. Nerv. Ment. Dis.* 90:569.

Bradley, W. G. 1974. *Disorders of peripheral nerves.* Oxford: Blackwell.

Brain, W. K., Hunter, D., and Turnbull, H. M., 1929. Acute meningoencephalitis of childhood. *Lancet* 1:221.

Branch A., and Tonning, D. J. 1945. Acute methyl alcohol poisoning. Observation in some thirty cases. *Can. J. Public Health* 36:147.

Brierley, J. B. 1976. Cerebral hypoxia. In *Greenfield's Neuropathology.* eds. W. Blackwood and J. A. N. Corsellis, pp. 43–85. London: Edward Arnold.

Brierley, J. B., Brown, A. W., and Calverley, J. 1976. Cyanide intoxication in the rat: Physiological and neuropathological aspects. *J. Neurol. Neurosurg. Psychiatry* 39:129.

Brierley, J. B., Brown, A. W., Excell, B. J., and Meldrum, B. S. 1969. Brain damage in the rhesus monkey resulting from profound arterial hypotension. I. Its nature, distribution and general physiological correlates. *Brain Res.* 13:68.

Brierley, J. B., Brown, A. W., and Meldrum, B. S. 1971. The nature and time course of the neuronal alterations resulting from oligemia and hypoglycemia in the brain of Macaca mulatta. *Brain Res.* 25:483.

Brierley, J. B., and Nicholson, S. N. 1969. Neuropathological correlates of neurological impairment following prolonged decompression. *Aerospace Med.* 40:148.

Brown, A. W., Aldridge, W. N., Street, B. W., and Verschoyle, R. D. 1979. The behavioral and neuropathologic sequelae of intoxication by trimethyltin compounds in the rat. *Am. J. Pathol.* 97:59.

Brown, A. W., and Brierley, J. B. 1968. The nature, distribution and earliest stages of anoxic-ischemic nerve cell damage in the rat brain as defined by the optical microscope. *Br. J. Exp. Pathol.* 49:87.

Brown, I. A. 1954. Chronic mercurialism: A cause of the clinical syndrome of amyotrophic lateral sclerosis. *Arch. Neurol. Psychiatry* 72:674.

Brown, I. A. 1957. *Liver-brain relationships.* Springfield, Ill.: Charles C. Thomas.

Brucher, J. M. 1962. La Leucoencephalopathie de l'intoxication oxycarbonée. *Rev. Neurol.* 106:731.

Brucher, J. M. 1967. Neuropathological problems posed by carbon monoxide poisoning and anoxia. In *Carbon monoxide poisoning,* vol. 24, *Progress in brain research,* eds.

H. Bour and I. McA. Ledingham, pp. 75–100. Amsterdam: Elsevier-North Holland.

Brucher, J. M., and Laterre, E. C. 1962. Les aspects neuropathologiques de l'encephalopathie post-anesthetique, Étude de deux cas. In *Fourth International Congress of Neuropathology proceedings,* vol. 3, ed. H. Jacob, pp. 126–137. Stuttgart: Georg-Thieme Verlag.

Brückner, R., Hess, R., Pericin, C., and Tripod, J. 1970. Tierexperimentelle Untersuchungen bei langdauernder Verabreichung von hohen Dosen von Jodchlor-8-hydroxychinolin mit besonderer Berücksichtigung möglicher toxischer Augenveränderungen. *Arzneim. Forsch.* 20:575.

Brunch, J. M., Ginsberg, M. M., and Nixon, C. E. 1933. The 1932 thallotoxicosis outbreak in California. *J.A.M.A.* 100:1315.

Burhaus, E. C. 1930. Methylalcohol poisoning (a clinical and pathological study of 11 fatal cases). *Ill. Med. J.* 57:260.

Busse, O., and Merian, L. 1912. Ein Todesfall nach Neosalvarsaninfusion. *M.M.W.* 59:2330.

Byers, R. K. 1959. Lead poisoning. Review of the literature and report on 45 cases. *Pediatrics* 23:585.

Campbell, I. R., Cass, J. S., Cholak, J., and Kehoe, R. A. 1957. Aluminum in the environment of man. A review of its hygienic status. *Arch. Ind. Health* 15:359.

Canavan, M. 1931. Schilder's encephalitis periaxialis diffusa. Report of a child aged sixteen and one-half months. *Arch. Neurol. Psychiatry* 25:229.

Canavan, M. M., Cobb, S., and Drinker, C. K. 1934. Chronic manganese poisoning: Report of a case with autopsy. *Arch. Neurol. Psychiatry* 32:501.

Carlton, W. W. 1967. Studies on the introduction of hydrocephalus and spongy degeneration by cuprizone feeding and attempts to antidote the toxicity. *Life Sci.* 6:11.

Carlton, W. W., and Kreutzberg, G. 1966. Isonicotinic acid hydrazide-induced spongy degeneration of the white matter in the brains of Peking ducks. *Am J. Pathol.* 48:91.

Casamajor, L. 1913. An unusual case of mineral poisoning affecting the nervous system; manganese? *J.A.M.A.* 60:646.

Casey, E. B., Jeffife, A. M., LeQuesne, P. M., and Millett, Y. L. 1973. Vincristine neuropathy: Clinical and electrophysiological observations. *Brain* 96:69.

Castaigne, P., Buge, A., Cambier, J., Escourolle, R., and Rancurel, G. 1971. La maladie de Marchiafava-Bignami: Étude anatomoclinique de observations. *Rev. Neurol.* 125:179.

Cavanagh, J. B. 1964. Peripheral nerve changes in *ortho*-cresyl phosphate poisoning in the cat. *J. Pathol. Bacteriol.* 87:365.

Cavanagh, J. B. 1979. The "dying back" process. A common denominator in many naturally occurring and toxic neuropathies. *Arch. Pathol. Lab. Med.* 103:659.

Center for Disease Control 1982. National Surveillance for Reye Syndrome, 1981. Update, Reye Syndrome and Salicylate Usage. *MMWR* 31:53.

Chandra, S. V., and Srivastava, S. P. 1970. Experimental production of early brain lesions in rats by parenteral administration of manganese chloride. *Acta Pharmacol. Toxicol.* 28:177.

Chew, W. B., Berger, E. H., Brines, O. A., and Capron, M. J. 1946. Alkali treatment of methyl alcohol poisoning. *J.A.M.A.* 130:61.

Clasen, R. A. Cooke, P. M., Pandolfi, S., Boyd, D., and Raimondi, A. J. 1962. Experimental cerebral edema produced by focal freezing. I. An anatomic study utilizing vital dye techniques. *J. Neuropathol. Exp. Neurol.* 21:579.

Clasen, R. A., Hartman, J. F., Coogan, P. S., Pandolfi, S., Laing, I., and Becker, R. A. 1974. Experimental acute lead encephalopathy in the juvenile rhesus monkey. *Environ. Health Perspect.* 7:175.

Cohen, P. J. 1966. The effects of decreased oxygen tension on cerebral circulation, metabolism and function. In *Proceedings of the International Symposium on the Cardiovascular and Respiratory Effects of Hypoxia.* eds. J. D. Hatcher and D. B. Jennings, pp. 81–104. Basel: S. Karger.

Colon, A. R., Ledesma, F., Pardo, V., and Sandberg, D. H. 1974. Viral potentiation of chemical toxins in the experimental syndrome of hypoglycemia, encephalopathy, and visceral fatty degeneration. *Dig. Dis.* 19:1091.

Conger, J. D., McIntyre, J. A., and Jacoby, W. J. 1969. Central pontine myelinolysis associated with inappropriate antidiuretic hormone secretion. *Am. J. Med.* 47:813.

Cook, D. G., Fahn, S., and Brait, K. A. 1974. Chronic manganese intoxication. *Arch. Neurol.* 30:59.

Cooke, W. T., and Smith, T. 1966. Neurological disorders associated with adult coeliac disease. *Brain* 89:683.

Cooper, J. R., and Kini, M. M. 1962. Biochemical aspects of methanol poisoning. *Biochem. Pharmacol.* 11:405.

Cooper, J. R., Pincus, J. H., Itokawa, Y., and Piros, K. 1970. Experience with phosphoryl transferase inhibition in subacute necrotizing encephalomyelopathy. *N. Engl. J. Med.* 283:793.

Corey, L., Rubin, R. J., Hattwick, M. A. W., Noble, G., and Cassidy, E. 1976. A nationwide outbreak of Reye's syndrome. *Am. J. Med.* 61:615.

Cotzias, G. C., Papavasilion, P. S., Ginos, J., Steck, A., and Duby, S. 1971. Metabolic modification of Parkinson's disease and of chronic manganese poisoning. *Ann. Rev. Med.* 22:305.

Couper, J. 1837. On the effects of black oxide of manganese when inhaled into the lungs. *Br. Ann. Med. Pharmacol.* 1:41.

Courville, C. B. 1955. *Effects of alcohol on the nervous system of man,* Los Angeles: San Lucas Press.

Courville, C. B. 1957. The process of demyelination in the central nervous system. IV. Demyelination as a delayed residual of carbon monoxide asphyxia. *J. Nerv. Ment. Dis.* 125:574.

Courville, C. B. 1964. *Forensic neuropathology.* Mundelein, Ill.: Callaghan, pp. 216–217.

Courville, C. B. 1971. *Birth and brain damage.* Pasadena, Calif.: M. F. Courville.

Crapper, D. R., and Dalton, A. J. 1973. Alterations in short-term retention, conditioned avoidance response acquisition and motivation following aluminum induced neurofibrillary degeneration. *Physiol. Behav.* 10:925.

Crapper, D. R., Krishman, S. S., and Quittkat, S. 1976. Aluminum, neurofibrillary degeneration and Alzheimer's disease. *Brain* 99:67.

Crocker, J.F.S. (ed.) 1979. *Reye's syndrome,* vol. 2, Halifax, Nova Scotia, Canada, 1978. New York: Grune and Stratton.

Crocker, J. F. S., and Ozere, R. L. 1979. The incidence and etiology of Reye's syndrome in eastern Canada. In *Reye's syndrome,* vol. 2, ed. J. F. S. Crocker, pp. 3–11. New York: Grune and Stratton.

Cumings, J. N. 1959. *Heavy metals and the brain.* Oxford: Blackwell.

Curley, A., Hawk, R. E., Kimbrough, R. D.,

Nathenson, G., and Finberg, L. 1971. Dermal absorption of hexachlorophene in infants. *Lancet.* 2:296.

Davenport, J., Farrell, D. F., and Sumi, S. M. 1976. Giant axonal neuropathy caused by industrial chemicals: Neuroaxonal masses in man. *Neurology* 26:349.

Davis, P. J. M., and Wright, E. A. 1977. A new method for measuring cranial cavity volume and its application to the assessment of cerebral atrophy at autopsy. *Neuropathol. Appl. Neurobiol.* 3:341.

De la Pava, S., and Pickren, J. W. 1962. Cerebellar pressure cones, post mortem study. *N. Y. J. Med.* 62:3594.

Dennis, J. P., Rosenberg, H. S., and Alvord, E. C., Jr. 1961. Megalencephaly, internal hydrocephalus and other neurological aspects of achondroplasia. *Brain* 84:427.

Doobold, H. J., and Elvehjam, C. A. 1935. The effect of feeding high amounts of soluble iron and aluminum salts. *Am. J. Physiol.* 111:118.

Dhiensiri, K., Sinavatana, P., and Lertsookprasert, S. 1979. Reye's syndrome in notheastern Thailand. In *Reye's syndrome,* vol. 2 ed. J. F. S. Crocker. New York: Grune and Stratton.

Dobkin, B. H. 1977. Reversible subacute peripheral neuropathy induced by phenytoin. *Arch. Neurol.* 34:189.

Doherty, P. C., Barlow, R. M., and Angus, K. W. 1969. Spongy changes in the brain of sheep poisoning by excess dietary copper. *Res. Vet. Sci.* 10:303.

Donaldson, J., Cloutier, T., Minnich, J. L., and Barbeau, A. 1974. Trace metals and biogenic amines in rat brain. In *Advances in neurology,* vol. 5, eds. F. H. McDowell and A. Barbeau. New York: Raven Press.

Dyck, P. J., Thomas, P. K., and Lambert, E. H., eds. 1975. *Peripheral neuropathy,* vols. 1 and 2. Philadelphia: W. B. Saunders.

Ecker, A. D., and Kernohan, J. W. 1941. Arsenic as a possible cause of subacute encephalomyelitis. *Arch. Neurol. Psychiatry* 45:24.

Edelmann, F. 1921. Ein Beitrag zur Vergiftung mit gasformiger Blausäure insbesondere zu den dabei auftretenden Gehirnveränderungen. *Dtsch. Z. Nervenheilkd.* 72:259.

Edsall, D. L., Wilbur, F. P., and Drinker, C. K. 1919. The occurrence, course and prevention of chronic manganese poisoning. *J. Ind. Hyg.* 1:183.

Edwards, G. N. 1865. Two cases of poisoning by mercuric methide. *St. Bart's Hosp. Rep.* 1:141.

Egashira, Y. 1975. A short history of autopsy study of SMON in Japan and principal lesions of the spinal cord in 113 autopsied cases. *Jpn. J. Med. Sci. Biol.* (Suppl.) 28:63.

Eiben, R. M. 1967. Acute brain swelling (toxic encephalopathy). *Pediatr. Clin. North Am.* 14:797.

Elliott, H. L., Dryburgh, F., Fell, G. S., Sabet, S., and MacDougall, A. I. 1978. Aluminum toxicity during regular haemodialysis. *Br. Med. J.* 1:1101.

Emden, H. 1901. Über eine Nervenkrankheit nach Manganvergiftung. *M. M. W.* 48:1852.

Engleson, G., and Herner, T. 1952. Allkyl mercury poisoning. *Acta Paediatr. Scand.* 46:289.

Eto, K., Kojima, H., Sakai, H., Miyayama, H., Suko, S., Sakurama, N., Sato, K., Shigenaga, K., Tokumitsu, S., Iwamasa, T., and Takeuchi, T. 1974. Pathological study of Minamata disease 10 years after the first outbreak. Chronic occurrence and its autopsy cases. *J. Kumamoto Med. Soc.* 48:162.

Feigin, I., and Popoff, N. 1963. Neuropathological changes late in cerebral edema: The relationship to trauma, hypertensive diseases and Binswanger's encephalopathy. *J. Neuropathol. Exp. Neurol.* 22:500.

Ferraro, A., 1933. Experimental toxic encephalomyelopathy (diffuse sclerosis following subcutaneous injection of potassium cyanide). *Psychiatr. Q.* 7:267.

Ferraro, A., and Morrison, R. 1928. Illuminating gas poisoning. An experimental study of the lesions of the nervous system in acute and chronic stages. *Psychiatr. 2* 2:506.

Findlay, G. M. 1924. The experimental production of biliary cirrhosis by salts of manganese. *Br. J. Exp. Pathol.* 5:92.

Fine, R. N., Clarke, R. R., and Shore, N. A. 1966. Hyponatremia and vincristine therapy: Syndrome possibly resulting from inappropriate antidiuretic hormone secretion. *Am. J. Dis. Child.* 112:256.

Fisher, C. M., and Adams, R. D. 1956. Diphtheric polyneuritis: A pathological study. *J. Neuropathol. Exp. Neurol.* 15:243.

Fishman, R. A. 1975. Brain edema. *N. Engl. J. Med.* 293:706.

Foncin, J. F., and Gruner, J. E. 1979. Tin neurotoxicity. In *Handbook of clinical neurology,* vol. 36, eds. P. J. Vinken and G. W.

Bruyn, pp.279–290. Amsterdam, New York Oxford: Elsevier-North Holland.

Food and Drug Administration 1982. Salicylate labeling may change because of Reye syndrome. *FDA Drug Bulletin* 12:9.

Fortemps, E., Amand, G., Bomboir, A., Lauwerys, R., and Laterre, E. C. 1978. Trimethyltin poisoning: Report of 2 cases. *Int. Arch. Occup. Environ. Health* 41:1.

Friberg, L., and Vostal, J., eds. 1972. *Mercury in the environment. An epidemiological and toxicological appraisal.* Cleveland: CRC Press.

Friede, M. 1963. Cerebellar edema—a metabolic and cell statistical analysis. *J. Neuropathol. Exp. Neurol.* 22:344.

Friede, R. L. 1966. The histochemical architecture of the Ammon's horn as related to its selective vulnerability. *Acta Neuropathol.* 6:1.

Friend, M., and Trainer, D. O. 1970. Polychlorinated biphenyl: Interaction with duck hepatitis virus. *Science* 170:1314.

Fullerton, P. M. 1966. Chronic peripheral neuropathy produced by lead poisoning in guinea pigs. *J. Neuropathol. Exp. Neurol.* 25:214.

Fusner, J., Poplack, D. G., Pizzo, P. A., and DiChiro, G. 1977. Leukoencephalopathy following chemotherapy for rhabdomyosarcoma: Reversibility of cerebral changes demonstrated by computed tomography. *J. Pediatr.* 91:77.

Gagliano, R. G., and Costanzi, J. J. 1976. Paraplegia following intrathecal methotrexate. Report of a case and review of the literature. *Cancer* 37:166.

Gamper, E. 1928. Zur Frage der Polioencephalitis haemorrhagica der chronischen Alkoholiker: Anatomische Befund beim Alkoholischen Korsakow und ihre Beziehungen und klinischen Bild. *Dtsch. Z. Nervenheilkd.* 102:122.

Garland, H., and Pearce, J. 1967. Neurological complications of carbon monoxide poisoning. *Q. J. Med.* 36:445.

Ghatak, N. R., Santoso, R. A., and McKinney, W. M. 1976. Cerebellar degeneration following long-term phenytoin therapy. *Neurology* 26:818.

Gholz, L. M., and Arons, W. L. 1964. Prophylaxis and therapy of amebiasis and shigellosis with iodochlorhydroxyquin. *Am. J. Trop. Med. Hyg.* 13:396.

Gilger, A. P., and Potts, A. M. 1955. Studies on

the visual toxicity of methanol. V. The role of acidosis in experimental methanol poisoning. *Am. J. Ophthalmol.* 39:63.

Ginsberg, M. D., and Myers, R. E. 1974. Experimental carbon monoxide encephalopathy in the primate. *Arch. Neurol.* 30:202.

Glaser, M. A., Imerman, C. P., and Imerman, S. W. 1935. So-called hemorrhagic encephalitis and myelitis secondary to intravenous arsphenamine. Based on a review of 158 cases. *Am. J. Med. Sci.* 189:64.

Glezen, W. P. 1982. Aspirin and Reye's syndrome. *Am. J. Dis. Child.* 136:971.

Globus, J. H., and Strauss, I. 1928. Progressive degenerative subcortical encephalopathy (Schilder's disease). *Arch. Neurol. Psychiatry* 20:1190.

Greenfield, J. G. 1939. The histology of cerebral edema associated with intracranial tumors with special reference to changes in the nerve fibers of the centrum semiovale. *Brain* 62:129.

Greenfield, J. G., Blackwood, W., McMenemey, W. H., Meyer, A., and Norman, R. M. 1963. Intoxications. In *Neuropathology*, eds. J. G. Greenfield et al., p. 266. London : Edward Arnold.

Grinker, R. R. 1925. Übereinen Fall von Leuchtgasvergiftung mit doppelseitiger Pallidumerweichung und schwerer Degeneration des tieferen Grosshirnmarklager. *Z. Gesamte Neurol. Psychiatr.* 98:433.

Grinker, R. R., and Stone, T. T. 1928. Acute toxic encephalopathy in childhood: A clinicopathologic study of thirteen cases. *Arch. Neurol. Psychiatry* 20:244.

Grüstein, A. M., and Popowa, N. 1929. Experimentelle Manganvergiftung. Arch. Psychiatry 87:742.

Haq, I. U. 1963. Agrosan poisoning in man. *Br. Med. J.* 5335:1579.

Harada, M. 1978. Minamata disease as a social and medical problem. *Jpn. Q.* 25:20.

Harris, I. 1976. Lead encephalopathy. *S. Afr. Med. J.* 50:1371.

Hassin, G. B. 1921. The contrast between the brain lesion produced by lead and other inorganic poisons and those caused by epidemic encephalitis. *Arch. Neurol. Psychiatry* 6:268.

Hay, W. J., Rickards, A. G., McMenemey, W. H., and Cumings, J. N. 1963. Organic mercurial encephalopathy. *J. Neurol. Neurosurg. Psychiatry* 26:199.

Haymaker, W., Ginzler, A. M., and Ferguson,

R. L. 1952. Residual neuropathological effects of cyanide poisoning. A study of the central nervous system of 23 dogs exposed to cyanide compounds. *Milit. Surg.* 111:231.

Henry, L. D., and diMaio, V. J. 1974. A fatal case of hexachlorophene poisoning. *Milit. Med.* 139:41.

Herner, T. 1945. Poisoning from organic compounds of mercury. *Nord. Med.* 26:833.

Herter, W. B. 1959. Hexachlorophene poisoning. *Kaiser Found. Med. Bull.* 7:228.

Hess, R., Keberle, H., Koella, W., Schmid, K., and Gelzer, J. 1972. Cioquinol: Absence of neurotoxicity in laboratory animals. *Lancet* 2:424.

Hicks, S. P. 1950. Brain metabolism in vivo. II. The distribution of lesions caused by azide, malonitrile, plasmocid and dinitrophenol poisoning in rats. *Arch. Pathol.* 50:545.

Hildebrand, J., and Kenis, Y. 1971. Additive toxicity of vincristine and other drugs for the peripheral nervous system. *Acta Neurol. Belg.* 71:486.

Hirano, A. 1969. The fine structure of brain in edema. In *Structure and function of nervous tissue*, vol. 25ed. G. H. Bourne, p. 69. New York: Academic press.

Hirano, A., and Kochen, J. A. 1973. Neurotoxic effects of lead in the chick embryo. Morphological studies. *Lab. Invest.* 29:659.

Hirano, A., Levine, S., and Zimmerman, H. H. 1967. Experimental cyanide encephalopathy. Electron microscopic observations of early lesions in the white matter. *J. Neuropathol. Exp. Neurol.* 26:200.

Hoekelman, R. A. 1982. Take two aspirin and call me in the morning. *Am. J. Dis. Chil.* 13:973.

Hoffmann, W. W. 1958. Cerebellar lesions after parenteral Dilantin R. administration, *Neurology* 8:210.

Holland, J. F., Scharlau, C., Gailani, S., Krant, M. J., Olson, K. B., Horton, J., Snider, B. I., Lynch, J. J., Owens, A., Carbone, P.P., Colsky, J., Grob, D., Miller, S. P., and Hall, T. C. 1973. Vincristine treatment of advanced cancer: A cooperative study of 392 cases. *Cancer Res.* 33:1258.

Hook, O., Lundgren, K-D, and Swensson, A. 1954. On alkylmercury poisoning. *Acta Med. Scand.* 150:131.

Hornykiewicz, O. 1966. Dopamine (3-hydroxytyramine) and brain function. *Pharmacol. Rev.* 18:925.

Horwitz, S. J., Klipstein, F. A., and Lovelace, R. E. 1968. Relation of abnormal folate metabolism to neuropathy during anticonvulsant drug therapy. *Lancet* 1:563.

Houghton, G. W., and Richens, A. 1974. Phenytoin intoxication induced by sulthiame in epileptic patients. *J. Neurol. Neurosurg. Psychiatry* 37:275.

Howell, J. McCl, Blakemore, W. F., Gopinath, C., Hall, G. A., and Parker J. H. 1974. Chronic copper poisoning and changes in the central nervous system of sheep. *Acta Neuropathol.* 29:9.

Hunt, A. H., Parr, R. M., Taylor, D. M., and Trott, N. G. 1963. Relation between cirrhosis and trace metal content of liver with special reference to primary biliary cirrhosis and copper. *Br. Med. J.* 2:1498.

Hunter, D., Bomford, R. R., and Russell, D. S. 1940. Poisoning by methyl mercury compounds. *Q. J. Med.* 9:193.

Hunter, D., and Russell, D. S. 1954. Focal cerebral and cerebellar atrophy in human subject due to organic mercury compounds. *J. Neurol. Neurosurg. Psychiatry* 17:235.

Hurst, E. W. 1940. Experimental demyelination of the central nervous system. 1. The encephalopathy produced by potassium cyanide. *Aust. J. Exp. Biol. Med. Sci.* 18:201.

Hurst, E. W. 1942. Experimental demyelination of the central nervous system. 3. Poisoning with potassium cyanide, sodium azide, hydroxylamine, narcotics, carbon monoxide, et. *Aust. J. Exp. Biol. Med. Sci.* 20:297.

Hurst, E. W., and Hurst, P. E. 1928. The aetiology of hepatolenticular degeneration. Experimental liver cirrhosis: Poisoning with manganese, chloroform, phenylhydrazine, bile and guanidine. *J. Pathol. Bacteriol.* 31:303.

Igata, A., Hasegawa, S., and Tsuji, Y. 1970. On the green pigments found in SMON patients. Two cases excreting greenish urine. *Jpn. Med. J.* 2421:25.

Igata, A., and Toyokura, Y. 1971. Subacute myelo-optico-neuropathy (SMON) in Japan. *M. M. W.* 113:1062.

Ikuta, F., Makifuchi, T., Ohama, E., Koga, M., Yamamura, Y., Oyake, Y., Saito, H., Kanno, S., and Kitamura, S. 1974. Morphological alterations in the autopsy cases of chronic organic mercury intoxication with minimal does. *Adv. Neurol. Sci.* 18:49.

Imanari, T., and Tamura, Z. 1970. Detection of chinoform from green fur of the tongue of SMON patients. *Igaku no Ayumi* 75:547.

Ironside, R., Bosanquet, F. D., and Mc-Menemey, W. H. 1961. Central demyelination of the corpus callosum (Marchiafava-Bignami diesease) with a report of a second case in Great Britain. *Brain* 84:212.

Ishizaki, T., Chitanondh, H., and Lakanavicharn, U. 1970. Marchiafava-Bignami's disease. Report of the first case in an Asian. *Acta Neuropathol.* 16:187.

Ishmael, J., Gopinath, C., and Howell, McC. 1971. Experimental chronic copper toxicity in sheep. Histological and histochemical changes during the development of the lesions in the liver. *Res. Vet. Sci.* 12:58.

Jacob, H. 1939. Über die diffuse Hemisphärenmarkerkrankung nach Kohlenoxydevergiftung bei Fallen mit klinisch intervallarer Verlaufsform. *Z. Gesamte Neurol. Psychiatr.* 167:161.

Jacob, H. 1963. CNS tissue and cellular pathology in hypoxaemic states. In *Selective vulnerability of the brain in hypoxaemia* eds. J. P. Schade and W. H. McMeneme. Oxford: Blackwell.

Jacob, H., Mumme, C., and Solcher, H. 1962. Entmarkung bei cerebralen Odemschaden (Strangulationsmyelopathie). *Arch. Psychiatr. Nervenkr.* 303:311.

Jaksch, R. von. 1907. Über Mangantoxikosen und Manganophobie. *M. M. W.* 54:969.

Jalili, M. A., and Abbasi, A. H. 1961. Poisoning by ethyl mercury toluene sulphonanilide. *Br. J. Ind. Med.* 13:303.

Jenson, S., and Jernelov, A. 1969. Biological methylation of mercury in aquatic organisms. *Nature* 223:753.

Jervis, G. A. 1942. Early infantile "diffuse sclerosis" of the brain (Krabbe's type). Report of two cases with a review of the literature. *Am. J. Dis. Child.* 64:1055.

Johnson, E. S., and Ludwin, W. K. 1981. The demonstration of recurrent demyelination and remyelination of axons in the central nervous system. *Acta Neuropathol.* 53:93.

Joliffe, N., Wortis, H., and Fein, H. D. 1941. The Wernicke syndrome. *Arch. Neurol. Psychiatry* 46:589.

Jordi, A. W. 1952. Acute poisoning by triorthocresyl-phosphate. *J. Aviation Med.* 23:623.

Kaehny, W. D., Hegg, A. P., and Alfrey, A. C. 1977. Gastrointestinal absorption of aluminum from aluminum-containing antacids. *N. Eng. J. Med.* 296:1389.

Kaeser, H. E., and Wüthrich, R. 1970. Zur Frage der Neurotoxizität der Oxychinolin. *Dtsch. Med. Wochenschr.* 95:1685.

Kane, R. L., Talbert, W., Harlan, J., Sizemore, G., and Cataland, S. 1968. A methanol poisoning outbreak in Kentucky. A clinical epidemiological study. *Arch. Environ. Health* 17:119.

Kay, H. E. M., Knapton, P. J., O'Sullian, J. P., Wells, D. G., Harris, R. F., Innes, E. M., Stuart, J., Schwartz, F. C. M., and Thompson, E. N. 1972. Encephalopathy in acute leukemia assocated with methotrexate therapy. *Arch. Dis. Child.* 47:344.

Kean, B. H. 1972. Subacute myelo-optic neuropathy. A probable case in the United States. *J.A.M.A.* 220:243.

Keeney, A. H., and Mellinkoff, S. M. 1951. Methyl alcohol poisoning. *Ann. Intern. Med.* 34:311.

Kepes, J. J., Reece, C. A., and Oxley, D. K. 1965. Central pontine myelinolysis. *J. Neuropathol. Exp. Neurol.* 22:302.

Kidd, M. 1964. Alzheimer's disease—an electromicroscopic study. *Brain* 87:307.

Kimbrough, R. D., and Gaines, T. B. 1971. Hexachlorophene effects on the rat brain. *Arch. Environ. Health* 23:114.

King, L. S., and Meehan, M. C. 1936. Primary degeneration of the corpus callosum (Marchiafava's disease). *Arch. Neurol. Psychiatry* 36:547.

Klatzo, I. 1967. Neuropathological aspects of brain edema. *J. Neuropathol. Exp. Neurol.* 26:1.

Klatzo, I., and Seitelberger, F., eds. 1967. *Brain edema.* New York: Springer-Verlag.

Klatzo, I., Wisniewski, H., and Streicher, E. 1965. Experimental production of neurofibrillary degeneration. I. Light microscopic observation. *J. Neuropath. Exp. Neurol.* 24:187.

Klavins, J. V. 1963. Central pontine myelinolysis. *J. Neuropathol. Exp. Neurol.* 22:302.

Kodama, H., Egashira, Y., Ohtaki, S., and Ohkawa, T. 1973. Experiments to reproduce human neuropathology of SMON in monkeys and dogs by administration of clioquinol. *Trans. Sco. Pathol. Jpn.* 62:122.

Kokenge, R., Kutt, H., and McDowell, F. 1965. Neurological sequelae following Dilantin overdose in a patient and in experimental animals. *Neurology* 15:823.

Kolkman, F. N., and Ule, G. 1967. Tin poisoning edema. In *Brain edema,* eds. I. Klatzo and F. Seitelberger, p. 530. New York: Springer-Verlag.

Koller, W. C., Glatt, S. L., and Fox, J. H. 1980. Phenytoin-induced cerebellar degeneration. *Ann. Neurol.* 8:203.

Kono, R. 1975. Introductory review of subacute myelo-optic neuropathy (SMON) and its studies done by the SMON research commission. *Jpn. J. Med. Sci. Biol.* (Suppl.) 28:1.

Kopeloff, L., Barrera, S., and Kopeloff, N. 1942. Recurrent convulsive seizures in animals produced by immunologic and chemical means. *Am. J. Physiol.* 98:88l.

Környey, S. 1963. Patterns of CNS vulnerability to CO, cyanide and other poisoning. In *Selective vulnerability of the brain to hypoxaemia*, eds. J. P. Schade and W. H. McMenemey, p. 165. Oxford: Blackwell.

Korobkin, R., Asbury, A. K., Sumner, A. J., and Nielson, S. L. 1975. Glue sniffing neuropathy. *Arch. Neurol.* 32:158.

Korsakoff, S. S. 1887. Disturbance of psychic function in alcoholic paralysis and its relation to the disturbance of the psychic sphere in multiple neuritis of non-alcoholic origin. *Vestn. Psichiatrii* 4 (Fasc. 2).

Korsakoff, S. S. 1889. A few cases of peculiar cerebropathy in the course of multiple neuritis. *Ejenedelnoja Klinicheskaja Gazeta* (Nos. 5, 6, 7).

Krainer, L., Black, D. A. K., McGill, R. J., and Rao, N. Y. 1947. Arsenical encephalopathy in Indian troops. *J. Neurol. Neurosurg. Psychiatry* 10:171.

Kumamoto University Study Group of Minamata Disease. 1968. *Minamata disease.* Kumamoto, Japan: Kumamoto University Press.

Kusui, K., and Kamide, M. 1958. A cured case of hemorrhagic diarrhea accompanying polyneuritic syndrome. *Psychiatr. Neurol. Jpn.* 60:1220.

Kutt, H., Winters, W., Kokenge, R., and McDowell, F. 1964. Diphenylhydantoin metabolism, blood levels, and toxicity. *Arch. Neurol.* 11:642.

Lambert, S. W. 1919. Poisoning by hydrocyanic acid gas with especial reference to its effects upon the brain. *Neurol. Bull.* 2:93.

Lampert, P., O'Brien, J., and Garrett, R. 1973. Hexachlorophene encephalopathy. *Acta Neuropathol.* 23:326.

Lapresle, J., and Fardeau, M. 1967. The central nervous system and carbon monoxide poisoning. II. Anatomical study of brain lesions following intoxication with carbon monoxide (22 cases). In *Carbon monoxide poisoning*, vol. 24, *Progress in brain research*, eds. H. Bour and I. McA. Ledingham, p. 31. Amsterdam: Elsevier-North Holland.

Larson, D. L. 1968. Studies show hexachlorophene causes burn syndrome. *J. Am. Hosp. Assoc.* 42:63.

Lawrence, R. D., Meyer, A., and Nevin, S. 1942. The pathological changes in the brain in fatal hypoglycemia. *Q. J. Med.* 35:181.

Lee, J. C. 1955. Effect of alcohol injections on the blood–brain barrier. *Q. J. Stud. Alcohol* 23:4.

Lee, J. C., and Bakay, L. 1965. Ultrastructural changes in the edematous central nervous system. I. Triethyltin edema. *Arch. Neurol.* 13:48.

Leigh, D. 1951. Subacute necrotizing encephalomyelopathy in an infant. *J. Neurol. Neurosurg. Psychiatry* 14:216.

Leong, A. S. Y. 1979. Marchiafava-Bignami disease in a non-alcoholic Indian male. *Pathology* 11:241.

Levine, S., and Stypulkowski, W. 1959a. Experimental cyanide encephalopathy. *Arch. Pathol.* 67:303.

Levine, S., and Stypulkowski, W. 1959b. Effect of ischemia on cyanide encephalopathy. *Neurology* 9:407.

Levine, S., and Wenk, E. J. 1959. Cyanide encephalopathy produced by intravenous route. *J. Nerv. Ment. Dis.* 129:302.

Levy, L. L., and Fenichel, G. M. 1965. Diphenylhydantoin activated seizures. *Neurology* 15:616.

Lewey, F. H., and Drabkin, D. L. 1944. Experimental chronic carbon monoxide poisoning of dogs. *Am. J. Med. Sci.* 208:502.

Lindenberg, R. 1955. Compression of brain arteries as pathogenetic factor for tissue necroses and their areas of predilection. *J. Neuropathol. Exp. Neurol.* 14:223.

Lindenberg, R. 1963. General discussion of patterns of CNS vulnerability. *In Selective vulnerability of the brain in hypoxaemia*, eds. J. P. Schade and W. H. McMenemey, p. 269. Oxford: Blackwell.

Lindenberg, R. 1971. Systemic oxygen deficiencies. In *Pathology of the nervous system*, vol. 2, ed. J. Minkler, p. 1583. New York: McGraw-Hill.

Liu, J., Wang, C., Yu, J., Wang, M., Chang, C., and Cheng, S. 1963. Hexachlorophene in the treatment of chlonorchiasis sinensis. *Chin. Med. J.* 82:702.

Lockhart, J. 1972. How toxic is hexachlorophene? *Pediatrics* 50:229.

Lolli, G. 1941. Marchiafava's disease. *Q. J. Stud. Alcohol.* 2:486.

Lovelace, R. E., and Horwitz, S. J. 1968. Peripheral neuropathy in long-term diphenylhy-dantoin therapy. *Arch. Neurol.* 18:69.

Lowry, M. F. 1975. Reye's syndrome. Its rela-tionship to Jamaican vomiting sickness. In *Hypoglycemia*, ed. E. A. Kean, p. 45. New York: Academic Press.

Lund, O. E. 1956. Histologische Befunde bei ex-perimentellen, akuten Kohlenoxydvergif-tungen. *Arch. Gewerbepathol. Gewer-behyg.* 15:96.

Lustig, F. W. 1963. A fatal case of hexachloro-phene (pHisoHex) poisoning. *Med. J. Aust.* 50:737.

MacDonald, A. E. 1929. *Concilium ophthal-mologicum*, vol. 13. Amsterdam: van Roosen, p.440 (quoted by Cooper and Kini, 1962).

Magee, P. N., Stoner, H. B., and Barnes, J. M. 1957. The experimental production of oe-dema in the central nervous system of the rat by triethyltin compounds. *J. Pathol. Bacteriol.* 73:107.

Mahurkar, S. D., Dhar, S. K., Salta, R., Meyers, L., Jr., Smith, E. C., and Dunea, G. 1973. Dialysis dementia. Lancet 1:1412.

Makela, A., Lang, H., and Korpela, P. 1980. Toxic encephalopathy with hyperammo-naemia during high-dose salicylate therapy. *Acta Neurol. Scand.* 61:146.

Mallory, F. B. 1925. The relation of chronic poi-soning with copper to hemochromatosis. *Am. J. Pathol.* 1:117.

Mancleff, A. A., Koumides, O. P., Clayton, B. E., Patrick, A. D., Renwick, A. G., and Roberts, G. E. 1964. Lead poisoning in children. *Arch. Dis. Child.* 39:1.

Manz, H. J. 1974. The pathology of cerebral edema. *Hum. Pathol.* 5:291.

Marchiafava, E. 1933. The degeneration of the brain in chronic alcoholism. *Proc. R. Soc. Med.* 26:1151.

Marchiafava, E., and Bignami, A. 1903. Sopra unalterazione del corpo calloso osservata in soggetti alcoolisti. *Rev. di Pat. Nerv.* 8:544 (quoted in Lolli, 1941).

Martinez, A. J., Boehm, R., and Hadfield, M. G. 1974. Acute hexachlorophene encephalop-athy: Clinico-neuropathological correla-tion. *Acta Neuropathol.* 28:93.

Mathieson, G., and Olszewski, J. 1960. Central pontine myelinolysis with cerebral changes. *Neurology* 10:345.

Matsumoto, H., Koya, G., and Takeuchi, T. 1965. Fatal Minimata disease. A neuro-pathological study of two cases of intra-uterine intoxication by a methylmercury compound. *J. Neuropathol. Exp. Neurol.* 24:563.

Mayor, G. H., Sprague, S. M., Hourani, M. R., and Sanchez, T. V. 1980. Parathyroid hormone-mediated aluminum deposition and egress in the rat. *Kidney Int.* 17:40.

McCormick, W. F., and Danneel, C. M. 1967. Central pontine myelinolysis. *Arch. Intern. Med.* 119:444.

McKhann, C. F., and Vogt, E. C. 1933. Lead poisoning in children. *J.A.M.A.* 101:1131.

McLain, G. E., Sipes, I. G., and Brown, B. R. 1979. An animal model of halothane hepa-totoxicity. *Anesthesiology* 51:321.

McLain, L. W., Jr., Martin, J. T., and Allen, J. H. 1980. Cerebellar degeneration due to chronic phenytoin therapy. *Ann. Neurol.* 7:18.

McLaughlin, A. I. G., Kazantzis, G., King, E., Teare, D., Porter, R. J., and Owen, R. 1962. Pulmonary fibrosis and encephalopathy as-sociated with the inhalation of aluminum dust. *Br. J. Ind. Med.* 15:253.

McLean, D. R., Jacobs, H., and Mielke, B. W. 1980. Methanol poisoning: A clinical and pathological study. *Ann. Neurol.* 8:161.

McLeod, J. G., and Penny, R. 1969. Vincristine neuropathy: An electrophysiological and histological study. *J. Neurol. Neurosurg. Psychiatry* 32:297.

Meldrum, B. S., and Brierley, J. B. 1971. Circu-latory factors and cerebral boundary zone lesions. In *Brain hypoxia*, eds. J. B. Brierley and B. S. Meldrum, p. 20. London: Heine-mann.

Mella, H. 1924. The experimental production of basal ganglion symptomatology in Maca-cus rhesus. *Arch. Neurol. Psychiatry* 11:405.

Mena, I. 1979. Manganese poisoning. In *Hand-book of clinical neurology*, vol. 36, eds. P. J. Vinken and G. W. Bruyn, p. 217. Am-sterdam, New York, Oxford: Elsevier-North Holland.

Menne, F. R. 1938. Acute methyl alcohol poi-soning. A report of 22 instances with post-mortem examination. *Arch. Pathol.* 26:79.

Merritt, H. H., and Putnam, T. J. 1938. Sodium diphenylhydantoinate in the treatment of convulsive disorders. *J.A.M.A.* 111:1068.

Merritt, H. H., and Weisman, A. D. 1945. Pri-mary degeneration of the corpus callosum (Marchiafava-Bignami's disease). *J. Neuro-pathol. Exp. Neurol.* 4:155.

Mettler, F. A., and Sax, D. S. 1972. Cerebellar

cortical degeneration due to acute azide poisoning. *Brain* 95:505.

Meyer, A. 1932. Experimentelle Vergiftungs-studien. II. Vergleichende phylogenetische Untersuchungen über Kohlenoxydvergif-tung des Gehirns. *Z. Gesamte Neurol. Psychiatr.* 139:422.

Meyer, A. 1933. Experimentelle Vergiftungs-studien. III. Über. Gehirnveränderungen bei experimenteller Blausäurevergiftung. *Z. Gesamte Neurol. Psychiatr.* 143:333.

Milian, G. 1928. Apoplexic séreuse arsénicale. *Acta Derm. Venereol.* 9:149.

Miller, M. W., and Clarkson, T. W., eds. 1973. *Mercury, mercurials and mercaptans.* Springfield, Ill.: Charles C Thomas.

Moress, G. R., D'Agostino, A. N., and Jarcho, L. W. 1967. Neuropathy in lymphoblastic leukemia treated with vincristine. *Arch. Neurol.* 16:377.

Mortimer, E. A., and Lepow, M. L. 1962. Varicella with hypoglycemia, possibly due to salicylates. *Am. J. Dis. Child.* 103:91.

Mubashir, B. A., and Bart, J. B. 1972. Vincristine neurotoxicity. *N. Engl. Jr. Med.* 287:517.

Mullick, F. G. 1973. Hexachlorophene toxicity—human experience at the Armed Forces Institute of Pathology. *Pediatrics* 51:395.

Murphy, J. V., Craig, L. J., and Glen, R. H. 1974. Leigh disease. Biochemical characteristics of the inhibitor. *Arch. Neurol.* 31:220.

Mustafa, S. J., and Chandra, S. Y. 1971. Levels of 5-hydroxytryptamine, dopamine and norepinephrine in whole brain of rabbits in chronic manganese toxicity. *J. Neurochem.* 18:931.

Myers, R. E. 1979. A unitary theory of causation of anoxic and hypoxic brain pathology. *Adv. Neurol.* 26:195.

Myers, R. E., and Kahn, K. J. 1971. Insulin-induced hypoglycemia in the non-human primate. II. Long-term neuropathological consequences. In *Brain hypoxia*, eds. J. B. Brierley and B. S. Meldrum, p. 195. London: Heinemann.

Myers, R. E., and Yamaguchi, S. 1977. Nervous system effects of cardiac arrest in monkeys. *Arch. Neurol.* 34:69.

National Halothane Study. 1969. *A study of the possible association between halothane anesthesia and post-operative necrosis*, eds. J. P. Bunker, W. H. Forrest, F. Mosteller, and L. D. Vandem. Washington, D.C.: U.S. Government Printing Office.

Neff, N. H., Barrett, R. E., and Costa, E. 1969. Selective depletion of caudate nucleus dopamine and serotonin during chronic manganese dioxide administration to squirrel monkeys. *Experientia* 25:1140.

Nelson, J. S., Dahlgren, R., and Fischer, V. W. 1975. Effects of lead salts on the CNS microcirculation of recently hatched chicks. In *Neuroscience abstracts*, p. 701. Bethesda, Md.: Society for Neuroscience.

Nelson, R. B., McGibbon, C., and Glyn-Hughes, F. 1943. Arsenical encephalopathy: A complication occurring during the treatment of syphilis. *Br. Med. J.* 1:661.

Nelson, S. R., Mantz, M. L., and Maxwell, J. A. 1971. Use of specific gravity in the measurement of cerebral edema. *J. Appl. Physiol.* 30:268.

Nicholas, P. O. 1968. Food poisoning due to copper in the morning tea. *Lancet* 2:40.

Nicholson, A. N., Freeland, S. A., and Brierley, J. B. 1970. A behavioral and neuropathological study of the sequelae of profound hypoxia. *Brain Res.* 22:327.

Norenberg, M. D., Leslie, K. O., and Robertson, A. S. 1982. Association between rise in serum sodium and central pontine myelinolysis. *Ann. Neurol.* 11:128.

Okinaka, S., Yoshikawa, M., Mozai, T., Mizuno, Y., Terao, T., Watanabe, H., Ogihara, K., Hirai, S., Yoshino, Y., Inose, T., Anzai, S., and Tsuda, M. 1964. Encephalomyelopathy due to an organic mercury compound. *Neurology* 14:69.

Olsen, L. C., Bourgeois, C. H. Keschamras, N., Harikul, S., Sanyakorn, C. T., Grossman, R. A., and Smith, T. J. 1971. Encephalopathy and fatty degeneration of the viscera in Thai children. *Am. J. Dis. Child.* 120:1.

Ordonez, J. V., Carrillo, J. A., Miranda, M., and Gale, J. L. 1966. Estudio epidemiologico de una enfermedad considerada como encefalitis en la region de los altos de Guatemala. *Bol. Of. Sanit. Panam.* 60:510.

Orthner, H. 1953. Methylalkoholvergiftung mit besonderes schweren Hirnveränderungen. Ein Beitrag zur Permeabilitätspathologie des Gehirns. *Virchows Arch. Pathol. Anat.* 323:442.

Osetowska, E. 1971a. Gases. In *Pathology of the nervous system*, vol. 2, ed. J. Minkler, p. 1638. New York: McGraw-Hill.

Osetowska, E. 1971b. Metals. In *Pathology of the nervous system*, vol. 2, ed. J. Minkler, p. 1644. New York: McGraw-Hill.

Paguirigan, A., and Lefken, E. B. 1969. Central pontine myelinolysis. *Neurology* 69:1007.

Palmer, A. C., and Noel, P. R. 1965. Neuropathological effects of dosing dogs with isonicotinic acid hydrazide and with its methanosulphonate derivative. *Nature* 205:506.

Parkinson, I. S., Ward, M. K., Feest, T. G., Fawcett, R. W. P., and Kerr, D. N. S. 1979. Fracturing dialysis osteodystrophy and dialysis encephalopathy. *Lancet* 1:406.

Parnitzke, K. H., and Peiffer, J. 1954. Zur Klinik und pathologischen Anatomie der chronischen Braunsteinvergiftung. *Arch. Psychiatr. Nervenkr.* 192:405.

Partin, J. C., Partin, J. S., Schubert, W. K.,., and McLaurin, R. L. 1975. Brain ultrastructure in Reye's syndrome (encephalopathy and fatty alteration of the viscera). *J. Neuropathol. Exp. Neurol.* 34:425.

Pearson, J. K. L. 1956. Copper poisoning in sheep following the feeding of a copper-supplemented diet. *Vet. Rec.* 68:766.

Pekelharing, C. A., and Winkler, C. 1893. *Beriberi: Researches concerning its nature and cause and the means of its arrest,* trans. J. Cantile. London: John Bale Sons and Daniellson.

Pentchew, A. 1958. Intoxikationen, In *Handbuch der speziellen pathologischen Anatomie und Histologie,* vol. 12, no. 2B, eds. O. Lubarsch, F. Henke, and R. Rössle, p. 1907. Berlin: Springer-Verlag.

Pentchew, A. 1965. Morphology and morphogenesis of lead encephalopathy. *Acta Neuropathol.* 5:133.

Pentchew, A. 1971. Intoxications. In *Pathology of the nervous system,* vol. 2, ed. J. Minkler, p. 1618. New York: McGraw-Hill.

Pentchew, A., Ebner, F. F., and Kovatch, R. M. 1963. Experimental manganese encephalopathy in monkeys. A preliminary report. *J. Neuropathol. Exp. Neurol.* 22:488.

Pentchew, A., and Garro, F. 1966. Lead encephalopathy of the suckling rat and its implications of the porphyrinopathic nervous diseases with special reference to the permeability disorders of the nervous system's capillaries. *Acta Neuropathol.* 6:266.

Perl, D. P., and Brody, A. R. 1980. Detection of focal accumulations of aluminum (Al) and silicon (Si) within neurofibrillary tangle bearing neurons of Alzheimer's disease. *J. Neuropathol. Exp. Neurol.* 38:335.

Perlstein, M. A., and Attala, R. 1966. Neuro-

logic sequelae of plumbism in children. *Clin. Pediatr. (Phila.)* 5:292.

Petito, C. K., Pulsinelli, W. A., Jacobson, G., and Plum, F. 1982. Edema and vascular permeability in cerebral ischemia: Comparison between ischemic neuronal damage and infarction. *J. Neuropathol. Exp. Neurol.* 41:423.

Pfeifer, R. A. 1928. Die Angioarchitektonik der Grosshirnrinde. Berlin: J. Springer.

Photakis, B. A. 1921. Anatomische Veränderungen des Zentralnervensystems bei Kohlenoxydvergiftungen. *Vierteljahrischer. Gerichtl. Med.* 62:42.

Pierce, P., Thompson, J., Likosky, W., Nickey, L., Barthel, W., and Hinman, A. 1972. Alkylmercury poisoning in humans. Report of an outbreak. *J.A.M.A.* 220:1439.

Plum, F. 1973. The clinical problem: How much anoxia-ischemia damages the brain? *Arch. Neurol.* 29:359.

Plum, F. 1983. What causes infarction in ischemic brain? (The Robert Wartenberg Lecture). *Neurology* 33:222.

Plum, F., Posner, J. B., and Hain, R. F. 1962. Delayed neurological deterioration after anoxia. *Arch. Intern. Med.* 110:18.

Pochedly, C. 1979. Prophylactic CNS therapy in childhood acute leukemia. Review of methods used. *Am. J. Pediatr. Hematol. Oncol.* 1:119.

Poisson, M., Mashaly, R., and Lafforgue, B. 1979. Progressive dialysis encephalopathy. Role of aluminum toxicity. *Ann. Neurol.* 6:88.

Poisson, M., Mashaly, R., and Lehkiri, B. 1978. Dialysis encephalopathy: recovery after interruption of aluminum intake. *Br. Med. J.* 2:1610.

Pollack, J. (ed.) 1975. *Reye's syndrome: Proceedings of the Reye's Syndrome Conference.* Columbus, Ohio, 1974. New York, Grune and Stratton.

Popoff, N., Winberg, S., and Feigin, I. 1963. Patholic observation in lead encephalopathy; with special references to the vascular changes. *Neurology* 13:101.

Potts, A. M., and Johnson, L. V. 1952. Studies on the visual toxicity of methanol. I. The effect of methanol and its degradation products on retinal metabolism. *Am. J. Ophthalmol.* 35:107.

Powell, H., Swarner, O., Gluck, L., and Lampert, P. 1973. Hexachlorophene myelinopathy in premature infants. *J. Pediatr.* 82:976.

Press, M. F. 1977. Lead encephalopathy in neonatal Long-Evans rats: Morphological studies. *J. Neuropathol. Exp. Neurol.* 36:169.

Preziosi, T. J., Lindenberg, R., Levy, D., and Christenson, M. 1970. An experimental investigation in animals of the functional and morphologic effects of single and repeated exposures to high and low concentrations of carbon monoxide. *Ann. N.Y. Acad. Sci.* 174:369.

Price, R. A., and Jamieson, P. A. 1975. The central nervous system in childhood leukemia. II. Subacute leukoencephalopathy. *Cancer* 35:306.

Prickett, C. O. 1934. The effect of a deficiency of vitamin B_1 upon the central and peripheral nervous systems of the rat. *Am. J. Physiol.* 107:459.

Prineas, J. 1969. The pathogenesis of dying-back polyneuropathies. *J. Neuropathol. Exp. Neurol.* 28:571.

Rapport, R. L. II., and Shaw, C. M. 1977. Phenytoin-related cerebellar degeneration without seizures. *Ann. Neurol.* 2:437.

Reichardt, M. 1919. Hirnschwellung. *Allg. Z. Psychiatr.* 75:14.

Reye, R. D. K., Morgan, G., and Baral, J. 1963. Encephalopathy and fatty degeneration of the viscera: A disease entity in childhood. *Lancet* 2:749.

Reynolds, D. W., Riley, H. D., Jr., LaFont, D. S., Vorse, H., Stout, L. C., and Carpenter, R. L. 1972. An outbreak of Reye's syndrome associated with influenza B. *J. Pediatr.* 86:249.

Richardson, J. C., Chambers, R. A., and Heywood, P. M. 1959. Encephalopathies of anoxia and hypoglycemia. *Arch. Neurol.* 1:178.

Richardson, J. E., and Russell, R. S. 1952. Cerebral disease due to functioning islet-cell tumours with pathological reports. *Lancet* 2:1954.

Robbins, E., and Gonatas, N. K. 1964. Histochemical ultrastructural studies on HeLa cell cultures exposed to spindle inhibitors. With special reference to the interphase cell. *J. Histochem. Cytochem.* 12:704.

Røe, O. 1943. Clinical investigations of methyl alcohol poisoning with special reference to the pathogenesis and treatment of amblyopia. *Acta Med. Scand.* 113:558.

Røe, O. 1946. Methanol poisoning. Its clinical course, pathogenesis and treatment. *Acta Med. Scand.* (Suppl.)182:1.

Røe, O. 1969. Past, present and future fight against methanol blindness and death. *Trans. Ophthamol. Soc. U. K.* 89:235.

Roizin, L., Halpern, M., Baden, M., Kaufman, M., Hashimoto, S., Lin, J. C., and Eisenberg, B 1972. Neuropathology of drug dependence. In *Chemical and biological aspects of drug dependence*, eds. S. T. Mule and H. Brill, p. 389. Cleveland: CRC Press.

Romano, J., Michael, M., Jr., and Merritt, H. H. 1940. Alcoholic cerebellar degeneration. *Arch. Neurol. Psychiatry* 44:1230.

Rose, M. 1935. Cytoarchitektonik und Myeloarchitektonik der Grosshirnrinde. In *Handbuch der Neurologie*, vol. 1, eds. O. Bumke and O. Foerster, p. 588. Berlin: J. Springer.

Rosen, G., Marcove, R. C., Caparros, B., Nirenberg, A., Kosloff, C., and Huvos, A. G. 1979. Primary osteogenic sarcoma. Rationale for preoperative chemotherapy and delayed surgery. *Cancer* 43:2163.

Rosenthal, S., and Kaufman, S. 1974. Vincristine neurotoxicity. *Ann. Intern. Med.* 80:733.

Ross, A. I. 1955. Vomiting and diarrhea due to copper in stewed apples. *Lancet* 2:87.

Ross, W. T., Daggy, B. P., and Cardell, R. R., Jr. 1979. Hepatic necrosis caused by halothane and hypoxia in phenobarbital-treated rats. *Anesthesiology* 51:327.

Rubinstein, L. J., Herman, M. M., Long, T. F., and Wilbur, J. R. 1975. Disseminated necrotizing leukoencephalopathy: A complication of treated central nervous system leukemia and lymphoma. *Cancer* 35:291.

Russell, D. S. 1937. Changes in the central nervous system following arsephenamine medication. *J. Pathol.* 45:359.

Sachs, O., Brown, W. J., and Aguilar, M. J. 1965. Spongy degeneration of white matter, Canavan's sclerosis. *Neurology* 15:165.

Sandler, S. G., Tobin, W., and Henderson, E. S. 1969. Vincristine-induced neuropathy. A clinical study of fifty leukemia patients. *Neurology* 19:367.

Sayre, J. W., and Kaymakealan, S. 1964. Cyanide poisoning from apricot seeds among children in Central Turkey. *N. Engl. J. Med.* 270:1113.

Schade, J. P., and McMenemey, W. H., eds. 1963. *Selective vulnerability of the brain in hypoxaemia.* Oxford: Blackwell.

Scharrer, E. 1940. Vascularization and vulnerability of the cornu Ammon's in the opposum. *Arch. Neurol. Psychiatry* 44:485.

Scherp, H. W., and Church, C. F. 1937. Neurotoxic action of aluminum salts. *Proc. Soc. Exp. Biol. Med.* 36:851.

Schmidt, D. 1982. *Adverse effects of antiepileptic drugs.* New York: Raven Press.

Schmorl, G. 1913. Encephalitis hemorrhagica nach Salvarsaninjektionen. *M.M.W.* 60:1685.

Schmorl, G. 1920. Demonstrationen 3. Gehirn bei Blausäurevergiftung. *M.M.W.* 67:913.

Schneck, S. A. 1979. Methylalcohol. In *Handbook of clinical neurology,* vol. 36, eds. P. J. Vinken and G. W. Bruyn, p. 351. Amsterdam, New York, Oxford: Elsevier-North Holland.

Schochet, S. S., Lampert, P. W., and Earle, K. W. 1968. Neuronal changes induced by intrathecal vincristine sulfate. *J. Neuropath. Exp. Neurol.* 27:645.

Scholz, W. 1953. Selective neuronal necrosis and its topistic patterns in hypoxemia and oligemia. *J. Neuropathol. Exp. Neurol.* 12:249.

Schwedenberg, T. H. 1959. Leukoencephalopathy following carbon monoxide asphyxia. *J. Neuropathol. Exp. Neurol.* 18:597.

Selby, G. 1972. Subacute myelo-optico-neuropathy in Australia. *Lancet* 1:123.

Selhorst, J. B., Kaupman, B., and Horwitz, S. J. 1972. Diphenylhydantoin-induced cerebellar degeneration. *Arch. Neurol.* 27:453.

Shaprio, W. R., Chernik, N. L., and Posner, J. G. 1973. Necrotizing encephalopathy following intraventricular installation of methotrexate. *Arch. Neurol.* 28:96.

Shattuck, G. C. 1928. Relation of beriberi to polyneuritis from other causes. *Am. J. Trop. Med.* 8:539.

Shaw, C. M. 1978. Proportional morphometry in diagnostic neuropathology. *J. Neuropathol. Exp. Neurol.* 37:689.

Shaw, C. M., Mottet, N. K., Body, R. L., and Luschei, E. S. 1975. Variability of neuropathological lesions in experimental methylmercurial encephalopathy in primates. *Am. J. Pathol.* 80:451.

Shelanski, M. L., and Taylor, E. W. 1967. Isolation of a protein subunit from microtubules. *J. Cell Biol.* 34:549.

Shelanski, M. L., and Wisniewski, H. 1969. Neurofibrillary degeneration induced by vincristine therapy. *Arch. Neurol.* 20:199.

Shepard, D. A. E. 1976. Methylmercury poisoning in Canada. *Can. Med. Assoc. J.* 114:463.

Shigematsu, I. 1975. Summary of research findings in 1972–1975 and future problems. *Jpn. J. Med. Sci. Biol.* (Suppl.) 28:287.

Shiraki, H. 1979. Neuropathological aspects of organic mercury intoxication, including Minamata disease. In *Handbook of clinical neurology,* vol. 36, eds. P. J. Vinken and G. W. Bruyn, p. 83. Amsterdam, New York, Oxford: Elsevier-North Holland.

Shiraki, H. 1979. Neuropathological aspects of the etiopathogenesis of subacute myelo-optico-neuropathy (SMON). In *Handbook of clinical neurology,* vol. 36, eds. P. J. Vinken and G. W. Bruyn, p. 141. Amsterdam, New York, Oxford: Elsevier-North Holland.

Shiraki, H., and Oda, M. 1968. Neuropathology of hepatocerebral disease with emphasis on comparative studies. In *Pathology of the nervous system,* ed. J. Minkler, p. 1089. New York: McGraw-Hill.

Shiraki, H., and Takeuchi, T. 1971. Minamata disease. In *Pathology of the nervous system,* vol. 2, ed. J. Minkler, p. 1651. New York: McGraw-Hill.

Shragg, T. A., Albertson, T. E., and Fisher, C. J., Jr. 1982. Cyanide poisoning after bitter almond ingestion. *West J. Med.* 136:65.

Shuman, R. M., Leech, R. W., and Alvord, E. C., Jr. 1974. Neurotoxicity of hexachlorophene in the human. I. Clinicopathologic study of 248 children. *Pediatrics* 54:689.

Shuman, R. M., Leech, R. W., and Alvord, E. C., Jr. 1975. Neurotoxicity of hexachlorophene in the human. II. A clinicopathological study of 46 premature infants. *Arch. Neurol.* 32:320.

Smith, H. V., and Spalding, J. M. K. 1959. Outbreak of paralysis in Morocco due to *ortho*-cresyl phosphate. *Lancet* 2:1019.

Smith, J. F., McLaurin, K. L., Nicholes, J. B., and Asbury, A. 1960. Studies in cerebral edema and cerebral swelling. 1. The changes in lead encephalopathy in children compared with those in alkyltin poisoning in animals. *Brain* 83:411.

Smith, M. I., and Elvove, E. 1930. Pharmacological and chemical studies of the cause of so-called ginger paralysis. *Public Health Rep.* 45:1701.

Smith, M. I., and Lillie, R. D. 1931. Histopathology of triorthocresyl phosphate poisoning. *Arch. Neurol. Psychiatry* 26:976.

Sobue, I., Ando, K., Iida, M., Takayanagi, T.,

Yamamura, Y., and Matsuoka, Y. 1971. Myeloneuropathy with abdominal disorders in Japan. A clinical study of 752 cases. *Neurology* 21:168.

Sommer, W. 1880. Erkrankung des Ammonhorns als aetiologisches Moment der Epilepsie. *Arch. Psychiatr. Nervenkr.* 10:631.

Spencer, P. S., and Schaumburg, H. H. 1976. Central-peripheral distal axonopathy: The pathology of "dying back neuropathy." In *Progress in neuropathology,* vol. 3, ed. H. M. Zimmerman, p. 253. New York: Grune and Stratton.

Spencer, P. S., Schaumberg, H. H., Raleigh, R. I., and Terhaar, C. J. 1975. Nervous system degeneration produced by the industrial solvent methyl *n*-butyl ketone. *Arch. Neurol.* 32:219.

Spielmyeyer, W. 1925. Zur pathogenese ortlich electiven Gehirnveränderungen. *Z. Gesamte Neurol. Psychiatr.* 99:756.

Spielmeyer, W. 1930. The anatomic substratum of the convulsive state. *Arch. Neurol. Psychiatry* 23:869.

Stadler, H. Z. 1936. Zur Histopathologie des Gehirns bei Manganvergiftung. *Zbl. Gesamte Neurol. Psychiatr.* 154:62.

Steegman, A. T. 1939. Encephalopathy following anesthesia. Histological study of four cases. *Arch. Neurol. Psychiatry* 41:955.

Stender, A., and Lüthy, F. 1931. Über Spätatrophie der Kleinhirnrinde bei chronischen Alcoholisms. *Dtsch. Z. Neurol.* 119:602.

Stewart-Wallace, A. M. 1939. A biochemical study of cerebral tissue and of the changes in cerebral edema. *Brain* 62:426.

Stokes, J. H. 1934. *Modern clinical syphilology* 2nd ed. Philadelphia: W. B. Saunders.

Stoner, H. B., Barner, J. M., and Duff, J. I. 1955. Studies on the toxicity of alkyltin compounds. *Br. J. Pharmacol.* 10:16.

Strauss, M. B. 1935. Etiology of "alcoholic" polyneuritis. *Am. J. Med. Sci.* 189:378.

Sullivan, M. P., and Windmiller, J. 1966. Side effects of amethopterin (methotrexacte) administered intrathecally in the treatment of meningeal leukemia. *Med. Rec. Ann.* 50:92.

Suzuki, K., and Kikkawa, Y. 1969. Status spongiosus of CNS and hepatic changes induced by cuprizone (biscyclohexanone oxalyldihydrazone). *Am. J. Pathol.* 54:307.

Takasu, T., Igata, A., and Toyokura, Y. 1970. On the green tongue observed in SMON patients. *Igaku no Ayumi* 72:539.

Takeuchi, T., and Eto, N. 1976. Neuropathology of Minamata disease with apallic syndrome—from the observation of 4 autopsied cases. *Adv. Neurol. Sci.* 20:880.

Takeuchi, T., and Eto, K. 1977. Pathology and pathogenesis of Minamata disease. In *Minamata disease,* eds. T. Tsubaki and K. Irukayama, pp. 103–141. Tokyo: Kodanska.

Takeuchi, T., Eto, K., Okabe, M., Katsuragi, S., and Miyajima, H. 1977a. Grade and distribution of pathological lesions in the nervous system in Minamata disease from observations of 72 autopsy and 6 biopsy cases. *J. Kumamoto Med. Soc.* 51:216.

Takeuchi, T., D'Itri, F. M., Fischer, P. V., Annett, C. S., and Okabe, M. 1977b. The outbreak of Minamata disease (methylmercury poisoning) in cats on Northwestern Ontario reserves. *Environ. Res.* 13:215.

Takeuchi, T., Tanoue, M., Kambara, T., Matsumoto, H., Morikawa, N., Murano, M., and Hara, Y. 1957. Pathology of central nervous system disorder of unknown etiology in the Minamata area (first report). *J. Kumamoto Med. Assoc.* (Suppl. 1) 31:34.

Tanaka, T. 1934. So-called breast milk intoxication. *Am. J. Dis. Child.* 37:1286.

Tateishi, J., Kuroda, S., Saito, A., and Otsuki, S. 1973. Experimental myelo-optic neuropathy induced by clioquinol. *Acta Neuropathol.* 24:304.

Tatetsu, S., Murayama, S., Harada, M., and Miyakawa, T. 1969. Sequelae of acquired Minamata disease. *Adv. Neurol. Sci* 13:76.

Terry, R. D., and Peña, C. 1965. Experimental production of neurofibrillary degeneration. (2) Electron microscopic, phosphatase histochemistry and electron probe analysis. *J. Neuropathol. Exp. Neurol.* 24:200.

Testa, U. 1929. Lesioni del corpo calloso nel l'alcoholisme subacut sperimentale. *Riv. Sper. Freniat.* 52:559 (quoted in Lolli, 1941).

Thienes, C. H. 1940. *Clinical toxicology.* Philadelphia: Lee and Febiger.

Thomas, A. 1905. Atrophic lamellaire des cellulas des Purkinje. *Rev. Neurol.* 13:917.

Thomas, J. A., Dallenbach, F. D., and Thomas, M. 1973. Distribution of radioactive lead (^{210}P) in the cerebellum of developing rats *J. Pathol.* 109:45.

Todd, J. R. 1969. Chronic copper toxicity of ruminates. *Proc. Nutr. Soc.* 28:189.

Toyokura, Y., Tsukagoshi, H., Tsubaki, T., Ito, U., and Furukawa, H. 1964. Pathology of so-called myelitis following abdominal symptoms—3 cases in Kushiro City. *Clin. Neurol.* 4:506.

Trey, C., Lipworth, L., Chalmers, T. C., Davidson, C. S., Gottlieb, L. S., Popper, II., and Saunders, S. J. 1968. Fulminant hepatic failure. *N. Engl. J. Med.* 279:798.

Troupin, A. S., and Ojemann, L. M. 1975. Paradoxical intoxication—a complication of anticonvulsant administration. *Epilepsia* 16:753.

Tsubaki, T. 1968. Organic mercury intoxication in the Agano river area studied by Niigata University research group. *Clin. Neurol.* 8:511.

Tsubaki, T. 1974. Recent problems for the diagnosis of Minamata disease. *Adv. Neurol. Sci.* 18:882.

Tsubaki, T., Honma, Y. and Hoshi, M. 1971. Neurological syndrome associated with clioquinol. *Lancet* 1:696.

Tsubaki, T., and Irukayama, K. 1977. Minamata disease; methylmercury poisoning in Minamata and Niigata, Japan. Tokyo, Kodansha; Amsterdam, New York: Elsevier.

Tsubaki, T., Sato, T., Kondo, K., Shirakawa, K., Kambayashi, K., Hirota, K., Yamada, K., and Murone, I. 1967. Outbreak of intoxication by organic mercury compounds in Niigata prefecture: An epidemiological and clinical study. *Jpn. J. Med.* 6:32.

Tsubaki, T., Toyokura, Y., and Tsukagoshi, H. 1965. Subacute myelo-optic-neuropathy following abdominal symptoms. A clinical and pathological study. *Jpn. J. Med.* 4:181.

Tsutsui, J., and Okamura, R. 1974. Neuroophthalmological investigations on methylmercury poisoning. *Adv. Neurol. Sci.* 18:100.

Tsutsumi, A. 1976. Clinicopathology of subacute myelo-optico-neuropathy (SMON). *J. Karyopathol.* 16:1.

Turel, A. P., Jr., Levinsohn, M. W., Derakhshan, I., and Gutierrez, Y. 1975. Reye's syndrome and cerebellar intracytoplasmic inclusion bodies. *Arch. Neurol.* 32:624.

Uchimura, J. 1928. Zur Pathogenese der ortlich elektiven Ammonshornerkrankung. *Z. Gesamte Neurol. Psychiatr.* 114:567.

van Bogaert, L., and Bertrand, I. 1949. Sur une idiotie familiale avec dégénérescence spongieuse du névraxe. *Acta. Neurol. Belg.* 49:572.

van Bogaert, L., and Dallemagne, M. J. 1943. Approaches expérimentales des troubles nerveux du manganisne. *Monatsschr. Psychiatr. Neurol.* 111:60.

van Bogaert, L., Dallemagne, M. J., and Wegria, R. 1938. Recherches sur le besoin d'oxygène chronique et aigu chez Macacus Rhesus. *Arch. Interr. Med. Exp.* 13:335.

Verhaart, W. J. C. 1941. Lead encephalopathy simulating diffuse sclerosis in a Chinese infant. *Am. J. Dis. Child.* 61:1246.

Victor, M., Adams, R. D., and Collins, G. H. 1971. *The Wernicke-Korsakoff syndrome.* Philadelphia: F. A. Davis.

Victor, M., Adams, R. D., and Mancall, E. L. 1959. A restricted form of cerebellar cortical degeneration occurring in alcoholic patients. *Arch. Neurol.* 1:579.

Vogel, F. S. 1959. The deposition of exogenous copper under experimental conditions with observations in its neurotoxic and nephrotoxic properties in relation to Wilson's disease. *J. Exp. Med.* 110:801.

Vogel, F. S., and Evans, J. W. 1961. Morphologic alterations produced by copper in neural tissues with consideration of the role of the metal in the pathogenesis of Wilson's disease. *J. Exp. Med.* 113:997.

Vogt, C., and Vogt, O. 1922. Erkrankungen der Grosshirnrinde in Lichte der Topistik, Pathoklise und Pathoarchitektonik. *J. Psychiatr. Neurol.* 28:1.

Vora, D. D., Dastur, D. K., Braganea, B. M., Parihar, L. M., Iyer, C. G. S., Fondekar, R. B., and Prabhakaran, K. 1962. Toxic polyneuritis in Bombay due to *ortho*-cresylphosphate poisoning. *J. Neurol. Neurosurg. Psychiatry* 25:234.

Voss, H. 1939. Progressive bulbar Paralyse und amyotrophische Lateralsklerose nach chronischer Manganvergiftung. *Arch. Gewebepathol. Gewebehyg.* 9:464.

Walton, J. N. 1968. Classification of the neuromuscular disorders. *J. Neurol. Sci.* 6:165.

Wardle, E. N. 1973. Dialysis dementia. *Lancet* 1:1412.

Wear, J. B., Jr., Shanahan, R., and Ratliff, R. K. 1962. Toxicity of ingested hexachlorophene. *J.A.M.A.* 181:587.

Weiden, P. L., and Wright, S. E. 1972. Vincristine neurotoxicity. *N. Engl. J. Med.* 286:1369.

Weiner, W. J., Nausieda, P. A., and Klawans, H. L. 1978. The effect of levodopa, lergotrile, and bromcriptine on brain iron, manganese, and copper. *Neurology* 28:734.

Weller, R. O., and Cervós-Navarro, J. 1977. *Pa-*

thology of peripheral nerves. London and Boston: Butterworth.

Wells, G. A. H., Howell J. McC., and Gopinath, C. 1976. Experimental lead encephalopathy of calves. Histological observations on the nature and distribution of the lesions. *Neuropathol. Appl. Neurobiol.* 2:175.

Wender, M. 1963. Studies of cerebral lipids in a relapsing case of carbon monoxide poisoning. *Acta Neuropathol.* 2:371.

Wernicke, C. 1881. *Lehrbuch der Gehirnkrankheiten für Ärzte und Studierende,* vol. 2. Kassel, Germany: Theodor Fischer, pp. 229–242.

Wheatley, B., Barbeau, A., Clarkson, T. W., and Lapham, L. W. 1979. Methylmercury poisoning in Canadian Indians—The elusive diagnosis. *Can. J. Neurol. Sci.* 6:417.

Wheeler, R. H., and Votaw, M. 1974. Vincristine and quadriparesis. *Ann. Intern. Med.* 81:709.

Wilson, G., and Winkelman, N. W. 1925. An unusual cortical change in carbon monoxide poisoning. *Arch. Neurol. Psychiatry* 13:191.

Wilson, J. T., and Brown, R. D. 1982. Reye syndrome and aspirin use: The role of prodromal illness severity in the assessment of relative risk. *Pediatrics* 69:822.

Wisniewski, H., Terry, R. D., and Hirano, A. 1970. Neurofibrillary pathology. *J. Neuropathol. Exp. Neurol.* 39:163.

Wood, C. A., and Buller, F. C. 1904. Poisoning by wood alcohol. Cases of death and blindness from Columbian spirits and other methylated preparations. *J.A.M.A.* 43:972.

Wyllie, J. 1957. Copper poisoning at a cocktail party. *Am. J. Public Health* 47:617.

Yamamura, Y. 1969. *n*-Hexane polyneuropathy. *Folia Psychiatr. Neurol. Jpn.* 23:45.

Yoshioka, M., and Tamura, Z. 1970. On the nature of the green pigment found in SMON patients. *Igaku no Ayumi* 74:320.

Zimmerman, H. M. 1943. Pathology of vitamin B group deficiencies. *Res. Publ. Assoc. Res. Nerv. Ment. Dis.* 22:51.

Zülch, K. J., and Behrend, R. C. H. 1961. The pathogenesis and topography of anoxia, hypoxia and ischemia of the brain in man. In *Cerebral anoxia and the electroencephalograms,* eds. H. Gastaut and J. S. Meyers, pp. 144–163. Springfield, Ill.: Charles C Thomas.

Zu Rhein, G. H., Eichman, P. L., and Puletti, F. 1960. Familial idiocy with spongy degeneration of the central nervous system of van Bogaert-Bertland type. *Neurology* 10:998.

Index